AF615808

DR. H. GROSS'

COMPARATIVE

MATERIA MEDICA

EDITED BY

CONSTANTINE HERING

SECOND EDITION

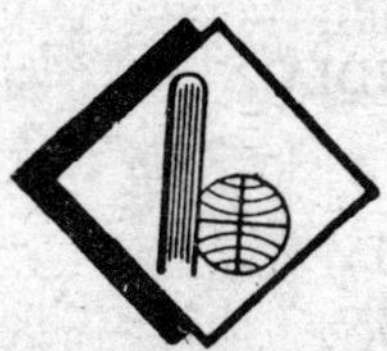

B. JAIN PUBLISHERS PVT. LTD.
NEW DELHI - 110 055

Price : Rs. 120.00

Reprint Edition : 1996

Published by:
B. Jain Publishers (P) Ltd.
1921, Street No. 10th Chuna Mandi,
Paharganj, New Delhi-110055 (INDIA)

Printed in India by :
J.J. Offset Printers
7, Printing Press Area, Ring Road,
Wazirpur, Delhi-110052

ISBN 81—7021—084—4

BOOK CODE B-2256

INTRODUCTION.

BY R. H. GROSS

In comparison to that which is not known, the knowledge of all physicians in this world is certainly small. But we should never be able to enlarge upon the existing basis, did we deny, as do the skeptics upon principle, the general *certainty of cognition* in medical science, or, to speak practically, the reliability of *experience* in the medical art *

True, there are many trifles connected with the demeanor of the physician, either winning or destroying confidence. without the observance of which even the most distinguished experience and ability cannot captivate the public. Such a boon is usually somewhat dependent upon innate individuality, though sometimes acquired or developed. It would be unjust to denounce bluntly the use of these outward expedients by the cheap name of "charlatanry;" they deserve this designation only when not based upon a solid, scientific foundation, — a foundation which, however, cannot be present, or at least not apparent, where skepticism is raised to a dogma; or, where no connection has yet been found between theory and *practice*.

But to return: in accordance with his experience, every physician cures as best he is able. In this respect we are in favor of the widest toleration, claiming the same for ourselves. No one is justified in marking out purely arbitrary paths in science, because these are mutually opposed as much as are anarchy and rational liberty.

Hohenheim's doctrine did not become the common property of all physicians, because it was enveloped by a mysterious obscurity.† ‡

Homœopathy has no such fate to fear since she has a widely diffused "Press" as an ally.—Great, but not insurmountable, are the difficulties which, until now, have prevented her universal recognition and practical application.

In so far as these difficulties lie in the Materia Medica, which, indeed. to the novice appears a chaos, I hope to remove them in a great measure by the present work.

Our treasury of remedies has grown so much, both extensively and intensibly, that the publication of further provings of new remedies seems only exceptionally desirable.

---

* Every practitioner who derives his support from the patronage of the public will admit that this "Experience" is his greatest ally and at the same time his best passport to confidence on the part of society. M.

† *Hohenheim*—more generally known and slandered under the name *Paracelsus*—did not do this himself; it was done by his followers and the editors of his writings. With them it was a kind of fashion to puff up everything by surrounding it with clouds of mysteriousness. Exactly as in our age crinolines are worn, disgusting to every man of the slightest cultivation of taste. C.Hg.

‡ Often, in past ages, has medical truth, departing from the paths marked out by the dogmatism of the schools after briefly glimmering before the vision of those who refused to seize upon it, vanished into oblivion. M.

On the other hand, the proving of (old) remedies on ourselves is indispensable to self-instruction. — But we would have to confine ourselves to the treatment of only some particularly acute diseases, in order to be able to move within the small circle of* our own personal proving. I mean, that it is impossible to have proved on *ourselves* all the remedies at our disposal for the treatment of *chronic* diseases.

It is therefore necessary to find and smooth a path which, without being arbitrary, shall be correct, and by which we may discover and appropriate, without much difficulty, the results of the hitherto known provings. I believe I have taken this path by exhibiting the DIFFERENTIAL DIAGNOSIS *of such remedies as are similar in their effects.*

Fichte (the father) has already observed, that every honest work leads the author beyond his original purpose. When I undertook this work, I had no idea of the wide reach of its results, because it has incidentally yielded the following:

A. The *characteristic effects* of such remedies as are herein compared; what is wanting in one diagnosis is found in others. The differential points delineate the character of the effects of the medicine as distinctly as microscopic objects appear under polarized light. This predominating character of the remedy must be useful even to the generalizing physician, for whom, in fact, this book has not been written; and who, since he will never fully make use of it by earnest study, is therefore also not competent to judge it.

B. Irrefragable proof is herein furnished that, in their fullest compass, the collective effects of a remedy agree with each other, under physiological laws, and that they have therefore their own intrinsic physiological explanation, by which at once all *theoretical* elaborations of single remedies become for the future unnecessary, and again, through which even those who hitherto have been strangers to Homœopathy may convince themselves, without further exertion, of Nature's truth in regard to "physiological" provings of remedies. The most important principle for testing the genuineness of every proving of a remedy is thereby also produced.

Further, this work will help to preserve for all time the results of the labors of the first half century of Homœopathy, as well as give new life to the study of remedies, inasmuch as thus far very little has been done to enable the medical profession to find its way through our Materia Medica, and thereby to liberate itself from indolent Scepticism and to make use of our treasure of remedies by individualizing in practice.

That of which "Non-Homœopaths" have accused us as triviality, they will find herein in a desirable lapidary style. In fact, it is also a sort of generalization, but one which does not extinguish the effective character of the object; for one can easily conceive that every agent is distinguished from another by definite traits.

All physicians take more or less notice of a relation of medical effects; particularly so the friends of Doctor *Rademacher* (the founder of a peculiar medical school in 1845), as well as the followers of the so-called "specific" healing art; — but the discovery of modalities, of conditions under which an agent discloses its specific powers, is thus far exclusively the merit of the homœopathicians.† Whosoever maintains that these mo-

---

* It is certain that one succeeds better with a *few* well-known remedies than with *many* whereof he knows little. But the practitioner who strives to reduce the number of his remedies more and more must necessarily generalize, — whereas, a true follower of individualizing homœopathy, commencing his practice with but a few articles, gradually learns the application of more and more. R.H.Gr.

† Homœopathy urges the difference of effects in separate remedies, and knows, therefore, no surrogate. R.H.Gr.

dalities are of trifling moment, proclaims indirectly the whole doctrine of Hahnemann to be charlatanism. To those who work in our field, the diagnosis of remedies, as it is before us, will help to designate more minutely the separate modalities of effects, because one of them frequently conditions the other. (Compare China—Ferr.; Carb. an.—Calc., and others.)

Wherever in such respects the new provings differ from the old ones, the cause will be found in the more massive and crude form of the drugs employed in the former; (which, being more subject to *alternative* phenomena, are therefore less characteristic. M.)

Those who reject all repertories and similar works as an obstacle to a collective and unitary comprehension of the features of a disease, natural or artificial, can be refuted by the unitary physiological character which any single remedy shows in such a collection of its separate symptoms. The misunderstood so-called symptomatic treatment of diseases in Homœopathy is thereby once for all justified, because it combats with the *total character* of the remedy the *total features* of the disease.

The study of this work, which may always be more entertaining than a calculation of logarithms, ought, with equal perseverance, to be gone through with; the more so as it is more satisfactory than that of mere repertories, since in the latter the symptoms of remedies must of necessity be *analyzed*, whilst here they are *synthetically compiled*. Our diagnosis must also have the preference to a repertory with beginners, who, although not familiar with it, can nevertheless always find in a moment the matter searched for.

To the skeptics I will yet observe that the statements in this book are mostly known to every practised Homœopathician, but not always present to his mind; it would require a prodigious memory; and further, that the doubt about authenticity may be cleared up by the internal evidence of truth, recognizable by every competent judge. These comparisons can be looked upon as the first step towards a mathematical method of elaborating the Materia Medica, which was first suggested by *Const. Hering*, and which is at the same time a statistical one.

The diagnostics of one remedy offer here a supplement and correction to another,* and also show one and the same remedy in different lights. They are based, not upon mere abstractions, new stand-points, and the like, but upon provings and *clinical observations*, i. e. upon *facts* of medicine according to Nature's laws, and are gained by the rules of the *art of observation;* and it is interesting to follow up the laws of Nature which reflect themselves in these facts. We quote only a few of the most prominent:

Sexual passion, often combined with jealousy, is intimately related on the one hand to cruelty, on the other to affected devoutness. In anger and sexual passion the secretion of saliva is increased; in a paroxysm of fear diminished.

The remedies in which hunger is predominant, produce an increased salivary secretion, and often a delicate taste (Camph., China, Coffea), while with a diminished saliva the appetite is wanting.

In Aconit., Chamom., China, Coff., we find predominantly a delicate sense of smell; and, correspondingly, *never dryness of the nose*, which would make a delicate smell impossible.

Those drugs which cause appetite fer beer, as well as those which generally cause scentless flatus, are at the same time remedies for the liver.

The position of those sleeping with the arms crossed over the head usually indicates

*** In such a work it can hardly be otherwise than that some errata shall remain unnoticed. R.H.Gr.**

liver complaint, and our remedies, the symptoms of which have been observed as containing such a position, have in fact a decided relation to the liver.

The condition "compression of teeth" is identical with that of pressure in general, as well as with the lying on the painful side.

Such analogies are everywhere illustrated. Thus, there is an analogy between the influence of stooping, retention of breath, expiration, retraction of abdomen, tension of abdomical muscles, of tightness of clothing around the hips, as well as bodily exertion.

While standing, the body is not completely at rest, but offers quite the same passive resistance as while riding in a carriage, particularly if on rough roads;—therefore, the analogous influence of both conditions.

Wine is usually analogous to the effects of warm diet; vinegar and vegetable acids to cold diet.

Those remedies the complaints of which are ameliorated by eructations have *mostly* also amelioration when the stomach is empty.

If the thirsty drink little at a time, there is either an instinctive repugnance to fluids, *or* the thirsty one has already experienced that drink is hurtful to him.

Dryness of the tongue indicates an affection of the brain; this we find confirmed by those of our provings in which dryness of tongue predominantly occurs.

Under Arsenic is found an inclination for the use of alcoholic drinks and aversion to sweets, and correspondingly also an irritable, malicious temper;—on the other hand there is, under Rhus, inclination for sweets and aversion to alcoholic drinks, and correspondingly a depressed mood.

We find under China, Lachesis, Acid. fluor. and Acid. sulphuric. appetite for spirituous liquors, and correspondingly mental excitement, ecstasies, &c.; under Mercury and Sabadilla (aversion to wine, but) appetite for beer, which produces sluggishness of thought, and, corresponding with it, stupidity. (Compare the different influences of wine and beer under the head of Camph., Apis.)

Mental excitement (ecstasy) is usually combined with insensibility of disposition, while a sensitive disposition is not unfrequently combined with a depression of intellect.*

In imbecile persons (as well as in children whose faculties are not yet roused) the pupils are mostly dilated (and often the urine pale); in insanity they are contracted.

In mania-à-potu we find certain optical illusions, while mental disturbances produced by venereal excesses are connected with hallucinations of hearing and smell. These relations are a true copy of the corresponding remedies in our medical treasury; particularly is there an augmented sexual desire wherever hallucinations of smell have been observed. It is evident that by the sense of smell (fragrancy) sexual desires are excited; and it is known that even the development of scent in the blossoms accompanies the sexual process of plants—that the development of the vocal organs is coincident with puberty—and that the free singing-bird suspends its song as soon as the sexual desire has been gratified.

In clear-sightedness the pupils are predominantly dilated and the optical illusions appear in bright colors; in dim-sightedness in dark colors.

The remedies which have a specific direction to the hard palate act at the same time on the inner nose and inner ear (second branch of the Nerv. trigem.); on the other hand,

* Analogously, we frequently find, during predominating polar currents of air, a diminished irritability of the nervous system and a vascular erethism (Mexico, Hungary), while during an equatorial direction of winds there is nervous erethism with synchronous torpor of the vascular system. R.H.Gr.

those remedies which act principally on the soft palate generally affect at the same time the external ear and external nose (connection of the Nerv. facial. with the Nerv. lingual.)

Persons inclined to constipation are usually of an irritable and vexatious disposition; and those who have a strong inclination to diarrhœa are commonly anxious and sad.

Such medicines as produce (and cure) painless diarrhœa are also remedies for internal hæmorrhages.

Remedies which augment the secretion of urine also usually increase thirst, reduce sexual desire, produce a depressed disposition of mind (and often weak-mindedness), while with increased sexual desire there is generally combined a diminished urinary secretion, and mostly also disposition to constipation. Ant. cr., Apis, Aur., Camph., Canth., Carb. veg., China, Colch., Con., Dig., Dulc., Iod., Mez., N. vom., Op., Plumb., Puls., Ruta, Staph., &c.

Women menstruating abundantly have usually strong sexual desires, and vice versa.

Leucorrhœa, in women who menstruate profusely, is frequently of marked consistency, while it is fluid in such as have their periods rarely with a scanty flow.

It is but rarely that we find in our provings a fluent coryza at night, because every fluent coryza is apt to cease during sleep and by the warmth of the bed.

In the so-called narcotics, dry coryza predominates over fluent coryza, and dry cough over the moist. Those few narcotics which have coryza more frequently of a fluent nature, and a moist cough, have also oftener diarrhœa than constipation.

Præcordial anguish is often one of the first symptoms of insanity; while an anxious feeling in the head or in the hypochondriac regions is rarely followed by insanity. (Our experience with the remedies corresponds to this observation. C.Hg.)

The remedies which create a cold breath are also capable of producing moist respiratory rales, while with a hot breath they are usually dry.

If a remedy produces moist respiratory rales it is nearly always also capable of exciting cough with expectoration. If the latter be not the case, then the cough is either wanting, as in cholera (Colch., Cupr.), or else the matter which is loosened by the cough is swallowed (Caust.),—or lastly, the secretion is not raised on account of the half-paralyzed state of the lungs (oedema, emphysema, &c.—Colch., Cupr., Ipec., Op., Antim. tartar.)

If a remedy has chill on one side of the body and heat on the other, the chill is always on the side on which the respective remedy is also otherwise predominant; on the other hand, the heat (and mostly also the perspiration) on the opposite side. It appears, therefore, that the chill is more characteristic of the remedy than the heat, which is rather the reaction.

Those remedies which, in moderate doses, produce no nausea, have the character of constitutional non-irritability; the same is true of those where itching of the skin is never, or only rarely, changed by scratching. Compare Colch., Helleb., Iod., Ipec., Op., Stramon.

Arsenic has the character of constitutional non-irritability, and, with it, predominant complaints in internal parts; we find, therefore, in this remedy the feeling of numbness or insensibility to be in internal or suffering parts; on the other hand, sensibility (to the touch, &c.) almost exclusively on external parts.

Such remedies as act specifically on the fore part of the arm (predominantly on flexion) affect mostly also the flexors and adductors of the lower extremities.

The muscles of the upper and fore-arm are, as regards gymnastics, in reciprocal relation to each other. By this only we can explain why the proved medicines, which act specifically on the upper arm, leave the fore-arm almost untouched, and vice versa.

Whenever a remedy acts predominantly on the interior or posterior side of the thigh, it acts also on the sole of the foot (Nerv. sciatic.); and if it acts predominantly on the exterior and anterior side of the thigh, it does so also on the dorsum of the foot, (Nerv. crural.) But, as a general rule, the whole course of the nerve is not attacked at one and the same time, nor in one and the same prover, but sometimes one and then again another part of the course and distribution of such nerve.

In this respect the contrast of the calf to the shin seems to make an exception, in so far as such remedies as affect the anterior and exterior sides of the *thigh* and the dorsum of the foot are often also specific for the calf. The explanation of this seeming anomaly is clear in the fact that the anterior plane of the tibia is not covered with muscles and cannot, therefore, contain any large branches of nerves.*

From what has been said it is apparent that we can judge of the purity of the provings by the physiological coincidence of their symptoms. If a thoroughly proved medicine contains contradictory symptoms, is has either been proved by different observers with different doses, *or* one of the two observations is erroneous, and it was no effect of the remedy. Of course we do not speak here of the so-called "alternative symptoms," therefore not of the agreement and disagreement of symptoms contained in one and the same relation of effects, but in regard to the *different* directions or drift which the effects of medicines take.

These diagnoses of remedies may be objected to on the ground that by further provings many of the antitheses may lose force; this may certainly be possible, but it will not occur often, because most of the modalities have already been *confirmed by manifold cures.*

All individualizing physicians, whether they call themselves homœopaths or otherwise, can use these diagnoses to advantage, provided they are acquainted with the range of the symptoms of the remedies referred to.† Without such knowledge they are of course useless; I have therefore no fear that my work will be abused by the ignorant.

Undoubtedly, diseases are also cured by physicians who pay no regard to modalities of symptoms, because they find it too inconvenient to individualize. They declare, without having ever applied the high potencies scientifically, such cures attained by the latter as spontaneous, simply because such high dilutions have proved ineffectual in their generalizing applications. Their success is explained by the habitual exhibition of massive doses which frequently force the disease to accept the symptoms of the applied remedy and to change the conditions under which its symptoms appeared before the use of the medicine.—Nature has her peculiar means of defence against every sort of attack, to wit, reaction; but to heal "surely, quickly and mildly" cannot be expected with massive doses.‡ It is therefore dangerous to use the reports of cures of such homœopathic physicians, because such cures, frequently followed not according to, but in spite of, the modalities of symptoms of the remedy in question, i. e. they followed antipathically. Even

---

* And the sciatic nerve, in its final distribution, supplies the calf and shin, and also the sole and dorsum of foot. M.

† Those who wish to have the most important symptoms of very nearly all the best proved remedies are referred to the Text-Book of Materia Medica by Adolphus Lippe. Published by A. J. Tafel, No. 48 North 9th Street, Philadelphia. Now completed. C.Hg.

‡ Still less, what is the most important: *permanently! never* done by massive doses. C.Hg.

if we consider it from the stand-point of the materialists, the application of massive doses is not contradictory, because the lower dilutions of our remedies are (not always, but generally) too large a dose for a homœopathic, and too small a dose for an antipathic effect. Medicines which have improved a sickness by traditional doses have not been prescribed accurately according to the law of similars, else they would have made the state of the patient worse instead of better.

When the law of Nature, as it has lately been laid down by *Grauvogl* in harmony with Hahnemann's doctrines, shall have once been universally acknowledged, then the latter can be no more pushed aside as antiquated (although truth never grows old) by those who, out of selfishness, abuse the name of homœopathy by applying it to the extremest eclectic empiricism. It is easy for any one to flatter himself with the assumption that he is a great genius if he rejects, as prejudice and delusion, all such phenomena as, not being plain upon the surface, cannot be immediately taken hold of. A physician of this category, particularly if he considers his practice merely as a lucrative business, fares very well, and it is not necessary for him to oppose the opinion of the masses.—The roughly naturalizing physician ignores contradictions and difficulties; he who bases his proceedings upon science solves the first and conquers the last, benefits always and injures never. Withal, there remains this advantage in Homœopathy, that the learned and the ignorant, the honest worker and the indolent, can all participate in its blessings. Homœopathy is that individualizing healing art which, like all her true disciples, seeks to exclude more and more all accident and chance. The generalizing physicians, who concede a large part of their success in healing to chance, just save to themselves the *appearance* of being scientific by their rampant skepticism; and greatly do they need this appearance, because with those chances they open the door to routinism as well as to charlatanry; they move therefore, provided they know better, on immoral ground.

The diagnoses not found in this work, such as Mercurius and Sepia (Mercurius and Stannum), Pulsat. and Silicea, Camph. and Ipec., &c., can be made up in the mean time by the comparison of those given. Of Gelseminum nitidum and Glonoïn there follows only a sample, the diagnosis from Belladonna.* Whenever the medical effects of these remedies shall have been more verified, then will Gelsem. have to be compared with Arsen., Puls., Veratr., &c., and Glonoïn, with Aconit., Camph., Digit., Op., &c.

One of the difficulties of the present work consisted in its limits. In order not to make it too extensive, and thereby unpractical, I was obliged to select from the pharmacodynamic affinities the most interesting and practically most important antitheses, and to generally leave out such symptoms as both have in common. In order to confine myself to the diagnosis, I usually had to leave all such symptoms of remedies unconsidered as were based upon single observations, and I have gained thereby in clearness and general survey.

I acknowledge thankfully that, without *Bœnninghausen's* previous efforts, my labors would have been above the power of a single individual. Bœnninghausen's diagnosis of Calcarea and Causticum (*Allg. h. Ztg.* 63, p 86 seq.) encouraged me to persevere in what I had reluctantly begun. No intelligent person can reproach me with having trodden in Bœnninghausen's footsteps, since in what he has done no one will be able to rival, much less surpass him.

The antitheses of remedies which have thus far been incompletely proved, or only rarely applied, and the symptoms of which could therefore have received but little con-

* Dr. J. C. Morgan has added a comparison of Gelseminum and Aconitum. C.Hg.

firmation in practice, are of course but meagre and uninteresting. This is one of the reasons why these diagnoses must for the present remain incomplete; but it is left to a succeeding generation to correct what is doubtful, and to complete what is deficient. What there is yet to do, in this respect, will become partially obvious when we observe that, in spite of all provings and counter-provings, the modalities of symptoms of some efficient and often used remedies, as Bellad., Bryon., Arnica, &c., have remained comparatively uncertain.

I hope that this work will, by all, be — not lauded, but — what would be to me the most acceptable acknowledgment — *used;* used even by those whose approbation would be of no benefit to a book of this kind. If it exposes to many a reader his own deficiency of knowledge, it is at the same time ready to fill up any such gap with fidelity and discretion.

The difference of the principal polychrest-remedies are partly familiar to all, but had to be referred to for completeness' sake.

It is true that the so-called naturally related or cognate remedies are not quite suitable as successive or alternate* remedies, but I could not omit them entirely, as the object of these pages is to facilitate the differential diagnosis of (also such) remedies, and because, as *Hering* has already shown, such remedies are especially diagnosed by the conditions under which their symptoms are either improved or aggravated. — Compare Carbo anim. et veg., Sulph. and Hep., Ant. crud. and Tart. emet., Phosph. and Acid. Phosph., &c., &c.

---

* The last appearing symptoms always being the most important (Hahnemann, Chron. Diseases, p. 171; Hahnemannean Monthly, vol. 1, n. 1, p. 7), for instance, after a medicine ceases to improve a case, the reappearing symptoms, or still more so the *new symptoms*, become the principal indicative in the next selection; we are never able to decide *a priori* what will be the next medicine suitable in a given case.

Close observation, however, had shown to Hahnemann himself, and to many of his followers, that after certain medicines (for instance Calcarea) certain others (for instance Lycopodium) are oftener indicated and follow each other well; hence the very important doctrine of *successive remedies* sprung up, i. e. there are some medicines which may often be given with peculiarly good results after each other. Of course never without consulting the changed state of the case, as we never know, and never can know, how a case may have become altered, and never know beforehand what medicine will be the next indicated.

In some cases (spoken of in the Organon, § 169 & 170) where two medicines appear to correspond to a case, one of them to one group, the other to another group, we may suggest that after the one has been given and overcame one part of the complex of symptoms, the other might be given next to overcome the others.—This may be sometimes the case, but it may also not; the chances are equal. We have first to see, inquire, and observe, as Hahnemann urges in § 170, before we decide. There are cases where, after such an indicated succession, the first medicine of the two appears to be indicated again, the symptoms having so changed, or the former group of symptoms indicating it being returned, and after it the second again, for the same reason, neither of the two being fully indicated, only both seem to cover the case. Such cases have been the offspring of the doctrine of *alternate medicines*. Both together being out of question as, then, they ought to have been proved together.

After a certain succession has been of a good effect more than once, it may be considered excusable to suppose a repetition might be of a similar good result, but never have we the slightest excuse to suppose such a thing *a priori*. As an example of the worst kind we may mention the alternation of Aconit. and Belladonna in scarlet fever, which has proved to be the most absurd and most injurious in innumerable cases, because Aconit. rarely, if ever, is indicated in scarlet fever, even not in the beginning, when it may lessen the fever, and the fever being of course beneficial, spoil the case. Belladonna and Rhus have been really indicated in scarlet fever and have been given one after the other, and in many cases with benefit alternately; but since we know when to give Calcarea or when Ammonium, we do not depend any more on such miserable makeshifts. *Alternation* is thus among true Homœopathicians to be understood as Hahnemann understood it, and never to be decided on *a priori*. C.Hg.

It is self-evident that many of the modalities mentioned are to be understood merely as prevailing and predominant, which would not exclude solitary deviations; for it is well known that, with several remedies (Nux vom., Rhus, Sil., Staph.), the complaints in the scalp constitute an exception to the other circumstances, partly in regard to the time of aggravation, and partly as to the predominant influence of warmth of bed.—Under Argent., Coloc., Rhus, &c., we find a contrast between trunk and extremities in so far as the complaints are at one time increased by extension, at another diminished by the same circumstance.—In Argent. and Sulph. the pains in the joints differ frequently from the muscular pains by the varied influence of rest and warmth of bed.—Aconit., of which most of the (inflammatory, congestive, catarrhal) symptoms are aggravated by a warm room (and by wine), has, on the other hand, the rheumatic pains ameliorated under the same conditions, while they are worse in cold open air.—As a general thing, congestive complaints are nearly always better in open air, even with remedies whose other symptoms are aggravated by cold free atmosphere. However, see: Chamom. and Nux vom.

In the separate comparisons are to be found not only what the one remedy has *opposite* to the other, but also what the one has in *preference*, or much *oftener* than the other, or when the same symptoms appear under different conditions. The relative differences I have tried to designate partly by their expression and partly by different type;—it lies, in fact, in the character of comparative observations, that the prominent type here used can have only a relative significance, not an absolute one: as in Bönninghausen's books. Where single words are not marked by different type, the sequence of different conditions is sometimes pointed out by the position of the words; if, for instance, under Rhus there is, "after rising from a seat," aggravation *or* amelioration, then the former refers to the commencement of the motion, the latter to its continuance

These general statements are intended for the comprehension of *all* the variety of complaints answering to a remedy, never for one and the same case; otherwise it could not be explained why under one remedy sometimes two quite opposite symptoms have been mentioned; as for instance under Merc., "itching, better *or* worse by scratching."

Wherever in any one diagnosis some headings have been omitted, it was because no notable phenomena had been observed under that heading, or only such as belonged to both remedies.

It should be understood, also, that on account of the general character of these notes, for instance, the term "aggravation" embraces all predisposing and exciting influences. It is, therefore, needless to explain in particular that, for instance, under Sulphuric acid the "aggravation by the use of brandy" refers to the consequences of a deleterious, habitual use of this beverage, while "amelioration after the use of wine," in the same remedy, signifies that it is simply a palliation of the symptoms produced by the medicine.

As a general thing, the *amelioration* of symptoms by the respective influences (motion, exertion, &c.) means that these influences are of a *moderate* degree; for example, Rhus has: "better on *moderate* pressure," on the other hand "worse on *deep* pressure,"—Ars., Bell., Cham., Rhus. t., "better from warmth of room," but "worse near a fire or hot stove,"—Cannab., Ipec., Thuya, "better in the room," but "worse when the same is too warm."

I need scarcely remark that no extreme inferences should be drawn from the statements in these diagnoses; to explain: if Pulsatilla has many complaints "better after eating," while Bryonia many "better with an empty stomach," it is not to be concluded that aggravation after eating does not occur in both remedies.

In order to gain in compass of expression, I have worded the *time* of aggravation or remission of symptoms in such a manner that conclusions can be drawn from either as to the other. If, for instance, Calcarea has "remission before midnight," we know that during any other time of the night or day aggravations occur, which, however, need evidently not be present in every corresponding case of disease. We can, thence, also surmise the extent of time of the remission and aggravation, respectively, to which the different symptoms of a remedy are subject On the other hand, we do *not* include, in the time of general remission or aggravation, attacks of *chills, fevers*, &c., nor *sleeplessness*, which often predominate just at the period when most of the other symptoms of a remedy show a remission, and vice versa.

With a similar brevity I have stated the relation of *thirst* to the different stages of febrile attacks The expression of "rarely" or "very rarely" presupposes the corresponding symptom in the opposite remedy to occur frequently —The "want of physical irritability" and "increased irritability" refer always to the (at the time present) material conditions of the entire individual constitution. It is therefore not to be understood that these phrases correspond with "over-sensitiveness," or "insensibility," or "feeling of numbness" (comp. Fluor, Merc., Staph.), which latter refer only to the condition of single or several nerve-branches, and which designates only the peripheral relation to external irritations. During a peripheral numbness or insensibility the central sensitiveness of some separate nervous trunks may be heightened, as we find it to be the case in many neuralgic affections. (Compare the note to Camph., Veratr.) *Dryness of skin* is not placed in antithesis to sweat, which is mostly found in the same remedy, but to *disposition to sweat* or *sweating easily*, in so far as both occur in feverless conditions.

The difference between *nervous* and *sanguineous apoplexy* is of little value to the pathologist, but remains important in relation to its phenomena and in therapeutics.

With the remarks on the coagulability of the blood it will have to be remembered that the same often depends on the dose and repetition of the drug, according to which it varies.

Wherever bright and dark hæmorrhages are differently stated, it refers also to the menses

I suppose there is no vindication needed for having placed the influences of the moon* and sun in contrast, as it is known that the influences of either exclude those of the other more or less, and, for instance, that a thunder-storm is not likely to occur while the moon is above the horizon. Besides, there are but few remedies which represent the influences of both equally. It is true that the electrometer has scarcely been used, thus far, in the provings of remedies, the state of the atmosphere during a thunder-storm being only a phenomenon of *dynamic* electricity, measurable by the galvanometer.

---

* Some doctors get into a condemnation fit if they see the "moon" mentioned in a medical work. With the most miserable superficiality they call it a superstition. But aggravations of symptoms, apparently synchronous with certain phases of the moon, have been observed and, indeed, noted by observers like Hahnemann himself, Bœnninghausen, and a few others. And they proceeded with such care that only from a very few medicines, about five per cent. of the whole number, such observations exist, and that is all that has been collected during the time of half a century! It is very cheap to sneer at it. But such "critics" have no right to call an easy process of this kind "reasoning." C.Hg.

It may not be superfluous to remark that the wordings "*first right, then left*" and "*first left, then right*," also "*from above downward*" and "*from below upward*" are applied according to the maxim of *Contraria contrariis*, by virtue of the law of inverse directions.*

The diagonal "*upper right, lower left*" implies in man and quadrupeds the stronger, while "*upper left, lower right*" signifies the weaker power. These formulæ are characteristic and important, because they contain, by implication, the principle of *motion;* while we mean, by a simple "*right* or *left*," no reference to rest or motion of the body.

The expression "*inner ear*" includes the middle portion, i. e. Tympanum and Eustachian tube.

Several remedies have the excretion of urine increased, *or also* diminished. Such an increased excretion is due, either to excessive doses of the medecine (Acon., Coloc., Op., Sassap., Sulph.), or to a spasmodic or paralytic state inherent in the symptoms of the remedy (Op., Bell., Canth., Hyosc., Stram.); or else the diminished excretion is conditioned by a simultaneous (watery) diarrhœa (Veratr., Phosph. acid., Arsenic). With Arsenic the stages of fever are also of various influence, as the excretion of urine during the chill is more copious than during the hot and sweating stage. — Besides, the assertions in regard to the urinary seeretion may suffer modification by considering the presence of a local disease of the urinary organs. Whenever, in the appendix, under the term "while urinating" the locality of the sensation is not stated, it is understood to mean the urethra.

Where simply the word "expectoration" is used, we understand always an "*expectoration by coughing.*" — "Expectoration rare" or "constant" refers not to the time of day (which is usually mentioned in connection with it), but to the *statistic relation* of the expectoration to the cough of the respective drug. It has concerned me more, as a general thing, to express the relative statistic significance of a symptom objectively, than to make sharp antitheses.

I am well aware that the allusions to antidotal symptoms are by no means exhausted, because every remedy which bears a symptomatic affinity to another one—i. e. which is similar in its form of symptoms, that is to say, which is alike in many and opposed in some actions—may also be its antidote; but I did not wish to let the opportunity pass of giving the reader an inducement to interesting comparisons. — At any rate, antidotes are effectually found only by the law of similars; and I wish to observe on this occasion that cases of chronic poisoning can frequently be recognized only by the aid of Homœopathy.

A few words on the disputed *primary* and *secondary effects* of medicines. Even though this conception be problematic (relative), still it is of importance; for should we drop such a distinction of effects entirely we would be obliged to admit all characteristic symptoms of a remedy to be capable of perversion to the contrary, such as contraction

---

* Compare note to Ammon. and Bell., and others. The formula "R. ⟶ L." or "L. ⟶ R." has been given only in eight of our comparisons, with such medicines only where it was considered sufficiently corroborated. More about it will be given in the Journals and in the "Analytical Therapeutics."

The formula "Upper right, lower left," or "Upper left, lower right" in the effects of a drug has to be exactly alike in the case, but the formula "right" or "left" is rarely to be considered exclusive; it may be the opposite side in the case, if only sufficiently similar otherwise; the formula "right to left" or "left to right," if it is a true characteristic of the drug, ought to be the opposite with the patient. C.Hg.

of pupil to dilation, ecstasy to dullness of mind, &c., which would be, to say the least, a venturous boldness. This distinction can be justified indirectly by Grauvogl's fundamental laws, in which it is affirmed that abstraction of water produces cold (on the other hand, supply of water—heat). Now, in accordance with this fact, all water-abstracting remedies produce *first cold and then heat;* at least, among the salts there is not one which has *first heat and then cold.* I would like to know what else this heat, following cold, could be, but a secondary effect; for it cannot be proved that abstraction of water produces heat just as well as cold. This is evidently no ground for striking out the "heat," following cold, from the register of symptoms, but we simply take note of the fact that it appeared *after* the cold (chill).

It is of course necessary to note, with the pathogenic symptoms, the dose which has been used; or else one would, like Hahnemann, have to confine oneself to a narrower scale of doses in provings and to experiment only with molecular quantities; because, if we take into account not only these, but also large and even poisonous doses, the result would be indefinite; but if, on the contrary, we follow the wise and measured path which Hahnemann has prescribed, then the relation of primary to secondary effects will be confined to a narrow limit, and it will be apparent how the inevitable characteristics of medical effects rest on just such a difference.

PHARMACEUTICAL KEY.

Added by C.Hg.

Aconitum—Tincture of the *herb* of Aconitum Napellus Stœrk, now *A. Störkianum, Reichenb.* (Hayne XII. t. 15, Schkuhr t. 145; Reichenbach t. 71; Ratzeburg Aconitum Cammarum t. 39. The root is stronger, and the seed the most uniform in strength; the symptoms of the herb, root and seed have not been separated, not even those of somewhat different species.

Agaricus—A trituration of part of the cap of the *Agaricus muscarius L.*, Amanita Persoon according to Hahnemann, or the tincture of the whole mushroom.

Alumina—A trituration of the Sesqui oxide of *Aluminum* $Al_2 O_3$ prepared from natural alum according to Hahnemann.

Ammonium carbonicum—The trituration of Sesqui carbonate of *Ammonia* $2 H_4NO$, $3 CO_2$ prepared from the Sal ammoniac of the shops, according to Hahnemann.

Ammonium muriaticum—The trituration of the *Chloride of Ammonium* H_4N, Ci_2, purified according to Hahnemann.

Anacardium—The trituration of the drug imported from the East-Indies, the seed of the *Semecarpus Anacardium.*

Antimonium crudum—A trituration of the mineral, the native Tersulphide of Antimony, taking the purest kind, according to Hahnemann.

Antimonium tartaricum—Trituration or solution of the old chemical preparation called Tartar emetic, Tartarus stibiatus, Antimonii and Potassæ tartras.

Apis—A solution in alcohol of the poison of the common honey-bee, *Apis mellifica*; a tincture of bees is an imperfect preparation, a trituration is the most objectionable.

Argentum—A trituration of the foil of the metal (Ag.) was used by Hahnemann; much better is the precipitate of the pure metal in the form of a fine dust.

Argentum nitricum—A trituration or solution of Nitrate of silver, Ag.O, NO_5.

Arnica—The tincture of the fresh root, according to Hahnemann, and not of the dried flowers of *Arnica montana*, a plant growing on high dry meadows in northern Europe, on mountains, or the Alps of middle Europe.

The flowers almost always contain the eggs or pupas of the Atherix maculatus, an insect of similar properties with Canthar.

Arsenicum—A solution in boiling water of the Arsenious acid $A_5 O_3$, the Arsenicum album of the shops. Later the trituration has been preferred.

Asa fœtida—A trituration or tincture of the drug, a gum-resin of the *Ferula Asa fœtida*, a plant found on the mountains of Persia.

Aurum—A trituration of the foil or the leaf-gold (aurum foliatum) of the shops, later the pure metal (Au) precipitated in the form of the finest dust.

Baryta—A trituration of the Carbonate of Baryta, BaO, CO_2, prepared from the Chloride of barium, according to Hahnemann.

Belladonna—A tincture of the juice of the leaves of *Atropa Belladonna*, a plant of the (calcareous) mountains of middle Europe. The tincture of the berries, from which most poisonings have been observed, is sometimes preferable.

Borax—A trituration of the Biborate of Soda of the shops Na O, $_2BO_3 + 10$ HO.

Bromium—A solution in pure water of the Bromine (Br.), prepared by the chemists from sea-water, saline springs, etc.

Bryonia—The tincture of the root of *Bryonia alba*, a plant of northern or middle Europe, growing in bushes along fences, near cultivated soil.

Calcarea—A trituration of the whitest deposite in the middle of broken oyster-shells, mostly Carbonate of lime CaO, CO_2, according to Hahnemann.

Camphora—An alcoholic solution of the Camphora of the shops, a solid volatile oil obtained by distillation from the *Laurus camphora*, a tree of the East-Indies.

Cannabis—A tincture of the juice of the hemp-plant, *Cannabis sativa*, cultivated all over the world. The Cannabis Indica, the inspissated juice of the same plant, prepared in the East, is always impure.

Cantharides—The tincture of the Spanish fly, *Lytta vesicatoria*, of the shops, obtained from southern Europe; substitutes act similarly, but not the same as Canth.

Capsicum—The tincture of the dry fruit of *Capsicum annuum*, the Cayenne pepper of the shops, best obtained from Africa.

Carbo animalis—A trituration of animal char-coal, prepared according to Hahnemann from a piece of thick neat's leather.

Carbo vegetabilis—A trituration of the vegetable char-coal, prepared, according to

Hahnemann, from the wood of the Betula alba; some provers used the wood of the Fagus sylvatica.

Causticum — According to Hahnemann: A very peculiar product of the distillation of slaked lime and bisulphate of potash, not acknowledged by the chemists of our day, but of a very marked chemical and dynamical effect. No spectrum has been obtained as yet.

Chamomilla—The tincture of the flowers and tops of *Matricaria Chamomilla*, a European plant, growing as a weed on cultivated soil.

China—The tincture or trituration of the bark of *Cinchona condaminea*, or other species, imported from Peru; the China regia or Cinchona rubra of the shops.

Cicuta—The tincture of the root of *Cicuta virosa*, growing in swampy places in northern Europe.

Cina—The tincture of a drug imported from Palestine; the dry tops and flowers (not seeds) of *Artemisia glomerata*; the Santonicum barbaricum of the shops, or Artemisia Vahliana, the Santonicum levanticum of the shops.

Clematis—The tincture of the leaves of *Clematis erecta*, a plant of the middle and southern part of Europe.

Cocculus—The tincture of the dried fruits of *Cocculus lacunosus* (Menispermum), a shrub found on the rocky shores of the Molukian islands, the Cocculus Indicus of the shops.

Coffea—The trituration or tincture of the unroasted coffee, the dry seeds of *Coffea Arabica*, cultivated in the tropics.

Colchicum—The tincture of the cormus of *Colchicum autumnale*, a plant growing on meadow-grounds in middle Europe. Seed preferable.

Colocynthis—A tincture or trituration of the dry fruit of *Cucumis Colocynthis*, a plant of the Levant.

Conium—The tincture of the herb of *Conium maculatum*, a plant growing near roads and in waste places of middle and southern Europe.

Cuprum—The trituration of the metal (Cu.) precipitated by galvanism in the form of the finest dust.

Cyclamen—The tincture of the root of *Cyclamen Europæum*, a plant found on the mountains of middle and southern Europe.

Digitalis—Tincture of the tops and leaves of *Digitalis purpurea*, a plant on the mountains of southern and western Europe; found also in America.

Drosera—A tincture of the whole plant, *Drosera rotundifolia*, growing in the swamps of Europe; also in N. America.

Dulcamara—A tincture of the stipites of *Solanum Dulcamara*, a European plant, growing on the banks of creeks and rivulets; also in N. America.

Euphrasia—A tincture of the whole plant, *Euphrasia officinalis*, found on dry meadows and pastures of northern Europe.

Ferrum—The original provings having been made with a solution of the acetate of iron, Hahnemann substituted afterwards a trituration of the finest filings of iron as pure as it was to be had, (Fe.) The Philadelphia Provers' Union used a powder of metallic iron prepared from the pure oxide by heating, passing a current of hydrogen over it until reduced.

Fluor. acid.—The solution in water of the fluohydric acid (HF.) in phials turned out of fluor spar.

Gelseminum—The tincture of the root of *Gelseminum nitidum*, Michaux or Gelseminum sempervirens P., a climbing shrub of the southern states of N. America.

Glonoinum — Glycerine $C_6\ H_3\ O_6$, acted on by Nitric acid, undergoing the same process which changes cotton into Pyroxyline (gun cotton), whereby the three equivalents of hydrogen are replaced by three of nitrous acid; becomes an explosive oil, which ought to be dissolved in alcohol to prevent explosion or decomposition. The name Gl-O-NO ine is formed according to the custom of the chemists (viz: Aldehyde) and the manner of the Rabbins for divisions of the Old Testament.

Graphites—A trituration of the mineral called black lead, graphite or plumbago, a slightly ferruginous carbon. (C.)

Helleborus—The tincture of the root of *Helleborus niger*, a plant of the Alpine woods of southern Europe.

Hepar sulphuris calcareum—The trituration of a chemical compound of Calcium and Sulphur. Calcium sulphuratum Ca S. According to the usual simple preparation adopted by Hahnemann, it contains to 3 Ca S one Ca O, SO^3; to prepare it in a different way, would give an essentially differing preparation.

Hyoscyamus—Tincture of the herb of *Hyoscyamus niger*, growing in all Europe, particularly about church-yards.

Ignatia—Tincture or trituration of the seed of *Ignatia amara*, a climbing shrub on the Philippine islands of the East.

Iodium—Alcoholic solution of Iodine, a so-called element of the chemists (I), prepared from saline springs or sea plants; some prefer a trituration.

Ipecacuanha—Tincture or trituration of the Ipecac of the shops, the dried root of *Cephaëlis Ipecacuanha*, imported from Brazil.

Kali carbonicum—The trituration of Carbonate of Potash of the shops, KO, CO_2. According to Hahnemann that prepared from common Tartar or Cream of Tartar, a bitartrate of Potash, is preferable to all others.

Kali bichromicum — Trituration of the Bichromate of Potash of the shops, KO, $_2CrO_3$.

Kreosot—Alcoholic or watery solution of a peculiar combination formed by dry distillation of wood, prepared according to Reichenbach, its discoverer, differing, according to Miller (Elements of Chemistry,

p. III, page 553), from the Carbolic or Phenic acid, which often passes for it.

Lachesis—Trituration of the poison of the *Trigonocephalus Lachesis*, a snake only found in the interior of South America.

Lycopodium—Trituration of the pollen-like sporules (seed) of *Lycopodium clavatum*, a fern in the higher European woods; here, in Michigan.

Magnesia carbonica—Trituration of the carbonate of Magnesia, prepared according to Hahnemann's prescription; 4 Mg O, 3 CO_2 + 4 Aqu.

Magnesia muriatica—The trituration of the chloride of Magnesium, Mg Cl, HO, prepared according to Hahnemann.

Mercurius—The trituration of the pure metal (Hg) or of Mercurius solubilis Hahnemanni.

Mezereum—The tincture of the bark of *Daphne Mezereum*, a shrub of northern and middle Europe.

Moschus—The tincture or trituration of the Musk of the shops, imported from Asia: the dried contents of a sac found near the genitals of the *Moschus moschiferus*, an animal of the deer-tribe.

Mur. acid; acidum muriaticum—The watery solution of the chloro-hydric acid (hydro chloric, muriatic acid). (HCl.)

Natrum carbonicum—The trituration of the Carbonate of Soda, Na O, CO_2 + 10 HO, prepared from the soda of the shops, according to Hahnemann's directions.

Natrum muriaticum—The trituration of the Chloride of Sodium, Na Cl, the common table-salt, purified according to Hahnemann's directions.

Nitr. ac.; acidum nitricum—The solution of the Nitric acid NO_5, the aqua fortis of the chemists, prepared according to Hahnemann's directions.

Nitrum—Trituration of the Nitrate of Potash KO, NO_5. The nitre or saltpeter of the shops, purified according to Hahnemann's directions.

Nux moschata—The trituration of the seed of the *Myristica moschata*, a tree cultivated at its home, the Moluccan islands; the common nutmeg of the shops.

Nux vomica—Trituration or tincture of the seed of *Strychnos Nux vomica*, a tree of the East Indies, the vomit-nut of the shops.

Opium—The dried juice of the *Papaver somniferum*, cultivated at its home, the Levant, and imported from the Mediterranean, particularly from Smyrna; all other kinds are objectionable.

Petroleum—The trituration of mineral oil, a natural combination of Carbon and Hydrogen, C_5 H_5. Only the purest transparent product of the depth ought to be taken, but neither the Seneca oil nor the Barbadian tar, nor any other substitute, nor that which has been purified, distilled, or altered by the chemists.

Phosphorus—The trituration of the vitreous, wax-like form of this elementary body (P) has been used by Hahnemann for provings as well as cures, and as during the trituration a part of the Phosphorus unites with Oxygen, an alcoholic solution has been substituted; also the solution in ether.

Experiments on the healthy, with other forms, particularly with the red amorphorus, might settle the question of the proper way of preparing it.

Phosph acid.; acidum phosphoricum—The trituration or watery solution of the glacial phosphoric acid, pyrophosphoric acid PO_5, 2HO, prepared from bones according to Hahnemann's direction.

Platina—The trituration of the metal (Pl.) precipitated in the form of dust, either according to the method of Stapf, the first who introduced these fine metallic precipitates, or according to later methods.

Plumbum—The solution or trituration of the acetate of lead. The sugar of lead of the shops was at first proved and used; later the trituration of the finest powder of the pure metal (Pb.) has been preferred by some.

Pulsatilla—The tincture of the upper part of the flowering herb *Pulsatilla pratensis*, a plant found on sunny hills and plains in middle and northern Europe.

Rheum—The trituration or tincture of the rhubarb of the shops, a dried root of the *Rheum australe*, or other species, imported from the interior of Asia; the so-called "Russian" is preferable.

Rhododendron—The tincture or trituration of the dried leaves and flowers of the *Rhododendron chrysanthemum*, imported from Siberia and Kamtschatka.

Rhus—The tincture of the juice of the leaves of *Rhus toxicodendron*, or the variety called *Rhus radicans* (poison-ivy), a shrub of North America.

Ruta—The tincture of the juice of the herb of *Ruta graveolens* (rue), growing on sunny, rocky soil in southern Europe, and cultivated in gardens.

Sabadilla—The tincture or trituration of the seed of the *Veratrum Sabadilla*, growing in swampy woods of Mexico. The semen sabadillæ of the shops is generally very impure and mixed with parts of the flowers of other plants

Sabina—The tincture of the leaves and tops of the *Juniperus Sabina*, the Savin, a tree of shady mountains in middle and southern Europe; cultivated.

Sambucus—The tincture of the flowers and leaves—or, separately, a tincture of the bark—of the *Sambucus nigra* (Elder), on moist places all over Europe; cultivated.

The Sambucus Canadensis of this country cannot be substituted, differing essentially in its effects.

Sassaparilla—The tincture or trituration of the dried root of a *Smilax*, the species not being known with certainty; but it is not the Sassaparilla of the southern states. Hahnemann used the root imported from Hayti, very likely the same as that imported from Essequibo. The common drug of the shops from Honduras seems not to be the same, and is very much inferior in its effects. If the drug be genuine, chewing must cause a great nausea in the fauces, extending upwards and remaining a long while.

Secale cornutum—The tincture or trituration of the Ergot of the shops, a morbid alteration of the grains of Secale cereale, frequently seen in damp summers. Whether it is a cryptogamic growth, or whether an insect causes it or follows it, is unsettled.

Sepia—The trituration of the dried juice contained in a bladder of the cuttle fish, *Sepia officinalis*, of the Mediterranean, imported from Rome. It is the poison of this mollusk which benumbs the small fish.

Silicea—The trituration of the Silica, the oxide of Silicon or Silicic acid ($Si\ O_3$), prepared, according to Hahnemann, from crystals of pure quartz.

Spigelia—The tincture of the dried herb of the *Spigelia anthelmia*, a plant of the West Indies and South America. The Spigelia Marilandica, the pink root of the shops, cannot be substituted.

Spongia—The tincture or trituration of the toasted common sponge of the shops, imported from the Mediterranean; the dried and washed-out solid body of a zoophyte, *Spongia officinalis*. Hahnemann used for his provings and cures the best sponge carefully roasted like coffee until brown and (friable) not burnt to a coal.

Stannum—The trituration of tin, (Sn.) Hahnemann used tin-foil of the purest kind, as the precipitates were not then known and had first to be invented by the Homœopathicians, but the latter preparations are decidedly better.

Staphisagria—The tincture or trituration of the seed of *Delphinium Staphisagria*, a plant of desolate places in southern Europe.

Stramonium—The tincture of the leaves and unopened flowers of *Datura Stramonium*, a native of Asia, now spread all over the world, growing on waste places. Tincture of the seed is preferable.

Sulphur—The trituration of the flowers of Sulphur of the shops, prepared according to Hahnemann; one of the different forms of this elementary body, (S.) The milk of Sulphur seems to differ somewhat. Also the solution in Alcohol called by Hahnemann Tinctura sulphuris.

Sulph. ac.; acidum sulphuricum—The solution in water of the Sulphuric acid SO_3; the oil of Vitriol of the shops.

Thuya—The tincture of the tops of the branches of *Thuya occidentalis*, a North American tree, the American arbor-vitæ, cultivated in Europe.

Valeriana—The tincture of the dried root of *Valeriana officinalis*, a plant of Europe, growing in damp shady and in dry sunny places; the plant from the latter location ought to be preferred.

Veratrum—The tincture of the dried root of *Veratrum album*, a plant of moist meadows of the Alps; the white Hellebore of the shops.

Zincum—The trituration of pure metallic zinc, an elementary body (Zn), formerly prepared from the filings, now of the precipitates in the form of dust.

REMARKS BY THE EDITOR.

Dr. R. H. Gross worked at his differential comparisons a great many years. When he had taken up a pair of "related" medicines, i. e. such as had a predominating similarity in their effects, or such as might be indicated in the same or similar diseases, he considered it a matter of complete indifference which one be placed on the left column of the page and which on the right-hand column. The two columns were to him like a pair of scales. He did not pay any attention to the doctrine of groups, the least of all to Teste's notions. After the collection was made, he arranged them alphabetically. The Index of this translation has been arranged exactly in the same way, and the reader can find at a glance what is contained in the book.

To compare all our proved medicines with each other, (if we calculate that there are about three hundred, more or less proved and applied), and to compare, respectively, each one with the other, would require about 50,000 diagnoses! But, of course, the greatest number of them, if worked out, would be useless in practice and a burden to our literature. Still a beginning had to be made in order to find out which are useful and which not, and to know which comparisons we had to make only in our own mind (as we do in other natural sciences.) This is our great aim, and to come nearer to it the work of Gross is a stepping-stone, a transition. As a selection had to be made, it seems that Dr. Gross took Aconitum and Pulsatilla on the one hand, and Sulphur and Arsenicum on the other, and added gradually what he considered next to most important. Here are about *five hundred* comparisons of *one hundred* of our most generally used drugs. Another similar volume, as a continuation of this present one, is ready if wanted by the profession, and that would satisfy all the demands of theory as well as of practice for the rest of this age

Such a result is certainly encouraging, since, although we are still a decided minority among physicians, we have proved already nearly all the elements of chemistry and about one-hundredth part of all that is offered by nature! This gigantic work had to be done by a few slandered men, within fifty years. It is by far more than any other natural science can boast to have accomplished in so short a time, and, as our increase in number is equally satisfactory, our sons and grandsons may reach the climax.

In advising how to use this book, we will address the students first and the practitioners next.

The student of Materia Medica has now a better chance than he ever had before to become familiar with the very essence of our knowledge of drugs. The bewildering awe overcoming every one entering into our dominion disappears with every step forward, if he takes *Gross* as his leader. Begin by first studying one medicine. Read what is given in the Text-Book of Dr. Lippe, or any other Extract you have on hand, and, immediately after it, its different comparisons, and you will at once get a clearer idea of its character. Of this you will convince yourself by reading, for a second time, what is given in the Text-Book.

The first impression the newcomers heretofore received was the perplexing *similarity* in our collection of symptoms, and it often led to the very absurd remark, particularly with our opponents, that the different drugs acted all alike, and had nearly all the same symptoms over and again. Here now, through Gross, the query will be reversed, and some will ask, "Where is the similarity?" Only here and there a few hints have been given regarding the similarity of the compared drugs, and, if more is required, refer to the Repertories; look to the Materia Medica itself, even to the Extracts; examine the Therapeutical Works, and you will find concordances enough.

The book is furthermore of the greatest value to show the necessity of a true, sharp *individualisation*, and will enable you to learn whether your examination of the sick has been imperfect. You may often return to the sick-bed and examine again and closer after having consulted the Comparative Materia Medica.

The practitioner may consult our work every day, at least in all cases where he is not perfectly certain in his choice. It may happen, and, indeed, often *will* happen, that we cannot at once decide between two medicines, and then we can go to find the very same remedies compared in the book; such a case requires no further advice, a single glance will decide the most important questions and save a great deal of time, except in some cases where a further, and better, and more complete examination will be required; but even in such cases we obtain instruction from the book, and a good advice into the bargain. If only one of the two drugs we have in view appears in the book, we have to look over such other comparisons as come nearest, or, what is very important, over comparisons with such drugs as either were the last given in the case, or had been given, with good result, to the same individual before; or else compare with a medicine which "rules the day," i. e. corresponds to the predominating *genius epidemicus* If both medicines are to be found in the book, but not compared, for instance *Mercurius* and *Stannum*, look to the index, and you will find that each of them is compared with Pulsatilla and with Sulphur. Study both, and you cannot fail finding the advice you wish. If it happens that we are undecided about several different medicines, we have to look over several comparisons. If neither of them is among the first hundred in the book, there is nothing else to be done than to make the wanted comparison yourself, and find out, at the same time, what a great undertaking it is to make one such comparison only, which, we sincerely hope, will impress upon you the importance to send in your subscription for a second volume, and not to forget to promote, as much as you can, the sale of this book; for a continuation of it will, as a matter of course, never appear if it does not meet with a ready sale.

The order in the arrangement of symptoms, which our author has adopted for satisfactory reasons, is only partly Hahnemann's plan. He commences with generalities mostly looked for by the practitioner, and the symptoms of the skin, with those of fever, following next. These are then divided from the other symptoms by means of a rule. Below this rule the symptoms of the mind were placed first, head next, and so on, according to Hahnemann's plan. A third division is again formed by another rule; it contains the Aggravations and Remissions during the day, and all other modalities and conditions. The fourth division points out the contrast of such conditions which are predominant in one remedy and the reverse in the other: one of the most difficult, but also most useful parts of the whole comparison. Here it is where we hope to obtain many additional corroborating, or, if necessary, correcting remarks by the practitioners.

According to the author every comparison had to fill a page, arranged in strictly alphabetical order, which is of great advantage in consulting the book. As a few of his comparisons could be printed together on one page, without disturbing the order, it was concluded to give others two pages, provided they could be arranged in such a way as to place them invariably opposite each other. Additions were also made to some of them, extending the limits adopted by Dr. Gross, in order to make them still more instructive for beginners.

There are *eight* such two-page medicines: Aconitum and Coffea—Bryonia and Pulsatilla—Coffea and Pulsatilla—Cuprum and Ferrum—Cyclamen and Pulsatilla—Rheum and Chamomilla—Rheum and Nux vomica—Veratrum and Belladonna. Thus *twelve* of our polychrests are more fully compared: nine times with one, twice with two, once with three others.

Beginners may find it very useful in learning by them what great practical use all such comparisons have, particularly if they are able to add observations of cured cases of their own, and know, as the Germans say, how to read "between the lines."

The translation has been made with the greatest care and the best intentions for *utmost accuracy*, trying, with due piety towards the author, to render his peculiarities and his own variations. The edition and revision has absorbed all the spare hours of a whole year. Some incongruities of language have undoubtedly slipped our notice. All remarks about such will be thankfully received, ackowledged, and made use of. The editor begs to be excused, in particular, for some Germanisms, most of which, it is hoped, will not hinder the use of the book; a few of them might even be permanently adopted, like the word "proving," and others.

"Fever," in the German language, means the whole attack in all its three stages.

Eastwind, in middle Europe, is a *land*wind, and, consequently, had to be translated by "Westwind," and *vice versa.*

Technical terms have been preferred whenever the author preferred them; otherwise they have not had the sole sweep as in other books, but the true, clear anglo-saxon was put in its place. For instance: "sweat" is generally used instead of the mock-modest "perspiration;" "bellyache" has taken the place of its real meaning; "*unpainful,*" philosophically (as used by Locke), is to be distinguished from "painless," and has been regularly used where it ought to have the preference. Several other expressions, not of daily use in the newspapers, have been preferred after a cautious consultation with American and German scholars.

Abridgments had to be resorted to so as to make the work less extensive and expensive. They will not puzzle the reader if he consults the opposite line or other places where there was space to spell the word out in its full length. *"Pred., Predom., Predominantly,"* is explained by the author in his introduction; it always means that the respective medicine has the respective symptom or modality far more than its opposite and is therefore to be preferred if the same is the case with the patient; but it is not to be used exclusively, i. e. the opposite may also come in use, being not a contra-indication, provided there are enough of other characteristics besides to confirm the choice.

R. ⟶ L. and L. ⟶ R. means that some symptoms, *with the provers*, have been observed to go from the right side to the left, or *vice versa* It has been supposed that in cases to be cured by such a drug the "drift" *with the sick* ought to be *the reverse*. Observations of this kind ought not to be lost, but carefully collected and communicated, as they may lead us to a greater certainty, in theory and practice, much more than any other proposed exclusive rule ever has done.

We cannot omit, at the close of this great undertaking, to express our thanks to all who aided us, as without such aid it would have been impossible for Editor and Publisher to succeed.

The first thing requisite was to have the manuscript, as left by the author, copied in more legible German. This was done, with the greatest exactness and in an incredibly short time, by DOCTOR L. KNABE.

To mention all who aided in the collection of a Glossarium, and in the translation of the text according to it, is inadmissible; but we say, with our thanks, that the translation of the Introduction — a most difficult task — was done by DR. R. KOCH, and a careful revision was made by DR. MORGAN. The Pharmaceutical Key was revised by DR. ZUMBROCK. The whole Appendix has been translated by DR. CONRAD WESSELHŒFT. The very interesting observations regarding cures of horses, in our work, have been translated with the aid of MR. TEGTMEYER of this city, a veterinary surgeon and a true Homæopathician.

Numerous *additions* by our Colleagues have been duly credited.

Finally our particular thanks are due to *Mr. John H. Schwacke*, who superintended the setting in type of a manuscript which would have been refused in most all other Printing offices, as the execution, according to the plan of the Author, offered such uncommon difficulties, that it required great skill, experience and ingenuity to overcome them. We ought to likewise mention the compositors, and thank them for their skill, their patience, and the great interest they have taken in the correct and tasteful typical arrangement of the work.

PHILADELPHIA, October 18th, 1866.

Constantine Hering.

LIST
OF THE
COMPARED REMEDIES.

To facilitate the understanding and use of this list, we premise that each remedy found in the left-hand column has for its opposite the respective heading under which it appears, leaving, of course, a blank in the right-hand column to indicate where the respective heading comes in.

ACONITUM.

	Apis.
	Arnica.
	Belladonna.
	Bryonia.
	Cantharides.
	Chamomilla.
	China.
	Coffea.
Gelseminum.	
	Ignatia.
	Nux vomica.
	Opium.
	Phosphor.
	Pulsatilla.
	Rhus.
Sepia.	
	Veratrum.

AGARICUS.

	Nux vomica.

ALUMINA.

	Calcarea.
	Lycopodium.
	Natr. mur.
	Plumbum.
	Silicea.

AMMON. CARB.

	Bellad.
Brom.	
	Phosphor.

AMMON. MURIAT.

	Arsenicum.
	Phosphor
	Pulsatilla.

ANACARDIUM

	Belladonna.
	Pulsatilla.

ANTIMON. CRUD.

	Antimon. tart.
	Pulsatilla.
	Sulphur.

ANTIMON. TART.

Antimon. crud.	
Ipecacuanha.	
Opium.	
	Pulsatilla.
	Rhus.
	Veratrum.

APIS.

Aconitum.	
	Arsenicum.
	Belladonna.
Camphora.	
	Cantharides.
Colchicum.	
	Lachesis.
	Phosphor.
	Pulsatilla.
	Rhus.
	Sepia.
Sulphur.	
Thuya.	

ARGENTUM.

	Mercurius.
	Pulsatilla.
	Sepia.

ARGENTUM NITRICUM.

	Kali bichrom.
	Natr. mur.
	Pulsatilla.
Thuya.	

ARNICA.

Aconitum.	
	Belladonna.
	China.
	Ipecacuanha.
	Nux vomica.
	Pulsatilla.
	Rhus.
	Veratrum.

ARSENICUM.

Ammonium muriat.	
Apis.	
Aurum.	

ARSENICUM.

	Belladonna.
	Calcarea.
Carbo anim.	
	Carbo veget.
	Causticum.
	Chamomilla.
	China.
Cuprum.	
Digitalis.	
	Ferrum.
Helleborus.	
	Hepar s. c.
	Iodium.
	Ipecacuanha.
Kali bichrom.	
Kali carb.	
Kreosot.	
	Lachesis.
	Lycopodium.
Muriat. acid.	
	Natr. mur.
	Nux vomica.
	Opium.
	Petroleum.
	Phosphor.
Phosph. acid.	
	Pulsatilla.
	Rhus.
Sambucus.	
	Secale.
	Sepia.
	Silicea.
	Staphisagria.
	Sulphur.
Thuya.	
	Veratrum.

ASA FŒTIDA.

	Calcarea.
	Mercurius.
	Phosphor.
	Pulsatilla.
	Silicea.

AURUM.

	Arsenicum.
	Belladonna.
	Calcarea.
	Lycopodium.
	Mercurius.
	Nitr. acid.
	Phosphor.
	Platina.
	Pulsatilla.
	Rhus.
	Sepia.
	Silicea.
	Sulphur.

BARYTA.

	Calcarea.
	Phosphor.
	Pulsatilla.
	Silicea.
	Sulphur.

BELLADONNA.

Aconitum.	
Ammon. carb.	
Anacard.	
Apis.	
Arnica.	
Arsenicum.	
Aurum.	
	Bryonia.
	Calcarea.
	Cantharides.
Carbo anim.	
Carbo veget.	
Chamomilla.	
	China.
Cicuta.	
Coffea.	
Colchicum.	
Colocynthis.	
	Conium.
	Cuprum.
Digitalis.	
Dulcamara.	
Gelseminum.	
Glonoinum.	
Helleborus.	
Hepar s. c.	
	Hyoscyamus.
	Lachesis.
	Mercurius.
	Mezereum.
	Moschus.
Nitrum.	
	Nux vomica.
	Opium.
	Phosphorus.
	Phosph. acid.
	Pulsatilla.
	Rhus.
Secale c.	
Sepia.	
Spigelia.	
	Stramonium.
	Sulphur.
Veratrum.	

BORAX.

	Nux vomica.

BROM.

	Ammon. c.
	Hepar s. c.
	Iodium.
	Spongia.

BRYONIA.

Aconitum.	
Belladonna.	
	Lycopodium.
Muriat. acid.	
	Nux vomica.
	Phosphor.
	Pulsatilla.
	Rhododendron.
	Rhus.
Spongia.	
	Sulphur.
Veratrum.	

CALCAREA.

Alumina.
Arsenicum.
Asa fœtida.
Aurum.
Baryta.
Belladonna.
Carbo anim.
Carbo veget.
Causticum.
China.
Cina.
Cuprum.
Ferrum.
Fluor acid.
Graphites.
Ipecacuanha.
Kreosotum.
Lycopodium.
Magnesia c.
Magnesia mur.
Mercurius.
Natrum carb.
Natr. mur.
Nitr. acid.
Nux vomica.
Petroleum.
Phosphor.
Pulsatilla.
Rhus.
Sassaparilla.
Sepia.
Silicea.
Sulphur.
Zincum.

CAMPHORA.

Apis.
Cantharides.
Opium.
Veratrum.

CANNABIS.

Cantharides.
Euphrasia.
Opium.
Pulsatilla.
Thuya.

CANTHARIDES.

Aconitum.
Apis.
Belladonna.
Camphora.
Cannabis.
Lycopodium.

CAPSICUM.

Nux vomica.
Pulsatilla.

CARBO ANIM.

Arsenicum.
Belladonna.
Calcarea.
Carbo veget.
Graphites.
Phosphor.
Pulsatilla.
Sepia.
Sulphur.

CARBO VEGET.

Arsenicum.
Belladonna.
Calcarea.
Carbo anim.
China.
Ferrum.
Graphites.
Lycopodium.
Mercurius.
Nux vomica.
Phosphor.
Pulsatilla.
Sepia.
Sulphur.

CAUSTICUM.

Arsenicum.
Calcarea.
Clematis.
Lachesis.
Phosphor.
Pulsatilla.
Rhus.
Sepia.
Sulphur.

CHAMOMILLA.

Aconitum.
Arsenicum.
Belladonna.
Coffea.
Cocculus
Ignatia.
Mercurius.
Nux vomica.
Pulsatilla.
Rheum.
Sambucus.

CHINA

Aconitum.
Arnica.
Arsenicum.
Belladonna.
Calcarea.
Carbo veg.
Cina.
Digitalis.
Ferrum.
Helleborus.
Ipecacuanha.
Lachesis.
Mercurius.
Natr. muriat.
Nux vomica.
Phosphor. acid.
Pulsatilla.

CHINA.

Sepia.
Sulphur.
Veratrum.

CICUTA.

Belladonna.
Ignatia.
Nux vomica.
Pulsatilla.

CINA.

Calcarea.
China.
Ignatia.
Nux vomica.
Pulsatilla.

CLEMATIS.

Mercurius.
Causticum.
Sulphur.
Thuya.

COCCULUS.

Chamomilla.
Cuprum.
Ignatia.
Nux vomica.
Phosphor.
Pulsatilla.
Rhus.

COFFEA.

Aconitum.
Belladonna.
Chamomilla.
Colocynthis.
Ignatia.
Nux vomica.
Pulsatilla.

COLCHICUM.

Apis.
Belladonna.
Nux vomica.
Pulsatilla.
Rhus.
Sepia.

COLOCYNTHIS.

Belladonna.
Coffea.
Nux vomica.
Pulsatilla.
Staphisagria.

CONIUM.

Bellad.
Nux vomica.
Pulsatilla.
Sulphur.

CUPRUM.

Arsenicum.
Belladonna.
Calcarea.
Cocculus.
Ferrum.
Mercurius.
Pulsatilla.
Sulphur.
Veratrum.

CYCLAMEN.

Pulsatilla.
Spigelia.

DIGITALIS.

Arsenicum.
Belladonna.
China.
Nux vomica.
Pulsatilla.
Sulphur.

DROSERA.

Ipecacuanha.
Nux vomica.
Pulsatilla.
Sulphur.

DULCAMARA.

Belladonna.
Lycopodium.
Mercurius.
Rhus.
Sepia.
Sulphur.

EUPHRASIA.

Cannabis.
Nux vomica.
Phosphor.
Pulsatilla.
Sulphur.

FERRUM.

Arsenicum.
Calcarea.
Carbo veget.
China.
Cuprum.
Iodium.
Lycopodium.
Pulsatilla.
Sulphur.

FLUOR. ACID.

Calcarea.
Nitr. acid.
Pulsatilla.
Silicea.
Sulphur.

GELSEMINUM.

Aconitum.
Belladonna.

GLONOINUM.

Belladonna.

GRAPHITES.

Calcarea.
Carbo anim.
Carbo veget.
Lycopodium.
Natr. carbon.
Petroleum.
Sepia.
Silicea.
Sulphur.

HELLEBORUS.

Arsenicum.
Belladonna.
China.
Lachesis.
Pulsatilla.
Veratrum.

HEPAR S. C.

Arsenicum.
Belladonna.
Bromum.
Iodium.
Lachesis.
Mercurius.
Silicea.
Spongia.
Sulphur.
Zincum.

HYOSCYAMUS.

Belladonna.
Nux vomica.
Pulsatilla.
Stramonium.

IGNATIA.

Aconitum.
Chamom
Cicuta.
Cina.
Cocculus.
Coffea.
Nux vomica.
Phosphor. acid.
Pulsatilla.
Rhus.
Sulphur.
Zincum.
Valeriana.

IODIUM.

Arsenicum.
Bromum.
Ferrum.
Hepar s. c.
Mercurius.
Sulphur.

IPECACUANHA.

Antim. tart.
Arnica.
Arsenicum.
Calcarea.
China.
Drosera.
Nux vomica.
Pulsatilla.
Veratrum.

KALI BICHROMICUM.

Argent. nitric.
Arsenicum.
Mercurius.
Natr. muriat.
Nitric. acid.
Pulsatilla.

KALI CARBON.

Arsenicum.
Lycopodium.
Nitr. acid.
Phosphor.
Pulsatilla.
Sepia.
Sulphur.

KREOSOTUM.

Arsenicum.
Calcarea.
Nux vomica.
Sulphur.

LACHESIS.

Apis.
Arsenicum.
Belladonna.
Causticum.
China.
Helleborus.
Hepar. s. c.
Lycopodium.
Mercurius.
Phosphorus.
Phosph. acid.
Pulsatilla.
Rhus.

LYCOPODIUM.

Alumina.
Arsenicum.
Aurum.
Bryonia.
Calcarea.
Cantharid.
Carbo veg.
Dulcamara.

LYCOPODIUM.

Ferrum.
Graphites.
Kali carbon.
Lachesis.
Magn. muriat.
Muriat. acid.
Natrum.
Petroleum.
Phosphor.
Phosph. acid.
Platina.
Plumbum.
Pulsatilla.
Sepia.
Silicea.
Stannum.
Staphisagria.
Sulphur.

MAGNESIA CARB.

Calcarea.
Phosphor.
Pulsat.
Sepia.
Silicea.

MAGN. MURIAT.

Calcarea.
Lycopodium.
Phosphor.
Pulsatilla.
Sepia.

MERCURIUS.

Argentum.
Asa fœtida.
Aurum.
Belladonna
Calcarea.
Carbo veget.
Chamom.
China.
Clematis.
Cuprum.
Dulcamara.
Hepar.
Iodium.
Kali bichrom.
Lachesis.
Mezereum.
Nitr. acid.
Opium.
Pulsatilla.
Sassaparilla.
Staphisagria.
Sulphur.
Thuya.
Zincum.

MEZEREUM.

Belladonna.
Mercurius.
Nitr. acid.
Phosphor.

MEZEREUM.

Pulsatilla.
Rhus.
Thuya

MOSCHUS.

Belladonna.
Phosphorus.

MURIATICUM ACIDUM.

Arsenicum.
Bryonia.
Lycopodium.
Pulsatilla.

NATR. CARBON.

Calcarea.
Graphites.
Lycopodium.
Natr. muriat.
Phosphorus.
Pulsatilla.
Sepia.
Sulphur.

NATR. MURIAT.

Alumina.
Argent. nitr.
Arsenicum.
Calcarea.
China.
Kali bichrom.
Natr. carb.
Phosphorus.
Sepia.
Sulphur.
Thuya.

NITR. ACID.

Aurum.
Calcarea.
Fluor. ac.
Kali bichrom.
Kali carb.
Mercurius.
Mezereum.
Petroleum.
Pulsatilla.
Sepia.
Sulphur.
Thuya.

NITRUM.

Belladonna.
Phosphor.
Rhus.
Sepia,
Sulphur.

NUX MOSCHATA.

Nux vomica.
Pulsatilla.
Rhus.

NUX VOMICA.

Aconitum.
Agaricus.
Arnica.
Arsenicum.
Belladonna.
Borax.
Bryonia.
Calcarea.
Capsicum.
Carbo veget.
Chamom.
China.
Cicuta.
Cina.
Coccul.
Coffea.
Colchicum.
Colocynth.
Conium.
Digitalis.
Drosera.
Euphrasia.
Hyoscyamus.
Ignatia.
Ipecacuanha.
Kreosot.
Nux mosch.
Phosphorus.
Pulsatilla
Rheum.
Rhus.
Sabad.
Staphisagria.
Sulphur.
Valeriana.
Veratrum.

OPIUM.

Aconitum.
Antim. tart.
Arsenicum.
Belladonna.
Camphor.
Cannabis.
Mercurius.
Plumbum.
Stramonium.
Veratrum.

PETROLEUM.

Arsenicum.
Calcarea.
Graphites.
Lycopod.
Nitric. acid.
Sepia.
Sulphur.
Thuya.

PHOSPHORUS.

Aconitum.
Ammonium c.
Ammon. mur.
Apis.
Arsenicum.
Asa fœtida.
Aurum.
Baryta.
Belladonna.
Bryonia.
Calcarea.
Carbo anim.
Carbo veget.
Causticum.
Cocculus.
Euphrasia.
Kali carb.
Lachesis.
Lycopodium.
Magn. carb.
Magn. mur.
Mezereum.
Moschus.
Natr. carb.
Natr. muriat.
Nitrum.
Nux vomica.
Phosph. acid.
Pulsatilla.
Rhus.
Spongia.
Sulphur.
Sulph. acid.
Thuya.

PHOSPHOR. ACID.

Arsenicum.
Belladonna.
China.
Ignatia.
Lachesis.
Lycopodium.
Phosphor.
Pulsatilla.
Sepia.
Sulphur.

PLATINA.

Aurum.
Lycopodium.
Pulsatilla.
Rhus.
Sepia.

PLUMBUM.

Alumina.
Lycopodium.
Opium.
Pulsatilla.
Stramon.
Sulphur.

PULSATILLA.

Aconitum.
Ammon. mur.
Anacard.
Antim. crud.
Antim. tart.
Apis.
Argentum.
Argent. nitr.

PULSATILLA.

Arnica.
Arsenicum.
Asa fœt.
Aurum.
Baryta.
Belladonna.
Bryonia.
Calcarea.
Cannabis.
Capsicum.
Carbo anim.
Carbo veg.
Causticum.
Chamom.
China.
Cicuta.
Cina.
Cocculus.
Coffea.
Colchicum.
Colocynth.
Conium.
Cuprum.
Cyclamen.
Digitalis.
Drosera.
Euphrasia.
Ferrum.
Fluor. acid.
Helleborus.
Hyoscyamus.
Ignatia.
Ipecacuanha.
Kali bichrom.
Kali carbon.
Lachesis.
Lycopodium.
Magnesia c.
Magn. mur.
Mercurius.
Mezereum.
Muriat. acid.
Natr. carb.
Nitr. acid.
Nux mosch.
Nux vomica.
Phosphor.
Phosphor. acid.
Platina.
Plumbum.
Rhodod.
Rhus.
Ruta.
Sabad.
Sepia.
Spigelia.
Spongia.
Stannum.
Staphisagria.
Stramonium.
Sulphur.
Sulph. acid.
Thuya.
Zincum.

RHEUM.

Chamomilla.
Nux vomica.

RHODODENDRON.

Bryonia.
Pulsatilla.
Rhus.

RHUS.

Aconitum.
Ant. tart.
Apis.
Arnica.
Arsenicum.
Aurum.
Belladonna.
Bryonia.
Calcarea.
Causticum.
Cocculus.
Colchicum.
Dulcamara.
Ignatia.
Lachesis.
Mezereum.
Nitrum.
Nux mosch.
Nux vomica.
Phosphor.
Platina.
Pulsatilla.
Rhododendron.
Sabadilla.
Sambucus.
Sepia.
Silicea.
Sulphur.
Veratrum.

RUTA.

Pulsatilla.
Sulphur.

SABADILLA.

Nux vomica.
Pulsatilla.
Rhus.

SAMBUCUS

Arsenicum.
Chamomilla.
Rhus.

SASSAPARILLA.

Calcarea.
Mercurius.

SECALE. C.

Arsenicum
Belladonna.
Veratrum.

SEPIA.

Aconitum.
Apis.
Argentum.
Arsenicum.

SEPIA.

Aurum.
Belladonna.
Calcarea.
Carbo anim.
Carbo veget.
Causticum.
China.
Colchicum.
Dulcamara.
Graphites.
Kali carb.
Lycopodium.
Magnesia c.
Magnesia mur.
Natrum carb.
Natr. mur.
Nitr. acid.
Nitrum.
Petroleum.
Phosph. acid.
Platina.
Pulsatilla.
Rhus.
Silicea.
Sulphur.
Sulph. acid.
Zincum.

SILICEA.

Alumina.
Arsenicum.
Asa fœtida.
Aurum.
Baryta.
Calcarea.
Fluor. acid.
Graphites.
Hepar s. c.
Lycopodium
Magnesia.
Rhus.
Sepia.
Sulphur.

SPIGELIA.

Belladonna.
Cyclamen.
Pulsatilla.

SPONGIA.

Bromium.
Bryonia.
Hepar s. c.
Phosphor.
Pulsatilla.

STANNUM.

Lycopodium.
Pulsatilla.
Sulphur.

STAPHISAGRIA.

Arsenicum.
Colocynthis.

STAPHISAGRIA.

Lycopodium.
Mercurius.
Nux vomica.
Pulsatilla.
Sulphur
Thuya.

STRAMONIUM.

Belladonna.
Hyoscyamus.
Opium.
Plumbum.
Pulsatilla.

SULPHUR.

Antim. crud.
Apis.
Arsenicum.
Aurum.
Baryta.
Belladonna.
Bryonia.
Calcarea.
Carbo anim.
Carbo veget.
Causticum.
China.
Clematis.
Conium.
Cuprum.
Digitalis.
Drosera.
Dulcamara.
Euphrasia.
Ferrum.
Fluor. acid.
Graphites.
Hepar s. c.
Ignatia.
Iodium.
Kali carb.
Kreosotum.
Lycopodium.
Mercurius.
Natr. carb.
Natr. muriat.
Nitr. acid.
Nitrum.
Nux vomica.
Petroleum.
Phosphor.
Phosph. acid.
Plumbum.
Pulsatilla.
Rhus.
Ruta.
Sepia.
Silicea.
Stannum.
Staphisagria.
Sulphur. acid.
Thuya.

SULPHUR.

Valeriana.
Veratrum.

Zincum.

SULPHUR. ACID.

Phosphor.

Pulsatilla.

Sepia.
Sulphur.

THUYA.

Apis.
Argent. nitric
Arsenicum.

Cannabis.
Clematis.
Mercurius.
Mezereum.
Natr. mur.
Nitr. acid.
Petroleum.

Phosphor.

Pulsatilla.
Staphisagria.
Sulphur.

VALERIANA.

Ignatia.
Nux vomica.

Sulphur.

VERATRUM.

Aconitum.
Antim. tart.
Arnica.
Arsenicum.

Belladonna.
Bryonia.

Camphora.
China.
Cuprum.
Helleborus.
Ipecacuanha.

Nux vomica.

Opium.

Rhus.

Secale.
Sulphur.

Calcarea.
Hepar s. c.
Ignatia.

ZINCUM.

Mercurius.
Pulsatilla.
Sepia.
Sulphur.

Aconitum.	Apis.
Complaints (tension, etc.) predominate in internal parts.	Complaints (tension, etc.) predominate in external parts.
Complaints predominate on the soft palate, in the liver and on the patella.	Complaints predominate on the roof of mouth, in the spleen and in the hollow of the knee.
The part affected is hot—Thirst	The part affected is chilled—Thirst seems to be wanting only during the sweat.
Chills in streaks	Burning in small spots, (subjective heat.)
Fear of loss of reason	Fear of apoplexy.
Fear and sadness predominant—Despair of recovery—Anxious feeling in the præcordia.	Eccentric cheerfulness or hopelessness — Wavering inconsistency — Jealousy — Anxious feeling in the head.
Ecstasies—Fancies	Dullness of mind.
Ailments following fear	Ailments following jealousy or hearing bad news
Saliva predominantly diminished	Saliva predominantly increased.
Inguinal hernia, small and of recent origin.	Inguinal hernia, large and of long standing.
Infrequent discharge of urine	Frequent discharge of urine.
Catamenia too late	Catamenia generally too soon.
Increase of milk	Decrease of milk.
Cough, especially in the evening and after midnight; expectoration very seldom; morning and during day.	Cough awakens from the first sleep before midnight, and ceases as soon as the least particle is loosened which is swallowed.
With HORSES: Inflammation of brain; putting the head firmly against the wall.	With HORSES: Inflammation of brain; runs the head furiously against the wall.
REMISSION during the day and before midnight.	REMISSION of complaints during the day.
Worse when looking down.	Worse when looking fixedly at any object.

Predomin. worse — **Predomin. better**

When rising from bed, from cold, and when assuming an erect position.

Predomin. better — **Predomin. worse**

From warmth, on expiration, after rising from bed, and also when sitting down.

Aconitum.	Arnica.
Complaints (tension) predominate in internal parts.	Complaints (tension) predominate in external parts.
Numbness in the suffering (gouty) limbs	Sensation of deadness in the bruised parts.
Itching, generally unchanged by scratching.	Itching lessened or unchanged by scratching.
Perspiration of the parts lain on	Coldness, sometimes confined to the parts lain on.
Heat with inclination to uncover	Heat, with aversion to uncover.
Thirst during all stages	Thirst sometimes wanting during heat and sweat; constant during and *before* the chill.
Sleeplessness predominant after midnight .	Sleeplessness prevailing before midnight.
Complaints predominate in upper part of chest and in the palms of hands.	Complaints predominate in lower part of chest and on the back of hands.
Fear of loss of reason	Fear of apoplexy.
Ailments following fright or vexation with fright, fear or anger.	Ailments following fright or anger.
Nausea in œsophagus, stomach or throat .	Nausea in the stomach.
Urine seldom and scanty, only exceptionally copious.	Urine seldom and scanty, only exceptionally frequent.
Catamenia generally too late	Catamenia generally too soon.
Expectoration seldom; in the morning and during the day.	Expectoration seldom; is loosened during the day and evening and is generally swallowed.
Remission during the day and before midnight.	**Remission** during the day and after midnight.
More frequently benefited than harmed by wine.	Worse from spirituous liquors.
Better with head lying high	Better in a horizontal position.
Better lying on the back	Better lying on the side *or* back.
Better when lying on the unpainful side .	Better when lying on the painful *or* on the unpainful side.
Worse when riding	Worse *after* riding.

Prevalently worse — **Prevalently better**

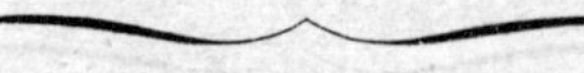

When swallowing, after lying down, in bed, being wrapt up and when opening the eyes.

Predomin. better — **Predomin. worse**

When walking in the open air *, being uncovered and when closing the eyes.

* The open air, without reference to the influence of motion, predominantly causes improvement with both remedies.

Aconitum.	Belladonna.
Left side, especially the lower left and upper right.	Right side, especially the lower right and upper left.
Arterial system dominant	Venous system dominant.
Pulse sometimes accelerated, sometimes retarded.	Pulse sometimes large, sometimes small.
The suffering parts are hot	The suffering parts are often cold.
Cold creeping upwards	Cold creeping downwards.
Thirst during all stages	Thirst not frequent during the chill; generally not constant.
Heat, or perspiration, with inclination to uncover.	Heat or perspiration, with aversion to uncover.
Sleeplessness predominant after midnight.	Sleeplessness before midnight
Complaints predominate on the soft palate and on the fore-arm.	Complaints predominate on the roof of mouth and on the upper arm.
Ecstasies	Mental dullness more frequent than ecstasies.
Sensibility of disposition	Predominant insensibility of disposition.
Fear of loss of reason	Fear of poisoning or apoplexy.
Ailments following fright, or vexation with fright, with fear, or with vehemence.	Ailments following fright, anger, mortification or vexation.
Pupils first *contracted*, then dilated	Pupils first *dilated*, then contracted.
Aversion to light, particularly sunlight.	Aversion to light, particularly candlelight.
Nausea in œsophagus or stomach.	Nausea in the throat or abdomen.
Retention of urine more frequent than incontinence.	Involuntary discharge of urine more frequent than retention.
Catamenia generally too late	Catamenia prevalently too soon.
Voice tremulous	Voice often nasal or raised.
Predominantly loud respiration.	Predominantly low respiration; only sometimes the expiration blowing.
REMISSION during the *day* and before midnight.	REMISSION during the *forenoon* and after midnight.
More frequently improved than aggravated by wine.	Prevalently aggravated by spirituous liquors.
Worse when standing.	Predominantly better when standing.
Better when lying on the back, *worse* when lying on the side.	Better when lying on the side *or* back.
Better when lying on the unpainful side.	Better when lying on the painful *or* on the unpainful side.
Worse when looking down	Worse when looking sideways or at running water.

Predomin. worse ——— **Predomin. better**

When stooping and sitting bent forward, after lying down, in bed, being wrapped up, from change of position, in the room *, and when opening the eyes.

Predomin. better ——— **Predomin. worse**

When sitting erect, from being uncovered, when walking in the open air, when closing the eyes.

---

* This aggravation in the room has particular reference to congestive and catarrhal complaints of Aconitum, while the opposite is the case with its rheumatic pains.

Aconitum.	Bryonia.
Left side. Dark hair	Right side. Light hair.
Constriction of internal parts	Constriction of external parts
Complaints predominant on upper lip, in upper part of chest and on fore-arm.	Complaints predominant on the under lip. in lower part of chest and on the upper arm.
Itching, unchanged by scratching	Itching, lessened *or* unchanged by scratching.
Heat on the suffering part	Cold *or* Heat on the suffering part.
Sensation of coldness in the veins.	Burning in the veins.
Perspiration increased after stool	Perspiration lessened after stool.
Thirst during all stages of the fever.	Thirst not constant, but predominant.
Sleeplessness prevalent after midnight	Sleeplessness prevalent before midnight.
Optical illusions, black or in dark colors	Optical illusions in bright or prismatic colors.
Smell acute, sensitive	Loss of smell.
Nausea in the throat, œsophagus, or stomach.	Nausea in the abdomen, not often in stomach, nor in the œsophagus.
Urine infrequent and scanty, only exceptionally copious.	Urine frequent, but scanty, only exceptionally copious.
Voice tremulous.	Voice nasal or raised.
Respiration quick and superficial	Respiration quick and deep, but without motion of the ribs.
Expectoration infrequent; in the morning and during the day.	Expectoration not constant; in the morning and evening, more rarely during the day.
REMISSION during the day and before midnight.	REMISSION of complaints during the day.
Worse when opening, better when closing the eyes.	Worse (better) when opening *or* when closing the eyes.
Worse when assuming an erect position.	Worse *or* better when assuming an erect position.
Worse when lying on the painful, better when lying on the unpainful side.	Most frequently better when lying on the painful, worse when lying on the unpainful side.
Worse from touch	Worse *or* better from touch.
Worse when growing cold and in cold weather, better when growing warm or in warm air.	Worse (better) when growing cold and in cold weather, *or* when growing warm and in warm air.

Predomin. worse —— **Predomin. better**

When standing, after lying down, in bed, and from the warmth of the bed.

Predomin. better —— **Predomin. worse**

After arising from bed, from washing and moistening the diseased part, and when walking in the open air.

Aconitum.	Cantharides.
Predominantly *left side*, tension in internal parts.	*Right side*, tension in external parts.
Complaints predominate on the soft palate and on fore-arm.	Complaints predominant on the roof of mouth and on upper arm.
Apoplexy more frequent than paralysis . .	Paralysis—No apoplexy.
Paralysis frequently one-sided	Paralysis generally of both sides.
Itching, generally unchanged by scratching.	Itching better *or* worse after scratching.
Dryness of skin.	Disposed to perspire easily.
Chills creeping upwards	Chills creeping downwards.
Heat with thirst and inclination to uncover.	Heat with thirst and aversion to uncover.
Thirst during all stages	Thirst during heat, not during chill; often between the cold and hot stage.
Sadness—Maliciousness—Absent-mindedness—Ecstasies.	Amativeness—Rage with convulsions, excited by touching the throat or by the sight of water.
Nausea in throat, œsophagus or stomach .	Nausea in the stomach.
Vomiting slime	Vomiting of food.
Catamenia retarded; oftener scanty than profuse; suppressed.	Catamenia generally too soon and too profuse.
Breathing generally audible.	Breathing inaudible.
REMISSION *during the day* and before midnight.	REMISSION in the morning and evening, until midnight.
Worse *or* better from pressure.	Better from pressure.
Better when lying on the back; worse lying on the side.	Worse (better) when lying on the back *or* on the side.
Better or worse after drinking wine . . .	Better from spirituous liquors.

Predomin. worse — **Predomin. better**

In the room, after lying down *, in bed, from the warmth of the bed, from being wrapt up, and while standing.

Predomin. better — **Predomin. worse**

In the open air and while walking in the open air, after arising from bed, from uncovering, from washing and moistening the suffering part.

*** This aggravation in the room is less applicable to the rheumatic than to the congestive and catarrhal complaints of Aconite.**

Aconitum.	Chamomilla.
Dark hair.	Light hair.
Skin and muscles rigid	Skin and muscles lax.
Numb sensation predominant in internal parts.	Sensitiveness in internal parts.
Apoplexy—Paralysis.	No apoplexy—Very rarely paralysis.
Convulsions of children, with heat, starting and single twitches.	Spasms of children, during dentition without fever.
Pulse generally quick, full and hard . . .	Pulse generally quickened, small and tense.
Ecstasies	Serious mood and wrapt in thought—Mental dullness.
Nausea in throat, œsophagus or stomach .	Nausea in stomach.
Galactorrhœa, with increased secretion of milk.	Galactorrhœa, with decreased or spoiled milk and consequent complaints of infants.
Nasal secretion thick	Nasal secretion watery.
Catarrh worse in-doors	Catarrh better in-doors, worse in open air

---

Aconitum.	Chamomilla.
REMISSION *during the day* and before midnight.	REMISSION *during the day* and after midnight.
Worse when growing cold; better when growing warm.	Better (worse) when growing cold *or* when growing warm *.
Worse from wrapping up; better from being uncovered.	Better (worse) from wrapping up *or* being uncovered.
Predominantly better after rising from bed.	*Worse or* better after rising from bed.
While assuming an erect position, almost always aggravated.	Better *or* worse while assuming an erect position.
Worse or better after drinking	Worse after drinking.

Predomin. worse ——— **Predomin. better**

From cold, but also in the room, when sitting bent forward, lying on the side, particularly lying on the painful side, from change of position, while opening the eyes, and on an empty stomach.

Predomin. better ——— **Predomin worse**

From warmth †, out of doors, while sitting erect, lying on the back or on the unpainful side, when closing the eyes, from washing and moistening the suffering part, and after breakfast.

---

* Both remedies have aggravations predominant in ***cold weather;*** **improvement in warm air.**

† This amelioration of Aconite symptoms out of doors is **particularly applicable** to congestive and catarrhal complaints, while the opposite is often the case with rheumatic complaints.

Aconitum.	China.
Most frequently aversion to motion . . .	Inclination to motion.
Itching, unchanged by scratching	Itching, relieved by scratching.
Complaints predominant on the lower jaw, in the upper part of chest, in the liver and on the fore-arm.	Complaints predominant on upper jaw, in lower part of chest, in the spleen (more frequently than in the liver) and on the upper arm.
Sanguineous apoplexy	Nervous apoplexy.
Pulse quick, hard and full	Pulse quick, hard, but small; more quiet after meals.
Thirst constant during all stages	Thirst is constant only during perspiration, but also between the chill and heat, and between the heat and sweat and *before* the chill.
Sleeplessness prevailing after midnight . .	Sleeplessness before midnight.

Aconitum.	China.
Sensitiveness of disposition—Irritability—Boldness.	Insensibility of disposition predominant—Indifference—Diffidence—Amativeness.
Perspiration on the head, better out of doors.	Perspiration on the head, particularly while walking out of doors.
Eyes protruding	Eyes most frequently sunken.
Saliva generally diminished	Saliva increased.
Nausea in the throat, œsophagus and stomach.	Nausea in the throat or stomach.
Catamenia too late—diminished	Catamenia too soon and profuse.
Nasal secretion thick	Nasal secretion watery.
Breath oftener hot than cold	Breath cold.
Cough and expectoration not frequent; in the morning and during the day.	Expectoration not constant; during the day and evening.

Aconitum.	China.
REMISSION *during the day* and before midnight.	REMISSION in the afternoon and evening.
Worse during inspiration and when taking a deep breath; *better* during expiration.	Most frequeutly better during inspiration and breathing deeply; thus *worse* during expiration.
Prevalently worse when assuming an erect position.	Better *or* worse when assuming an erect position.
Prevalently worse when rising from bed. .	Better *or* worse when rising from bed.
Prevalently worse when rising from a seat .	Better *or* worse when rising from a seat.
Worse from wrapping up; better from being uncovered.	Better *or* worse from wrapping up and from being uncovered.
Better when lying on the unpainful side. .	Better when lying on the painful *or* on the unpainful side.
More frequently better than worse after wine.	Worse after spirituous liquors.

Predomin. worse ——— **Predomin. better**

After sleeping,* in the room,† in dry weather, bending the diseased part backwards, and lying on the left side.

Predomin. better ——— **Predomin. worse**

After perspiring, while walking out of doors, during hot weather, from washing with cold water, while sitting, during expiration, and lying on right side.

---

* But yet, "on awaking," China has aggravation at least quite as often as amelioration—the first on awaking after being disturbed from sleep, the latter after sufficient sleep.

† Compare the note to Acon. and Canthar.

Aconitum.	Coffea.
L. ⟶ R.	**R. ⟶ L.***
Pain pressing from within outward . .	Pains pressing from without inward.
Pains steady or in attacks, with short intermissions; intolerable, most violent; restlessness, with agony even to furious despair, fainting fits; coincident with inflammatory symptoms.	Pains remit or increase; often in attacks, with longer intermissions; seem to be exquisite, insufferable; patients are beside themselves, whining, crying, anxious; with other nervous symptoms.*
Lameness; H.Gr. Paralysis of limbs . .	Great motor agility.*
Day and night, continuous pains in the joints, worse from the least motion, with swelling and exceeding sensibility to the touch.	Ischias (rending, shooting) or N. cruralis in attacks, inc. by walk'g; rel. by pressure, except on foramen; worse aftern. and night.*
Complaints in joints; rending, shooting, cramp-like or cracking; loss of power.†	No pain in joints.*
Pulse changed; frequent, full and hard, or quick and irregular; intermitting. H.Gr.	Pulse, if changed, more frequent, but less vigorous, even small and infirm. Grauvogl.*
Chills creeping upward; heat, with thirst; thirst constant during all stages.	Chills creeping downw.; heat without thirst; no thirst during chill, constant after the heat and during the sweat.
Feels cold or hot in the suffering part; when hot or sweating, likes to be uncovered.	Affected parts sensitive to warmth or cold air: cannot bear uncover'g.*
In red miliary fever: Increasing restlessness, agonizing anxiety and heat of body.	In the same: Increasing pains in head and throat, combined with a dispos. to weep.*
Measles: Dry, barking cough; painful hoarseness; eyes red; cannot bear light; jerks of left leg or l. arm, or grinding of teeth; restless moaning and lamenting; lying in a comatose state.	Measles: Frequent, short, and dry cough, hoarse when crying; skin and all senses over-sensitive; spasmodic motions, trembling, grinding of teeth; over-wakefulness, with heat and sweat in face.
Sleeplessness, more after midnight; from fear, fright or anxiety; with *fear of the future*; sometimes in consumptives.	Sleepl.; children want to play; before and at midnight; from being kept awake, or *after typhoid fevers*.*
Anxious dreams (with mental exertion*) .	Pleasant dreams (even merry.*)
Foreboding of death, predicting the day .	Fear of death during the suffering.*
Clairvoyance, perception of distant things.	Vivid imagination, ecstatic or sentimental.*
Easily frightened and startled by things outside of himself, particularly by noise.	Slight passive motions (rocking, etc.) startle him; are perceived as enormous.*
Tossing himself about, the limbs, head, etc.	Throws things about, away, down, etc.*
Dejection — Hopelessness — Fretfulness — Malice — Absent-mindedness — Fancies.	Joyousness; ailments after excessive joy or disappointed love; easy comprehension.
Answers only with Yes or No	Answer short, not disposed to talk, *or* endless volubility when describing his ailments.*
Weakness of memory predom.	Memory active.
Threatenings of apoplexy; burning pain in the brain; pressing, contracting pain above root of nose, red eyes, face red and puffed, pulse hard, either full and strong or small and quick.	Threatenings of apoplexy; over-excited, exalted; talkativeness; full of fear, pangs of conscience, discouraged, complaining, aversion to the open air, sleepless, convulsive grinding of teeth.*
Crackling (crepitation) in temples, forehead and nose; worse towards evening and from motion; better from sitting.	Crackling noise, synchronous with the pulse, in one side of the head; worse in the morning and out of doors, better within doors.*
Headache from talking	Congest. fr. talking; headache fr. thinking.*
Aversion to noise; it startles him	Aversion to noise; it hurts him.*

† It seems in all organs surrounded by serous membranes the capillaries are injected, reddening their surface, with shooting, piercing pains, an over-action of their function to rarify the air. On the other hand, Coffea promotes the change of matter in bones; hence, as a dietetic, is injurious to children, palliative in old age.*

Aconitum. | Coffea.

(Continued.)

Aconitum.	Coffea.
Nose bleeds, blood bright red, coagulating, with feverish heat, eyes injected; particularly during the climacteric years.	Nose bleeds, with heaviness of head, exaltation preventing sleep; as in nervous, irritable persons.*
Excessive hunger and thirst, but eats slowly.	Eating and drinking hastily.*
Diarrhœa, from getting wet; slimy, bloody, with violent pains in bowels; tenesmus also between the discharges, the hypochondriac regions are sore to the touch.	Diarrhœa from too much thought and care about domestic affairs; watery, painless, very weakening, with over-sensibility and great irritability.*
Urine infrequent and scanty, only exceptionally copious—(Scrotum drawn up.)	Urinating too often, rather copious—(Scrotum relaxed.*)
Catamenia oftener scanty than profuse	Catamenia too profuse.
During pregnancy, and particularly in childbed, foreboding of death.	During parturition or the afterpains, extreme *fear of death*.*
Violent labor-pains, following in rapid succession, partic. with a large child (head seems immovable), contractions insufficient, pains overwhelming; shrieking; red, sweating face; *thirsty*.†	Labor-pains unbearable, *ineffectual*; constant whining, crying, lamenting; violent moving of limbs; head hot, red; face puffed, eyes glittering; complete despair, great *fear of death*.*
Childbed-fever after suppression of lochia, mammæ lax, no milk; dry, hot skin, hard, frequent pulse; or tensive, contracted; fearful, wild, staring, glittering eyes, dry tongue, great thirst, inflated abdomen, sensitive to the slightest touch.	Childbed-fever from mental excitement; frequent crawling with feverish warmth; tongue moist, no thirst; delirium, talking with open eyes, eyes shining, violent abdominal pains, with over-sensitiveness; despair; sleeplessness.*
Larynx sensitive to the touch; voice croaking; cough whistling, barking, hollow.	Larynx as if covered with a dry phlegm.*
Cough; always taking cold; worse after drinking, troublesome all the evening, but particularly after midnight; shooting pain also in side, hypochondria, back and small of back, or with a suffocating feeling.	Cough; single, sudden shocks, quickly follow'g each other; from irritation in throat, phlegm in back part of throat, with dimness before the eyes, dur'g even'g and midnight, when falling asleep or soon after *
Palpitation of heart, sometimes intermitting, or with difficult respiration, great anxiety.	Palpitation of heart violent, irregular, with trembling of limbs.*
REMISSION during the day (except the forenoon**) and evening.	REMISSION in the forenoon and midnight, (except the cough *)
Warmth lessens the pains, particularly warm air; coldness aggravates.	In distressing toothache the only relief is obtained by holding the coldest water or ice in the mouth.* ‡
Complementary to Arnica, partic. after hurts	Complementary to Colocynthis in pains.*

Predomin. worse — **Predomin. better**

While standing, and also in the room.§ H.Gr.—When assuming an erect position.*

Predomin. better — **Predomin. worse**

While walking out of doors, and when sitting down. H.Gr.—Children from being rocked or moved about.*

N.B. All that is marked with * has been added by C.Hg.

† This observation was made by Dr. W. Wesselhöft, 1835. Even resolute, enduring women, who had born several children, tossed about in agony. Coffea was first given by Dr. Kallenbach, in cases of excessive pains, without a perceptible cause; frequent, weak, empty pulse; great pain in small of back, in nervous women, who get into a state of over-excitement or hysteric sensibility, who wished to be killed. The *fear of death*, as a characteristic, was discovered by Dr. Jäger. The same in afterpains, particularly with primiparæ, or after a mole.*

‡ For this observation of Dr. Blair, of Ohio, we have to thank Dr. Hale, of Chicago, who confirmed and communicated it afterwards; also Dr. Fanning (H. Rev. 5,161 and 214.) In all cases potences, even 200th were given.

§ Compare note to Aconit. and Cantharides.

** Dr. J. C. Morgan.

Aconitum.	Ignatia.
Plethora—Sanguineous apoplexy. . . .	Anæmia—Nervous apoplexy.
Thirst during all stages of the fever. . .	Thirst only during cold stage.
Complaints predominant on the upper lip, on soft palate, in the liver, on the fore-arm, and in the hip-joint.	Complaints predominant on the unuer lip, on the roof of mouth, in the spleen (more frequently than in the liver), on the upper arm and in the shoulder-joint.
Itching, unchanged by scratching. . . .	Itching, relieved or changing place by scratching.
Sleeplessness predominant after midnight.	Sleeplessness before midnight.
Maliciousness—Ecstasies	Gentleness—Mental dulness—Rarely unconsciousness.
Ailments after rage	Ailments after shame, mortification, hearing bad news, grief, jealousy or disappointed love.
Saliva predominantly decreased	Saliva increased.
Appetite for wine or brandy	Aversion to wine or brandy.
Urine infrequent and scanty, only exceptionally copious; dark.	Urine too often and copious; pale.
Retention of Urine more frequent than incontinence.	Involuntary discharge of urine.
Catamenia too late—Milk increased—Galactorrhœa.	Catamenia too soon—Milk decreased.
Expectoration infrequent; in the morning and during the day.	Expectoration infrequent; in the evening.
REMISSION *during the day* and before midnight.	REMISSION of complaints before midnight.
Worse during pregnancy	Worse *or* better during pregnancy.
Worse when assuming an erect position. .	Better *or* worse when assuming an erect position.
Worse when rising from bed	Better *or* worse when rising from bed.
Better *after* rising from bed	Worse *or* better after rising from bed.
Worse *or* better after drinking	*Worse* after drinking.
Worse from bodily exertion	More frequently improved than aggravated by bodily exertion.

Predomin. worse ——— **Predomin. better**

During respiration, particularly inspiration and taking a deep breath, drawing in the abdominal muscles*, when rising from a seat, lifting the affected limb, change of position, lying on the painful side, and when swallowing†, in the room and sitting bent forward.

Predomin. better ——— **Predomin. worse**

Between breathing and during expiration, when letting the diseased limb hang down, when lying on the unpainful side, out of doors ‡, and when sitting erect.

---

* Corresponding to this, Ignat. has aggravation from puffing up the abdomen.

† Corresponding to this, Ignat. has aggravation when not swallowing. Besides this, we find with Ignat. aggravation when swallowing liquids.

‡ Compare note to Aconite and Cantharides.

Aconitum.	Nux vomica.
Prevalent *left side*	Prevalent *right side*.
Heat on the diseased part	Perspiration on the suffering side.
Heat, with inclination to uncover. . . .	Heat, with aversion to uncover.
Thirst during all stages of the fever . . .	Thirst most frequently during the chill, and also between the heat and sweat.
Complaints predominant on the soft palate and on the patella.	Complaints predominant on the roof of mouth and in the hollow of knee.

Aconitum.	Nux vomica.
Ecstasies	Mental dullness — Amativeness—Ailments after being insulted, indignation, grief, disappointed love or jealousy.
Predominant dimness of sight.	Predominant clearness of sight.
Optical illusions in black or dark colors. .	Optical illusions in bright colors.
Saliva predominantly diminished	Saliva most frequently increased.
Desire for beer	Desire *or* aversion to beer.
Nausea in the throat, œsophagus or stomach.	Nausea in *stomach* or œsophagus.
Urine dark	Urine generally pale.
Catamenia too late, generally diminished .	Catamenia too soon or too profuse.
Recent, small inguinal hernia, also with bitter vomiting.	Inguinal hernia, particularly when large and of long duration, also with sour vomiting.
Nasal secretion thick.	Nasal secretion watery.
Expectoration infrequent; in the morning and during the day.	Expectoration not constant; in the morning, during the day and evening.

Aconitum.	Nux vomica.
Remission *during the day* and before midnight.	**Remission** in the evening, until midnight.
Prevalently *better* after rising from bed. .	Worse *or* better after rising from bed.
Worse when stooping	Better *or* worse when stooping.
Worse when swallowing.	Better *or* worse when swallowing.
Worse while standing	*Better or* worse while standing.
Worse while in a perspiration.	Worse *or* better while in a perspiration.
Prevalently better when lying on the back, worse lying on the side.	*Worse or* better when lying on the back *better or* worse lying on the side.
Better when lying on the unpainful side .	Better when lying on the *unpainful or* or the painful side.
Most frequently aggravated by bending the diseased part backwards.	Most frequently improved by bending the diseased part backwards.
Worse from the heat of the sun	Worse in snowy air.

Predomin. worse — **Predomin. better**

In the room, after lying down, in bed, from warmth of the bed *, lying on the left side, being wrapt up and when standing.

Predomin. better — **Predomin worse**

Out of doors †, when walking in the open air, lying on right side, from uncovering, and durin expiration ‡.

---

* it is only exceptionally that we find an aggravation with Nux vomica from the warmth of the bed.
† Compare note to Aconitum and Cantharides.
‡ Corresponding to this we find aggravation during inspiration with Aconitum.

Aconitum.	Opium.
Left side. Dark hair	*Right side.* Light hair.
Oversensitiveness*—Increased irritability .	Predominantly no pain—Want of bodily irritability.
Thirst during all stages of the fever. . .	Thirst almost only between the heat and sweat.
The pulse is sometimes accelerated, sometimes retarded, in the same person.	Pulse sometimes large, sometimes small, in the same person.
Apoplexy with staring eyes, hot head, cold extremities, and paralysis of the left side of the body.	Apoplexy with somnolency (snoring , half-closed eyes, heat with sweat, and paralysis of the right side of the body.
Pulse quick and hard.	Pulse full and slow
Sleeplessness more frequent than somnolency.	Somnolency more frequent than sleeplessness.
Anxious dreams	Dreams predominantly pleasant.
Sensibility of disposition	Insensibility of disposition.
Sadness—Despondency—Irritable mood—Peevishness—Maliciousness.	Joyousness — Indifference — Gentleness—Ailments after shame or excessive joy.
Memory oftener weakened than active . .	Memory oftener active than weakened.
Acute, sensitive smell	Loss of smell.
Complaints on the upper lip	Complaints on the under lip.
Grinding the teeth—Trismus	Lameness of jaw more frequent than grinding the teeth or trismus.
Nausea, particularly in œsophagus or stomach.	Nausea very rare.
Catamenia predominantly too scanty. . .	Catamenia too profuse.
Respiration most frequently quick . . .	Respiration most frequently slow.
Expectoration infrequent; in the morning and during the day.	Expectoration infrequent; during the day.
Remission *during the day* and before midnight.	Remission during the day and evening.
More frequently improved than aggravated by wine.	More frequently aggravated than improved by wine.
Worse when looking down	Worse when looking sideways.

Predomin worse ——— **Predomin. better**

From cold and during cold weather, when opening the eyes, and from sitting bent forward.

Predomin. better ——— **Predomin worse**

From warmth and in warm air, when closing the eyes, while sitting, particularly sitting erect.

---

* But yet a sensation of numbness, particularly in internal parts, occurs with both remedies.

Aconitum.	Phosphor.
Left side. Often indicated with children .	*Right side.* Often indicated with old people.
Sensation of numbness predominant in internal and generally also in external parts.	Sensitiveness in internal and numbness in external parts *.
Complaints predominant in the upper lip and in the patella.	Complaints predominant in the under lip and in the hollow of the knee.
Apoplexy more frequent than paralysis . .	Paralysis more frequent than apoplexy.
Itching, unchanged by scratching	Itching more frequently relieved than aggravated by scratching.
Sensation of coldness in the veins. . . .	Burning in the veins.
Constant thirst	Constant want of thirst.
Sleeplessness predominant after midnight .	Sleeplessness before midnight.
Sensibility of disposition	Insensibility *or* sensibility of disposition.
Mood sad and desponding—Malice—Rarely amativeness.	Mood changeable, joyous or despondent; indifferent; haughty; ailments after grief.
Memory oftener weak than active	Memory oftener active than weak.
Eyes protruding	Eyes sunken.
Nausea in throat, œsophagus or stomach .	Nausea in stomach.
Urine infrequent and scanty	Urine frequent, but scanty.
Retention of urine more frequent than incontinence.	Involuntary discharge of urine.
Catamenia too late, diminished, but of long duration.	Catamenia prevalently too soon; profuse *or* scanty, of long *or* short duration.
Expectoration infrequent	Expectoration not constant.
REMISSION *during the day* and before midnight.	REMISSION of complaints after midnight.
Worse while in a perspiration	Worse *or* better while in a perspiration.
Prevalently worse in bed	Worse *or* better in bed †.
Worse when lying on the side, better when lying on the back.	Most frequently ameliorated when lying on the side, aggravated when lying on the back.
Worse during and after sleep	Worse *or* better during sleep; better *after* sleep, except the siesta.
Prevalently better after rising from bed . .	Worse *or* better after rising from bed.
Worse while standing	Predominantly better while standing.
Worse from mental exertion	Worse *or* better from mental exertion.
Worse from riding.	More frequently aggravated than improved by riding.
Most frequently aggravated after drinking .	Most frequently better after drinking.
Worse (better) from cold *or* warm diet . .	Worse from warm and better from cold diet.
Better *or* worse from wine	Better from wine.

Predomin. worse ——— **Predomin. better**

During dry weather, from sweet-meats, from the touch, when lifting or resting the diseased limb, when standing, and after sleep.

Predomin. better ——— **Predomin worse**

During wet weather, from washing with cold water, after perspiring, during expiration, and letting the diseased limb hang down.

* We find over-sensitiveness to pain with both remedies.
† The warmth of the bed aggravates with both remedies.

Aconitum.	Pulsatilla.
Left side, particularly *lower left* and *upper right* side.	*Right side*, particularly *lower right* and *upper left side*.
Sanguineous apoplexy — Thirst during all stages of the fever.	Nervous apoplexy—Thirst only during and before the heat, more rarely after the heat
Pulse often quicker than the beat of heart, rarely the opposite; most frequently quick, full, and hard.	Pulse frequently suppressed, with strong beat of heart; generally quick, small and weak
Itching generally unchanged by scratching.	Itching changed *or* aggravated by scratching.
Sleeplessness predominant after midnight.	Sleeplessness before midnight.
Complaints predominant on the upper lip, on the soft palate, in the upper part of chest, on the fore-arm, in the palm of hand, on the patella.	Complaints predominant on the under lip, on the roof of the mouth, in the lower part of chest, on the upper arm, on the back of hand, and in the hollow of the knee.
Maliciousness — Irritable mood	Good-naturedness — Gentleness — Indifference — Embarrassment — Amativeness — Greediness.
Ailments following fright, anger or vexation, with vehemence.	Ailments following mortification, grief or excessive joy.
Ecstasies.	Sometimes weakness of reasoning powers.
Eyes protruding	Eyes sunken.
Pupils most frequently dilated.	Pupils most frequently contracted.
Optical illusions in black or dark colors. .	Optical illusions in bright colors.
Acute, sensitive smell	Predominant loss of smell.
Saliva predominantly decreased	Saliva most frequently increased.
Nausea in œsophagus or stomach, less frequently in throat.	Nausea in throat, stomach, or abdomen.
Retention of urine more frequent than incontinence.	Incontinence more frequent than retention of urine.
Catamenia frequently of too long duration.	Catamenia most frequently of too short duration.
Cough generally dry	Cough most frequently with expectoration.
Aggravation from evening until morning.	Aggravation from noon until midnight.
Better in the dark	Better *or* worse in the dark.
Worse while in a perspiration, better after it.	Worse *during and after* perspiring.
Worse when swallowing.	Worse *or* better when swallowing.
Better from eructation	Most frequently aggravated by eructation.
Worse *or* better from cold (resp. warm) diet.	Predominantly better from cold and worse from warm diet.
Worse when rising from bed	*Better or worse* when rising from bed.
Worse when rising from a seat	*Worse or better* when rising from a seat.
Better when sitting down	Worse *or* better when sitting down
Worse *or* better from motion (resp. rest.).	Worse when resting and in the beginning of motion, better during continued and moderate motion.
Worse when looking down.	Worse when looking up.

Prevalently worse — **Prevalently better**

From cold, growing cold, during cold dry weather, when opening the eyes, on inspiration, from tying the clothes tight, from bodily exertion, when lifting or resting the diseased limb on something, when lying on the painful side, and when rising from bed.

Predomin. better — **Predomin. worse**

From warmth, from growing warm, in warm, moist air, when closing the eyes, on expiration, from loosening the clothes, when sitting, letting the diseased limb hang down, and when lying on the unpainful side, after perspiration, and from eructation.

Aconitum.	Rhus.
Left side; particularly *lower left, upper right side*—Dark hair.	*Right side*, particularly *lower right, upper left side*—Light hair.
Complaints (tension) predominant in internal parts.	Complaints (tension) predominant in external parts.
Over-sensitiveness to pain *.	Insensibility and sensation of numbness predominant.
Itching unchanged by scratching	Itching relieved by scratching.
Torpor of the left side of the body . . .	"Gone to sleep" of the right side of body.
Pulse generally quick, full, hard	Pulse irregular, generally quick, faint, weak or soft.
Heat on the suffering part	Cold perspiration on the diseased part.
Heat, with inclination to uncover	Heat, with aversion to uncover.
Thirst during all stages of the fever . . .	Thirst not constant.
Sleeplessness predominant after midnight .	Sleeplessness predominant before midnight.
Apoplexy more frequent than paralysis . .	Paralysis more frequent than apoplexy.
Mood peevish, irritable, malicious . . .	Mood almost exclusively depressed, dejected.
Fear of loss of reason	Fear of being poisoned.
Absentmindedness – Ecstasies	Difficult comprehension.
Complaints predominant on the soft palate, in the upper part of chest, and in the palms of the hands.	Complaints predominant on the roof of the mouth, in the lower part of chest, and on the back of the hand.
Acute, sensitive smell	Loss of smell.
Saliva predominantly decreased	Saliva most frequently increased.
Desire for wine or brandy	Aversion to wine.
Recent and small inguinal hernia	Inguinal hernia, especially old and large ones, with flatulent distention.
Urine infrequent and scanty, only exceptionally copious; dark; red sediment.	Urine frequent and copious; pale; white sediment.
Retention of urine more frequent than incontinence.	Involuntary discharge of urine predominant.
Catamenia too late and diminished . . .	Catamenia too soon and profuse.
Expectoration infrequent; in the morning and during the day.	Expectoration not constant; in the morning.
REMISSION *during the day* and before midnight.	REMISSION of complaints during the day.
Worse in bed	Better in bed (warmth) *or* (rest) worse †.
Prevalently better after rising from bed.	Worse *or* better after rising from bed.
Worse on rising from a seat	*Worse or* better on rising from a seat.
Predominantly better when sitting down .	Worse *or* better when sitting down.
Worse when stretching out the diseased limb.	Most frequently better when stretching out the diseased limb.
Worse *or* better from motion (resp. rest.) .	Worse in the beginning of motion and during rest, better during continuous moderate motion.
Worse *or* better from cold (resp. warm) diet.	Worse from cold, better from warm diet.
Worse from the heat of the sun	Worse from snowy air.

Predomin. worse — **Predomin. better**

During dry weather, in the room, from wrapping up, lying on the side, especially lying on the painful side, from being overheated, and when stretching out the diseased limb.

Predomin. better — **Predomin. worse**

During wet weather, out of doors, from uncovering, lying on the back, lying on the unpainful side, when sitting, from washing with cold water and moistening the diseased part, and when drawing up the diseased limb.

* Yet we find "sensation of numbness predominant in internal parts" with Aconitum, "sensitiveness predominant in external parts" with Rhus.

† With Rhus we also find aggravation from the warmth of the bed; but these cases are not at all frequent.

Aconitum.	Veratrum.
L. → R.	**R. → L.**
Left side, particularly *lower left and upper right side.*	*Right side*, particularly *lower right and upper left side.*
Dark hair	Light hair.
Skin and muscles rigid	Skin and muscles lax.
Apoplexy more frequent than paralysis.	Paralysis more frequent than apoplexy.
Pulse changed, quick, large, hard, sometimes irregular, intermitting or quicker than the pulsation of the heart, (rarely the opposite).	Pulse changed in quality and strength, generally slower, even slower than the pulsation of the heart, sometimes irregular or intermitting, often imperceptible.
Chills creeping upwards	Chills creeping downwards.
Thirst constant	Thirst not constant.
Sleeplessness prevalent after midnight	Sleeplessness prevalent before midnight
Fear of loss of reason	Fear of being poisoned or of apoplexy.
Fretfulness	Haughtiness—Amativeness—Consequences of grief.
Ecstasies	Insanity.
Eyes protruding	Eyes most frequently sunken.
Pupils most frequently dilated	Pupils most frequently contracted.
Optical illusions in black or dark colors	Optical illusions in bright colors.
Acute, sensitive smell	Loss of smell.
Nausea in œsophagus or stomach, rarely in the throat.	Nausea in the stomach.
Expectoration infrequent; in the morning and during the day.	Expectoration not constant; during the day.
Complaints predominant on fore-arm	Complaints predominant on upper arm.
Remission *during the day* and before midnight.	Remission of complaints during the day and evening.
In bed, predominantly worse	In bed, worse *or* better.
Worse when rising from bed	When rising from bed, better *or* worse.
Prevalently better *after* rising from bed	*After* rising from bed, worse *or* better.
Worse when rising from a seat	When rising from a seat, better *or* worse.
Better *or* worse from motion (resp. rest.)	Predominantly better when moving, worse during rest.
Worse on inspiration, better on expiration.	Worse on inspiration *or* on expiration.
Predominantly worse when growing cold; predominantly better when growing warm.	When growing cold, better *or* worse; when growing warm, better *or* worse.
Better *or* worse from cold (resp. warm) diet.	Worse from cold, better from warm diet.
Worse in dry, cold weather	Worse in damp, cold weather.

Predomin. worse ⟵ ⟶ **Predomin. better**

In dry weather, when ascending, when sitting down, and while sitting.

Predomin. better ⟵ ⟶ **Predomin. worse**

In wet weather and when descending.

N. B. As a general rule, Veratrum has not the over-sensitiveness to pain of the Aconit-patient.

Agaricus.	Nux vomica.
Left side.—Light hair. Skin and muscles lax.	*Right side.*—Dark hair. Skin and muscles rigid.
Complaints predominate (cold, sensation as of a plug &c.) in external parts.	Complaints predominate (cold, sensation as of a plug &c.) in internal parts.
Obesity—Pain pressing inward . . .	Emaciation—Pain pressing outward.
Clonic spasms predominant	Tonic spasms predominant. Apoplexy.
Pulse at times intermitting the 10—30th beat; very unequal.	Pulse at times intermitting the 4—5th beat; oftener quick, full and hard.
Thirst rather rare; particularly no thirst during chill.	Thirst mostly during chill and between the fever and sweat.
Perspiration often only on the front part of the body.	Perspiration often only on the back part of the body.
Partial chill on the upper part of body . .	Partial chill on lower part of body.
Silly merriness—Taciturnity	Sadness—Loquacity.
Complaints in consequence of anger . .	Consequences of anger, fright, mortification, grief, disappointed love and jealousy, and also of vexation with fright, fear, indignation or vehemence.
Mental excitability and ecstacies	Difficult comprehension — Absent-mindedness—Fancies.
Short-sightedness—Dim-sightedness . . .	Far-sightedness — Predominant clear-sightedness.
Optical illusions in dark colors	Optical illusions in bright colors.
Very rarely nausea	Nausea, particularly in the stomach.
Diarrhœa	Predomin. costiveness.
Fluent coryza	Dry coryza, oftener; especially in the open air. Fluent coryza, on the contrary, in doors.
Cough generally with expectoration . . .	Cough *often* dry, but *sometimes* with expectoration.
Complaints most frequent on the shin . .	Complaints predom. on the calf of the leg.
AGGRAVATION in the morning and afternoon.	REMISSION of complaints evening till midnight.
Worse on awakening	On awakening better *or* worse.
More frequently aggravated than improved by pressure.	More frequently improved than aggravated by pressure.
Predominantly aggravated by eructations.	Most frequently better after eructation.
Worse when stooping	More frequently improved than aggravated by stooping.
Better *or* worse from spirituous liquors.	Almost always aggravated by spirituous liquors.
After stool better *or* worse	Worse after stool.

Predomin. worse ——— **Predomin. better**

In wet weather, during rest, when standing, sitting, and lying, when closing the eyes, and on inspiration.

Predomin. better ——— **Predomin. worse**

In dry weather, when walking, and generally from motion, when opening the eyes and on expiration.

Alumina.	Calcarea.
Upper left, lower right side	Upper right, lower left side.
Complaints chiefly in exterior parts . . .	Complaints particularly in internal parts.
Inclination for the open air	Aversion to the open air.
Heat right side	Heat of the left side.
Pulse often unchanged	Pulse changed, trembling—Apoplexy.
First chill, then heat	First heat, then chill.
Thirst seldom—Perspiration abating when walking out of doors.	Thirst constant, except during the chill—Perspiration increased when walking out of doors.

Alumina.	Calcarea.
Seriousness—Changeable mood	Sadness or silly merriness—Irritable mood—Amativeness—Hopelessness—Fancies—Imbecility—Consequences of vexation with fear or fright; of hearing disagreeable news.
During sleep, lying on the side	During sleep, lying on the back with the arms over the head—sometimes lying on the belly.
Complaints from carrying on the back . .	Complaints from carrying on the head.
Complaints oftener on the external than internal ear.	Complaints oftener on internal than external ear.
Urine pale, copious	Urine dark, too frequent.
Catamenia too soon, scanty, of short duration.	Catamenia predom. too soon, too profuse, of long duration.
Leucorrhœa acrid	Leucorrhœa mild.
Sexual desire lessened, and still erections.	Sexual desire increased, but impotent.
Complaints from pollutions	Complaints predominant from coition.
Complaints on outside of thigh	Complaints prevalent on the *inner* side of thigh.
Cough generally dry	Cough oftener loose.

Alumina.	Calcarea.
Aggravation of symptoms during the day.	Remission before midnight.
Better *while* eating	Often better *after* eating.
Ailments after poisoning with lead . . .	Ailments after abuse of Mercury or Cinchona, from Phosphor, Digitalis or Nitric acid.

Predomin. worse —— **Predomin. better**

In the room, when resting, when standing, sitting or lying, in dry weather, and when lying on the right side.

Predomin. better —— **Predomin. worse**

Out of doors, when in motion, in wet weather, from washing, from moistening the diseased part, when swallowing, in the evening twilight, and lying on the left side.

Alumina.	Lycopodium.
Upper left, lower right side	Upper right, lower left side.
When asleep, lying on the side – Paralysis more frequent one-sided.	When asleep, lying on the back—Paralysis more frequent of both sides.
Jerks in the muscles or joints	Jerks in internal parts.
Pulse full and somewhat accelerated; often unchanged.	Pulse accelerated only after meals and in the evening.
One-sided heat, predom. right side . . .	One-sided heat, predom. left side.
Thirst seldom	Thirst is wanting only during the chill.
Seriousness	Gentleness—Depression—Distrustfulness—Irritable mood—Haughtiness—Absent-mindedness—Fancies—Delirium—Insanity—Imbecility—Apoplexy—Consequences of fright, rage, grief, mortification, or of vexation with vehemence, fear, or of reserved displeasure.
Complaints chiefly on the *external* ear and on the under lip.	Complaints particularly on the internal ear and on the upper lip.
Urine too copious	Urine frequent, but scanty.
Catamenia too soon and of too short duration.	Catamenia too late and of too long duration.
Audible respiration, and cough generally dry.	Respiration generally with moist sound; therefore cough with expectoration, the latter particularly in the morning and evening.
Complaints on the outside of thigh . . .	Complaints on the inner side of thigh.
AGGRAVATION of symptoms in fore- and afternoon.	REMISSION of complaints after midnight and in *forenoon.*
Better when swallowing, particularly when swallowing saliva or liquids; while swallowing solids is sometimes inconvenient.	Worse when swallowing.

Predomin. worse —— **Predomin. better**

On an empty stomach, when ascending, when stooping.

Predomin. better —— **Predomin. worse**

After breakfast, while eating, when descending, from the touch and pressure, from washing and from moistening the diseased part.

Alumina.	Natr. mur.
Throbbing in internal parts—Paralysis, particularly of extensors.	Throbbing in external parts—Paralysis, particularly of the flexors.
Complaints predom. on wrist, on the *back part* of thigh, and on the patella.	Complaints predom. on ankle, on the *front part* of thigh, and in the hollow of the knee.
Pulse full and somewhat accelerated; often unchanged.	Pulse very irregular; sometimes quick and weak, sometimes full and slow.
Thirst seldom	Thirst during the fever and apyrexia.

Alumina.	Natr. mur.
Seriousness — Irritability — Fear — Very seldom unconsciousness — No delirium.	Indifference — Sadness *or* cheerfulness — Amativeness—Irritable mood—Absent-mindedness — Imbecility — Consequences of fright, anger, vexation, mortification, or reserved displeasure.
Apoplexy has not yet been observed. . .	Apoplexy.
Complaints chiefly on the *external* ear, on the lower teeth, and on the *back part* of the thigh.	Complaints particularly on the *internal* ear, on the upper teeth, and on the *front part* of the thigh.
Catamenia too soon and of too short duration.	Catamenia too late and too long.
Fluent coryza—Upper part of the chest .	Dry coryza—Lower part of the chest.
Expectoration, not confined to any particular time.	Expectoration particularly in the morning.

Alumina.	Natr. mur.
Aggravation of symptoms during the day.	Remission of complaints in the afternoon.
Better when walking out-doors; cold cannot be borne well, nor a warm room.	Improved by sitting still in mild, open air; feeling better where it is cool than where it is warm, and in warm rooms.
Better when swallowing, particularly swallowing saliva and liquids; while swallowing solids is sometimes inconvenient.	Worse when swallowing, particularly when swallowing liquids.
Worse from the pressure of the hat . . .	Better from tying the clothes tight.
Worse from cold, better from warm diet .	Better sometimes from cold, sometimes from warm diet.
Lead-diseases	China-cachexy.

Predomin. worse — **Predomin. better**

On an empty stomach, when dancing, after lying down, while resting, standing, sitting, lying, in bed, stretching out the diseased limb, and lying on the right side.

Predomin. better — **Predomin. worse**

After breakfast, while eating, after rising from bed, from motion, from drawing up the diseased limb, from the touch and pressure, and from lying on the left side.

Alumina.	Plumbum.
Upper left, lower right side.	Upper right, lower left side.
Complaints chiefly in external parts, (burning, etc.)	Complaints particularly in internal parts, (burning, etc.)
Inclination for the open air.	Aversion to the open air.
Distention of the veins	Throbbing in the veins.
Pulse often unchanged; generally full and somewhat accelerated.	Pulse very unequal; most frequently slow, small and contracted.
Heat descending	Heat ascending.
Thirst seldom	Thirst constant.
Sleeplessness predom.—Lying on the side during sleep.	Somnolence predom.—Lying on belly.
Complaints from bodily exertion	Complaints from mental exertion.
Paralysis often one-sided; painless . . .	Often paraplegia; predom. painful—Apoplexy.
Fear—Irritability—changeable mood . .	Gentleness—Distrust—Delirium—Imbecility.
Far-sightedness	Short-sightedness.
Urine increased	Urine decreased.
Catamenia and sexual desire decreased . .	Catamenia and sexual desire increased.
Pollutions	Prostratorrhœa.
Nasal secretion thick	Nasal secretion watery.
Saliva increased	Saliva generally lessened.
Cough generally dry	Cough generally with expectoration.
Complaints on the *outer* side of the thigh, on the leg, on the fore-arm and sole of the foot.	Complaints on the *inner* side of the thigh, on thigh, upper arm, and on the top of the foot.
Aggravation of symptoms during the day.	Remission of complaints in the forenoon.

Predomin. worse ——— **Predomin. better**

When resting, standing, from the use of spirituous * liquors, and from bodily exertion.

Predomin. better ——— **Predomin. worse**

From motion, while walking, and in the (evening) twilight.

* Lead-colic is relatively prevented by alcoholic drinks; Alumina sometimes cures it.

Alumina.	Silicea.
Upper left, lower right side — Want of bodily irritability.	Upper right, lower left side — Increased irritability.
Aversion to motion — Inclination for open air.	Inclination for motion — Aversion to the open air.
Pulse often unchanged; generally full and somewhat accelerated.	Pulse changed; most frequently accelerated, hard, small or imperceptible.
Thirst seldom	Thirst particularly during the heat.
Paralysis oftener one-sided	Paralysis oftener of both sizes — Apoplexy.
Itching relieved by scratching	Itching unchanged or aggravated by scratching.
Predom. humid eruptions	Predom. dry eruptions.
Fear — Seriousness — Changeable mood.	Gentleness — Depression — Indifference — Amativeness — Fancies.
Complaints predom. on the under lip and on the *upper* part of chest.	Complaints predom. on the upper lip and on the *lower* part of chest.
Urine increased in quantity	Urine too frequent.
Fluent coryza predom.	Coryza more frequently dry than fluent.
Cough generally dry	Cough generally loose.
Sexual desire decreased	Sexual desire increased.
Catamenia too soon and short	Catamenia predom. too late and of long duration.
Remission of complaints from evening till morning.	Remission of complaints before midnight.
Lead-diseases	Ailments after abuse of Sulphur or Mercury, and from the sting of insects.

Predomin. worse ——— **Predomin. better**

On an empty stomach, in the room, when dancing, letting the diseased limb hang down, and lying on the right side.

Predomin. better ——— **Predomin. worse**

After breakfast, when swallowing, in the open air, from washing, from moistening, rubbing, lifting the diseased limb or resting it on something, and lying on left side.

Ammon. carb.	Belladonna.
Hæmorrhages of dark blood	Hæmorrhages of bright-red blood.
Sweat on lower part of body	Partial sweat on the upper part of body.
Sleeplessness predom. after midnight . .	Sleeplessness before midnight.
Seriousness	Change of mood, sometimes gay and silly, sometimes sad, distrustful, or irritable and malicious.
	Ailments after fear, fright, rage, vexation or mortification.
	Imbecility—Insanity.
Apoplexy or Paralysis not yet observed .	Apoplexy and Paralysis.
Shortsightedness	Far-sightedness.
Painful diarrhœa	Painless diarrhœa.
Catamenia too late, scanty, of short duration.	Catamenia too soon, profuse and long.
Complaints in lower part of chest . . .	Complaints in upper part of chest.
Expectoration not constant;—in the morning and during the day.	Expectoration not constant; — from morning till evening.

Ammon. carb.	Belladonna.
Remission of complaints in the forenoon and at night.	Remission of complaints in the *forenoon* and after midnight.
Worse from bending the diseased part backward.	*Worse* when bending the diseased part to one side.
Worse during new moon	Worse during full moon.
Worse while sitting and from eructation .	*Generally better* when sitting (particularly when bending forward) and from eructation.

Predomin. worse — **Predomin. better**

In wet weather, when letting the diseased limb hang down, when stooping, sitting, and from eructation.

Predomin. better — **Predomin. worse**

In dry weather, when lifting or resting the diseased limb on anything.

N. B. The effects of both remedies principally begin on the right side, extending afterwards to the left, and both are only effective when the complaint of the patient develops in the opposite direction. For instance: the hardness of hearing, which indicates Ammon. carb., is cured more effectually by it, when the complaint began on the left side and extended or threatened to extend to the right side; — inflammations of the ears or earache, indicating Belladonna, are more certainly cured by it, when they appeared first on the left then on the right side. C.Hg.

Ammon. carb.	Phosphor.
Itching lessened by scratching	Itching *lessened* or increased by scratching.
Pulse quick, hard and tense	Pulse various, irregular; sometimes intermitting.
Chill increased in the open air, lessened in a warm room.	Chill less in the open air than in a warm room.
Sweat increased when eating	Sweat lessened when eating.
Sleeplessness after midnight	Sleeplessness before midnight.

Ammon. carb.	Phosphor.
Weak memory	Memory active.
Seriousness—Absent-mindedness . . .	Changing mood, sometimes gay, sometimes sad, sometimes irritable.—Haughtiness—Amativeness.
	Mental excitability—Ecstasies—Insanity.
Neither Apoplexy nor Paralysis . . .	Apoplexy—Paralysis.
Sweat, particularly around the joints . .	Sweat, particularly on one side; —vesicles around the joints.
Optical illusions, particularly in white and in bright colors.	Optical illusions, particularly in black, in dark (or in prismatic) colors.
Appetite for sweets	Aversion to sweets.
Complaints predom. in the spleen . . .	Complaints predom. in the liver.
Costiveness on account of hardness of the fæces.	Costiveness on account of inactivity of intestines.
Diarrhœa painful	Diarrhœa oftener painless than painful.
Urine with a whitish sediment	Urine with white, yellow or red sediment.
Catamenia too late	Catamenia oftener too soon than too late.
Sexual desire decreased	Sexual desire increased.
Nasal secretion watery	Nasal secretion thick or viscous.
Expectoration seldom	Expectoration not constant.
Coughing up dark blood	Coughing up bright red blood.

Ammon. carb.	Phosphor.
REMISSION of complaints, in the night and forenoon.	REMISSION after midnight.
Worse during sleep	During sleep generally *worse*, but often also better; still greater improvement *after* sleep *, with exception of the siesta.
Worse during new moon	Worse before a thunder-storm.
Ailments from sting of insects	Ailments after abuse of salt or of Iod.

Predomin. worse ——— **Predomin. better**

In wet weather, in the open air †, and when sitting.

Predomin. better ——— **Predomin. worse**

In dry weather, in the room, from the warmth of the bed, when turning over in bed, from pressure ‡, and assuming an erect position.

---

* This amelioration of Phosphor-complaints results undoubtedly from sufficient sleep, for "*on awakening*" in general Phosphor has aggravation quite as often as amelioration.

† *When walking in the open air*, Phosphor has sometimes improvement, and sometimes aggravation, but the latter is a consequence of the motion.

‡ Ammon. has an exception here in the case of pressure from *tight clothes*.

Ammon. mur.	**Arsenic.**
Tension or constriction in external parts .	Tension or constriction in internal parts
Very rarely paralysis	Paralysis.
Complaints predom. on fore-arm and in the hollow of the elbow.	Complaints predom. on upper arm and in the hollow of the knee.
Pulse unaltered, and, when changed, continuously accelerated.	Pulse changed, irregular, small, soft, quick, trembling, or imperceptible.
Sweat on lower part of body	Chill on lower part of body.
Heat, with thirst *.	Heat, with desire for drink, without thirst †.
Chill or coldness increased after getting out of bed.	Chill, etc., lessened after getting out of bed.
Sweat increased by motion	Sweat lessened by motion.
Sleeplessness before midnight	Sleeplessness predom. after midnight.
Dreams of water, traveling, sickness, animals, falling, shooting, etc.	Dreams of fire or thunder-storms, of vexation or dead persons.

Fretfulness	Fear — Despondency — Irritability - Malice — Greediness.
No delirium	Delirium—Consequences of fear, fright or vexation.
Saliva increased	Saliva diminished.
Cough: expectoration not constant; in the night and morning.	Expectoration predom., but not constant; during the day.

REMISSION of complaints in the afternoon .	REMISSION *during the day* and before midnight.
Aggravation almost always on awakening .	Better *or* worse on awakening; better after sufficient sleep.
When assuming an upright position, almost always aggrav.	When assuming an upright position, more frequently improved than aggrav.
After rising from bed, almost always aggrav.	After rising from bed, more frequently improved than aggrav.
Better *or* worse when stretching out the diseased limb.	*Worse* when stretching out the diseased limb.
Better *or* worse when swallowing. . . .	*Worse* when swallowing.
Most frequently better after stool. . . .	Most frequently aggrav. after stool.

Predomin. worse —— **Predomin. better**

When sitting down, when descending, when standing, when bending the diseased part, and on an empty stomach.

Predomin. better —— **Predomin. worse**

When rising from a seat, when ascending, after lying down, during sleep, from rubbing, on expiration, and after breakfast.

N. B. Although insensibility is a constitutional characteristic of Arsenic, still we find over-sensitiveness to pain, with this remedy, a symptom not yet observed with Ammon. mur.

---

* Amm. mur. has more thirst between the cold and hot stage and between hot and sweating stage, also after sweat, than during hot stage. It is similar with Arsen., but the latter has more thirst *before* the chill than Amm. mur.

† The patient drinks often, but little at a time.

Ammon. mur.	Phosphor.
Gnawing sensation in internal parts . . .	Gnawing sensation in external parts.
Very rarely paralysis	Paralysis—Apoplexy.
Complaints predominate in the lower eyelids and in the spleen.	Complaints predominate in the upper eyelids and in the liver.
Pulse often unchanged; generally continuously accelerated.	Pulse generally accelerated, full, and hard; irregular; often intermitting.
Heat, with thirst — Perspiration, without thirst *.	Predom. lack of thirst.
Dreams of water, traveling, animals, of falling, shooting, etc.	Dreams of fire, quarrels and vexation, of dead persons, of the business of the day, or erotic, historical dreams, or with mental exertion.

Neither joyousness, haughtiness, amativeness, nor delirium, have yet been observed.	Mood changing—Fancies—Ecstasies—Insanity—Ailments after fright, anger or vexation. During fevers, often unconsciousness or delirium.
Painful diarrhœa	Diarrhœa most frequently painless.
Expectoration during the night and in the morning.	Expectoration in the morning and during the day.

REMISSION of complaints in the afternoon .	REMISSION after midnight.
Improvement oftener than aggrav. after stool.	Worse after stool.
Better in bed	In bed (warmth of bed), worse or (rest) better.
After getting out of bed, almost always aggrav.	*After* getting out of bed, better *or* worse.
Predom. aggrav. on an empty stomach; but also nearly always after eating; must often eat a little, but not enough to satisfy the hunger.	On an empty stomach, predom. better; after eating, worse *or* better; particularly better after a satisfying meal.
From light (in the dark) worse *or* better.	Worse from light; better in the dark.

Predomin. worse —— **Predomin. better**

In the open air †, in the twilight, when resting, standing, sitting and lying, particularly lying on right side, lifting or resting the diseased limb on anything, when descending, and from drinking wine.

Predomin. better —— **Predomin. worse**

In the room, when moving ‡, when walking, lying on the left side, letting the diseased limb hang down, ascending, from external pressure, washing and moistening the suffering part, and *while* getting out of bed.

N.B. The over-sensitiveness to pain, of the Phosphor-patient, does not occur with Amm. mur.

---

* Compare note to preceding diagnosis of Amm. mur. and Arsen.
† When "*walking* in the open air," Amm. mur. has predom. improvement; Phosphor aggravation *or* improvement.
‡ The "improvement from motion," which sometimes occurs with Ph sphor. seems to refer only to pain in the joints.

Ammon. mur.	Pulsatilla.
Aversion to the open air	Desire for the open air.
Pulse generally unaltered, but when changed, continuously accelerated.	Pulse most frequently *quick*, small and weak, particularly in the evening.
Sweat on lower part of body	Chill on lower part of body.
Thirst not constant; thirst during hot stage.	Thirst *only* during hot stage.
Sweat, without thirst *	
Mood irritable, malicious—Neither unconsciousness nor delirium—No apoplexy.	Mood changing: gentle, sad, greedy—Apoplexy—Rarely delirium or unconsciousness—Ailments after excessive joy, fright or vexation with fright, dread or fear.
Optical illusions in dark colors.	Optical illusions in bright colors.
Catamenia too soon and profuse	Catamenia too late and scanty, rarely profuse; suppressed.
Expectoration night and morning . . .	Expectoration, morning and during the day.
Complaints predom. in fore-arm and in the palm of the hand.	Complaints predom. in upper arm and on the back of the hand.
REMISSION of complaints in the afternoon.	AGGRAVATION afternoon and evening, after sunset, till midnight.
Worse *or* better from light	Worse from light; better in the dark.
Worse when taking a deep breath . . .	Better *or* worse when taking a deep breath.
Predom. worse when lying on the back; better when lying on the side.	Most frequently better when lying on the back; worse when lying on the side.
Nearly always aggrav. after rising from bed.	Improved oftener than aggrav. after rising from bed.
Better when bending or moving the diseased part.	Better *or* worse when bending or moving the diseased part.

Predomin. worse — **Predomin. better**

In the open air †, on inspiration, lifting or resting the diseased limb, lying on the right side, lying on the painful side, and after rising from bed.

Predomin. better 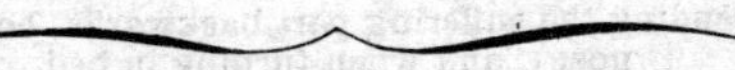 **Predomin. worse**

In the room, on expiration, letting the diseased limb hang down, lying on left side, lying on the unpainful side, after lying down generally, in bed, during sleep, and from rubbing the diseased part.

N. B. Amm. mur. has not the over-sensitiveness to pain of the Pulsatilla-patient.

*** Amm. mur., like China, has the most thirst *between* the different stages of the fever; Pulsatilla also has much thirst between the chill and heat, but less between the heat and sweat, and none at all *after* the sweating stage.**

† From "walking in the open air," both remedies have predom. improvement.

Anacardium.	Belladonna.
Left side—Complaints of external parts predom.	Right side—Complaints of internal parts predom.
Emaciation—Painless eruptions	Obesity—Painful eruptions.
Paralysis more frequent than apoplexy . .	Apoplexy more frequent than paralysis.
Complaints predom. in the spleen, on the fore-arm, in the hollow of the elbow.	Complaints predom. in the liver, on the upper arm, and in the hollow of the knee.
Pulse often unchanged, generally accelerated.	Pulse quick or slow, sometimes trembling or irregular.
Thirst, particularly during the heat . . .	Thirst most rare during chill.

Imbecility of will—Maliciousness. C.Hg.	Waywardness – Lacrymosity. C.Hg.
The mental symptoms have the character of dull insusceptibility more exclusively than those of Belladonna—No Ecstasies.	Mood changing—Fancies—Mental dullness, but also ecstasies.
Consequences of fright or mortification . .	Consequences of fright, anger, mortification, or of vexation with dread, fear, or vehemence.
Eyes sunken.	Eyes protruding.
Pupils generally contracted.	Pupils more frequently dilated than contracted.
Diarrhœa predom. painful	Diarrhœa predom. painless.
Voice hoarse or deep.	Voice hoarse or raised.
Expectoration seldom; during the day . .	Expectoration seldom; in the morning, during the day or in the evening.

REMISSION after midnight and during the day.	REMISSION after midnight and in *forenoon*.
Worse when assuming an erect position .	When assuming an erect position, generally worse, sometimes better.
Worse when bending the diseased part . .	Better *or* worse when bending the diseased part.
Better *or* worse from touch.	Almost always aggrav. by touch.

Predomin. worse —— **Predomin. better**

From warmth, in the room, bending the suffering part backwards, boring with the finger (in the ear or nose), and when turning in bed.

Predomin. better —— **Predomin. worse**

From cold, in the open air, in the sunshine, when eating, and from weeping.

N. B. Anacardium rarely has the over-sensitiveness to pain of the Belladonna-patient, Belladonna rarely the numb sensation in the suffering parts so frequent with Anacardium.

Anacardium.	Pulsatilla.
Left side -- Want of bodily irritability *	*Right* side.—Increased irritability.
Complaints predom. in external parts	Complaints predom. in internal parts.
Pains pressing inward	Pain pressing outward.
Complains predom. in the inner nose, in upper part of chest, in the spleen, on fore-arm, in palms of hands, and on the top of the foot.	Complaints predom. on the external nose, in lower part of chest, in the liver, on upper-arm, back of the hand, and of the sole of the foot.
Paralysis more frequent than apoplexy	Apoplexy more frequent than paralysis.
Itching *aggrav.*, or ameliorated, *or* changing its location, by scratching.	Itching, aggrav. *or* unchanged by scratching.
Painless eruptions	Painful eruptions.
Pulse often unchanged, generally accelerated.	Pulse changed, intermitting, &c., generally quick, small, and weak.
Thirst most frequent during the heat	Thirst, almost only during the hot stage of the fever, and between the cold and hot stages; less frequently after the hot stage.
One-sided heat; left side	One-sided heat; right side.
Chill increased in the open air. — Sweat lessened while eating.	Chill lessened in the open air — Sweat increased while eating.
Insensibility of disposition	Sensitiveness of disposition.
Maliciousness — Excited mood	Goodnature—Gentleness—Calm sadness—Greediness.
Consequences of fright	Consequ. of fright, excessive joy, grief, mortification, and of vexat. with fear or fright
Imbecility—Insanity	Absent-mindedness—Melancholy.
Memory weak *or* active	Weakness of memory.
Optical illusions in dark colors	Optical illusions in bright colors.
Urine frequent, but scanty	Urine infrequent and scanty.
Dry coryza	Fluent coryza, (sometimes only one-sided,) more frequent than dry coryza.
Expectoration infrequent; during the day.	Expectoration predom., but not constant; in the morning and during the day.
AGGRAVATION *in the morning* and evening until midnight.	AGGRAVATION in the afternoon and evening till midnight.
Worse after sleep	After sleep *worse or* better.
Worse when assuming an erect position	When assuming an erect position, *worse or* better.
Better when sitting down	When sitting down, *worse or* better.
Worse when rising from a seat	When rising from a seat, *worse or* better.
Better *or* worse from the touch	*Worse* from the touch.
Most frequently improved by pressure	Worse *or* better from pressure.
Rubbing and scratching generally aggravates, but sometimes improves.	*Worse* from rubbing and scratching.
Worse from moving the diseased part	*Better or* worse fr. moving the diseased part.
Worse when bending the diseased part	Bett. *or* worse when bend'g the diseased part.
Worse when swallowing	Worse *or* better when swallowing.
Worse after meals	After meals worse, but sometimes better.
Better while eating; worse *afterwards*	Better while drinking; worse *afterwards.*

Predomin. **worse** — Predomin. **better**

While moving, walking, lifting the diseased limb, during inspiration, lying on the painful side, and when sitting erect.

Predomin. **better** — Predomin. **worse**

During rest, after lying down, in bed, when lying, sitting, and standing, particularly when lying on the unpainful side, sitting bent forward, stooping, letting the diseased limb hang down, during expiration, when eating, and in sunshine.

* Hence Anacard. has not the oversensitiveness to pain of the Pulsatilla patient.

Antimon. crud.	Antimon. tartar.
Oversensitiveness predom*.	Insensibility, sensation of numbness (not want of irritability).
Hæmorrhages of dark blood predom. . .	Hæmorrhages of bright red blood.
Pulse often unchanged, sometimes slow, sometimes quick.	Pulse changed *too quick* or too slow, or both in alternation or intermitting.
Thirst not constant	No thirst during the chill, is not constant during the hot stage, but between the hot and sweating stage.
Sleeplessness†, particularly after midnight.	Sleeplessness particularly before midnight.
Pleasant dreams predom.	Anxious dreams predom.

Sentimental mood (particularly in the moonlight).	Changeable mood—Dullness of mind.
Mental excitability (ecstasies) *or* stupor .	Unconsciousness.
Delirium—Amativeness	
Consequences of disappointed love . . .	Consequences of anger or vexation.
Pressing or tearing in external parts . .	Pressing or tearing in internal parts.
Bitter vomit.	Predom. sour vomit.
Dry coryza	Fluent coryza.
Expectoration seldom; — in the *morning* and evening.	Expectoration not constant; in the *morning* and during the day.

REMISSION undecided	REMISSION during the day.
Ailments from Arsenic or the sting of insects.	Ailments after the abuse of China.

Predomin. worse — **Predomin. better**

From washing or moistening the diseased part, when stooping, from cold diet, eructations, and when stretching out the diseased limb.

Predomin. better — **Predomin. worse**

When drawing up the diseased limb, sitting down, and from warm diet.

---

* We find in both remedies, sensitiveness predom. "*in internal parts.*"

† It is well known that both remedies have *somnolency* more frequently than sleeplessness.

Antimon. crud.	Pulsatilla.
Left side predom.; particularly the *lower left* and upper right side.	*Right* side; particularly *lower right* and *upper left* side.
Pulse often unchanged; very unequal . .	Pulse generally quick; small and weak.
Sleeplessness after midnight	Sleeplessness before midnight.
Mood sentimental, (particularly in the moonlight.)	Mood changing; fear; irritability; calm sadness of gentle dispositions; greediness.
Mental excitability — Ecstasies—Imbecility —Consequences of disappointed love.	Absent-mindedness — Melancholy—Unconsciousness — Ailments from fright, joy, mortification, grief, or from vexation with dread or fear.
Complaints oftener on the inner than external nose.	Complaints oftener on the external than inner nose.
Complaints of the upper lip predom. . .	Complaints of the under lip predom.
Thirst not constant.	Thirst almost only during the fever, but sometimes before the chill, between chill and fever, and between fever and sweat.
Heat increased by motion	Heat abated by motion.
Disgust for food	Ravenous hunger.
Urine frequent, but scanty	Urine infrequent and scanty, often with inefficient urging to urinate.
Catamenia too profuse, or suppressed by having been over-heated.	Catamenia oftener too weak than profuse: suppressed from getting wet feet, with painful, vain urging to urinate.
Dry coryza	Fluent coryza (particularly of the right side) more frequent than stoppage of nose.
Irritation to cough is felt in abdomen . .	Irritation for cough is felt in pit of stomach. Raue.
Cough generally dry; when there is expectoration, it appears particularly in the morning.	Cough, most frequently with expectoration, which is loosened in the morning and during the day.
AGGRAVATION of symptoms at all times of the day and night.	AGGRAVATION from noon till midnight.
Complaints predom. in upper part of chest.	Complaints predom. in lower part of chest.
Complaints from moonlight	Complaints before a thunder-storm.
Ailments from sting of insects, or from Arsenic.	Ailments from copper-vapors, Sulphur or Cinchona.

Predomin. worse — **Predomin. better**

From vinegar and sour things in general, from cold diet and drinking water, from bathing and washing, from moistening the diseased part, uncovering, lifting or stretching out the diseased part, lying on the painful side, and from pressure.

Predomin. better — **Predomin. worse**

From warm diet, rubbing and scratching, wrapping up warm, from letting the diseased limb hang down as well as drawing it up, and when lying on the unpainful side.

Antimon. crud.	Sulphur.
Inclination for the open air	Aversion to the open air.
Painful eruptions — External parts turn black.	Painless eruptions — Parts naturally red grow white.
No paralysis of the limbs	Paralysis of the limbs.
Pulse often unchanged; very unequal	Pulse often accelerated and hard, sometimes intermitting or imperceptible.
Chill increased in the warm room	Chill abating in the warm room.
Heat or sweat, with aversion to uncover	Heat or sweat, with inclination to uncover.
Thirst not constant	Thirst mostly during heat; during the chill most frequently no thirst.
Somnolence predom.	Sleeplessness predom., particularly before midnight.

Antimon. crud.	Sulphur.
Mood distrustful; sentimental, particularly in the moonlight; amorous.	Mood changing; serious solemn, indifferent, gentle, depressed, vexed and irritated.
Consequences of disappointed love	Consequences of hearing bad news, shame, mortification, or of vexation with fright or fear.
Mental excitability—Ecstasies	Difficult comprehension — Absent-mindedness — Fancies — Mental dullness — Insanity—Unconsciousness.
Imbecility more frequent than insanity	Insanity more frequent than imbecility.
Saliva predom. increased	Saliva most frequently lessened.
Bitter vomit	Predom. sour vomit.
Urine frequent, but scanty	Urine frequent, but scanty; sometimes, however, profuse.
Sediment red	Sediment *white* or red.
Expectoration; in the morning	Expectoration not constant; in the morning and during the day, more rarely at night.

Antimon. crud.	Sulphur.
REMISSION of complaints undecided	REMISSION in the *afternoon* and before midnight.
Predom. better after rising from bed	Worse *or* better after rising from bed.
Worse from eructation	Almost always improved by eructation.
Worse from the heat of the sun	Worse from snowy air.
Ailments from sting of insects, or from Arsenic.	Ailments from abuse of metallic preparations: Nitric acid, Jod., Sepia, Rhus, or Cinchona.

Predomin. **worse** — Predomin. **better**
From eructation, external pressure, and from uncovering.

Predomin. **better** — Predomin. **worse**
From wrapping up, and from walking in the open air *

N. B. We very rarely find with Sulphur the over-sensitiveness to pain of the Antimon.-patient; on the other hand, Antimony has not the sensation of numbness in suffering parts of the Sulphur-patient.

---

* Both remedies generally have improvement of complaints '*in the open air;*" the Antimony complaints are aggrav. by the heat of stoves, and Sulphur symptoms are predominantly improved by it, while the latter are aggravated in crowded rooms.

Antimon. tart.	Pulsatilla.
Predom. *left* side, particularly *lower left* and *upper right side.*	*Right* side, particularly *lower right and upper left side.*
Hæmorrhages bright-red—Disposition to perspire easily.	Hæmorrhages dark—Dryness of the skin.
Perspiration on the suffering part . . .	Heat on the suffering part.
During all stages of the fever: pulse quick, full, strong; at times trembling when it abates, often slow and weak.	Pulse accelerated, small and weak,—rarely slow.
Thirst between hot and sweating stage . .	Thirst, particularly between chill and heat; not so often between heat and sweat.
Heat increased by motion	Heat abated by motion.
Pressure-pains from outside inward . . .	Pressing from inside outward.
Hypochondriasis, with inclin. to violence .	Hypochondriasis with calm sadness.
Hopelessness—Indolence	Changing mood—Fear—Indifference.
Mental dulness—Imbecility . . .	Hastiness—Calm sadness of gentle dispositions—Distrust—Amativeness—Greediness.
No delirium	Absent-mindedness—Fancies—Melancholy.
Consequences of vexation	Consequences of fright, joy, mortification, grief, or of vexation with fear or reserved displeasure.
Diphtheritis with plastic exudations . .	Catarrhal croup in the fauces.
Respiration with great rattling of mucus .	Respiration generally without rattling of mucus, but with a dry sound.
Short gasping inspirations and long slow expirations.	Difficult expiration.
Voice hollow	Voice hoarse and rough.
Expectoration in the morning	Expectoration in the morning and during the day.
No thirst	Thirst only during the heat.
Sour vomit predom.	Oftener bitter than sour vomit.
Remission during the day	**Remission** from midnight until noon.
Worse while perspiring;—*after* perspiration rather better than worse.	*Worse* during and after perspiration.

Predomin. worse ——— **Predomin. better**

From motion, and when lying on the painful side.

Predomin. better ——— **Predomin. worse**

When resting, standing, lying on the painful side, from rubbing, eructation, when stooping* and after perspiring.

N. B. With Antimon. tart. we rarely find the numb feeling in suffering parts that is so frequently found with Pulsatilla.

---

* Both remedies have aggrav. as well as amelioration from "assuming an erect position."

Antimon. tart.	Rhus.
Left side, particularly *lower left and upper right side.*	*Right* side, partic. *lower right and upper left side.*
Complaints (pressing, tension, tearing, &c.) predom. in internal parts.	Complaints (pressing, tension, tearing, &c.) predom. in external parts.
Pain pressing inward—Oligæmie	Pain pressing outward—Most frequently plethora.
Predom. somnolence—Pulse predom. strong.	Predom. Sleeplessness—Pulse pred. weak.
Only during the heat sometimes thirst and between the heat and perspiration.	Thirst not constant.
Heat increased by motion	Heat lessened by motion.
Rarely Apoplexy—No Paralysis of the limbs.	Paralysis—Apoplexy.

Hopelessness—Consequences of anger . .	Fear—Dejectedness. Consequences of vexation with dread or fear.
Mental dulness	Difficult comprehension—Fancies—Unconsciousness.
Nausea in stomach or abdomen, less frequently in the throat.	Nausea in œsophagus or stomach, less frequently in the throat.
Urine scanty; predom. dark	Urine often and copious; —pale.
Respiration with a moist sound	Respiration with dry sound.

Worse when rising from bed	*Worse or* better when rising from bed.
After rising from bed almost always better.	*After* rising from bed *worse or* better.
Predom. worse when sitting down . . .	Better *or* worse when sitting down.
Worse when rising from a seat	*Worse or* better when rising from a seat.
Better after rising from a seat	Better *or* worse after rising from a seat.
Worse in bed	Better *or* worse in bed.
Worse after drinking	*Worse or* better after drinking.
Ailments from Baryt. and Sepia	Ailments from Bryonia, Rhododendron or Antimon. tart.

Predomin. worse — **Predomin. better**

From warmth and in warm air, from warm diet, motion *, when walking, and during expiration.

Predomin. better — **Predomin. worse**

From cold, growing cold and in cold weather, from cold diet, when resting, standing, during inspiration from eructation, when stooping and rising, and from washing and moistening the diseased part.

N. B. We rarely find the numb sensation in the suffering parts so frequently occuring in Rhus. with Antimon. tart.

---

* **Both remedies have aggrav. in the *beginning of motion*.**

Antimon. tartar.	Veratrum.
Left side, particularly *lower left and upper right side.*	*Right* side, particularly *lower right and upper left side.*
Crawling or tearing in internal parts . .	Crawling or tearing in external parts.
Rarely apoplexy	Paralysis of the limbs.
Pulse accelerated, full and strong	Pulse irregular; most frequently slow, small and weak.
Only during and after the heat sometimes thirst.	Thirst not constant.
Hopelessness	Joyousness or dejection—Haughtiness—Irritable, malicious mood.
Consequences of vexation	Consequences of fright, anger, *grief*, or of vexation with dread or fear.
Mental dullness—Imbecility	Mental excitability, rarely dullness—Absentmindedness—Fancies—Insanity predom.
Saliva predom. increased	Saliva oftener lessened than increased.
Nausea in stomach or abdomen, less often in the throat.	Nausea in stomach.
Predom. sour vomit	Predom. bitter vomit.
Urine decreased	Urine *decreased or* increased.
Fluent coryza predom.	Dry coryza predom.
Expectoration not constant; in the morning.	Expectoration not constant; chiefly during the day.
AGGRAVATION from evening until morning.	AGGRAVATION night and *morning.*
Almost always aggravated in bed	Worse *or* better in bed.
Worse also when rising from bed	*Better or* worse when rising from bed.
After rising from bed, nearly always better.	*After* rising from bed, worse *or* better.
Worse when rising from a seat	Better *or* worse when rising from a seat.
Ailments from Baryta or Sepia	Ailments from Ferrum, Arsenic, or Cinchona.

Predomin. worse	**Predomin. better**

In warm air, from warm diet, drinking milk, sitting bent forward, from motion *, and while walking.

Predomin. better	**Predomin. worse**

In cold weather, from cold diet, drinking cold water, sitting erect, while resting, standing, stooping, and assuming an erect position.

N. B. We rarely find in Antimon. tart. the numb sensation in suffering parts not infrequent with Veratrum.

---

* Both remedies have aggravation when *beginning* to move.

Apis.	Arsenic.
Left side predom.	*Right* side.
Bodily irritability	Want of bodily irritability.
Hæmorrhages dark	Hæmorrhages bright-red.
Bodies of the poisoned decompose rapidly .	Bodies of the poisoned decompose very slowly.
Complaints predom. in external parts . .	Complaints predom. in internal parts.
Apoplexy oftener than paralysis; — the latter generally only one-sided.	Paralysis (generally of both sides) oftener than apoplexy.
Predom. somnolence	Predom. sleeplessness.
Pulse most frequently accelerated and full .	Pulse very quick, small and weak.
Heat generally with thirst and inclination to uncover, the latter is agreeable.	Heat generally without thirst and with aversion to uncover; improv. by wrapping up.
Dropsy without thirst	Dropsy with unquenchable thirst.
Eccentric mirth *or* hopelessness — Fickle inconsistency — Jealousy — Absent-mindedness — Dread of apoplexy.	Melancholy—Greediness.
Consequences of fright, hearing bad news, rage, vexation or jealousy.	Consequences of grief, fright, or of vexation with dread, fear, reserved displeasure, or vehemence.
Anxious feeling in the head.	Anxious feeling in the præcordia.
Complaints predom. on the upper eye-lids and on the *external* ear.	Complaints on the lower eye-lids and on the inner ear.
Saliva increased	Saliva diminished.
Thirst seems wanting only during the sweat.	Thirst, particularly during sweat and before and after the attack.
Urine frequent, but scanty; only exceptionally copious.	Urine scanty (with diarrhœa) *or* copious.
Cough with difficult expectoration, which wakens the patient before midnight; ceases as soon as the least particle is loosened.	Expectoration not constant; is loosened only during the day.
REMISSION of complaints during the day .	REMISSION *during the day* and before mid night.
Worse *or* better from pressure	Better from pressure.
After sleep oftener aggrav. than ameliorated.	After sleep better, that is, after sufficient sleep; but on awaking generally aggravation quite as often as improvement.
Worse from light, better in the dark . .	Worse (better) from light *or* in the dark.
Ailments from the sting of insects (or Iod.).	Ailments from Plumbum, Strychnine, Cinchona, Digitalis (Iod), Phosphor.

Predomin. worse — **Predomin. better**

From wrapping up, warmth and warmth of the bed, in warm rooms, when moving, partic. moving the suffering part, and after sleep.

Predomin better — **Predomin. worse**

From uncovering, from cold*, spirituous liquors, after perspiration, and when assuming an erect position.

* Both remedies have aggravations in cold weather.

Apis.	Belladonna.
Left side	*Right side.*
Complaints of external parts predom. . .	Complaints of inner parts predom.
Inclination for open air—Emaciation . .	Disinclination to open air—Obesity.
Chills on the suffering part.	Coldness on the suffering part.
Chill with thirst	Chill without thirst.
Heat with inclination to uncover; the latter is agreeable.	Heat with aversion to uncover, and improved by wrapping up warm.
Perspiration increased in the room . . .	Perspiration diminished in the room
Rarely paralysis	Paralysis.

Sensitiveness of disposition.	Insensibility of disposition predom.
With children stiffening of the body on being touched or moved (with inflammation of the brain).	With children stiffening of the body during attacks of spasmodic coughs.
Blood taken from the veins is black, viscous, does not coagulate.	The blood is most frequently bright and coagulates quickly, is therefore often already coagulated when discharged.
Horses kick, and show inclination to run off.	Horses stare and have a restless look; refuse to have their front-feet examined, or to be mounted; overturn themselves.
Unsteadiness—Jealousy—Consequences of hearing bad news.	Changing mood—Distrust—Fancies—Insanity.
Anxious feeling in the head	Anx. feeling in the region of the heart.
Complaints predom. in the spleen, and on the inner side of thigh.	Complaints predom. in the liver and on the outer side of thigh.
Thirst is wanting only during sweat. . .	Thirst most rare during the chill.
Appetite for sour things.	Aversion to sour things.
Milk diminished with nursing women . .	Milk most frequently increased.

Remission of complaints during the day .	Remission after midnight and in the *forenoon.*
Worse *or* better from pressure	Better from pressure.
Better when assuming an erect position .	*Worse or* better when assuming an erect position.

Predomin. worse — **Predomin. better**

After lying down, in bed, from warmth, when stooping, sitting down; as also from holding the breath, warmth of the bed, and wrapping up.

Predomin. better — **Predomin. worse**

In the open air, from cold, from washing, and from wet applications, when rising from bed, and from uncovering.

Apis.	Cantharides.
Left side predom.	*Right* side predom.
Skin and muscles rigid	Skin and muscles lax.
Complaints predom. in external parts	Complaints predom. in internal parts.
Dryness of skin	Disposition to sweat, (perspires easily.)
Blood does not coagulate (after being pricked with a needle, etc.)	Blood coagulates quickly.
Heat, with inclination to uncover, with or without thirst.	Heat, with aversion to uncover and with thirst; rarely with aversion to drink.
No thirst during the sweat	Thirst is wanting only during the chill, but appears between the cold and hot stage and during the heat.
Somnolence	Sleeplessness, particularly after midnight.
Apoplexy; rarely paralysis; the latter generally one-sided, (hemiplegia.)	Paralysis generally of both sides, (paraplegia.)

Jealousy—Absent-mindedness—Imbecility.	Amativeness—Fancies—Insanity.
Consequences of rage, vexation, or hearing bad news.	
Complaints predom. on the *upper* eyelids, on the *inner* side of the thigh, in the hollow of the knee.	Complaints on the *lower* eyelids, on the *outer* side of the thigh, and in the hollow of the elbow.
The patient drinks often, but little at a time.	The patient does not drink often, but much at a time.
Urine frequent, but scanty; only exceptionally copious.	Urine infrequent and scanty; only exceptionally (with paralysis) copious.
Sexual desire increased *or* diminished	Sexual desire increased.

Remission of complaints during the day	Remission of complaints in the morning and evening, until midnight.
Worse *or* better from pressure	Ameliorated by pressure.

Predomin. **worse** — Predomin. **better**

From warmth, in warm rooms, after lying down, and when growing warm in bed.

Predomin. **better** — Predomin. **worse**

In the open air, from cold, from washing with cold water and moistening the suffering part.

Apis.	Lachesis.
Complaints (burning, etc.) predom. in *external* parts.	Complaints (burning, etc.) predom. in *internal* parts.
Complaints predom. *left* side, excepting the genitals.	Complaints predom. *right* side, excepting the genitals.
Inclination for open air	Aversion to open air (predom.)
Skin and muscles rigid—Gang. ene . . .	Skin and muscles lax—Sphacelus.
Suppurations do not occur	Suppuration, particularly in internal parts.
Pulse predom. accelerated and full . . .	Pulse unequal; generally quick, small, and weak; often alternating with full and strong beats.
Heat, with (or without) thirst and inclination to uncover.	Heat, *without* thirst, and with aversion to uncover.
Thirst is generally wanting only during perspiration.	Thirst is wanting during the chill, and not frequent during the heat, but appears before the chill.
Chill increased in the warm room. . . .	Chill lessened in the warm room.
Somnolence predom.—Anxious dreams. .	Sleeplessness predom.—Dreams generally pleasant.
Cheerfulness *or* despondency—Indifference—Difficulty of thinking—Imbecility.	Cheerfulness—Distrust—Easy comprehension—Mental excitability—Insanity.
Ailments from rage or vexation with fright.	Ailments from disappointed love or grief.
Complaints predom. on the *upper* eyelids and in the spleen.	Complaints predom. on the *lower* eyelids and in the liver.
Catamenia too soon	Catamenia too soon *or* too late.
Coryza, dry in the morning, fluent in the evening.	Fluent coryza predom.
Respiration prevalently quick	Respiration prevalently slow.
Cough wakes the patient before midnight, and ceases as soon as the least particle is loosened, which is swallowed.	Expectoration in the morning and during the day.
Difficulty of breathing, particularly when bent forward (and when leaning back.)	Difficulty of breathing less when sitting bent forward.
REMISSION of complaints during the day .	AGGRAVATION from noon until midnight.
Poisoning by contagious Anthrax or Jodine.	Ailments from abuse of Mercury.

Predomin. worse ——— **Predomin. better**

In a warm room, from motion, shaking the head, after rising from a seat, when swallowing food *, in cold weather, and during inspiration.

Predomin. better ——— **Predomin. worse**

In the open air, when holding the suffering part bent, when assuming an erect position, and when rising from bed.

N. B. The over-sensitiveness to pain of the Apis-patient is found only very rarely with Lachesis.

* When swallowing drink, both remedies have predom. aggrav.; Lachesis also when swallowing saliva.

Apis.	Phosphor.
Left side—Dark hemorrhages.	*Right side*—Bright-red hemorrhages.
Complaints (sensitiveness, etc.) predom. in external parts.	Complaints (sensitiveness, etc.) predom. in internal parts.
Apoplexia sanguinea—Apoplexia serosa .	Apoplexia nervosa.
Rarely paralysis of the limbs	Apoplexy less frequent than paralysis.
Pulse more equal than with Phosphor . .	
Want of thirst seemingly only during the sweating stage.	Want of thirst.
Complaints predom. on the upper lip, on the pylorus, and in the spleen.	Complaints predom. on the lower lip, on the cardia, and in the liver.
Anxious feeling in the head	Anxious feeling in the præcordia.

Apis.	Phosphor.
Sensitiveness of disposition—Loquacity—Fear of apoplexy.	Insensibility *or* sensitiveness of disposition—Taciturnity—Fear of loss of reason.
Consequences of hearing bad news, or of jealousy.	Consequences of grief. (?)
Absent-mindedness — Difficulty in thinking—mental dullness—Imbecility.	Fancies — Mental excitability—Ecstasies—Insanity.
Pupils most frequently dilated	Pupils generally contracted.
Vomiting of bile	Most frequently sour vomit.
Retention of urine.	Involuntary discharge of urine.
Cough, with difficulty to raise, awakens before midnight, and ceases as soon as the least particle is loosened, which is swallowed.	Expectoration not constant; in the morning and during the day.
Beating of heart and pulse intermittent . .	Palpitation of the heart, with equal, generally accelerated beating.
Milk diminished	Milk most frequently increased.

Apis.	Phosphor.
Remission of complaints during the day .	**Remission** after midnight.
Worse when awaking and after rising from bed.	Better *or* worse when awaking and after rising from bed.
Worse in bed	Worse *or* better * in bed.
Ailments from sting of insects, poisoning by contagious Anthrax, or abuse of Cinchona.	Ailments from abuse of table-salt.

Predomin. worse 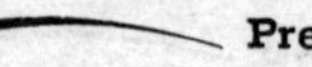 **Predomin. better**

From warmth, when lifting up the diseased limb, after sleep †, when sitting down, leaning back, and from the touch.

Predomin. better —— **Predomin. worse**

From cold, when letting the diseased limb hang down, after perspiration, from cold applications, when assuming an erect position, and rising from bed.

---

* The warmth of the bed aggravates with both remedies.

† After the siesta, Phosphor also has aggravation; the same on awaking when roused from sleep; therefore, better after sufficient sleep.

Apis.	Pulsatilla.
Left side—Inclination to wash with cold water.	*Right side*—Disinclination to wash with cold water.
Complaints predom. on external parts . .	Complaints predom. in internal parts.
Complaints most frequent on exterior ear, on the upper lip, and in the spleen.	Complaints most frequent in the inner ear, on the under lip, and in the liver.
Apoplexia sanguinea—Apoplexia serosa—Blood coagulates slow.	Apoplexia nervosa — Blood coagulates quickly.
Pulse most frequently accelerated and full .	Pulse most frequently quick, small and weak.
Thirst seems to be wanting only during the sweat.	Want of thirst — Thirst only during the heat and before and after the chill, rarely after the heat.
Chill increased by motion	Chill lessened by motion.
Chill on the suffering part	Heat on the suffering part.
Nettlerash all over the body, except the feet.	Eruption all over the body, except the face.
Overstrained merriness — Fickle unsteadiness - Excitability and irascibility (more rarely dejection)—Jealousy.	Predom. lacrymose mood — Gentleness — Distrust—Greediness—Amativeness.
Anxious feeling in the head	Anxious feeling in the præcordia.
Consequences of rage, jealousy, or hearing bad news.	Consequences of excessive joy, grief, mortification, or vexation with dread or fear
Imbecility	Melancholy.
Horses kick, and show an inclination to run off.	Horses sensitive to the touch, particularly on the ears, and, therefore, cannot be bridled.
Pupils most frequently dilated	Pupils most frequently contracted.
Diarrhœa (with exception of dysentery) generally painless.	Diarrhœa most frequently painful.
Urine frequent, but scanty; only exceptionally copious—Retention of urine.	Urine infrequent and scanty—Incontinence more frequent than retention of urine.
Cough, with difficulty to raise, awakens before midnight and ceases as soon as the least particle is loosened, which is swallowed.	Expectoration predom., but not constant; in the morning and during the day.
Milk diminished	Milk most frequently increased.
REMISSION of complaints during the day .	REMISSION from midnight until noon.
Worse on awaking	*Worse or* better on awaking.
Worse after rising from bed	*Better or* worse after rising from bed
Worse when sitting down	*Worse or* better when sitting down.
Worse when rising from a seat	*Worse or* better when rising from a seat.
Worse *after* rising from a seat	*Better or* worse *after* rising from a seat.
Worse from moving the diseased limb . .	*Better or* worse when moving the diseased limb.
Worse when swallowing, particularly food and *drink*.	*Worse or* better when swallowing, particularly worse when swallowing saliva.
Better when assuming an erect position.	Worse *or* better when assuming an erect position.

Predomin. worse —— **Predomin. better**

From bodily exertion, while moving, lifting the diseased limb, in cold weather, from drinking cold water* from vinegar, and from sour things generally, during inspiration and after rising from bed or a seat.

Predomin. better —— **Predomin. worse**

During rest, when letting the diseased limb hang down, in warm air, and from drinking wine.

* Drinking water ameliorates the already existing Pulsatilla complaints: on the other hand, new complaints frequently arise in consequence of cold drink, which Pulsatilla cures.

Apis.	Rhus.
L. —> R.	**R. —> L.**
Particularly affections of the ovaries, and eruptions go from l. to r.	Eruptions and pain from r. to l. C.Hg.
Left side predom.	Right side predom.
Sensitiveness to pain predom.	Insensibility or sensation of numbness predom.*
Hæmorrhages dark—Blood incoagulable .	Hæmorrhages light-colored, serous—Blood coagulates easily.
Inclination for open air	Aversion to the open air.
Cutting pain in internal parts	Cutting pain in external parts.
Burning, with piercing pain.	Burning pain, with itching.
Pulse most frequently accelerated and full .	Pulse irregular; generally accelerated, faint, weak and soft.
Heat, with inclination to uncover	Heat, with aversion to uncover, which aggrav.; while wrapping up, ameliorates.
Chill on the suffering part	Sweat on the suffering part.
Thirst seems to be wanting only during sweat.	Thirst not constant.
Somnolence predom.	Sleeplessness predom.
Overstrained gaiety—Fickle unsteadiness—Irritable and irascible mood; more rarely dejection—Jealousy.	Dejection.
Fear of apoplexy	Fear of being poisoned.
Consequences of fright, rage, vexation, jealousy, or of hearing *bad news*.	Consequences of vexation with fear.
Apoplexy more frequent than paralysis . .	Paralysis more frequent than apoplexy.
Diarrhœa (with the exception of dysentery) predom. painless.	Diarrhœa most frequently painful.
Secretion of urine oftener diminished than increased, but yet urinating oftener than usual; urine dark.	Secretion of urine increased; urine pale, frequently copious.
Retention of urine.	Involuntary discharge of urine.
Respiratio abdomalis	Respiratio thoracica.
Cough, with difficulty to raise, awakens before midnight and ceases as soon as the least particle is loosened which is swallowed.	Expectoration not constant; is raised chiefly in the morning.
Milk diminished	Milk most frequently increased.
Worse when swallowing food, and particularly *drink*.	Worse when swallowing food and saliva.
Worse from the heat of the sun.	Worse in snowy air.

Predomin. worse ——— **Predomin. better**

From wrapping up, warmth, warmth of the bed †, and in warm rooms, also from motion ‡.

Predomin. better ——— **Predomin. worse**

From uncovering, from cold and washing with cold water, in the open air, from eructation, spirituous liquors, during rest, and when assuming an erect position.

* Yet we find, with Rhus as well as with Apis, "sensitiveness of external parts."

† We also find aggrav. in bed, with Rhus, probably more as a consequence of rest than of the warmth of the bed-clothes; this applies chiefly to the scalp.

‡ Rhus has aggrav. during rest and in the beginning of motion, amelioration during continued moderate (not exerting) motion.

Apis.	Sepia.
Itching, relieved by scratching	Itching aggrav. by scratching.
Inclination for open air and washing with cold water.	Aversion to open air and washing with cold water.
Phlebitis	Distention of the veins—Throbbing in the veins.
Apoplexy more frequent than paralysis; the latter generally one-sided.	Paralysis more frequent than apoplexy: generally of both sides.
Pulse most frequently accelerated and full .	Pulse is accelerated, partic. by vexation and motion; at night quick and full; during the day slow.
Chill on the suffering parts	Sweat on the diseased parts.

Apis.	Sepia.
Morbid merriness — Fickle unsteadiness — Delirium.	Mood serious, sad, irritable — Avarice — Fancies.
Pupils most frequently dilated	Pupils contracted.
Puffiness around (under) the eyes, and predom. on the upper lip.	Puffiness above the eyes, and predom. on the underlip.
Complaints predom. on pylorus, in the spleen, and in the hollow of the knee.	Complaints predom. on the cardia, in the liver, and in the hollow of the elbow.
Retention of urine; discharge often, but scanty, sometimes copious.	Discharge of urine involuntary; too seldom.
Catamenia too soon	Catamenia generally too late.
Sexual desire too strong; less frequently too weak, the latter more with women.	Sexual desire changeable, with less potency.
Respiratio abdominalis	Respiratio thoracica.
Cough wakens before midnight, and ceases as soon as the least particle is loosened, which is swallowed.	Expectoration not constant; is loosened in the night and morning, and is generally swallowed.

Apis.	Sepia.
REMISSION of complaints in the fore- and afternoon.	REMISSION in the afternoon.
WORSE from bodily exertion	Much oftener amelioration than aggravation by exertion; on the other hand aggravation by mental exertion. CHg.
Better in the open air, worse in a warm room.	Sometimes better, and sometimes worse out doors, particularly in *cold* open air.
Worse when swallowing warm *drink or food.*	Worse when swallowing food.
Better after sweating	*Worse* during and after sweat.
Worse from being over-hurried	Worse when idle.
Worse in the heat of the sun	Worse in snowy air.

Predomin. worse ——— **Predomin. better**

From warmth, wrapping up, after* sleep, from motion, partic. moving the diseased part, from bodily exertion, sitting down as well as rising from a seat.

Predomin. better ——— **Predomin worse**

From cold, uncovering, during rest, and from scratching and rubbing.

---

* Here the improvement of the Sepia symptoms is, no doubt, in consequence of sufficient sleep; for in general *on awaking* this remedy has aggravation at least quite as often as amelioration.

Argent.	Mercur.
Pressing or pinching pain in external parts.	Pressing or pinching pain in internal parts.
Pain pressing inwards	Pain pressing outwards.
Inclination for the open air.	Aversion to the open air.
No Apoplexy	Apoplexy.
Pulse often unchanged; accelerated in the evening after lying down; slow in the morning.	Pulse irregular; generally full and accelerated; quick at night, slow during the day.
Coldness on small spots	Sweat on small spots.
Want of thirst, particularly during the hot stage of the fever.	Thirst during all stages of the fever, but not constant.

Argent.	Mercur.
Fear of apoplexy, particularly with palpitation of the heart.	Fear of loss of reason—Consequences of mortification—Unconsciousness.

Argent.	Mercur.
Itching, unchanged by scratching . . .	Itching, relieved *or* aggrav. by scratching.
Complaints predom. in lower part of chest, on the front side of the thigh, on the patella, and on the calf of the leg.	Complaints predom. in the upper part of chest, the back part of thigh, in the hollow of the knee, and on the shin.
Most frequently hunger	Most frequently loss of appetite.
Expectoration almost constant; during day and evening.	Expectoration not constant; during the day.

Argent.	Mercur.
REMISSION evening and *night*	REMISSION of complaints during the day.
Worse when swallowing	Worse *or* better when swallowing; particularly worse when swallowing saliva or liquids.
Ailments from abuse of Mercury	Ailments from the sting of insects, Sulphur, Calcarea, or Cinchona; also from Arsenic or Copper vapors.

Predomin. worse — **Predomin. better**

During rest, while * lying down, sitting, and standing, particularly when lying on the back, sitting bent forward, leaning against anything, when descending, in doors, and from smoking.

Predomin. better — **Predomin. worse**

During motion, while walking, lying on the side, assuming an erect position, ascending, and in the *open air*.

---

* Both remedies have aggravation "in bed."

Argent.	Pulsatilla.
Left side; particularly *lower left, upper right side.*	*Right* side; particularly *lower right, upper left side.*
Complaints (pinching pain, etc.) predom. in external parts.	Complaints (pinching pain, etc.) predom. in internal parts.
Pain pressing inwards	Pain pressing outwards.
Itching, unchanged by scratching	Itching, aggrav. *or* unchanged by scratching.
Pains increase gradually and disappear suddenly.	Pains come on suddenly and disappear gradually.
Complaints predom. on external ear, soft palate, and on the patella.	Complaints most frequently in the inner ear, on the roof of the mouth, and in the hollow of the knee.
No apoplexy	Apoplexy.
Pulse accelerated in the evening, after lying down.	Pulse generally small, weak, and quick, partic. in the evening; slower in the morning.
Sweat sometimes only on the front part of the body.	Sweat sometimes only on the back part of the body.
Want of thirst, even during the heat . .	Thirst *only* during the hot stage of the fever, *before* and *after* the chill, and after the hot stage.
Fear of apoplexy, particularly with palpitation of the heart.	Consequences of excessive joy, of fright, grief, mortification, or of vexation with fear, fright, dread, reserved displeasure.
Neither unconsciousness nor delirium . .	Unconsciousness—Delirium.
Urine often and copious	Urine infrequent and scanty.
Expectoration almost constant; during the day and evening.	Expectoration predom., but not constant; in the morning and during the day.
Remission of complaints in the evening and *night*.	Remission from midnight till noon.
Worse when lying on the back, *better* when lying on the side.	More frequently aggrav. by lying on the side than the back; often improved by the latter position.
Better while and after rising from bed, and after rising from a seat.	*Better or* worse while and after rising from bed, or from a seat.
Worse when swallowing	Worse *or* better when swallowing.
Worse when drawing a deep breath . . .	Better *or* worse when drawing a deep breath.
Worse when looking at running water . .	Worse when looking up.

Predomin. worse — **Predomin. better**

From cold, uncovering, when lying on the painful side, when lifting, resting on anything, stretching out or bending the diseased limb sideways, as well as when running, and from pressure.

Predomin. better — **Predomin. worse**

From warmth, wrapping up, when lying on the unpainful side; when letting the diseased limb hang down, or when drawing it up.

N.B. Argent. lacks the over-sensitiveness to pain as well as the sensation of numbness in the suffering parts which characterizes Pulsatilla.

Argent.	Sepia.
Inclination for open air	Aversion to the open air.
Pain pressing inwards	Pain pressing outwards.
Rending pain in internal, pinching pain in external parts.	Tearing pain in external, pinching pain in internal parts.
Itching, generally unchanged by scratching.	Itching aggravated by scratching — Apoplexy.
Pulse accelerated in the evening, after lying down; slow in the morning.	Pulse quick and full at night; slow during the day.
Want of thirst, even during the hot stage of the fever.	Thirst is constant only during the chill, and is entirely wanting during sweat.

Argent.	Sepia.
Fear of apoplexy, particularly with palpitation of heart.	Consequences of vexation with fear.
Vacancy of mind, but only with vertigo or headache.	Vacancy of mind and thoughtlessness, with desire to work. C.Hg.
Most frequently hunger	Most frequently want of appetite.
Discharge of urine too often and copious .	Discharge of urine too seldom.
Expectoration nearly constant; during the day and evening.	Expectoration predom., but not constant; is loosened particularly in the night and morning, and is generally swallowed.
Complaints predom. on the front part of the thigh.	Complaints predom. on the back part of the thigh.

Argent.	Sepia.
REMISSION evening and *night*	REMISSION of complaints in the afternoon.
Predom. worse after lying down and in bed.	Better *or* worse after lying down and in bed.
Better while and after rising from bed . .	Worse *or* better while and after rising from bed.
Better when rising from a seat.	Worse *or* better when rising from a seat.
Predom. better during expiration, worse during inspiration.	Most frequently aggrav. during expiration, and then better during inspiration.
Predom. better when walking in the open air.	Worse *or* better when walking in the open air.
Worse when walking fast or running . .	*Better or* worse when walking fast or running.
Worse when looking at running water . .	Worse when looking up or over a large surface.

Predomin. worse — **Predomin. better**

While lying on the painful side, descending, sitting down, or when assuming an erect position.

Predomin. better — **Predomin. worse**

When lying on the unpainful side, when ascending, and from rubbing.

N.B. Argent. lacks the over-sensitiveness to pain of the Sepia-patient.

Argent. nitr.	Kali bichrom.
Upper left, lower right side.	Upper right, lower left side.
Complaints predom. in internal parts . .	Complaints predom. in external parts.
Pain pressing inwards	Pain pressing outwards.
Paralysis—Sensation of numbness in external parts.	Sensitiveness in external parts.
Gloomy, dull; wishes to do nothing . . .	Aversion to all occupation, but without laziness.
Scrupulousness—Want of self-confidence .	Indifferent, or low-spirited after the least annoyance. C.Hg.
Inclination to motion	Aversion to motion — Inclination to lie down.
Want of thirst	Thirst.
Dry cough (without expectoration.) . . .	Expectoration is not constant.
Collection of viscous thick mucus in the choanæ and in the throat, compels to gag and retch; small greasy, round lumps of mucus in the larynx, which are removed by light coughs.	Mucus so viscid that it draws out like a long thread from the gullet and throat; continually a troublesome retching and cough. C.Hg.
Pustulous ecthyma—Erysipelas	Measles—Ulcers. C.Hg.
AGGRAVATION of symptoms after midnight, in the morning and afternoon.	AGGRAVATION in the morning and at noon.
General feeling better in the open air, particularly catarrhs (eyes, stomach), while vertigo and headache are aggrav. in the open air.	General feeling better out-doors, particularly vertigo improved while walking in the open air; chilliness and complaints of the stomach are aggravated in the open air.
Chill from being uncovered; wrapping up causes a smothered feeling.	Uncovering aggravates; wrapping up ameliorates.
Worse after vomiting.	*Better* after vomiting *
Squeamishness in the stomach, improved by eating; but acute pains in the stomach aggrav. by eating.	The gastric pains are diminished by eating; the rheumatic pains are increased or renewed by it.

*** It is true that with K. bichr. an eruption breaks out in the face *after vomiting*, but in reference to the general state this must be regarded as an improvement quite as much as the breaking out of eruptions *in hot weather*. The subjective symptoms are aggravated *in cold weather*.**

Argent. nitr.	Natrum mur.
Left side	*Right side.*
Complaints predom. in internal parts	Complaints predom. in external parts.
Want of feeling and sensation of numbness in external parts.	Want of feeling and numbness in internal parts*.
Inclination for motion — Aversion to the open air †.	Aversion to motion — Inclination for the open air.
Awaking too early	Generally awaking too late.
Reserve—Sadness	Loquacity—Cheerfulness *or* sadness.
Fear of apoplexy	Fear of loss of reason.
Apoplexy has not yet been observed	Unconsciousness—Delirium—Apoplexy.
Vertigo, inclining to fall sideways	Vertigo, inclining to fall forwards.
Complaints predom. on the upper eyelids	Complaints predom. on the lower eyelids.
Want of thirst	Thirst during the fever and when there is no fever.
Urine frequent and scanty	Urine frequent and generally copious.
REMISSION of complaints in the *forenoon* and evening, till midnight.	REMISSION in the afternoon.
Complaints from the pressure of the clothes ‡.	Often improved by tying the clothes tight.
Chill from being uncovered; but difficult respiration is increased by being wrapped up.	Uncovering aggravates—Wrapping up ameliorates.
Worse from cold, *better* from warm diet	*Better* sometimes from cold, sometimes from warm diet.
Better from wine	*Worse* from spirituous liquors.
Worse while drinking.	*Worse after* drinking.
Nausea, lessened by sour things	Sour things disagree with the patient.
Worse from opening or spreading out the hands.	*Worse* when closing the hands.

* With Natr. mur. we also find *sensitiveness* in internal and external parts.

† Yet the catarrhal complaints of Arg. nitr. are improved in the open air.

‡ But yet the headache of Arg. nitr. is ameliorated by tying something tightly around the head, by the pressure of the hat, etc.

Argent. nitr.	Pulsatilla.
Predom. *left side* of the body	Complaints predom. on the *right side*.
Inclination for motion	Aversion to motion.
Aversion to the open air	Inclination for the open air.
Pressing pain from outside inward	Pressing from inside outward.
Itching, aggrav. by scratching	Itching unchanged *or* aggrav. by scratching
Heat without thirst	Heat with thirst.

Argent. nitr.	Pulsatilla.
Embarrassment—Scrupulousness—Lack of self-confidence.	Boldness (*or* embarrassment; precipitancy, rashness. C.Hg.).
Vertigo inclining to fall sideways	Vertigo inclining to fall backwards—Apoplexy.
Farsightedness	Shortsightedness.
Want of thirst	Thirst only during the heat*.
The stream of urine spreads asunder	The stream of urine thin.
Urine often, but scanty	Urine infrequent and scanty.
Sexual desire diminished—Impotence	Sexual desire increased.
Cough without expectoration	Expectoration not constant; in the morning and during the day.
Complaints predominate on *fore*-arm	Complaints predom. on *upper*-arm.
Emaciation, particularly of the legs	Emaciation, particularly of the suffering parts.

Argent. nitr.	Pulsatilla.
Aggravation in the afternoon, after midnight and in the morning.	AGGRAVATION in the afternoon and after sunset until midnight.
Aggravation when drinking (difficult respiration).	Aggravation *after* drinking.

Predomin. **worse**	Predomin. **better**

From motion, when lifting the diseased limb, from tying the clothes tight, and from cold diet.

Predomin. **better**	Predomin. **worse**

During rest, while standing, from scratching and rubbing, letting the diseased limb hang down, lying on a cold cushion, from warm diet, drinking wine, and loosening the clothes.

---

* Puls. has thirst, (which is not constant even during the heat,) more between the stages of the fever, that is, *before* and *after* the chill, and after the heat.

Arnica.	Belladonna.
Left side—Complaints predom. in external parts.	*Right side*—Complaints predom. in internal parts.
Inclination for motion and open air . . .	Aversion to motion * and open air.
Complaints predom. in the lower part of the chest, and on the inner side of the thigh.	Complains predom. in the upper part of the chest, and on the outer side of thigh.
When the pulse grows slow, it is weak . .	When the pulse grows slow, it is strong.
Cold on the side lain on	Sweat on the side lain on.
Thirst constant, particularly during chill .	Thirst most rare during chill.

Arnica.	Belladonna.
Weak memory	Memory very active *or* very weak.
Ailments from fright or anger	Consequences of fright, anger, mortification, or of vexation with fright, dread, fear or vehemence.
Pupils oftener contracted than dilated . .	Pupils oftener dilated than contracted.
Shortsightedness	Farsightedness.
Appetite for sour things.	Aversion to sour things.
Nausea in the stomach	Nausea in the throat or in the abdomen; less frequently in the stomach.
Fœtid flatus	Scentless flatus.
Voice deep	Voice raised.
Audible respiration predom.	Respiration predom. low.
Expectoration infrequent; is loosened during the day and evening; is generally swallowed.	Expectoration infrequent; in the morning, during the day or evening.

Arnica.	Belladonna.
REMISSION after midnight and *during the day*.	REMISSION after midnight and in the *forenoon*.
Worse during increase of moon	Worse during full moon.
Better in a horizontal position.	Predom. better with the head lying high.
Worse when assuming an erect position .	*Worse or* better when assuming an erect position.
Worse when leaning against anything . .	Worse *or* better when leaning against anything, particularly better when leaning against something hard (and from lying on something hard).
Worse when bending the diseased part . .	Better *or* worse when bending the diseased part.
Worse or better when moving the diseased part.	Worse when moving the diseased part.
Ailments from charcoal vapors	Ailments from poisoning with contagious Anthrax, Iodine, Plumbum, or abuse of Mercury.

Predomin. worse —— **Predomin. better**

In doors, from stooping, and lying with the heat high.

Predomin. better —— **Predomin. worse**

In the open air †, when swallowing, and in a horizontal position.

---

* We also find inclination for motion in single or suffering parts with Belladonna.

† Both remedies have aggrav. "when walking in the open air."

Arnica.	China.
Inflammation and other complaints predom. in external parts.	Inflammation and other complaints predom. in internal parts.
Tearing pain upwards	Tearing pain generally downwards.
Inclination for the open air.	Aversion to the open air.
Complaints from charcoal vapors.	Complaints from mercurial vapors.
Itching, relieved *or* unchanged by scratching.	Itching, relieved by scratching.
Pulse most frequently accelerated; hard and full.	Pulse quick, hard, but small; more quiet after meals.
Coldness sometimes confined to the side lain on.	Sweat on the side lain on.
Heat on upper part of body (lower part cold.)	Sweat on the upper part of body.
Partial sweat on the front part of body.	Partial sweat on the back part of body.
Thirst constant only during the chill.	Thirst constant only during sweat*.
Congestion predom. to the eyes	Congestion of blood to the ears.
During sleep, lying with head low	During sleep, sitting posture.
Complaints predom. on the lower jaw and teeth, on the back part of thigh, and in the hollow of the elbow.	Complaints predom. on the upper jaw and teeth, on the front side of the thigh, and in the hollow of the knee.
Consequences of fright or anger	Consequences of vexation.
Unconsciousness	Rarely unconsciousness in fevers.
Eyes protruding	Eyes generally sunken.
Saliva generally diminished.	Saliva increased.
Nausea in the stomach	Nausea in the throat or stomach.
Afterpains return when suckling the child.	Cough, with bloody expectoration when suckling the child.
Inspiration quick, expiration slow	Inspiration slow, expiration quick.
Expectoration infrequent; is generally swallowed.	Expectoration not constant.
Remission after midnight and *during the day*	Remission of complaints in the afternoon and evening.
Worse *when* perspiring	Worse, particularly *after* perspiring.
Worse when closing eyes, better when opening them.	When closing the eyes (or opening them), *better or* worse.
Better in a horizontal position.	Better when lying with the head high.
Better *or* worse when lying on the painful (or unpainful) side.	Predom. worse when lying on the painful, better when lying on the unpainful side.
Worse on awaking.	Worse *or* better on awaking.
Worse when assuming an erect position	Better *or* worse when assuming an erect position.
Worse when bending the diseased limb	Better *or* worse when bending the diseased limb.
Predom. worse after meals	Worse *or* better after meals.
Worse on inspiration, better on expiration.	Most frequently better on inspiration, worse on expiration.
Worse when taking a deep breath	Improved oftener than aggrav. when taking a deep breath.
Worse from sleeping too long	Worse from being awake all night.

Predomin. worse (Arnica) — **Predomin. better** (China)

In the room, from warm applications, from uncovering the head, lying on the left side and with the head high.

Predomin. better (Arnica) — **Predomin. worse** (China)

In the open air †, when wrapping up the head, after lying down, in bed, when sitting, when swallowing, from eructation, lying on the right side, and in a horizontal position, or with the head low.

* Cinchona has thirst more frequently before and between the different stages of fever.

† Both remedies have aggrav. "when *walking* out-doors;" it appears, therefore, to be caused more by motion than by the open air.

Arnica.	Ipecacuanha.
Left side.—Muscles predom. rigid—Dark hair.	*Right* side.—Muscles lax—Light hair.
Increased irritability—Inclination for the open air.	Want of bodily irritation—Aversion to the open air.
Inflammation and other complaints predom. in external parts.	Inflammation and other complaints predom. in internal parts.
Ailments from charcoal vapors	Ailments from Arsenic or copper vapors.
Itching, relieved or unchanged by scratching	Itching, unchanged by scratching.
Pulse unequal; most frequently quick, full, and hard.	Pulse very much accelerated, but weak.
Chill increased by drinking	Chill moderated by drinking.
Predom. *external chill*, with internal heat.	Predom. *internal chill*, with external heat.
Heat of the upper part of body; coldness of lower part of body.	Upper part of body cold.
Thirst constant only during the chill. . .	Thirst not constant.
Ailments from fright or anger	Ailments from vexation and reserved displeasure.
Fancies	No delirium—Very rarely unconsciousness in fevers.
Paralysis	Very rarely paralysis.
Eyes protruding	Eyes sunken.
Optical illusions in dark colors.	Optical illusions in bright colors.
Urine scanty and infrequent; sometimes frequent.	Urine scanty.
Labor-pains, weak or ceasing	Spasmodic labor-pains.
Expectoration infrequent; is loosened during the day and evening, and is generally swallowed.	Expectoration infrequent; in the *morning* and during the day.
Complaints predom. on the back of the hand	Complaints predom. in the palms of the hands.
Remission *during the day* and after midnight.	Remission of complaints during the day.
Better when lying on the back *or* on the side.	Better when lying on the back; worse when lying on the side.
Worse on awaking	Worse *or* better on awaking.
	Better after sufficient sleep.
Aggrav. oftener than improved after sleep.	Better after sleep.
Better in the open air*; worse in the room.	Predom. worse in the open air; better in the room, if it is not too warm.
Worse after sleeping too long.	Worse from being awake all night.

Predomin. worse — **Predomin. better**
When closing the eyes, from cold, after drinking, after sleeping, and in the room.

Predomin. better — **Predomin. worse**
When opening the eyes, from warmth, after rising from bed, and in the open air.

* Both remedies have aggrav. "when *walking* in the open air;" therefore, motion decides in this case.

Arnica.	Nux vomica.
Left side; partic. *upper left and lower right.*	*Right side;* partic. *upper right and lower left.*
Inclination for motion and open air . . .	Aversion to motion and open air.
Complaints (sensation of cold, pinching, &c.) predom. in external parts — Cold, left side.	Complaints (sensation of cold, pinching, &c.) predom. in internal parts — Cold on the right side of the body.
Pulse sometimes intermitting the 7th beat.	Pulse sometimes intermit. the 4th or 5th beat.
Thirst constant only during the chill . .	Thirst mostly during the chill, and between the heat and sweat.
Perspiration on front part of body . . .	Perspiration on back part of body.
Ailments from charcoal vapors	Ailments from Arsenic or copper vapors.
Compl. predom. in the hollow of the elbow.	Complaints predom. in hollow of the knee.
Paralysis predom. in the arms	Paralysis predom. in the legs.
With horses compl. partic. pastern joints .	With horses, complains partic. of the hocks.
Sleeplessness before midnight	Sleeplessness predom. after midnight.

Arnica.	Nux vomica.
No malice, &c.	Maliciousness—Amativeness.
Ailments from fright or anger	Ailments from fright, anger, mortification, grief, disappointed love, jealousy, or from vexation with fright, dread, fear, indignation, or vehemence.
Short-sightedness—Dim-sightedness	Far-sightedness — Pred. clear-sightedness.
Optical illusions in dark colors	Optical illusions in bright colors.
Saliva predom. diminished	Saliva most frequently increased.
Appetite for sour things.	Predom. aversion to sour things.
Diarrhœa predom.	Constipation predom.
Expectoration infrequent; is loosened during day and evening, and is generally swallowed.	Expectoration not constant; in the morning, during the day and evening.

Arnica.	Nux vomica.
Aggravation in the morning and evening until midnight.	Remission of complaints in the evening until midnight.
Better in a horizontal position	Better lying with the head high.
After sleep most frequently aggravation .	After sleep most frequently amelioration.
Worse on awaking	On awaking *better or* worse*.
Worse after drinking	After drinking *worse or* better.
Better when swallowing	When swallowing *worse or* better.
Better from eructation	*Worse or* better from eructation.
Worse or better when moving the diseased part.	Worse when moving the diseased part.
Worse from being overhurried	Worse when idle, *or* fr. being overhurried †.

Predomin. worse (Arnica) — **Predomin. better** (Nux vomica)

In the room, lying with the head high, lying on the left side, when closing the eyes, lifting or resting the diseased limb on anything, on inspiration, on expiration, eating, and after sleep.

Predomin better (Arnica) — **Predomin. worse** (Nux vomica)

In the open air ‡, lying in an horizontal position, or with the head low, lying on the right side, when opening the eyes, letting the diseased limb hang down, on expiration §.

---

* Improvements of Nux. vom. complaints here follow after sufficient sleep; for after sleeping too long, this remedy also has aggravation; on being roused from sleep pred. aggravation.

† This is only apparently a contradiction, and arises from the common cause of *the same* mental disposition.

‡ Both remedies have aggravation "when *walking* in the open air," and when moving.

§ Both remedies have aggravation when respiring deeply.

Arnica.	Pulsatilla.
Left side, even coldn. and other fever compl.	*Right* side, even chill, coldness, heat, &c.
Upper left, lower right side — Inclination for motion.	*Upper right, lower left* side—Aversion to motion.
Complaints (pinching pain &c.) predom. in external parts.	Complaints (pinching pain, &c.) predom in internal parts.
Ailments frequently on the *external* ear, on the upper lip.	Complaints frequent *in the inner* ear and on the underlip.
Dropsy of *internal* parts	Dropsy predom. in *external* parts.
Paralysis, generally painful	Paralysis generally painless.
Prevents suppuration	Cures suppuration.
Ailments from charcoal vapors	Ailments from copper or mercurial vapors.
With horses: Spasmodic ischurie with hot hoofs, and the excrements in small balls.	With horses: Spasmodic ischurie with cold feet and the excrements in large balls.
Itching, unchanged *or* reliev'd by scratching.	Itching, unchanged *or* aggrav. by scratching.
Pulse often more frequent than the beat of the heart; inequal; generally quick, full and hard.	Pulse often suppressed, with strong beat of the heart; generally quick, but small and weak.
Thirst constant only during the chill—Perspiration on the front side of body.	Thirst only during the hot stage of fever—Perspiration on the back part of body.
During sleep prefers to lie with the head low or horizontal.	During sleep prefers to lie with the back high; often throws the arms over the head; sometimes lying on the belly.
Irritable mood—Fear of apoplexy . . .	Gentleness—Calm sadness—Peevishness—Boldness—Distrust—Greediness.
Ailments from fright or anger	Ailments from excessive joy, fright, grief, mortification, or from vexation with fright, dread, fear, or reserved displeasure.
Eyes protruding	Eyes sunken.
Optical illusions in dark colors	Optical illusion in bright colors.
Saliva predom. diminished	Saliva most frequently increased.
Predom. loss of appetite	Most frequently hunger.
Nausea in the stomach	Nausea in the throat, stomach and abdomen.
Generally retention of urine from exertion.	Incontinentia urinæ from exertion.
Catamenia too soon	Catamenia too late.
Expectoration infrequent; during day and evening; is generally swallowed.	Expectoration predom., but not constant; in the morning and during the day.
Remiss. during the day and after midnight.	Remission from midnight until noon.
Worse when assuming an erect position, and when rising from a seat.	Worse *or* better when assuming an erect position, and from rising from a seat.
When swallowing almost always improved.	When swallowing *worse or* better.
Better from eructation	*Worse or* better from eructation.
Worse when taking a deep breath . . .	*Better or* worse when respiring deeply.
Most frequently aggravated wher moving the part.	Most frequently improved when moving the diseased part.
Worse when bending the diseased part . .	Bett. *or* worse wh. bending the diseased part.
Complaints after bodily exertion	Complaints more aft. mental exertion. C.Hg.

Predomin. worse — **Predomin. better**

From cold, uncovering, on inspiration, when moving, walking, running, walking in the open air *, from bodily exertion, when stretching, lifting, or resting the diseased limb on anything, lying with the head high, from weeping, and after drinking cold water †.

Predomin better — **Predomin worse**

From warmth, wrapping up, on expiration, during rest, after lying down, in bed, when lying, sitting, and standing, drawing up the diseased limb, or letting it hang down, lying with the head low, or in a horizontal position, and from rubbing and scratching.

N.B. Arnica has not the sensation of numbness in suffering parts, which is not infrequ. with Pulsatilla

---

* Both remedies have amelioration "in the open air," aggravation in the room.

† Compare note to Apis and Pulsatilla.

Arnica.	Rhus.
Left side—Dark hair	*Right side*—Light hair.
Inclination for open air—Cutting pain internally.	Aversion to open air—Cutting pain in external parts.
Apoplexy more frequent than paralysis . .	Paralysis more frequent than apoplexy.
With Horses: Hydrocephalus, with a stubborn posture.	With Horses: Hydrocephalus, with jerkings of the head.
Painful ulcers	Painless ulcers.
Pulse most frequently quick, full, and hard.	Pulse generally accelerated, but weak, faint, and soft.
Heat on the upper part of body, (lower part cold.)	Chill or heat on upper part of body.
Thirst constant only during the chill . . .	Thirst not constant.
In Typhus: Thinks is well; putrid breath, (and stool); yellow-greenish spots as large as the tip of a finger on the skin, like those appearing after death; are unchanged by pressure.	In Typhus: Complains of great weakness or violent pain in the limbs; stools smelling like carion; small red spots, disappearing when pressed; rarely ecchymosis or violet spots of the size of an inch. C.Hg.
Irritable mood—Fear of apoplexy . . .	Low-spirited—Fear of being poisoned.
Absent-mindedness—Ailments from fright or anger.	Ailments from vexation with fear.
Discharge of blood from the ear	Discharge of pus from the ears.
Saliva predom. diminished	Saliva most frequently increased.
Desire for spirituous liquors	Aversion to wine.
Nausea in the stomach	Nausea in œsophagus or stomach, less frequently in the throat.
Urine scanty and infrequent; in some cases frequent urging; sediment generally red.	Urine frequent and copious; sediment white.
Expectoration infrequent; is loosened during the day and evening, and is generally swallowed.	Expectoration not constant; during the day.
Complaints predom. in the hollow of the elbow, and on the soles of the feet.	Complaints predom. in the hollow of the knee, and on the top of the foot.
Remission during the day and after midnight.	Remission of complaints during the day.
Worse when leaning against anything . .	*Worse or* better when leaning against anything; particularly *better* when leaning against anything hard, and from pressure.
More frequently aggravated than ameliorated by moving the diseased part.	More frequently ameliorated than aggravated by moving the diseased part.
Worse when bending the diseased part . .	Worse or better when bending the diseased part.
Predom. worse after meals	Worse *or* better after meals.
Worse after drinking	Worse *or* better after drinking.

Predomin. worse ——— **Predomin. better**

In the room, during continuous moderate motion, when walking*, and when stretching out the diseased limb.

Predomin. better ——— **Predomin. worse**

In the open air†, during rest, after lying down, when lying, sitting and standing, when drawing up the diseased limb, and from eructation.

N.B. Rhus has not the over-sensitiveness to pain that the Arnica-patient has; on the other hand, Arnica has not the sensation of numbness in the suffering parts which is not infrequent with Rhus.

* Both remedies have aggravation from walking fast, and running, and from exertion in general.

† "When *walking* in the open air," Arnica has preval. aggravation; Rhus predom. amelioration; therefore motion, and not the open air, must decide the choice.

Arnica.	Veratrum.
Left side.—Dark hair—Muscles predom. rigid.	*Right side.*—Light hair—Muscles predom. lax.
Rending pain upwards—Painful paralysis.	Rending pain downwards—Painless paralysis.
Apoplexy more frequent than paralysis.	Paralysis more frequent than apoplexy.
Complaints (pinching pain, etc.) predom. in external parts.	Complaints (pinching pain, etc.) predom. in internal parts.
Congestion of blood predom. to the extremities.	Congestion of blood to the head.
Pulse most frequently accelerated, full, and hard; sometimes *quicker than the beat of the heart.*	Pulse most frequently slow, small, and weak; even *slower than the beat of the heart;* often imperceptible.
Heat or sweat, with aversion to uncover.	Heat or sweat, with inclination to uncover.
Dry heat predom., particularly on the upper part of the body.	Sweat predom., particularly on the upper part of body.
Thirst predom., but constant only during the chill.	Thirst not constant.
Fear of apoplexy	Fear of being poisoned, or of apoplexy—Cheerfulness or dejection—Amativeness—Haughtiness—Malice.
Consequences of fright or anger	Consequences of fright, anger, *grief,* or of vexation with dread or fear.
Mental excitability	Ecstasies *or* mental dullness—Insanity.
Hot spots on the top of the head	Cold spots on the top of the head.
Eyes protruding	Eyes most frequently sunken.
Optical illusions in dark colors.	Optical illusions in bright colors.
Urine scanty and infrequent; sometimes frequent urgency.	Urine infrequent and scanty; but sometimes copious.
Labor-pains weak or ceasing	Spasmodic labor-pains.
Expectoration infrequent; is loosened during the day and evening, and is generally swallowed.	Expectoration not constant; during the day.
Remission during the day and after midnight.	Remission during the day and evening.
Worse when growing cold; better when growing warm.	Worse *or* better when growing cold (or warm.)
Predom. better in bed	*Worse or* better in bed.
Predom. worse after eating.	Worse *or* better after eating.
Worse from being overhurried.	Worse when idle.

Predomin. worse — **Predomin. better**

From being uncovered, from motion, while walking, and when ascending.

Predomin. better — **Predomin. worse**

From wrapping up, during rest, after lying down, while lying, sitting and standing, when descending, and when swallowing.

N.B. Arnica has not the sensation of numbness in suffering parts which we often find with Veratrum; the latter generally has not the over-sensitiveness to pain of the Arnica-patient. But, notwithstanding this, both remedies have the predom. characteristic of increased constitutional irritability.

Arsenic.	**Belladonna.**
Itching, aggrav. by scratching — Eruptions generally dry.	Itching, unchanged *or* relieved by scratching—Eruptions humid.
Emaciation—Paralysis after neuralgia, with atrophy of muscles—Rarely apoplexy.	Obesity—Nervous lameness, also after apoplexy—Apoplexy.
Ulcers, with much discharge or proud flesh.	Ulcers, with little discharge of pus.
Hæmorrhages; blood coagulates slowly. .	Hæmorrhages; blood coagulates quickly.
Pulse predom. weak	Pulse predom. strong.
Sleeplessness predom. after midnight . .	Sleeplessness before midnight.
Fear of being alone—Sensitiveness of disposition.	Love of being alone—Predom. insensibility of disposition.
Satiety of life, with fear of death; also with inclination to stab himself.	Satiety of life, with longing for death; also with inclination to throw himself out of the window.
Greediness—Mental dullness	Changing mood—Distrust—Amativeness.
In nervous conditions, unconsciousness is never so complete as with Belladonna.	Absent-mindedness – Fancies—Mental excitability and ecstasy, *or* mental dullness.
Consequences of grief and sorrow . . .	Consequences of mortification or anger.
Weakness of memory	Memory active *or very* weak.
Desire to drink without thirst	Thirst, with aversion to drink
Pulse weak — Partial sweat on lower or back part of body.	Pulse predom. strong — Partial sweat on upper or front part of body.
Appetite for milk, coffee, beer, sour things.	Aversion to milk, coffee, beer, or sour things.
Unconquerable desire for brandy	Unconquerable desire for the acid of lemons. C.Hg.
Nausea predom. in the throat	Nausea in the throat or abdomen.
Fetid flatus	Scentless flatus.
Fluent coryza	Dry coryza.
Respiration audible—Voice trembling . .	Respiration predom. low—Voice nasal or raised.
Cough most frequently *with* expectoration; expectoration only during the day.	Cough predom. dry; when there is expectoration, it appears in the morning, during the day and evening.
Milk diminished	Milk generally increased.
Complaints predom. on the *inner* side of the thigh and on the calf.	Complaints predom. on the outer side of thigh and on the shin.
AGGRAVATION evening and after midnight—REMISS. before midnight and *during day.*	REMISSION of complaints after midnight and during forenoon.
Worse in the Fall	Worse in the Spring.
Ailments from Strychnine or Digitalis . .	Ailments from the sting of insects, or from abuse of Mercury.
Ailments from sleeping on damp ground .	Ailments from sleeping in the sun or in the moonlight.
Worse, especially when swallowing food .	Worse, especially when swallowing drink.

Predomin. worse — **Predomin. better**

During rest, after lying down, while lying, standing and sitting, particularly sitting bent forward, from cold diet*, after sweat, and when turning in bed.

Predomin. better — **Predomin. worse**

From motion, after† sleep, from washing, sitting erect, from warm diet.

* From drinking *cold water* Bellad. also has aggrav., because one of its effects is that of swallowing *drink*.

† The improvement of the Arsen symptoms here follow after sufficient sleep; for on awaking (when roused) from sleep, this remedy has aggrav. oftener than improvement. In this respect N. vom., Phosphor., Pulsat., Sepia, Cinchona, and Ipec. are very similar.

Arsenic.	Calcarea.
Muscles (and skin) rigid	Skin and muscles lax.
Itching, aggravated by scratching	Itching, *lessened or* aggrav. by scratching.
Eruption predom. on the upper lip	Eruption predom. on the under lip.
Ulcers even with the surface; sometimes with proud flesh (pred. with copious discharge.)	Deep ulcers (pred. with scanty discharge.) C.Hg.
Swollen glands, cold	Swollen glands, hot.
Emaciation, particularly of the feet, and atrophy of the tips of the fingers.	Obesity (particul. with children and young people) or emaciation, partic. of the face—Swelling of the tips of the fingers.
Pulse small and weak	Pulse predom. full.
During heat desire for drink, without thirst, and with aversion to uncover.	Heat, with thirst and inclination to uncover.
First chill, then heat	First heat, then chill.
Chill lessened after rising from bed	Chill increased after rising from bed.
Perspiration lessened when walking in the open air.	Perspiration increased when walking in the open air.
Sleeplessness predom. after midnight	Sleeplessness predom. before midnight.
Rarely apoplexy	Apoplexy.
Hopelessness—Malice—Insanity—Loquacity.	Sadness—Amativeness—Fancies—Taciturnity.
Consequences of grief, sorrow, reserved displeasure, and of vexation with vehemence.	Ailments from hearing bad news.
Numb sensation of the teeth	Sensitiveness of the teeth. C.Hg.
Most frequently loss of appetite	Most frequently hunger.
Desire for coffee	Aversion to coffee.
Thirst mostly during the sweat	Thirst during all stages of the fever.
Nausea in the throat	Nausea in the stomach.
Urine scanty (with diarrhœa) *or* copious	Urine too frequent.
Acrid leucorrhœa	Mild leucorrhœa.
Voice trembling	Voice strange, singing, or nasal.
Expectoration only during the day	Expectoration in the morning and during the day.
Spinal complaints, with gressus gallinacus	Spinal complaints, with gressus vaccinus.
Complaints predom. on upper arm, and in the hollow of the knee.	Complaints predom. on the fore-arm, and on the patella.
Paralysis of the legs predom.	Paralysis of the arms predom.
REMISSION before midnight and during the day.	REMISSION before midnight.
Ailments from poisoning by contagious Anthrax., Jodine, Lead, Strychnine (or Phosphor.)	Ailments from abuse of Mercury, Nitric acid, or Phosphor.

Predomin. worse —— **Predomin. better**

In dry weather, from the touch, during rest, when standing, sitting and lying, particularly lying on the back, when lifting up or resting the diseased limb on anything, from uncovering, after breakfast and from rubbing and scratching.

Predomin. better —— **Predomin. worse**

In wet weather, from washing and moistening the diseased limb, or when letting it hang down, when moving generally and particularly the painful limb, from wrapping up warm and from the warmth of the bed, from lying on the side, after* sleep, on an empty stomach.

* Compare note to diagnosis of Arsenic and Belladonna.

Arsenic.	Carb. veget.
Rending or piercing pain upwards . . .	Rending or piercing pain downwards.
Cutaneous eruptions, most frequently dry .	Eruptions most frequently humid.
Flat ulcers, with copious discharge . . .	Deep ulcers, with scanty discharge.
Burning sensation of scares	Scares burn; become painful on change of weather; break open. C.Hg.
Partial sweat on lower part of body. . .	Partial sweat on upper part of body.
Least thirst during chill, most with sweat .	Thirst is constant only during the chill.
Sweat less when and after rising from bed, and lessened by motion.	Sweat increased when and after rising from bed, and by motion.
Sleeplessness, particularly after midnight; therefore, awaking too early.	Sleeplessness before midnight; awaking too late.
Complaints predom. on the pylorus and on the leg.	Complaints predom. on the cardia and on the thigh.
Weakness of reasoning powers	Fancies—Excited imagination.
Saliva decreased	Saliva increased.
Predom. loss of appetite	Predom. hunger.
Appetite for milk	Aversion to milk.
Diarrhœa predom.; is generally painless .	Costiveness predom.; when there is diarrhœa, it is generally painful.
Urine scanty (with diarrhœa), or copious (during the cold stage of fever.)	Urine infrequent and scanty.
Expectoration predom., but not constant; during the day.	Expectoration rather infrequent; in the morning.
Bad effects of putrid animal matter, particularly when changed by disease (pus, etc.); from inhalation, or from contact with wounds.	Bad effects of putrid vegetable matter; from inhalation or contact with wounds. C.Hg.
Consequences of sausage-poison	Ailments from putrid fish*. C.Hg.
REMIS. before midnight and *during the day*.	REMIS. after midnight and in the afternoon.
Aggrav. more *during* than *after* the sweat.	Aggrav., particularly *after* the sweat.
Worse after lying down; but in bed (rest) worse or (warmth) better.	Better after lying down; but worse in bed and from the warmth of the bed.
Worse or better on awaking	Worse on awaking.
Better after sleep, that is after sufficient sleep.	Worse after sleeping.
Worse in cold, better in warm weather . .	Better *or* worse in cold (resp. warm) air.
Worse in dry, better in moist air	Worse *or* better in dry (resp. wet) air.
Worse in the Autumn	Worse in the Spring.
Worse (better) from light *or* in the dark .	Better from light, worse in the dark.

Predomin. worse — **Predomin. better**

When growing cold, from uncovering, cold diet, after lying down, during rest, while sitting, particularly sitting bent forward.

Predomin. better — **Predomin. worse**

When growing warm, from wrapping up, warm diet, coffee†, after a satisfying meal, from the warmth of the bed, after sleeping, from motion, when rising from bed, after rising from a seat, when assuming an erect position, from external pressure, riding, washing and moistening the diseased part.

N.B. The *burning pain* which both remedies have, and both more in the night, predom. in Arsenic in the stomach and abdomen; and in Carb. veg. in the chest, while coughing; we find it in Arsenic predom in external parts and the skin; in Carb. veg. internally; however, Arsen. has a burning sensation in all the veins, and Carb. veg. sometimes externally, as for instance on the umbilicus. Arsen. has burning pain in the eyes, on the external ear, on the tongue, in the mouth, throat, pit of the stomach, the loins, bladder, urethra, breast-bone, the third finger; Carb. veg. has it in the head, on the ear-lap, cheeks, roof of mouth, fauces, in the neck, on the back, shoulders, upper arm, elbow, fore-arm, thigh, knee, and soles of the feet. C.Hg.

* Both remedies cured the bad effects from drinking ice-water because these are similar to those of putrid matter. C.Hg.

† Probably only because coffee is generally drank *warm* This remark is applicable also to Causticum Phosphor Sepia; less to Belladonna, Pulsatilla, and Mercury because narcotics, in general, are a simile to coffee, and Mercury symptoms are quite as often aggrav. by cold as by warm diet.

Arsenic.	Causticum.
Upper left, lower right side	Upper right, lower left side.
Complaints (sensat. of cold, heaviness, &c.) predom. in internal parts.	Complaints (cold, heaviness) predom. in external parts.
Itching aggrav. by scratching	Itching lessened *or* aggrav. by scratching.
Discharge from ulcers predom. too copious.	Discharge from ulcers predom. too scanty.
Pulse quick, small, weak, intermitting; quicker in the morning, slower in the evening.	Pulse often unchanged; quicker in the evening, slower in the morning.
First heat, then sweat	First chill, then sweat.
Least thirst during the chill; most during sweat; besides this, thirst before and after the fever, and between the chill and heat.	Predom. want of thirst; partic. during the chill and sweat.
Chill increased by drinking and in bed . .	Chill lessened by drinking and in bed.
Sweat lessened by motion and walking in the open air.	Sweat increased by motion and walking in the open air.
Paralysis, particularly of the Extensores	Paralysis, particularly of the Flexores.
Want of reserve	Taciturnity.
Malice — Greediness — Delirium — Mental dullness—Imbecility—Insanity.	Distrust — Haughtiness — Absent-mindedness — Fancies.
Consequences of dread or fear	Ailments from mortification or disapp. love.
Insensibility of internal parts	Sensitiveness in internal parts.
Eruption around the eyes	Eruption in the eye-brows.
Horizontal half-sight	Perpendicular half-sight.
Thirst, unquenchable by drinking; desire for drink without thirst.	Thirst easily quenched; thirst with aversion to drink.
Urine scanty (with diarrhœa), or copious (during the cold stage of fever.)	Urine frequent, but scanty.
Sexual desire increased	Sexual desire decreased.
Catamenia too soon and too copious . .	Catamenia too late and scanty.
Cough most frequently with expectoration.	Cough most frequently dry.
Expectoration *only* during the day . . .	Expectoration is loosened from evening till morning; rarely during the day; is generally swallowed.
Complaints predom. on *upper* arm and on the sole of the foot.	Complaints predom. on *fore*-arm and on the *top of* the foot.
Vesicles containing blood on the tips of the fingers; ulcerous scabs under the nails.	Warts on the tips of the fingers.
Aggravation in the evening, *after midnight*, and in the morning.	Aggravation in the *evening*, during the night and morning.
Remiss. during the day and before midnight.	Remission during the day.
Worse from drinking cold water, generally also in cold open air, from running and bodily exertion.	*Better* from drinking cold water, in the open air, from running and bodily exertion; in some cases worse from exertion.
Worse from eating bread	More frequently improved than aggravated after eating bread.
Better from warm diet	Worse from warm diet.
Better when standing and when crouching down.	*Worse* when standing and when crouching down.
Worse (better) from the light *or* in the dark.	Worse from the light; better in the dark.
Ailments from (China) (Plumbum) Veratrum, Strychnine, Ipecacuanha, Lachesis, Carb. veg., Graphites, Phosphor, Digitalis, Iodine, or contagious Anthrax.	Ailments from (China) (Plumbum) Asa fœt. Euphrasia, or Colocynthis.

N. B. Although Arsen. has the characteristic of constitutional irritability, yet we also find oversensitiveness to pain with this remedy, which Causticum has not.

Arsenic.	Chamomilla.
Right side—Predom. want of irritability .	*Left* side—Increased bodily irritability.
Muscles rigid, (skin the same.)	Skin and muscles lax.
Gnawing, sensation of weight, etc., in external parts.	Gnawing, sensation of weight, etc., in internal parts.
Oftener indicated with old people than children.	Often indicated with children and women.
Blood coagulates slowly or not at all . .	Blood coagulates quickly.
Pulse very quick, small and weak, or intermitting.	Pulse accelerated, small, but tensive.
Partial sweat on the lower part of body .	Partial sweat on upper part of body.
Chill or sweat lessened after rising from bed.	Chill or sweat *increased* after rising from bed.
Sweat lessened by motion . . .	Sweat increased by motion.
Sweat often disappears while falling asleep, often on awaking.	Sweat often disappears on awaking.
Heat, with desire for drink without thirst; least thirst during the chill, most during sweat.	Heat (chill or sweat), with thirst.
Itching aggrav. by scratching	Itching unchanged by scratching, rarely aggravated.
Loquacity—Imbecility—Insanity	Taciturnity—Seriousness—Absent-mindedness.
Children do not want to be spoken to . .	Children do not want to be touched. C.Hg.
Consequences of grief and sorrow, or of vexation with reserved displeasure.	Consequences of anger, or of vexation with vehemence.
Complaints predom. on the *lower* eyelids and on the upper lip.	Complaints predom. on the *upper* eyelids and on the *under* lip.
Nausea in the throat	Nausea in the stomach.
Expectoration predom. with the cough, but not constant.	Expectoration rather infrequent.
AGGRAVATION in the evening and night, particularly *after midnight.*	AGGRAVATION in the evening and night, particularly *before midnight.*
Better when moving the diseased limb . .	More frequently aggrav. than ameliorated when moving the diseased limb.
Predom. worse during and after sweat . .	*Worse* during sweat; better after it.
Better from drinking coffee.	Worse *or* better after drinking coffee.
Worse *or* better after stool.	*Better* after stool.
Ailments from contagious Anthrax, Jodine, Plumbum, Phosph. Strychnine, Digitalis, Ipecacuanha.	Ailments from Coffea, Colocynth, Ignatia, Nux vom., Pulsatilla, or Valeriana.
Worse (better) from light *or* in the dark .	Worse from light, better in the dark.
Children sometimes feel easier when carried about very quickly.	Children feel easier when carried about slowly. C.Hg.

Predomin. worse — **Predomin. better**

From cold and cold diet, when lying on the painful side, sitting, particularly sitting bent forward, on expiration, change of position, and after perspiring.

Predomin. better — **Predomin. worse**

From warmth and from warmth of the bed, warm diet, washing and moistening the diseased part, after* sleep, lying on the unpainful side, sitting erect, and on inspiration.

* Compare note to Arsen. and Bellad.

Arsenic.	China.
Generally aversion to motion	Inclination for motion.
Right side predom.—Muscles (and skin) rigid.	*Left* side—Skin and muscles lax.
Want of irritability—Rarely apoplexy . .	Increased bodily irritability—Apoplexy.
Itching increased by rubbing and scratching.	Itching lessened by rubbing and scratching.
Cold swelling of the glands — Diseases of the bones.	Hot, painful swelling of the glands — Diseases of the periosteum.
Rending pain, upwards	Rending pain downwards.
Sphacelus more frequent than gangrene .	Gangrene.
Pulse very quick, small and weak; quicker in the morning, slower in the evening .	Pulse quick, small, but hard; more quiet after meals.
Partial sweat on lower part of body . . .	Sweat on upper part of body.
Distention of the veins of the feet . . .	Distention of the veins of the hands.
Heat, with desire for drink without thirst (see Arsen., Puls.).	Heat most frequently without thirst.
Thirst is wanting during the chill; but appears between chill and heat, and during the sweat.	Thirst during the chill, but not constant; appears particularly *between* the different stages of the fever, and during sweat.
Sweat lessened by motion and walking in the open air.	Sweat increased by motion and walking in the open air.
Sleeplessness preval. after *midnight* . . .	Sleeplessness *before midnight.*
Loquacity — Sensitiveness of disposition — Fear—Greediness.	Taciturnity—Predom. insensibility of disposition — Amativeness — Absent-mindedness — Fancies.
Mental dullness — Imbecility—Insanity . .	Mental excitability—Rarely delirium.
Consequences of fright, grief, or of vexation with dread, fear, reserved displeasure, or with vehemence.	Ailments from vexation.
Loss of taste	Delicate taste.
Desire for warm food	Aversion to warm food.
Aversion to sweets	Inclination for sweets.
Nausea in the throat	Nausea in the throat *or* stomach.
Urine scanty (with diarrhœa) *or* copious .	Urine infrequent and scanty.
Deep, quick inspiration, and difficult, interrupted expiration.	Difficult inspiration, and quick, blowing expiration.
Expectoration predom. with the cough, but not constant; during the day.	Expectoration not constant; during the day and evening.
With Horses: Swelling of the fore-feet; predominating ailments of the hoof or the cleft of the hoof.	With Horses: Swelling of fore-legs above the knee.
Remis. during the day and before midnight.	Remission in the afternoon and evening.
Uncovering aggravates, wrapping up ameliorates.	Uncovering ameliorates quite as often as it aggravates.
Worse from uncovering the head; *better* from wrapping it up.	*Better* from uncovering the head, *worse* from wrapping it up.
Washing and moistening improves oftener than aggravates.	Moisture aggravates.
Improved oftener than aggr. in wet weather.	Worse in wet weather.
Improved quite as often as aggravated by vomiting; likewise after passing urine.	Aggravation by vomiting, and also after passing urine.
Better from the warmth of the bed . . .	Generally worse from the warmth of the bed.
Predom. better from motion	Predom. worse from motion.
Ailm. from contag. Anthr., Digit., Phosph., Strychn., Plumb. or abuse of Cinchona.	Ailments from abuse of Sulphur or Mercury, and from helleborus niger.
Worse (better) from the light *or* in the dark.	Worse from the light; better in the dark.

Arsenic.	Ferrum.
Predom. *right* side; particularly *lower right and upper left side.*	Predom. *left* side; particularly *lower left and upper right side.*
Want of irritability	Increased bodily irritability.
Skin and muscles rigid	Skin and muscles lax.
Blood coagulates slowly, or not at all . .	Blood coagulates quickly.
Rending and piercing pain upwards . . .	Rending and piercing pain downwards.
Paralysis more frequent than apoplexy . .	Apoplexy more frequent than paralysis.
Pulse quick, small and weak	Pulse full and hard.
Heat, with aversion to uncover	Heat, with inclination to uncover.
Heat increased by motion	Heat abating when moving.
Chill without thirst	Chill with thirst.

Arsenic.	Ferrum.
Fear — Dejection — Indifference — Malice — Greediness.	Changing mood; sadness or cheerfulness; particularly cheerful one evening, sad the next — Haughtiness.
Insensibility – Delirium — Imbecility — Insanity.	Fear of apoplexy – Rarely delirium.
Ailments from fright, grief, or from vexation with dread, fear, reserved displeasure or vehemence.	Ailments from anger.
Vertigo when walking over an open space.	Vertigo when walking over water.

Arsenic.	Ferrum.
Complaints predom. on the *lower* eyelids .	Complaints predom. on the *upper* eyelids.
Catamenia too soon	Catamenia predom. too late.
Desire for sour things	Loathing sour things.
Difficult, interrupted expiration, with deep inspiration.	Difficult inspiration.
Expectoration predom., but not constant; only during the day.	Expectoration almost constant; only in the morning.
Straining the eyes aggravates	Straining the eyes improves oftener than aggravates.
Spirituous liquors aggravates	Improved by wine, except such as are termed: acid wines*.
Quite as often better as worse in bed† . .	Generally worse in bed.

Predomin. worse — **Predomin. better**

In dry weather, when lying on the back, from drinking cold water, from cold diet generally, being uncovered, from bodily exertion, after breakfast, from exerting the mind or the eyes.

Predomin. better — **Predomin worse**

In wet weather, when lying on the side, from warm diet, wrapping up, when standing, and on an empty stomach.

N.B. Are antidotes to each other, and follow each other well. C.Hg.

---

* Ferrum also cures mania-a-potu in conformable cases; but this is caused much less frequently by wine than beer or brandy. H.Gr. Even beer does not, if used without alternating it with alcoholic drinks. C.Hg.

† The *warmth of the bed* generally improves, while the *rest* in bed aggravates.

Arsenic.	Hepar. s. c.
Anæmie predom.—Tension in inward parts.	Plethora predom.—Tension in external parts.
Complaints predom. on the lower eyelids, in the inner ear, on the lower part of leg, and on the sole of the foot.	Complaints predom. on the upper eyelids, on the external ear, on the thigh, and on the instep.
Cutaneous eruptions, generally dry	Eruptions humid.
Ulcers even with the surface, with copious discharge of a carion-like odor; sometimes proud flesh.	Deep ulcers, generally with scanty discharge; also with an odor like rotten eggs.
Cold glandular swellings	Hot glandular swellings.
Pulse very quick, small and weak	Pulse accelerated, full and hard.
Pulse frequent in the morning, slow in the evening.	Pulse frequent at night, slow during the day.
Sweat less while and after getting out of bed; moderated by motion and walking in the open air.	Sweat increases while and after getting out of bed, by motion and walking in the open air.
Least thirst during the chill, most during sweat; appears also before and after the heat and after the chill.	Thirst predom., but not constant.
Fear—Indifference—Malice—Greediness—Want of reserve.	Reserve—Very rarely unconsciousness.
Imbecility more frequent than insanity	Insanity—Apoplexy.
Saliva generally decreased	Saliva predom. increased.
Urine scanty (with diarrhœa) *or* copious (during the chill.)	Urine not often and scanty.
Sexual desire increased	Sexual desire diminished.
Involuntary seminal emissions	Discharge of succus prostraticus.
Fluent coryza	Dry coryza.
Generally expectoration; during the day	Cough generally dry—Expectoration in the morning and during the day.
REMISSION *during the day* and before midnight.	REMISSION of complaints in the afternoon.
Better *or* worse after urinating	Worse after passing urine.
Predom. worse during and after sweat	Better after the sweat.
Worse or better on awaking; *better* after sufficient sleep.	Worse on awaking; worse after sleep.
Worse *or* better from light (in the dark.)	Worse from light; better in the dark.
Worse from chewing tobacco	Predom. better from smoking.
Worse while talking	Better *or* worse while talking.
Ailments from contagious Anthrax, Plumbum, Phosph., Strychnine, Cinchona, Digitalis, or Ipecacuanha.	Ailments from Mercury and other metals, Nitric acid, Silicea, or Belladonna.

Predomin. worse — **Predomin. better**

During rest, after lying down, while lying down, after perspiring, and after breakfast.

Predomin. better — **Predomin. worse**

From motion, when walking, when riding, on an empty stomach, when rising from bed, after sleeping, from drinking coffee, from eructation, from biting, from pressure, and when leaning against anything.

Arsenic.	Iod.
Upper left, lower right side	Upper right, lower left side.
Muscles and skin rigid	Skin and muscles lax.
Diseases of the bones	Diseases of the periosteum.
Itching, aggravated by scratching . . .	Itching, unchanged by scratching.
Generally dry eruptions	Eruptions predom. humid.
Scars burn	Scars itch, break open, or pimples break out on them.
Tension, sensation of heaviness, etc., in internal parts.	Tension, heaviness, etc., in external parts. C.Hg.
Pulse very quick, small and weak. . . .	Pulse accelerated; at the same time large and hard, or weak and like a thread.
Heat, with aversion of being uncovered .	Heat, with inclination for being uncovered.
Chill on lower part of body.	Sweat on lower part of body.
Least thirst during chill, most during sweat; appears also before and after the fever and between the chill and heat; during the hot stage desire for drink without thirst.	Thirst, particularly during the sweat.
Perspiration lessened by motion	Perspiration increased by motion.

Arsenic.	Iod.
Restlessness and haste	Phlegmatic temperament.
Fear—Irritability—Malice—Greediness—Imbecility—Insanity.	Changing mood; rarely delirium.
Ailments from fright, grief, or vexation with dread, fear, reserved displeasure, or with vehemence.	No unconsciousness.
Saliva decreased	Saliva predom. increased.
Generally want of appetite	Predom. hunger.
Aversion to meat	Desire for meat.
Urine scanty (with diarrhœa or hot stage of fever) *or* frequent and copious (during chill.)	Urine scanty.
Voice trembling	Voice nasal or deep.
Difficult, interrupted expiration	Undulating inspiration.
Expectoration predom., but not constant; during the day.	Expectoration rather constant; in the evening.
Spinal complaints, with gressus gallinaecus.	Spinal complaints, with gressus vaccinus.
With Horses: Emaciation, with want of appetite, rather aversion to food.	With Horses: Emaciation, although the animal takes more than sufficient food.

Arsenic.	Iod.
Remission during the day and before midnight.	Remission in the forenoon and before midnight.
Ailments from contagious Anthrax, Iodine, Plumbum, Digitalis, Phosphor, Ipecac., Strychnine, or from abuse of Cinchona.	Ailments from Arsenicum, Mercurius, Calcarea or Argentum nitricum.

Predomin. worse — **Predomin. better**

In cold weather, from cold and being uncovered, during rest*, after lying down, when sitting still, particularly when sitting bent forward, and after breakfast.

Predomin. better — **Predomin. worse**

In warm air, from warmth, warmth of the bed, and wrapping up, from motion, when assuming an erect position, on an empty stomach, and from external pressure

N.B. Follow each other well, sometimes in alternation Dr. G. Bute.

---

* Both remedies have improvement of symptoms "*when standing.*" There is no complete rest for the human body.

Arsenic.	Ipecacuanha.
Muscles rigid—Rarely apoplexy	Muscles lax—Rarely paralysis.
Anæmie	Plethora.
Itching aggravated by scratching . .	Itching unchanged by scratching.
Pus predom. copious	Pus scanty. C.Hg.
Partial chill or sweat on the lower part of body.	Partial cold or sweat on upper part of body.
Chill increased by drinking and in the open air.	Chill lessened by drinking and in the open air.
Perspiration lessened by motion	Perspiration increased by motion.
Least thirst during the chill, most during sweating stage.	Thirst not constant.
Delirium—Unconsciousness (in the fever.).	Very rarely unconsciousness or delirium.
Loquacity	Taciturnity.
A bluish circle around the cornea	A red circle around the cornea.
Aversion to sweets	Appetite for sweets.
Nausea in the throat	Nausea in the throat, rarely in the abdomen.
Urine scanty (with diarrhœa) or copious .	Urine scanty.
Fluent coryza	Dry coryza.
Cough most frequently with expectoration; during the day.	Cough predom. dry; expectoration in the morning and during the day.
Remission *during the day and before* midnight.	**Remission** during the day.
Worse (better) from light, *or* in the dark .	Worse from light, particularly candle-light; better in the dark.
Better *or* worse when stooping . .	Worse when stooping.
Ailments from contagious Anthrax, Iodine, Plumbum, Digitalis, Strychnine, Ipecac., or Phosphor.	Ailments from Arsenic or Copper vapors, from Arnica or Opium.

Predomin. worse —— **Predomin. better**

From cold, during* rest, while lying, when closing the eyes, lying on the back, on expiration, and after drinking.

Predomin. better —— **Predomin. worse**

From warmth, while moving, while walking, when bending the diseased limb, when opening the eyes, lying on the side, from the warmth of the bed, drinking coffee, when biting, and when sitting down.

N.B. Ipecacuanha and Lachesis lack the sensation of numbness in suffering parts which is frequent with Arsenic.

* Both remedies have predom. improvement "*while standing.*"

Arsenic.	Lachesis.
Want of bodily irritability—Skin and muscles rigid.	Increased irritability—Skin and muscles lax.
Anæmie predom.—Often indicated with men and old people.	Plethora—Is often indicated with women and children.
Sensation of numbness in internal parts . .	Sensitiveness of internal parts*.
Tension in internal parts	Tension predom. in external parts.
Paralysis more frequent than apoplexy . .	Apoplexy more frequent than paralysis.
Paralysis with atrophy of the muscles; generally painless.	Nervous lameness, originating in central organs; generally painful.
Eruptions most frequently dry	Eruptions humid.
Ulcers predom., with copious discharge . .	Ulcers, sometimes with scanty discharge.
Old scars burn	Old scars burn, break open, bleed. C.Hg
Chill or sweat, lessened after rising from bed.	Chill or sweat, increased after rising from bed.
Sleeplessness predom. after midnight . . .	Sleeplessness predom. before midnight.

Arsenic.	Lachesis.
Fear of being alone	Likes to be alone.
Satiety of life, with fear of death	Satiety of life, with longing for death.
Dejection—Indifference—Greediness . . .	Distrust—Haughtiness—Amativeness—Jealousy.
Difficult comprehension—Mental dullness .	Easy comprehension—Mental excitability.
Imbecility more frequent than insanity . .	Insanity more frequent than imbecility.
Consequences of grief, or vexation with dread, fear, reserved displeasure, or with vehemence.	Consequences of jealousy or disappointed love.
Desire for drink, without thirst	Thirst, with disgust for drink.
Urine scanty (with diarrhœa) *or* copious (during the chill.)	Urine too frequent.
Catamenia predom. too copious and of long duration.	Catamenia predom. too scanty and of short duration.
Respiration quick	Respiration slow.
Voice trembling—Cough most frequently *with* expectoration; expectoration only during the day.	Voice nasal—Cough generally dry; when there is expectoration, it is loosened in the morning and during the day, but is generally swallowed.
Complaints predom. on the calf of the leg .	Complaints predom. on the shin.

Arsenic.	Lachesis.
AGGRAVATION, particularly in the evening and *after midnight.*	AGGRAVATION in the afternoon and evening, till midnight.
Worse in dry (cold) weather	*Worse* in wet weather.
Worse in the Winter and Autumn . . .	*Worse* in the Summer and Spring.
Worse (better) from light *or* in the dark .	Worse from light, better in the dark.
Worse from touch, better from pressure .	Worse from touch and pressure.
Ailments from contagious Anthrax, Iodine, Plumb., Digitalis, Phosph., Strychnine, or Ipecac.	Ailments from the sting of insects, or from abuse of Mercury.

Predomin. worse (Arsenic) — **Predomin. better** (Lachesis)

In dry weather, from cold diet, and after breakfast.

Predomin. better (Arsenic) — **Predomin. worse** (Lachesis)

In wet weather, from warm diet, on an empty stomach, after† sleep, while and after rising from bed, from holding the diseased limb bent, and from pressure.

---

* Both remedies have sensitiveness oftener than insensibility in external parts.

† Compare note to Arsenic, Belladonna.

Arsenic.	Lycopodium.
Muscles rigid	Muscles lax.
Rending and piercing pain upwards	Rending, and piercing pain downwards.
Upper left, lower right side—Rarely apoplexy.	Upper right, lower left side—Apoplexy.
Complaints predom. on the lower eye-lids, and on the upper-arm.	Complaints predom. on the upper eye-lids and on the fore-arm.
Erysipelas around the joints	Perspiration around the joints.
Eruptions most frequently dry	Eruptions most frequently humid.
Pulse quick, small, weak, or intermitting	Pulse somewhat accelerated after eating, and in the evening.
Pulse quick in the morning, slow in the evening.	Pulse quick in the evening, slow in the morning.
Chill on the lower part of the body	Cold shudders on the upper part of the body.
Heat with aversion to uncover, and desire for drink without thirst.	Heat with inclination to uncover, and thirst.
More thirst before than after the fever	Thirst continues *after* the sweat.
Want of reserve—Greediness	Taciturnity—Changing mood—Gentleness—Amativeness—Haughtiness—Distrust—Absent-mindedness—Fancies.
Sleeplessness predom. after midnight	Sleeplessness predom. before midnight.
Desire for coffee and bread, particularly rye bread.	Aversion to coffee and bread, particularly rye bread.
Aversion to sweets	Appetite for sweets.
Nausea in the throat—Desire for drink without thirst.	Nausea in the stomach—Thirst with disgust for drink.
Fetid flatus. Diarrhœa predom.	Predom. scentless flatus and constipation.
Urine scanty (with diarrhœa) *or* copious	Urine frequent, but scanty.
Incontinence oftener than retention of urine.	Retent. of urine oftener than incontinence.
Catamenia predom. too soon	Catamenia predom. too late.
Fluent coryza	Coryza dry oftener than fluent.
Cough with predom. but not constant expectoration; during the day.	Expectorat. almost constant; in the morning and evening.
Remission during the day and before midnight.	Remission in the *forenoon* and after midnight.
Worse when growing cold and in cold weather, better when growing warm and in warm air.	Wor.e *or* better when growing cold, and in cold weather; likewise when growing warm and in warm air.
Better from the warmth of the bed	Worse *or* better from the warmth of the bed.
Worse or better on awaking, that is, better after sufficient sleep.	Worse on awakening and after sleeping.
Worse when alone; better in company	Worse *or* bett. when alone (or in company.)
Worse in the autumn	Worse in the spring.

Predomin worse —— **Predomin. better**

In dry weather, from cold, in cool open air, from being uncovered. lying on the back, when sitting bent forward, when ascending, when closing the eyes, and on expiration *.

Predomin. better —— **Predomin. worse**

In wet weather, from warmth, in warm rooms, from wrapping up, lying on the side, after sleep, when sitting erect, when descending, when opening the eyes, from drinking coffee, after a satisfying meal, when standing or leaning on anything, from pressure, and from washing, moistening, or bending the diseased part.

* Both remedies have aggrav. when respiring deeply.

Arsenic.	Natr. mur.
Complaints predom. in internal parts . .	Complaints predom. in external parts.
Paralysis, partic. of the extensors . . .	Paralysis, partic. of the flexores.
Rarely apoplexy	Apoplexy.
Dry skin—Eruptions most frequently dry—Scars burn.	Perspires easily—Eruptions most frequently humid—Scars become painful, redden.
Pulse generally very quick, small and weak.	Pulse very irregular; sometimes quick and weak, sometimes full and slow.
Sweat lessened after getting out of bed, and when moving.	Sweat increased after getting out of bed and when moving.
Fear—Dejection—Hopelessness—Greediness—Insanity.	Changing mood—Amativeness—Absent-mindedness.
Consequences of grief and sorrow . . .	Ailments from anger or mortification.
Fear of being alone	Likes to be alone.
Sleeplessness, partic. after midnight, therefore awaking too early.	Sleeplessness before midnight, and awaking too late.
Horizontal half-sight	Perpendicular half-sight.
Saliva decreased	Saliva increased.
Complaints pred. on the roof of the mouth.	Complaints predom. on the soft palate.
Most thirst during the sweating stage of fever*.	Thirst during all stages of the fever and during the apyrexia.
Desire for drink without thirst. . . .	Thirst with disgust for drink.
Appetite for coffee or rye bread . . .	Aversion to coffee or rye bread.
Aversion to farinaceous food	Appetite for farinaceous food.
Nausea in the throat	Nausea in the stomach.
Urine scanty (with diarrhœa), or copious (partic. during the chill).	Urine too frequent.
Catamenia predom. too soon	Catamenia predom. too late.
Fluent coryza	Dry coryza.
Cough most frequently with expectoration, which generally appears only during the day.	Cough predom. dry; when there is expectoration, it is loosened only in the morning.
REMISSION of complaints, *during* the day and before midnight.	REMISSION of complaints in the afternoon.
Aggrav. of many symptoms in the Winter and Autumn.	Aggrav. of many symptoms in the Summer and Spring.
Improvement after rising from a seat . .	After rising from a seat, quite as often aggravated as improved.
Better from loosening the clothes	Predom. better from tying the clothes tight.

Predomin. worse — **Predomin. better**

From cold, in cold open air, during rest, after lying down, while lying and sitting, lying on the back, during and after perspiration, and when stretching out the diseased limb.

Predomin. better — **Predomin. worse**

From warmth, and warmth of the bed, in a warm room, from motion, from riding, when bending the diseased part, lying on the side, from pressure, a satisfying meal, washing, moistening, after catamenia, and when drawing up the diseased limb.

N.B. Natr. mur. has not the oversensitiveness to pain often found with Arsenic.

---

* Arsen. also has thirst before and after the chill and after the sweat, but not during the chill; during heat, desire without thirst.

Arsenic.	Nux vomica.
Upper left, lower right side	Upper right, lower left side.
Want of irritability	Increased bodily irritability.
Insensibility of single parts predom . . .	Sensitiveness of single parts predom.
Paralysis, with atrophy of the muscles . .	Lameness, nervous (central); Apoplexy.
Predom. clonic spasms; sleep after sweat.	Pr. tonic spasms; sleep betw chill and heat.
Scars burn—Warts	Scars are sore to the touch—Corns. C.Hg.
Pulse soft—Chill without thirst; most thirst during sweat and between chill and heat.	Pulse hard—Most thirst during the chill; thirst between heat and sweat.
Partial sweat on the lower part of body .	Sweat on upper part of body.
Chill lessened after getting out of bed . .	Chill increased after getting out of bed.
Heat is increased when or after awaking .	Heat lessened when and after awaking.
Sweat less. by motion and walking out-doors.	Sweat incr. by motion and walking out-doors.
Greediness—Imbecility—Insanity.	Amativeness. Absent-mindedness. Fancies.
Consequences of vexation with grief and reserved displeasure.	Consequences of anger, mortification, or of vexation with indignation; likewise of disappointed love or jealousy.
Toothache makes him angry	Toothache drives to despair. C.Hg.
Dim-sightedness	Predom. clear-sightedness.
Saliva predom. diminished	Saliva most frequently increased.
Desire for drink, without thirst	Thirst, with disgust for drink.
Appetite for coffee, bread, particularly rye-bread, or for sour things and beer.	Aversion to coffee, bread, particularly rye-bread, and to sour things—Inclination for *or* aversion to beer.
Aversion to fatty things and sweets . . .	Appetite for fatty things or sweets.
Nausea in the throat	Nausea in stomach, rarely in œsophagus.
Diseases on the pylorus	Diseases of the cardia.
Diarrhœa predom.; is generally painless .	Costiveness; when diarrhœa, it is painful.
Urine scanty (with diarrhœa) *or* copious .	Urine infrequent and scanty.
Fluent coryza	Most frequently dry coryza, partic. out-doors; in the room fluent.
Difficult, interrupted expiration	Difficult inspiration.
Respiration mostly with a moist sound . .	Respiration with a dry sound.
Cough generally with expectoration . . .	Cough generally dry.
Expectoration generally only during the day.	Expect. in the morning and during the day.
Milk decreased	Milk increased.
Distention of the veins of the feet . . .	Distention of the veins of the hands.
Complaints predom. on the *upper* arm . .	Complaints predom. on the *fore*-arm.
Complaints after violent bodily exertion. .	Compl. after much mental exertion. C.Hg.
With Horses: Hip-shot from inflammation of the kidneys, standing crooked, legs drawn together.	With Horses: Hip-shot or lame in the back from inflammation of the kidneys, with legs spread far apart.
Remission of complaints *during the day* and before midnight.	Remission in the evening and before midnight.
Worse (better) from light *or* in the dark .	Worse from light, better in the dark.
Ailments from Strychnine, Digitalis, or from contagious Anthrax.	Ailments from Arsenic or copper vapors, or from Sulphur.

Predomin. worse — **Predomin. better**

During rest, after lying down, while lying and sitting.*

Predomin. better — **Predomin. worse**

When moving, particularly moving or bending the diseased part, when walking, getting out of bed,† and from drinking coffee.

* Both remedies have improvement when sitting *erect* and standing

† Both remedies have sometimes improvement, sometimes aggravation *after* getting out of bed.

Arsenic.	Opium.
Muscles rigid	Muscles lax.
Paralysis more frequent than apoplexy . .	Apoplexy more frequent than paralysis.
Bodies of the poisoned withstand decomposition.	Bodies of the poisoned decompose rapidly.
Complaints predom. on the upper lip and upper arm.	Complaints predom. on under lip and forearm.
Pulse predominantly quick, small and weak.	Pulse very different; full and slow, with snoring respiration; quick and hard, with heat and quick respiration.
Partial sweat on lower part of body . . .	Sweat on upper part of body.
Talkativeness during sweat	Dislikes to talk during the sweat. C.Hg.
Least thirst during the chill, most during sweat.	Want of thirst.
Thirst between chill and heat, and before and after the fever.	Thirst almost only between heat and sweat.
Dejection and despondency — Maliciousness.	Indifference — Gentleness — Amativeness — Mood bold, rarely peevish or irritable.
Mental dullness—Rarely unconsciousness .	Ecstasies or mental dullness—Fancies.
Weak memory	Memory active *or* weak.
Ailments from grief or vexation.	Ailments from excessive joy, from rage, shame, or vexation with fright.
Diarrhœa predom.	Constipation predom.
Urine scanty (with diarrhœa) or copious—Incontinence more frequent than retention of urine.	Urine infrequent and scanty; copious only after strong doses—Retention of urine more frequent than incontinence.
Expectoration predom., but not constant .	Expectoration infrequent.
REMISSION *during the day* and before midnight.	REMISSION during the day and evening.
Worse *or* better from light (resp. in the dark.)	Worse from light, better in the dark.
Worse in bed (rest) *or* better* (warmth.) .	Worse in bed and from the warmth of the bed.
Better *or* worse when assuming an erect position.	Worse when assuming an erect position.
Better or worse after getting out of bed .	Better after getting out of bed.
Worse *or* better on awaking; that is, better after sufficient sleep.	On awaking and after sleep most frequently aggrav.
Ailments from contagious Anthrax, Iodine, or abuse of Cinchona, from Phosphor, or Ipecac.	Ailments from charcoal vapors (or Mercury.)

Predomin. worse — **Predomin. better**

From cold and growing cold, in cold weather, in cool out-door air, from being uncovered, after the sweat, when lying on the back, when sitting bent forward, and from rubbing and scratching.

Predomin. better — **Predomin. worse**

From warmth and growing warm, in warm air, in a warm room, from wrapping up, after sleep, lying on the side, when sitting and standing, from riding, and when moving the suffering part.†

N.B. Although both remedies have the character of constitutional want of irritability, yet we often find over-sensitiveness to pain with Arsenic; predom. painlessness on the other hand with Opium. We find "sensation of numbness in internal parts" with both remedies.

* Both remedies have aggravation "after lying down."

† Both remed es have predom. improvement from motion in general.

Arsenic.	Petroleum.
Tension or constriction in internal parts .	Tension or constriction in external parts.
Ulcers predom. with too much discharge .	Ulcers with scanty discharge.
Pulse very quick, small and weak; or intermitting; quicker in the morning, slower in the evening.	Pulse made stronger, full, and accelerated by every motion.
Least thirst during the chill, most during the sweat *. Drinks often, but little at a time during the heat.	Thirst only during the heat.

Arsenic.	Petroleum.
Mood indifferent; hopeless; peevish; malicious—Greediness—Sitt'g lost in thought —Insanity.	Mental excitability—Absent-mindedness.
Most frequently loss of appetite	Most frequently hunger †.
Diarrhœa most frequently painless . . .	Diarrhœa predom. painful.
Urine scanty (with diarrhœa) *or* copious, (partic. during chill.)	Urine often, but scanty.
Sexual desire increased.	Sexual desire predom. decreased.
Catamenia predom. too soon and copious .	Catamenia predom. too late and scanty.
Fluent coryza	Dry coryza.
Cough generally with expectoration . . .	Cough predom. dry.

Arsenic.	Petroleum.
REMISSION *during the day* and before midnight.	REMISSION during the day and after midnight.
Worse *or* better from light, (or in the dark.)	Worse from light; better in the dark.
Worse or better on awaking, that is, better after sufficient sleep.	Worse on awaking.
Better or worse after getting out of bed	Better after getting out of bed.

Predomin. worse ——— **Predomin. better**

In dry weather, during rest, after lying down, while sitting, when alone,—and after breakfast.

Predomin. better ——— **Predomin. worse**

In wet weather, from motion, while walking and standing, after sleep, when getting out of bed, on an empty stomach, from biting, when bending the diseased part, when riding, and in company.

---

* Besides this, Arsenic has thirst *before* and *after* the chill, and after the sweat.

† The Petroleum hunger is a greedy appetite, insatiable at dinner, or ravenous hunger that causes nausea, awakes the patient at night from sleep; Arsenic also cures when the patient has great hunger not in accordance with other symptoms. C.Hg.

Arsenic.	Phosphor.
Upper left, lower right side.	Upper right, lower left side.
Want of bodily irritability, (torp. weakn.)	Increased irritability, (irritable weakness.)
Gnawing in internal parts, insensibility, or sensation of numbness in internal parts.	Gnawing in external parts — Sensation of numbness in external parts.
Sensitiveness of external parts	Sensitiveness of internal parts.
Itching aggrav. by scratching	Itching *lessened or* aggrav. by scratching.
Cold swelling of the glands — Scars burn .	Hot swelling of the glands—Contraction in the scars; they break open, bleed.
Paralysis with atrophy of the muscles . .	Paralysis seems nervous (central) Apoplexy.
Erysipelas around the joints	Vesicles in groups around the joints.
Distention of the veins of the feet . . .	Distention of the veins of the hands.
Emaciation, partic. of the feet and atrophy of the tips of the fingers.	Emaciation of the hands.
Pulse generally small and weak	Pulse generally full and hard.
Heat with aversion to uncover	Heat with inclination to uncover.
Chill lessened after getting out of bed . .	Chill incr. aft. get. out of bed, (& by motion.)
During the day chill, at night sweat . . .	In the morning cold, in the evening heat.
Chill on lower, sweat on back part of body.	Sweat on the lower front part of body.
Sweat disappears during sleep or on awak'g.	Sweat disappears on awaking.
Talkativeness during sweat	Dislikes to talk dur'g the sweat. stage. C.Hg.
Most thirst during sweat, least during chill.	Want of thirst.
Sleepless aft. midn't, th'fore awak'g too early.	Sleepless bef. midn't, th'fore awak'g too late.
Sensitiveness of disposition	Insensibil. of disp. oftener than sensitiveness.
Hopelessness — Malice — Greediness — Mental dullness.	Changing mood — Amativeness — Haughtiness — Mental excitability—Ecstacies.
Loquacity—Weakness of memory . . .	Taciturnity—Active memory.
Ailments from vexation with dread, fear or reserved mortification.	Consequences of rage or vexation with fright.
Ailm. from lead or abuse of China, fr. Ipec.	Ailments from abuse of common salt.
Changed expression of the face	Color of the face changes often. C.Hg.
Complaints of *inner* ear, *lower* eye-lids, pylorus, upper lip, and calf of the leg.	Complaints of *external* ear, *upper* eye-lids, *under* lip, cardia, and shin.
Appetite f. coffee, or bread, partic. rye bread.	Aversion to coffee and rye bread.
Nausea in throat—Fetid flatus	Nausea in stomach Scentless flatus.
Urine scanty (with diarrhœa) *or* copious .	Urine frequent, but scanty.
Expectoration predom., but not constant; during the day.	Expectoration not constant; in the morning and during the day.
Milk decreased	Milk most frequently increased.
Idiopathic heart-disease; skin-diseases d°.	Symptomatic heart-disease; skin-diseases d°.
Spine-disease with gressus gallinaceus . .	Spine-disease with gressus vaccinus.
Bodies of the poisoned withstand decompos.	Bodies of the poisoned decompose rapidly.
REMIS. before midnight and *during the day*.	REMISSION after midnight.
Wind-colic better when lying down, (and growing warm in bed.	Wind-colic, worse when lying down, (and growing warm in bed.)
Worse from cold drink; from cold diet in general; *better* from warm.	*Worse while* drinking, *better after* drinking — Warm diet aggrav., cold diet improves.
Worse in Winter	Worse in Summer. C.Hg

Predomin. worse — **Predomin. better**

In dry weather, in the open air, during rest, partic. when sitting, in the evening twilight, from being uncovered, drinking cold water, cold diet, after drinking in general, from the touch and from rubbing, and lifting up the diseased limb.

Predomin. better — **Predomin. worse**

In wet weather, in a warm room, from motion, from letting the diseased limb hang down, or from washing or moistening it, from wrapping up, and growing warm in bed, from warm diet, from riding, and after stool like diarrhœa.

Arsenic.	Pulsatilla.
Want of irritability	Increased irritability.
Cold swelling of the glands.	Hot, painful swelling of the glands.
Itching aggrav. by scratching.—Warts . .	Itch. aggr. *or* unchang'd by scratch'g.–Corns.
Pulse quick in the morn'g, slower in the ev'g.	Pulse slow in the morn'g, quicker in the ev'g.
Sensation of cold in internal parts . . .	Sensation of cold in external parts.
Cold or sweat on the diseased part . . .	Heat on the diseased part.
Sweat often disappears on falling asleep, often on awaking.	Sweat often disappears on awaking.
Chill increased out doors; heat by exercise.	Chill less'd out doors, heat less'd by exercise.
Least thirst during chill, most dur'g sweat; drinks often, but little during the heat; cold water does not agree with him.	Thirst only during the heat; cold water agrees well with the patient.
Blood coagulates slowly	Discharged blood coagulates rapidly.
Sleeplessness, partic. after midnight, and awaking too early.	Sleeplessness before midnight, and awaking too late.
With Horses: Verminous colic; the upper lip is drawn up.	With Horses: Colic; the mouth is wide open.
Paralysis more frequent than apoplexy . .	Apoplexy more frequent than paralysis.
Paralysis with atrophy of the muscles . .	Nervous lameness from central organs.
Dread of loneliness—Loquacity—Maliciousness—Irritable mood.	Likes to be alone—Taciturnity—Goodnaturedness—Calm sadness.
Ailments from vexation with grief, reserved displeasure, or vehemence.	Ailments from vexation with fright, from mortification or excessive joy.
Burning itching on the head, in the evening, when undressing, and growing cold.	Biting, pierc'g itch'g on head, partic. even'gs, when undress'g, & wh. grow'g warm in bed.
Complaints predom. on the upper lip .	Complaints predom. on the under lip.
Saliva predom. decreased	Saliva generally increased.
Food tastes as though salted too little . .	Food tastes too salty.
Most frequently loss of appetite	Most frequently hunger.
Appetite for milk	Aversion to milk.
Nausea in throat	Nausea in throat stomach, or abdomen.
Diarrhœa most frequently painless . . .	Diarrhœa most frequently painful.
Unine scanty (with diarrhœa) *or* copious .	Urine infrequent and scanty.
Catamenia too soon, profuse, of long durat'n.	Cat. pred. too late, scanty, & of short durat'n.
Expectoration during the day	Expectoration in the morn. & during the day.
Milk decreased	Milk most frequently increased.
Aggravation in the evening and at night, partic. after midnight and in the morning.	Aggravation from noon till midnight.
Children want to be carried about, quickly.	Child'n want to be carried but slowly. C.Hg.
Predom. better when getting out of bed .	When getting out of bed, *better or* worse.
Worse when rising from a seat	*Worse or* better when rising from a seat.
Better *after* rising from a seat	*After* rising from a seat *better or* worse.
Worse when swallowing	When swallowing better *or* worse.
Better from eructation	*Worse or* better from eructation.
Better *or* worse after passing urine . . .	Worse after passing urine.
Complaints from violent bodily exertion .	Complaints more after mental than bodily exertion. C.Hg.

Predomin. worse — **Predomin. better**

In cold dry weather, in cool open air, from cold, growing cold, and being uncovered, drinking cold water, and cold diet in general, vegetable diet, vinegar, acids in general, from walking fast, running, and exertion in general, tightening the clothes, lying on the back, lying on the painful side, and stretching out the diseased limb.

Predomin. better — **Predomin. worse**

In warm and moist air, in a warm room, from warmth, growing warm, wrapping up, and warmth of bed, from warm diet, eructation, drinking coffee, from biting, while standing, loosening the clothes, lying on the side, lying on the unpainful side, and when drawing up the diseased limb.

Arsenic.	Rhus.
Complaints (pressing, gnawing, tension, cutting, &c.) predom. in internal parts.	Complaints (pressing, gnawing, tension, cutting, &c.) predom. in external parts.
Disch'd blood coagul. either not, or slowly.	Discharged blood coagulates rapidly.
Itching increased by scratching	Itching lessened by scratching
Erysipelas around the joints	Itching around the joints.
Eruptions generally dry	Eruptions generally humid.
Flat ulcers, sometimes with proud flesh	Deep ulcers.
Cold swelling of the glands	Hot painful swelling of the glands.
Paralysis with atrophy of the muscles	Nervous lameness – Apoplexy.
Distention of the veins of the feet	Distention of the veins of the hands.
Heat increased by exercise, abating after drinking coffee.	Heat abated by exercise, increased by drinking coffee.
Pulse sometimes suppressed, with strong beat of the heart.	Pulse sometimes quicker than the beating of the heart.
Chill on lower part of body—Partial sweat on back of body.	Chill on upper part of body – Sweat on front of body.
Least thirst during chill, most during sweat.	Thirst not constant.
Sleeplessness predom. after midnight; awaking too early.	Sleeplessness pred. before midnight; awaking too late.
Mood irritable, malicious — Greediness — Dread of loneliness — Conseq. of vexation with reserved displeasure or vehemence.	Mood dejected—Fear of being poisoned—Fancies—Love of loneliness.
Saliva predom. decreased	Saliva most frequently increased.
Desire for brandy	Aversion to wine.
Aversion to sweets	Appetite for sweets.
Nausea in throat	Nausea in *œsophagus* or in stomach.
Diarrhœa, generally painless	Diarrhœa predom painful
Urine scanty (with diarrhœa) *or* copious	Urine often and copious.
Difficult, interrupted expiration	Difficult inspiration.
Exp. pred., but not constant; dur'g the day.	Expectoration infrequent; in the morning.
Milk decreased	Milk most frequently increased.
Compl'ts pred. on upper arm & sole of foot.	Complaints pred. on fore-arm & top of foot.
REMIS. during the day and before midnight.	REMISSION of complaints during day.
Worse *or* better from light (in the dark.)	Worse from light, better in the dark.
Improved by warmth of bed	*Better or* worse from warmth of bed.
On awaking worse *or* better, that is, better after sufficient sleep.	Worse on awaking – Most frequently aggr. after sleep.
Better or worse when assuming an erect position.	Almost always aggrav. when assuming an erect position.
Almost alw. improv'd when gett'g out of bed.	Worse *or* better when getting out of bed.
Worse when rising from a seat	Oftener aggrav. than improved when rising from a seat.
Better *after* rising from a seat	Worse or better after rising from a seat.
Better when bending the diseased part	Aggrav. oftener than improved when bending the diseased part.
Worse after drinking	After drinking *worse or* better.
Aggrav. oftener than improved after stool.	Improved oftener than aggrav. after stool.
Worse when looking up	Worse when looking down.

Predomin. worse ——— **Predomin. better**

In dry weather, lying on the painful side, stretching out the diseased limb, from rubbing and scratching, after sweat, on expiration after breakfast.

Predomin. better ——— **Predomin. worse**

In wet weather, lying on the unpainful side, drawing up the diseased limb, when washing and moistening it, standing, after sleep, on an empty stomach, drinking coffee, and from eructation.

N.B. Rhus has not the oversensitiveness to pain, so often found with Arsenic.

Arsenic. | Secale cornutum.

Arsenic	Secale cornutum
is often indicated with childless women . .	Is often indicated with women who have many children.
Intermitting of accelerated pulse	Intermitting of retarded pulse.
Partial sweat on back or lower part of body.	Sweat on front or upper part of body.
Retards the decomposition of the poisoned.	Hastens decomposition.
Sensation of coldness predom. in internal parts.	Sensation of coldness predom. in external parts.
Heat or sweat, with aversion to uncover .	Heat or sweat, with inclination to uncover.
Least thirst during chill, most during sweat.	Thirst during all stages of the fever.
Sensitiveness of skin	Insensibility of the skin. C.Hg.

Arsenic	Secale cornutum
Sensitiveness of disposition — Restlessness and haste—Fear—Consequences of grief and sorrow, or of vexation with vehemence.	Insensibility of disposition — Indolence — Fancies—Very rarely unconsciousness.
Most frequently loss of appetite	Predom. hunger.
Nausea in throat	Very rarely Nausea.
Urine scanty (with diarrhœa) *or* copious—Incontinence more frequent than retention of urine.	Urine infrequent and scanty—Predom. retention of urine.
Sleeplessness predom.	Somnolence predom.
Spine-disease, with gressus gallinaceus . .	Spine-disease, with gressus vaccinus.
Complaints predom. on upper arm.	Complaints predom. on fore-arm.

Arsenic	Secale cornutum
AGGRAVATION in the evening, *after midnight*, and in the morning.	AGGRAVATION, nocturnal.
REMISSION during the day and before midnight.	REMISSION from morning till evening.
Better or worse after getting out of bed	Better after getting out of bed.

Predomin. worse — **Predomin. better**

From cold, growing cold, uncovering, and in cold weather, during rest, after lying down, while lyin and sitting*, lying on the painful side, while sweating, from rubbing and scratching, and whe stretching out the diseased limb.

Predomin. better — **Predomin. worse**

From warmth† and warmth of bed, when growing warm, wrapping up, and in warm air, from exercise, walking, lying on the unpainful side, and from drawing up or bending the diseased limb.

N. B. Although both remedies have the character of constitutional want of irritability, yet we often find with Arsenic over-sensitiveness to pain, while Secale has "unpainfulness" predom. Both remedies sometimes have "sensitiveness of external parts."

---

* Both remedies have improvement "*when standing.*"

† In Secale, external warmth aggravates, particularly the pain of ulcers and in the limbs. C.Hg.

Arsenic.	Sepia.
Rending pain upwards—Complaints of internal parts predom.	Rending pain downwards—Complaints of external parts predom.
Sleeplessness predom. after midnight. . .	Sleeplessness predom. before midnight.
Pulse quick in the morning, slow in the evening.	Pulse quick at night, slow during the day.
Least thirst during chill, most during sweat.	Want of thirst, particularly during the sweat—Thirst only during chill.*
Partial sweat on lower part of body . . .	Partial sweat on upper part of body.
First chill, then heat	First heat, then chill.

Dread of loneliness	Likes to be alone.
Obstinacy—Malice—Delirium	Imbecility of the will — Absent-mindedness—Fancies.
Ailments from grief	Ailments from rage.
No Apoplexy	Apoplexy.
Swelling under the eyes	Swelling above the eyes.
Eruptions, etc., on the upper lip	Eruptions, etc., on the under lip.
Appetite for bread, particularly rye-bread; and also milk.	Aversion to bread and milk.
Diseases of the pylorus	Diseases of the cardia.
Leucorrhœa, thick	Leucorrhœa, watery.
Expectoration during the day	Expectoration is loosened at night and in the morning, and is swallowed.
Complaints predom. on upper arm and in hollow of the knee.	Complaints predom. on fore-arm and in hollow of the elbow.
Complaints from violent bodily exertion .	Better after bodily exertion, but worse after mental exertion. C.Hg.

REMISSION *during day* and before midnight.	REMISSION of complaints in afternoon.
Worse *or* better from light (or in the dark.)	Worse from light, better in the dark.
Worse in cold weather, better in warm air .	Worse *or* better in cold (or warm) air.
Worse after lying down	Worse *or* better after lying down.
Better from warmth of bed	*Better* or worse from warmth of bed.
Worse when rising from a seat.	*Better* or worse when rising from a seat.
Worse from exertion, walking fast, running.	Improved oftener than aggravated by exertion, etc.
Worse from chewing tobacco	Predom. better from smoking.
Better *or* worse after passing urine . . .	Worse after passing urine.
Worse in the Autumn	Worse in the Spring.

Predomin. worse — **Predomin. better**

When quite alone, closing the eyes, lying on the painful side, when turning in bed, drinking cold water, from cold diet in general, and after breakfast. (After bodily exertion. C. Hg.)

Predomin. better — **Predomin. worse**

In company, when opening the eyes, lying on the unpainful side, drinking coffee, from warm diet generally, after eating till satisfied, when biting, from pressure in general, leaning backwards, when washing, moistening or bending the diseased part, when standing, riding, from eructation, and on an empty stomach.

---

* Both remedies have thirst *before* and *after* the chill.

Arsenic.	**Silicea.**
Upper left, lower right side—Want of bodily irritability.	Upper right, lower left side — Increased bodily irritability.
Muscles rigid—Rending pain upwards . .	Muscles lax — Rending pain downwards.
Complaints (constriction &c.) predom. in internal parts.	Complaints (constriction, &c.) predom. in external parts.
Ulcers, discharge predom. too copious . .	Ulcers, discharge predom. too scanty. C.Hg.
Scars burn	Scars become painful, break open. C.Hg.
Pulse very quick, small, and weak; intermitting.	Pulse quick and small, but hard.
Pulse quick in the morning, slow in evening.	Pulse quick at night, slow during day.
Partial sweat on lower part of body . .	Partial sweat on upper part of body.
Distention of the veins of the feet . . .	Distention of veins of the hands.
Least thirst during chill, most during sweat.	Thirst predom.
Itching aggrav. by scratching	Itching, aggr. *or* unchanged by scratching.
Dreams of fire, thunderstorms, dead persons, misfortunes, embarrassments, &c.	Dreams of water, sickness, thieves, business of the day, also erotic dreams, &c.

Fear—Malice—Greediness—Irritability—Delirium.	Gentleness—Amativeness—Absent-mindedness—Fancies.
Ailments from fright or grief, or from vexation with vehemence.	Very rarely unconsciousness—Apoplexy.
Complaints of lower eyelids, and inner ear predom.	Complaints of upper eyelids and generally of *external* ear predom.
Secretion of saliva decreased	Saliva increased.
Nausea in throat	Nausea in stomach, less frequently in abdomen.
Diarrhœa predom.	Costiveness predom.
Urine scanty (with diarrhœa) or copious .	Urine too frequent.
Catamenia predom. too soon	Catamenia oftener too late than too soon.
Fluent coryza	Coryza dry oftener than fluent.
Expectoration, predom., but not constant.	Expectoration almost constant.

REMISSION *during day* and before midnight.	REMISSION of complaints before midnight.
Worse *or* better, from light, (or in the dark.)	Worse from light, better in the dark.
Worse *or* better on awaking, that is, better after sufficient sleep.	Worse on awaking and after sleep.
Worse during rest; better when exercising.	Worse or better when exercising, (resp. rest.)
Better or worse when assuming an erect position.	Better when assuming an erect position.
Worse after drinking	*Worse or* better after drinking.
Worse in the Autumn	Worse in the spring.
Ailments from contagious Anthrax, Iodine, Plumbum, Digitalis, Phosphor., Ipecac., Strychnine, or abuse of Cinchona.	Ailments from sting of insects, or abuse of Sulphur or Mercury.

Predomin. better —— **Predomin worse**

After eating till satisfied, from biting, pressure in general; from washing, moistening or bending the diseased limb, when standing and riding, getting out of bed and after sleep.

Arsenic.	Staphisagria.
Want of irritability—Complaints (gnawing, throbbing, sensation of cold &c.) predom. in internal parts.	Bodily irritability — Complaints (gnawing, throbbing, cold sensation, &c.) predom. in external parts.
Trembling of external parts	Internal trembling, trembling sensation.
Pain in the limbs jump'g from place to place.	Stationary pain in the limbs.
Rending piercing pain in the muscles . .	Rending piercing pain, partic. in the joints.
Itching, aggrav. by scratching	Itching, aggrav. *or* locality changed by scratching.
Erysipelas around the joints	Crusty eruption around the joints.
Paraplegia	Hemiplegia.
Chill increased out doors	Chill abating out doors.
Heat with aversion to being uncovered, and desire for drink without thirst.	Heat with inclination to uncover, and with thirst.
Thirst, partic. during sweat *	Want of thirst, partic. during the chill and sweat; more thirst during the heat.
Loquacity—Mood irritable and malicious—Avarice—Delirium—Insanity.	Taciturnity — Mood indifferent — Amativeness—Fancies.
Ailments from fright or vexation, with fear.	Ailments from the misbehavior of others, or from shame, disappointed love, mortification or indignation.
Losing the hair on front part of head .	Losing hair on back part or sides of the head.
Complaints predom. on *lower* eyelids and on upper arm.	Complaints predom. on *upper* eyelids and on *fore* arm.
Saliva predom. decreased, therefore most frequently want of appetite.	Saliva predom. increased, therefore predom. hunger.
Diarrhœa more frequent than constipation.	Costiveness predom.
Urine scanty (with diarrhœa) *or* copious .	Urine often, but scanty.
Involuntary seminal emissions	Predom. discharge of succ. prostat.
Catamenia predom. too soon & too copious.	Catamenia too late and too scanty.
Voice trembling — Expectoration not constant; during the day.	Voice nasal — Expectoration almost constant; is loosened partic. at night and generally swallowed.
Remis. *during the day* and before midnight.	**Remission** uncertain.
Worse when swallowing food	Better *or* worse when swallowing, partic. worse when swallowing drink.
Ailments from contagious Anthrax, Iodine, Plumbum, Digitalis, Phosphor., Ipecac., Strychnine, or abuse of Cinchona.	Ailments from abuse of Mercury and from Colocynth.

Predomin. worse — **Predomin. better**

In dry weather, during rest, after lying down, while sitting, particularly sitting bent forward, and after breakfast.

Predomin. better — **Predomin. worse**

In wet weather, from motion, particularly moving the suffering part, when walking and riding, getting out of bed, after sleep, on an empty stomach, from washing and moistening the diseased part, sitting erect, from pressure, and generally also after passing urine.

*** Both remedies have no thirst during the chill.**

Arsenic.	Sulphur.
Right side—Insensibil. of intern. parts pred.	*Left* side—Sensitiven. of intern. parts pred.
Rending pain upwards—Itching aggrav. by scratching.	Rending pain downwards—Itching lessened by scratching.
Erysipelas around the joints	Itching, erysip., or vesicles around the joints.
Cold swelling of the glands	Hot, but gener'y painless swelling of glands.
Chill or sweat on lower part of body . .	Heat or sweat on lower part of body.
Heat or sweat with avers. to being uncover'd.	Heat or sweat with inclination to uncover.
Most thirst during sweat	Most thirst during the hot stage.
Pulse quick, small, and weak	Pulse accelerated, but full and hard.
Chill lessened after getting out of bed . .	Chill increased after getting out of bed
Sweat lessened by motion	Sweat increased by motion.
Sleeplessness, partic. after midnight, awaking too early.	Sleeplessness before midnight; awaking too late.
Malice—Hopelessness—Greediness . . .	Gentleness—Sadness—Changing mood—Absent-mindedness—Fancies.
Ailments from grief, fright, or from vexation with reserved displeasure.	Ailments from shame, hearing bad news, mortification, or vexation with fright.
Compl'ts of lower eyelids & upper arm pred.	Compl'ts of upper eyelids & fore arm pred.
Appetite for milk & bread, part. rye bread.	Aversion to milk or bread, partic. rye bread.
Appetite for beer and spirituous liquors .	Inclination *or* avers. to beer & spirit. liquors.
Nausea in throat	Nausea in stomach, rarely in throat.
Urine scanty (with diarrhœa) *or* copious, partic. with chill.	Urine often, but scanty; sometimes copious, that is, after large doses.
Expectoration predom. but not constant; during day.	Expectoration not constant; in the morning and during day, rarely at night.
REMISSION *during day* and before midnight.	REMISSION after and before midnight.
Worse when alone, better in company . .	Most frequently better when alone, worse in company.
Worse *or* better from light, (or in the dark.)	Almost alw's worse fr. light, bett. in the dark.
Worse when looking up	Worse when looking down, partic. at running water.
Worse when lying on back, better when lying on the side.	Most frequently better when lying on the back, worse when lying on the side.
Worse or better on awaking, that is, better after sufficient sleep.	Worse on awaking, and after sleep.
Worse in cold weather, better in warm air.	In cold (resp. warm) air, better *or* worse.
Worse when growing cold, better when growing warm.	When growing cold (resp. warm) better *or* worse.
Better when standing.	Worse from standing a long time; but better when standing still after exercise.
Almost always improved when moving the diseased part.	Most frequently aggrav. by moving the diseased part.
Worse when stretching out the diseased limb.	Generally aggravated by stretching out the limb, sometimes improved.
Predom. better on an empty stomach . .	Worse *or* better on an empty stomach.
Worse in the Autumn	Worse in Spring.

Predomin. worse —— **Predomin. better**

In dry weather, in cool open air, from cold, uncovering, rubbing and scratching, lying on back, and being alone.

Predomin. better —— **Predomin. worse**

In wet weather, in warm rooms*, from warmth, wrapping up, warmth of bed, after sleep, lying on side, standing, riding, when washing, moistening or bending the diseased part, biting, drinking coffee, eating till satisfied, and in company.

N. B. We rarely find with Sulph. the oversensitiveness to pain of the Arsenic-patient.

*** Yet Sulphur, like Arsen., sometimes has improvement from warmth of stove.**

Arsenic.	Veratrum.
Want of bodily irritability—Rending pain upwards.	Bodily irritability — Rending pain downwards.
Skin and muscles rigid	Skin and muscles generally lax.
Ulcers, with copious discharge, sometimes proud flesh —(Warts.)	Ulcers, with scanty discharge—(Corns.) C.Hg.
Sleep in a half-sitting posture	Sleep, lying with head bent backwards.
Sleeplessness, particularly after midnight; therefore, awaking too early.	Sleeplessness before midnight; awaking too late, from a deep, stupefying morning-nap.
Pulse very much accelerated, small and weak.	Pulse irregular; most frequently slow, small and weak.
Sweat lessened by motion	Sweat increased by motion.
Talkative during sweating stage	Dislikes to talk during sweat. C.Hg
Internal sensation of coldness*	Sensation of cold predom. external.
Heat, with aversion to uncover	Heat, with inclination to uncover.
Heat, then sweat	Chill, then sweat.
Thirst, particularly during sweating stage of fevers.	Thirst not constant.
Thirst with the pain	Want of thirst with the pain.

Arsenic.	Veratrum.
Wrapt in thought — Want of reserve — Avarice — Mental dullness and imbecility more frequent than insanity — Rarely Apoplexy.	Being beside one's self—Taciturnity—Distrust — Gladness *or* sadness — Amativeness — Absent-mindedness — Mental excitability more frequent than mental dullness—Fancies—Insanity—Apoplexy.
Complaints predom. on *lower* eyelids . .	Complaints predom. on *upper* eyelids.
Desire for drink, without thirst	Thirst, with disgust for drink.
Nausea in throat	Nausea in stomach.
Intussusception with pains in abdomen, increased by motion; sensitive to pressure.	Intussusception with anxiety, forcing to pace the room, pressing abdomen with hands. C.Hg
Urine scanty (with diarrhœa) *or* copious, (particularly during the chill.)	Urine infrequent and scanty, only exceptionally copious.
Fluent coryza	Predom. dry coryza.
Cough, generally with expectoration . . .	Cough, generally dry.

Arsenic.	Veratrum.
REMISSION *during the day* and before midnight.	REMISSION during day and evening.
Worse (better) from light *or* in the dark .	Worse from light, better in the dark.
Ailments from Iodine, Plumb., Strychn., Digitalis, Phosph., Ipecac., or contagious Anthrax.	Ailments from Iron or Arsenic.

Predomin. worse — **Predomin. better**

In dry weather, from being uncovered, generally also after sweating, from ascending, drinking milk, and after salt food.

Predomin. better — **Predomin. worse**

In wet weather, from wrapping up, warmth of bed, after† sufficient sleep, when standing, and when descending.

---

* Chill, with synchronous or alternative heat, is found with both remedies.
† On awaking, when disturbed from sleep, Arsenic has aggravation.

Asa fœt.	Calcarea.
Left side	*Right* side.
Inclination for open air—Pain pressing outward.	Aversion to open air — Pain pressing inward.
Pain predom. piercing outward	Piercing outward *or* inward.
Itching, lessened *or* unchanged by scratching.	Itching, *lessened or* aggravated by scratching.
Ulcers, discharge too copious	Ulcers, discharge *scanty* or copious. C.Hg.
Pulse often unchanged; unequal; generally very much accelerated, but small.	Pulse quick and full, often trembling.
No chill—Want of thirst	Thirst.
Coma predom.; when sleeplessness, it is predom. after midnight.	Sleeplessness predom., particularly before midnight.

Changing mood—Neither unconsciousness, delirium, apoplexy, nor paralysis have as yet been observed.	Mood fearful; silly *or* despondent; irritable; amorous — Fancies—Imbecility—Consequences of hearing bad news and of vexation with fright, dread, or fear.
Diseases of the spleen predom.	Diseases of liver predom.
Urine of an ammoniacal smell	Urine re-acting acid.
Cough predominantly dry; expectoration during day.	Cough generally with expectoration; in the morning and during day.
Complaints predom. on upper arm and on front side of thigh.	Complaints predom. on fore-arm and on back part of thigh.

Aggravation afternoon and evening, more rarely after midnight.	Remission of complaints before midnight.
Most frequently aggrav. after lying down .	Most frequently improved after lying down.
Better after getting out of bed	Worse *or* better* after getting out of bed.
Worse from bodily exertion	Less frequently improved than aggrav. by exertion; partic. worse from exertion on an empty stomach.
Ailments from Pulsatilla or abuse of Mercury.	Ailments from Phosphor, Digitalis, Cinchona, Mercury, or Nitri acidum.

Predomin. worse — **Predomin. better**

During rest, when standing, sitting and lying, in-doors, and on expiration.

Predomin. better — **Predomin. worse**

From exercise, walking, out of doors, on inspiration, and after stool.

---

* Here, motion decides in the first case, and the cessation of warmth of bed in the second.

Asa fœt.	Mercur.
Inciinatior for open air—Rending pain upwards.	Aversion to open air—Rending pain downwards.
Sore pain in internal parts	Sore pain in external parts.
Discharge from ulcers too copious . . .	Suppuration too copious, or too scanty. C.Hg.
Coma predom.; when there is sleeplessness, it is predom. after midnight.	Sleeplessness predom., partic. before midnight.
Pulse often unchanged; small	Pulse changed in quality and strength, generally accelerated and full.
Want of thirst	Thirst predom.
Complaints predom. on under-lip, spleen, upper-arm, on front side of thigh, and on patella.	Complaints predom. on upper-lip, liver, fore-arm, back part of thigh, on tip of elbow, and in hollow of knee.

Changing mood — No unconsciousness — No apoplexy.	Mood fearful, dejected, irritable, malicious, amorous — Absent-mindedness — Fancies – Imbecility — Consequences of mortification.
Appetite for wine	Aversion to wine, but appetite for beer.
Urine smelling like ammoniac	Urine smelling sour.
Catamenia too soon	Catamenia too late.
Milk increased	Milk diminished *or* spoiled.

AGGRAVATION afternoon, evening, and after midnight.	AGGRAVATION from evening till morning.
Itching, lessened by scratching	Itching lessened *or* aggrav. by scratching.
Worse when swallowing	Better *or* worse when swallowing, partic. worse when swallowing saliva and drink.
Better *or* worse on inspiration.	Worse on inspiration.
Better when assuming an erect position .	When assuming an erect position worse *or* better.
Ailments from Pulsatilla or Mercury . .	Ailments from sting of insects, Arsenic-vapors, Cinchona or Sulphur, and from copper vapors.

Predomin. worse — **Predomin. better**

In the room, during rest, when lying, standing, and sitting, partic. sitting bent forwards, and on expiration.

Predomin. better — **Predomin worse**

Out of doors, and when walking out doors, from exercise in general; sitting erect, from the touch, rubbing and scratching; on an empty stomach, after stool, and on inspiration.

Asa fœt.	Phosphor.
Left side—Obesity	*Right* side—Emaciation more frequent than obesity; the latter only of single internal parts.
Coma predom.; when there is sleeplessness, it occurs particularly after midnight.	Sleeplessness before midnight, *or* Coma.
Itching, lessened by scratching	Itching oftener lessened than aggravated by scratching.
Ulcers discharge too copiously	Discharge of ulcers too copious, rarely scanty, or they bleed too much. C.Hg.
Complaints predom. in the spleen on front side of thigh, on patella, and top of foot.	Complaints predom. in the liver, on back part of thigh, in hollow of knee, and sole of foot.
Pulse often unchanged; generally quick and small.	Pulse changed in quality and strenght, generally accelerated, full, and hard.

Asa fœt.	Phosphor.
Mood changeable	Mood changing, cheerful *or* sad and fearful; indifferent or irritable; amorous; haughty, &c. — Ailments from fright, anger, vexation, (or grief.)
Unconsciousness, delirium, apoplexy, and paralysis have not yet been observed.	Mental excitability—Ecstacies—Fancies—Insanity.
Painful diarrhœa	Diarrhœa predom. painless.
Expectoration infrequent; during day . .	Expectoration not constant; in morning and during day.

Asa fœt.	Phosphor.
AGGRAVATION ofternoon, evening, and after midnight.	REMISSION of complaints after midnight.
Worse in bed*	In bed (rest) better or (warmth) worse.
Better after getting out of bed	Worse *or* better after getting out of bed.
Better when walking out doors†	When walking out doors (air) better *or* (exercise) worse.
Ailments from Pulsatilla or Mercury . .	Ailments from Iodine or abuse of salt.

Predomin. worse ——— **Predomin. better**

During rest, when standing, sitting, and lying, after sleep ‡, after eating till satisfied, after drinking, partic. beer, and on an empty stomach.

Predomin. better ——— **Predomin. worse**

During motion, **§ when walking, assuming an erect position, after stool, and after breakfast.**

N. B. Asa f. has not the oversensitiveness to pain of the Phosphor-patient.

---

* Asa f. sometimes has improvement, sometimes aggrav. "after lying down."

† Both remedies have predom. improvement "out of doors."

‡ To this Phosphor has, as an exception, aggrav. after the siesta; the improvement of the Phosphor-symptoms follows after *sufficient* sleep, and *not* after being roused from sleep.

§ An "improvement by motion," which sometimes occurs with Phosphor, seems to refer exclusively to pain in the joints, is therefore an improvement by moving the suffering part.

Asa fœt.	Pulsatilla.
Left side predom.—Itching, lessened by scratching.	*Right* side—Itching, aggravated or unchanged by scratching.
Burning or pressing piercing pain in the muscles.	Rending, piercing pain in muscles and joints.
Sensitive ulcers, with copious greenish, fetid, viscid, or thin, ichorous pus—Ulcers grow black.	Sensitive ulcers, with much yellow or milky pus, which sometimes causes soreness.
Diseases of the bones even to necrosis . .	Diseases of the bones even to caries.
Pulse often unchanged	Pulse changed, intermitting, etc.; quick in evening, slow in morning.
No chill	
Want of thirst, particularly heat without thirst.	Thirst *only* during heat, and even then not constant*.
Sleeplessness after midnight	Sleeplessness before midnight.
Changing mood	Calm sadness of gentle dispositions—Fear—Fretfulness—Distrust—Greediness—Amativeness—Absent-mindedness—Fancies—Unconsciousness—Delirium.
Apoplexy not observed as yet	
Diseases of spleen predom.	Disease of liver predom.
Catamenia too soon	Catamenia too late.
Expectoration infrequent; during day . .	Expectoration predom., but not constant; in the morning and during the day.
Complaints of patella and top of foot predom.	Complaints of hollow of knee and sole of the foot predom.

AGGRAVATION afternoon, evening and after midnight.	AGGRAVATION afternoon and evening, after sunset, until midnight.
Better when assuming an erect position. .	Worse *or* better when assuming an erect position.
Better after getting out of bed, or rising from a seat.	Generally better, sometimes worse, after rising from bed or a seat.
Worse when swallowing	*Worse or* better when swallowing.
Better after stool	*Better or* worse after stool.
Ailments from pulsatilla	Ailm. from Chamomilla, Cinchona, Sulph., Sulphuric acid, from Copper vapors, or Cantharides.
Worse after sleep	*Worse or* better after sleep.

Predomin. worse ——— **Predomin. better**

From bodily exertion.

Predomin. better ——— **Predomin. worse**

From the touch†, and from rubbing and scratching.

N.B. Asa fœt. has neither the pain jumping from place to place, nor the over-sensitiveness to pain of Pulsatilla.

---

* Besides this, Pulsatilla has thirst *before* and *after* the chill, and between the hot and sweating stage.

† Except the edges of carious ulcers, they are exceedingly sensitive to the slightest touch. C.Hg.

Asa fœt.	Silicea.
Left side—Inclination for open air . . .	*Right* side—Aversion to open air.
Constriction in internal parts	Constriction in external parts.
Rending pain upwards	Rending pain downwards.
Itching, lessened by scratching	Itching, aggrav. *or* unchanged by scratching.
Discharge of ulcers too copious	Suppuration scanty or copious. C.Hg.
Pulse often unchanged; generally quick and small.	Pulse quick and small, but hard; sometimes imperceptible.
Want of thirst	Thirst predom.
Coma predom.	Sleeplessness.

Asa fœt.	Silicea.
Mood changeable	Mood dejected; indifferent; gentle; amorous
Apoplexy or paralysis not yet observed .	Absent-mindedness—Fancies.
Complaints predominant on the under lip .	Complaints predom. on upper lip.
Saliva predominantly decreased	Saliva increased.
Generally diarrhœa	Generally constipation.
Catamenia too soon	Catamenia oftener too late than too soon.
Fluent coryza	Coryza dry oftener than fluent.
Cough predominantly dry	Cough predom. with expectoration.
Complaints predominant on shoulder-joint, upper arm, front side of thigh, and on shin.	Complaints predominant on hip-joint, fore-arm, back part of thigh, and on calf of leg.

Asa fœt.	Silicea.
Aggravation afternoon, evening, and after midnight—(Remiss. morning, forenoon, and before midnight.)	Remission of complaints before midnight.
Worse in bed	In bed (warmth) better *or* (rest) worse.
Better after getting out of bed	Worse *or* better after getting out of bed.
Worse after drinking	Worse *or* better after drinking.
Worse from exertion, walking fast, and running.	Worse *or* better from bodily exertion, etc.
Ailments from Pulsatilla	Ailments from Sulphur.

Predomin. worse — **Predomin. better**

In the room, and on an empty stomach.

Predomin. better — **Predomin. worse**

Out of doors, when walking out-doors, from touch*, rubbing and scratching, and after breakfast.

N.B. Asa fœt. has not the over-sensitiveness to pain which characterizes Silicea.

---

* Compare † to Asa and Pulsatilla.

Aurum.	Arsenic.
Increased bodily irritability	Want of bodily irritability.
Complaints predom. in external parts	Complaints predom. in internal parts.
Plethora	Anæmia.
Apoplexy more frequent than paralysis	Paralysis more frequent than apoplexy
Gnawing sensation in external parts	Gnawing sensation in internal parts.
Swollen glands painful	Swollen glands cold.
Itching unchanged by scratching	Itching aggrav. by scratching.
Deep ulcers	Flat ulcers.
Dropsy, with clear, gold-colored urine	Dropsy with turbid urine.

Aurum.	Arsenic.
Satiety of life, with longing for death, partic. in the evening — Taciturnity — Sanguine temperament.	Satiety of life, with fear of death, partic. at night — Want of reserve — Choleric temperament.
Mood changeable — Distrust — Consequences of disappointed love, contradiction or anger.	Mood indifferent; predom. malicious.
Active memory predom.	Weak memory—Unconsciousness.
Insanity more frequent than imbecility	Imbecility more frequent than insanity.
Hunger predom.	Generally loss of appetite.
Urine infrequent and scanty	Urine scanty (with diarrhœa) *or* copious.
Catamenia too late	Catamenia too soon.
Voice often nasal	Voice often trembling.
Cough predom. dry—Expectoration morning and evening.	Cough generally with expectoration, during day.
Complaints predom. on thigh, on outer side of tigh, and top of foot.	Complaints predom. on leg, on inner side of thigh and on sole of foot.

Aurum.	Arsenic.
Remission *during day* and evening till midnight.	Remission *during day* and before midnight.
Predom. worse in bed*	In bed (rest) worse *or* (warmth) better.
Improved oftener than aggrav. when closing the eyes.	When closing the eyes oftener aggrav. than improved.
When opening the eyes aggrav. oftener than improved.	When opening the eyes improved oftener than aggravated.
Worse on awaking	Worse *or* better on awaking, that is, better after sufficient sleep.
Better when assuming an erect position	*Better or* worse when assuming an erect position.
Better after getting out of bed	*Better or* worse after getting out of bed.
Better or worse when rising from a seat	Worse when rising from a seat.
Better *or* worse when talking	Worse when talking.
Ailments from abuse of Mercury	Ailments from abuse of Cinchona, Iodine, Plumb., Digital., Strychnine, Phosphor., Ipecac., or contagious Anthrax.

Predomin. worse — **Predomin. better**

In wet weather, from drinking coffee, standing, and riding, bending the diseased limb, in the room, and after sleep.

Predomin. better — **Predomin. worse**

In dry weather†, while eating, and out of doors.

---

* *Warmth* of bed improves, with both remedies.
† Cold weather aggrav., warm air improves with both remedies.

Aurum.	Belladonna.
Complaints of external parts predom. . .	Complaints of internal parts predom.
Inclination for open air—Often indicated with old people.	Aversion to open air—Often indicated with children and young women.
Pulse accelerated, but small	Pulse generally quick, full, hard, and tense.
Want of thirst predom., partic. during the chill.	Least thirst during the chill.
Very rarely paralysis — Sleeplessness after midnight.	Paralysis—Sleeplessness before midnight.

Aurum.	Belladonna.
Sensitiveness of disposition	Insensibility of disposition predom.
Does nothing but ask questions	Cannot express thoughts without first saying something foolish.
Unconsciousness not yet observed . . .	Indifference—Mental excitability *or* mental dullness.
Ailments from disappointed love, contradiction, or vexation with reserved displeasure.	Ailments from vexation with fright.
Pupils most frequently contracted . . .	Pupils most frequently dilated.
Discharge of fetid pus from ears	Predom. discharge of blood from ears.
Fetid flatus	Scentless flatus.
Catamenia too late	Catamenia too soon.
Fluent coryza predom.	Dry coryza predom.
Expectoration rather infrequent; morning and evening.	Expectoration infrequent; morning, during day, and evening.
Milk decreased	Milk most frequently increased.
Complaints predom. on top of foot . . .	Complaints predom. on sole of foot.

Aurum.	Belladonna.
Remission *during day* and evening till midnight.	**Remission** after midnight and *forenoon.*
Better when assuming an erect position .	*Worse or* better when assuming an erect position.
When getting up from a seat, better *or* worse.	Worse when getting up from a seat.
Worse when bending the diseased part, partic. bending it inwards.	When bending the part, (partic. inwards or backwards,) *better or* (sideways) worse.
Oftener improved than aggrav. when eating.	Oftener aggrav. than improved when eating.
Worse from drinking wine	Better *or* worse from drinking wine.

Predomin. **worse** — Predomin. **better**

When opening the eyes, in wet weather, in the room, during rest, after lying down in bed *, lying, sitting, and standing, when sitting down, stooping, bending the diseased part inwards, and stretching out the diseased limb.

Predomin. **better** — Predomin. **worse**

When closing the eyes, in dry † weather, out of doors, and walking out doors, from motion, particularly moving the diseased part, when assuming an erect position, getting out of bed, drawing up the diseased limb, and when walking.

---

* The Aurum-symptoms are improved quite as often as aggrav. by *warmth* of bed.

† Both remedies have aggrav. in *cold* weather.

Aurum.	Calcarea.
Increased bodily irritability.	Want of bodily irritability.
Complaints predom. in external parts . .	Complaints predom. in internal parts.
Inclination for open air—Often indicated with old people.	Aversion to open air—Often indicated with children and young women, rarely old people.
Itching, unchanged by scratching	Itching, oftener improved than aggravated by scratching.
Sleeplessness after midnight	Sleeplessness predom. before midnight.
Pulse accelerated, but small	Pulse quick, full, often trembling.
Chill, without thirst, (want of thirst predom.)	Chill, with thirst, (thirst predom.)
Sweat or heat, with aversion to uncover .	Sweat or heat, with inclination to uncover.
Satiety of life, with longing for death—Mood changing—Distrust.	Satiety of life, with fear of death—Amativeness.
Ailments from disappointed love, or from fright, anger, contradiction, mortification, or vexation with vehemence or reserved displeasure.	Ailments from hearing bad news, or from vexation with fright.
Active memory predom.	Weakness of memory.
Insanity more frequent than imbecility . .	Imbecility more frequent than insanity.
Pupils contracted	Pupils dilated.
Optical illusions generally in bright colors .	Optical illusions in black or dark colors.
Appetite for coffee	Predom. aversion to coffee.
Urine infrequent and scanty; retention of urine.	Urine too often; involuntary discharge of urine.
Complaints from pollutions	Complaints predom. after coition.
Catamenia too late	Catamenia generally too soon.
Expectoration rather infrequent; morning and evening.	Expectoration predom., but not constant; morning and during day.
Spine disease, with gressus gallinaceus . .	Spine disease, with gressus vaccinus.
Complaints predom. on thigh, particularly on outer and front side of thigh.	Complaints predom. on leg and on inner and back part of thigh.
REMIS. *during day* and even'g, till midnight.	REMISSION before midnight.
Improved quite as often as aggravated by warmth of bed.	Worse from warmth of bed.
Better after getting out of bed.	Worse *or* better after getting out of bed.
Worse when hungry	Worse after a satisfying meal.
Worse from exertion, walking fast, running, etc.	Exertion aggravates oftener than improves; particularly worse from exertion on an empty stomach.

Predomin. worse —— **Predomin. better**

From uncovering, in the room, during rest, after lying down, from sitting down, when lying, sitting, and standing.

Predomin. better —— **Predomin. worse**

From wrapping up, out of doors, and walking out-doors, from motion, walking, getting out of bed, pressure, when eating, and after stool.

N.B. We rarely find the over-sensitiveness to pain of Aurum with Calcarea; rarely with Aurum the sensation of numbness in suffering parts which is often found with Calcarea.

Aurum.	Lycopodium.
Rending pain upwards—Pain pressing inwards.	Rending pain downwards—Pain pressing outwards.
Rarely paralysis	Paralysis predominant.
Sleeplessness after midnight	Sleeplessness before midnight.
Pulse quick, but small	Pulse accelerated only after eating and in the evening; slower in the morning.
Heat or sweat, with aversion to uncover .	Heat or sweat, with inclination to uncover.
Want of thirst predominant, particularly during chill.	Thirst predominant, even after sweat, but none during chill.

Aurum.	Lycopodium.
Satiety of life, particularly in the evening, with longing for death—Ailments from disappointed love, or from contradiction.	Satiety of life, particularly in the morning, in bed—Malice—Haughtiness—Greediness—Amativeness—Absent-mindedness—Unconsciousness.
Active memory predominant	Weakness of memory.
Eyes protruding—Pupils contracted . . .	Eyes sunken—Pupils dilated.
Optical illusions in bright colors . . .	Optical illusions in dark colors.
Horizontal half-sight	Perpendicular half-sight.
Appetite for coffee	Aversion to coffee.
Fetid flatus	Scentless flatus predominant.
Urine infrequent and scanty	Urine often, but scanty.
Cough predominantly dry	Cough generally with expectoration.
Complaints predominant on thigh, particularly on outer and front side of it.	Complaints predominant on leg and on inner and back part of thigh.

Aurum.	Lycopodium.
REMISSION *during day* and evening, till midnight.	REMISSION after midnight and during *forenoon.*
Worse when growing cold, and in cold weather; better when growing warm, and in warm air.	Better *or* worse when growing cold and in cold weather, (or growing warm and in warm air.)
Worse when hungry	Worse after a satisfactory meal.
Better when assuming an erect position . .	Worse *or* better when assuming an erect position.
Better when getting out of bed	Worse *or* better when getting out of bed.
Worse when sitting down	Better *or* worse when sitting down.

Predomin. worse — **Predomin. better**

From cold, being uncovered, ascending, and when stooping.

Predomin. better — **Predomin. worse**

From warmth, wrapping up, descending, when eating, and from external pressure.

N.B. The sensation of numbness in the suffering parts, characteristic of Lycopodium, is rarely found with Aurum.

Aurum.	Mercur.
Inclination for open air — Often indicated with old people.	Aversion to open air—Often indicated with children and women.
Rending pain upwards—Pain pressing inwards.	Rending pain downwards — Pain pressing outwards.
Itching unchanged by scratching	Itching lessened *or* aggrav. by scratching.
Sleeplessness after midnight	Sleeplessness preval. before midnight.
Pulse accelerated and small	Pulse generally accelerated and full.
Chill lessened after getting out of bed . .	Chill increased after getting out of bed.
Chill without thirst—Want of thirst predom.	Chill with thirst — Thirst predom., but not constant.

Aurum.	Mercur.
Mood changing — Cheerfulness or despondency — Distrust — Ailments from grief, disappointed love, contradiction, anger, or from vexation with reserved displeasure, fear or vehemence.	Dejection—Malice—Amativeness—Absentmindedness—Very rarely delirium.
Active memory predom.	Weakness of memory.
Insanity more frequent than imbecility . .	Imbecility more frequent than insanity.
Pupils contracted — Optical illusions predom. in bright colors.	Pupils dilated — Optical illusions in dark colors.
Hunger predom.	Generally loss of appetite.
Appetite for wine	Aversion to wine; but appetite for beer.
Urine infrequent and scanty—Retention of urine.	Urine often and copious—Incontinence.
Nasal secretion thick	Nasal secretion generally watery.
Expectoration morning and evening . . .	Expectoration during day.
Complaints predom. on the outer and lower side of thigh.	Complaints predom. on the inner and back part of thigh.

Aurum.	Mercur.
REMISSION *during day* and evening till midnight.	REMISSION of complaints during day.
Worse when growing cold; better when growing warm.	Better *or* worse when growing cold, (resp. warm.)
Better or worse from warmth of bed . .	Worse from warmth of bed.
Ailments from abuse of Mercury	Ailments from Arsenic or copper vapors, from Calcarea or Sulphur; abuse of Cinchona or sting of insects.

Predomin. worse ——— **Predomin. better**

In doors, during rest, when standing, sitting, and lying.

Predomin. better ——— **Predomin. worse**

Out of doors, walking out doors, from motion generally, partic. moving diseased limb, from external pressure, and after stool.

N.B. We rarely find the oversensitiveness to pain of the Aurum-patient with Mercurius, although both remedies bear the character of increased constitutional irritability.

Aurum.	Nitr. acid.
Increased irritability	Want of bodily irritability.
Sore pain in external parts	Sore pain in internal parts.
Rending pain in internal parts	Rending pain in external parts.
Inclination for open air — Painful swelling of the glands.	Aversion to open air—Painless swelling of the glands.
Itching unchanged by scratching	Itching rather improved by scratching.
Pulse accelerated, but small	Pulse very unequal and irregular, double, intermitting.
Want of thirst predom., particularly during the chill.	Thirst is wanting during chill, and is not constant during heat.

Aurum.	Nitr. acid.
Satiety of life with longing for death . .	Satiety of life with fear of death.
Mood changing, cheerful *or* despondent; irritable; no unconsciousness.	Malice—Unconsciousness.
Ailments from grief or disappointed love, fright, anger, contradiction, mortification, or vexation with dread, fear, reserved displeasure, or vehemence.	Ailments from mental excitement in general.
Apoplexy	Apoplexy not yet observed.
Optical illusions predom. in bright colors .	Optical illusions in dark colors.
Hunger predom.	Want of appetite predom.
Retention of urine	Involuntary discharge of urine.
Sexual desire increased	Sexual desire predom. decreased.
Erections with desire	Erections without desire—Impotency.
Catamenia too late	Catamenia predom. too soon.
Expectoration infrequent; morning and evening.	Expectoration not constant; morning and during day.
Complaints predom. on outer side of thigh.	Complaints predom. on inner side of thigh.

Aurum.	Nitr. acid.
Remission *during day* and evening till midnight.	Remission of complaints during forenoon.
Worse in cold weather, better in warm air.	Oftener improv. than aggr. in cold weather. Oftener aggrav. than improved in warm air
Worse after drinking	*Worse or* better after drinking.
When rising from a seat better *or* worse .	Worse when rising from a seat.
Ailments from abuse of Mercury	Ailments from Mercur., Calc., or Digitalis.

Predomin. worse — **Predomin. better**

In doors, during rest, in * bed, when sitting down, being uncovered, when stooping, and riding.

Predomin. better — **Predomin. worse**

Out doors and when walking out doors, when walking, and from exercise generally, from wrapping up, when assuming an erect position, when and after getting out of bed, when eating, after stool, and from pressure.

N.B. The oversensiveness to pain of Aurum is rarely found with Nitr. acid.—This is quite in accordance with the constitutional character of both remedies.

---

* Aurum and Nitric acid both have predom. improvement from *warmth* of bed.

Aurum.	Phosphor.
Complaints (sensitiveness, etc.) predom. in external parts.	Complaints (sensitiveness, etc.) predom. in internal parts.
Pain pressing inwards — Apoplexia sanguinea.	Pain pressing outwards — Apoplexia nervosa.
Rarely paralysis	Paralysis more frequent than apoplexy.
Sleeplessness after midnight; awaking too early.	Sleeplessness before midnight; awaking too late.
Distention of veins of feet	Distention of veins of hands.
Pulse accelerated, but small	Pulse varying; most frequently quick, full, and hard.
Chill, lessened after getting out of bed . .	Chill, increased after getting out of bed.
Heat or sweat, with aversion to being uncovered.	Heat or sweat, with inclination to uncover.
Hopelessness—Distrust	Indifference—Haughtiness—Amativeness.
Hypochondriasis, with longing for death .	Hypochondriasis, with sensual frenzy, destructive rage, bloodthirstiness, hypocrisy; also with the idea of hanging or standing high.
Ailments from disappointed love, mortification, contradiction, or vexation with reserved displeasure.	Ecstasies — Unconsciousness — Ailments from vexation with fright.
Eyes protruding—Optical illusions generally in bright colors.	Eyes sunken—Optical illusions in black or rainbow colors.
Appetite for coffee	Aversion to coffee.
Fetid flatus	Generally scentless flatus.
Urine infrequent and scanty—Retention of urine.	Urine frequent, but scanty—Incontinence.
Catamenia too late	Catamenia generally too soon.
Milk decreased	Milk generally increased.
Voice often nasal	Voice often trembling or hissing.
Expectoration infrequent; morning and evening.	Expectoration not constant; in the morning and during day.
Spine disease, with gressus gallinaceus . .	Spine disease, with gressus vaccinus.
Complaints predom. on thigh, particularly on front side of it and on top of foot.	Complaints predom. on leg and on back part of thigh and on sole of foot.
AGGRAV. nocturnal; partic. *after midnight* and in the morning.	REMISSION of complaints after midnight.
Generally improved by warmth of bed . .	Generally aggravated by warmth of bed.
Worse on awaking	Worse *or* better on awaking; partic. worse after the siesta; better after sufficient sleep.
Better after getting out of bed	Better *or* worse after getting out of bed.
Oftener improved than aggravated when rising from a seat.	Almost always aggravated when rising from a seat.
Better from eructation	Worse *or* better from eructation.
Worse from mental exertion	Worse *or* better from mental exertion.
Ailments from abuse of Mercury	Ailments from abuse of table-salt or Iodine.

Predomin. worse — **Predomin. better**

From being uncovered, during rest, when sitting down, when sitting, standing, and lying, from the touch, drinking wine, after drinking in general, and after sleep.

Predomin. better — **Predomin. worse**

From wrapping up, from exercise and when walking, assuming an erect position, when getting out of bed, from pressure, and after stool.

Aurum.	Platina.
Apoplexy—Paralysis	Neither apoplexy nor paralysis has yet been observed.
Plethora—Heat, with aversion to being uncovered.	Anæmie — Heat, with inclination to uncover.
Want of thirst predom., particularly during chill.	Thirst predom., particularly during heat.
Satiety of life, with (taciturnity and) longing for death.	Satiety of life, with (taciturnity and) fear of death—Amativeness—Changing mood.
Ailments from disappointed love, or vexation with vehemence.	Ailments from shame or indignation.
Mental dullness	Mental excitability—Unconsciousness.
Active memory predominant	Weakness of memory.
Hunger predominant	Generally loss of appetite.
Catamenia too late and scanty	Catamenia too soon and profuse.
Expectoration rather infrequent	No expectoration with the cough.
Complaints predom. on front side of thigh.	Complaints predom. on back part of thigh.
AGGRAVATION night, particularly after midnight and in the morning*	AGGRAVATION after midnight and in the evening.
Worse in bed; yet oftener improved than aggravated by *warmth* of bed.	Worse in bed and from warmth of bed.
Ailments from abuse of Mercury	Ailments from abuse of Plumbum.

Predomin. worse — **Predomin. better**

From cold, growing cold, and being uncovered.

Predomin. better — **Predomin. worse**

From warmth, growing warm, from wrapping up, when assuming an erect position, when moving the diseased part, from external pressure, and after stool.

N.B. Although both remedies have the character of increased constitutional irritability, yet Platina has not the over-sensitiveness to pain of Aurum. On the other hand, Aurum very rarely has the sensation of numbness in suffering parts which is frequent with Platina.

---

* Aurum is very decidedly predom. in the morning. Platina in the evening. Aurum has decidedly more headache in the morning, which lasts until 3 o'clock P. M., or till evening; also the swelling of cheeks, lips, and particularly of the nose, only in the morning; on the other hand swelling of throat in the evening, 6 till 11 o'clock. Platina, on the contrary, has decidedly more headache in the evening, from afternoon 4 until evening 10 o'clock; burning heat of the face and redness, with quivering before the eyes, from 5 till 9 o'clock; particularly also increase of mental symptoms in the evening, before going to bed. Only gastric symptoms in the morning, and in consequence displeasure, ill humor, etc. C.Hg.

Aurum.	Pulsatilla.
Apoplexia sanguinea—Often indicated with old people.	Apoplexia nervosa — Often indicated with children and women.
Complaints of external parts predom. . .	Complaints of internal parts predom.
Pain pressing inwards	Pain pressing outward . . . .
Itching, unchanged by scratching	Itching, aggr. *or* unchanged by scratching.
Sleeplessness after midnight; awaking too early.	Sleeplessness before midnight; awaking too late.
Satiety of life with longing for death — Mood cheerful *or* sad; irritable.	Satiety of life with fear of death — Indifference—Calm sadness of gentle dispositions—Amativeness—Greediness.
Ailments from disappointed love, contradiction, anger, or vexation with vehemence.	Ailments from excessive joy or from vexation with fright — Absent-mindedness — Unconsciousness.
Eyes protruding	Eyes sunken.
Complaints on the outside of the gums . .	Complaints on the inside of gums.
Appetite for milk	Aversion to milk.
Retention of urine	Incontinence more frequent than retention of urine.
Cough preval. dry	Cough generally with expectoration.
Expectoration morning and evening . . .	Expectoration morning and during day.
Milk decreased	Milk most frequently increased.
Complaints predom. on palm of hand, thigh, and top of foot.	Complaints predom. on back of hand, leg, and sole of foot.
Remission *during day* and evening till midnight.	Aggravation afternoon and evening till midnight.
Generally improved by the warmth of bed .	Almost always aggrav. by warmth of bed.
Worse on awaking	*Worse or* better on awaking.
Better when assuming an erect position .	Worse *or* better when assuming an erect position.
Almost always improved when getting out of bed.	When getting out of bed, *generally* better, sometimes worse.
Better *after* getting out of bed	*Better* or worse *after* getting out of bed.
Predom. worse when sitting down . . .	Better *or* worse when sitting down.
Better after rising from a seat	*Better* or worse after rising from a seat.
Better from moving the diseased part . .	*Better or* worse from moving the part.
Worse when bending the diseased pa·t . .	Better *or* worse when bending the part.
Better from pressure	Worse *or* better from pressure.

Predomin. worse — **Predomin. better**

On opening the eyes, from cold, growing cold, and in cold weather, being uncovered, stretching out the diseased limb, when walking fast, running, and from bodily exertion in general.

Predomin. better — **Predomin worse**

On closing the eyes, from warmth, growing warm, and in warm air, wrapping up, when eating, from eructation, and when drawing up the diseased limb.

N.B. With Aurum we rarely find the sensation of numbness in the suffering parts, so frequent with Pulsatilla.

Aurum.	Rhus.
Inclination for open air—Very rarely paralysis.	Aversion to open air—Paralysis.
Pain pressing inward—Rending pain in internal parts.	Pain pressing outward—Rending pain in external parts.
Sleeplessness after midnight; awaking too early.	Sleeplessness predom. before midnight—Awaking too late.
Itching, unchanged by scratching . . .	Itching improved by scratching.
Distention of veins of feet—Congestion of blood to ears.	Distention of veins of hands—Congestion to eyes.
Want of thirst during cold stage	Thirst not constant.

Aurum.	Rhus.
Satiety of life with longing for death—Cheerfulness *or* dejection—Irritability—Distrust—Ailments from grief, disappointed love, mortification, anger, or vexation with reserved displeasure or vehemence.	Satiety of life with fear of death—Predom. sadness, dejection—Unconsciousness.
Active memory predom.	Weakness of memory.
Pupils contracted	Pupils dilated.
Hunger predom.	Loss of appetite predom.
Urine infrequent and scanty—Retention of urine.	Urine frequent and copious—Incontinence.
Catamenia too late	Catamenia predom. too soon.
Milk decreased	Milk generally increased.
Expectoration infrequent	Expectoration not constant.
Complaints predom. in palm of hands, and on front side of thigh.	Complaints predom. on back of hands, and on back part of thigh.
Dropsy with clear, gold-colored urine . .	Dropsy with turbid urine.

Aurum.	Rhus.
REMISSION *during day* and evening till midnight.	REMISSION of complaints during day.
Predom. *better* on and after getting out of bed, and after rising from a seat.	Worse *or* better on and after getting out of bed, and after rising from a seat.
Worse when moving the diseased part . .	*Generally* better, sometimes worse when moving the part.
Worse when bending the diseased limb . .	Worse *or* better when bending the diseased limb.
Worse after drinking	*Worse or* better after drinking.

Predomin worse ———— **Predomin. better**

In doors, and when stretching out the diseased limb.

Predomin. better ———— **Predomin. worse**

Out doors *, when drawing up the diseased limb, assuming an erect position, and from eructation.

N.B. Rhus has not the oversensitiveness to pain of Aurum. On the other hand, Aurum very rarely has the sensation of numbness in suffering parts, frequent with Rhus.

*** Both remedies have improvement "when *walking* out doors," therefore motion decides here.**

Aurum.	Sepia.
Inclination for open air—Pain pressing inwards.	Aversion to open air—Pain pressing outwards.
Rending pain upwards—Rending pain in internal parts.	Rending pain downwards—Rending pain in external parts.
Itching, unchanged by scratching . . .	Itching, aggravated by scratching.
Painful swelling of glands	Painless swelling of glands.
Pulse accelerated, but small	Pulse is accelerated, particularly by vexation and exercise; quick and full at night, slow during day.
Want of thirst predominant during chill .	Want of thirst predominant, particularly during sweat—Thirst only during chill.
Very rarely paralysis	Paralysis.
Complaints predominant on front side of thigh.	Complaints predominant on back part of thigh.

Aurum.	Sepia.
Taciturnity — Cheerfulness *or* dejection—Distrust—Delirium.	Loquacity — Predominant sadness — Indifference—Avarice—Absent-mindedness—Imbecility—Unconsciousness.
Does nothing but ask questions	Says something else than he intended.
Active memory predominant	Weakness of memory.
Generally optical illusions in bright colors .	Optical illusions in dark colors.
Discharge of fetid pus from ears	Predominant discharge of blood from ears.
Hunger predominant	Generally loss of appetite.
Appetite for milk	Aversion to milk.
Jaundice, with pain in liver and pit of stomach, greenish-brown urine, bad breath, and putrid taste.	Jaundice, with pain in liver.
Retention of urine	Involuntary discharge of urine.
Nasal secretion thick	Nasal secretion watery.
Expectoration infrequent; morning and evening.	Expectoration predominant, but not constant; is loosened night and morning, and generally swallowed.

Aurum.	Sepia.
Remission *during day* and evening, till midnight.	Remission of complaints afternoon.
Almost always aggrav.* after lying down .	Better *or* worse after lying down.
Worse on awaking	Worse *or* better on awaking; that is, better after sufficient sleep.
Better on and after getting out of bed .	Generally better, sometimes worse, on and after getting out of bed.
Worse from exertion, walking fast, running, etc.	Oftener improved than aggravated by exertion.
Worse when hungry	Worse after a satisfying meal.
Worse in cold weather, better in warm air .	Worse *or* better in cold (resp. warm) air.

Predomin. worse ——— **Predomin. better**

In wet weather, when sitting down, and after sleep.

Predomin. better ——— **Predomin. worse**

In dry weather, from pressure, when eating, from eructation, and after stool.

* Both remedies have improvement oftener than aggravation from *warmth of bed*.

Aurum.	Silicea.
Inclination for open air—Often indicated with old people.	Aversion to open air—Often indicated with children.
Constriction in inward parts—Pain pressing inwards.	Constriction in external parts—Pain pressing outwards.
Rending pain upwards — Apoplexia sanguinea—Very rarely paralysis.	Rending pain downwards—Apoplexia nervosa—Paralysis.
Itching, unchanged by scratching . . .	Itching, aggrav. *or* unchanged by scratching.
Distention of veins of feet	Distention of veins of hands.
Want of thirst predominant, particularly during chill.	Thirst predominant, particularly during heat.
Pulse quick and small	Pulse quick, small, but hard; irregular.
Mood irritable; distrustful; fearful; cheerful *or* sad.	Mood gentle; indifferent; dejected; amorous.
Active memory predominant — Delirium—Insanity.	Weakness of memory.
Optical illusions generally in bright colors .	Optical illusions in black or dark colors.
Hunger predominant	Generally loss of appetite.
Urine infrequent and scanty—Retention of urine.	Urine often, but scanty—Incontinence.
Coryza predominantly fluent	Coryza dry oftener than fluent.
Cough predominantly dry—Expectoration morning and evening.	Cough predominantly loose—Expectoration during day.
Complaints predominant in palm of hand, on thigh, and particularly on front side of thigh.	Complaints predominant on back of hand, leg, and on back part of thigh.
Remission *during day*, evening and before midnight.	Remission of complaints before midnight.
Better after getting out of bed	Worse *or* better after getting out of bed.
Better or worse when rising from a seat .	Worse when rising from a seat.
Worse from exertion, walking fast, running, etc.	Worse *or* better from exertion, etc.
Worse when blowing the nose	Worse when blowing the nose; but better *afterwards*.
Worse after drinking	Worse *or* better after drinking.
Worse when hungry	Worse after a satisfying meal.
Ailments from abuse of Mercury . . .	Ailments from Mercury, Sulphur, or sting of insects.

Predomin. worse — **Predomin. better**

In wet weather, in-doors, and when sitting down.

Predomin. better — **Predomin. worse**

In dry weather, out-doors and walking out-doors, when getting out of bed, when eating, and from external pressure.

N.B. Aurum very rarely has the sensation of numbness in suffering parts, which is quite frequent with Silicea.

Aurum.	Sulphur.
Increased bodily irritability.	Want of bodily irritability.
Inclination for open air—Pain pressing inwards.	Aversion to open air—Pain pressing outward.
Rending pain, upw'ds.—Itching unchanged by scratching.	Rending pain downwards—Itching lessened by scratching.
Painful eruptions	Painless eruptions.
Painful swelling of glands	Painless but hot swelling of glands.
Pulse quick, but small	Pulse accelerated, full and hard.
Chill lessened after getting out of bed	Chill increased after getting out of bed.
Heat with aversion to being uncovered	Heat with inclination to uncover.
Want of thirst predom., partic. during chill.	Thirst predom., mostly during heat.
Sleeplessness aft. midn't; awak'g too early.	Sleeplessness before midn't; awak'g too late.
Mood cheerful *or* sad—Distrust	Mood sad and despondent; indifferent.
Ailments from disappointed love, grief, contradiction, anger, or from vexation with reserved displeasure.	Ailments from hearing bad news, from shame or vexation with fright.
Does nothing but ask questions	Repeats words spoken to him, on account of difficult compheheension.
Active memory predom.	Weakness of memory.
Apoplexy more frequent than paralysis.	Paralysis more frequent than apoplexy.
Eyes protruding — Complaints predom. on inner angle of the eye.	Eyes generally sunken — Complaints predom. on external angle of eye.
Optical illusions predom. in bright colors.	Optical illusions in dark colors.
Complaints predom. on upper gum	Complaints predom. on lower gum.
Hunger predom.—Appetite for milk	Generally loss of appetite—Avers'n to milk.
Urine infrequent and scanty	Urine often and scanty; but sometimes copious.
Nasal secretion thick	Nasal secretion watery.
Expectoration infrequent; morning & evening.	Expectoration not constant; morning and during day, less frequent at night.
Complaints predom. on outer and front side of thigh and on top of foot.	Complaints frequent on inner and back part of thigh, and on sole of foot.
External parts become black	Red parts grow white.
Remis. *during day* & evening till midnight.	Remission afternoon and before midnight.
Worse when hungry	Worse after a satisfying meal.
Worse when growing cold, and in cold weather; better when growing warm, and in warm air.	Better *or* worse when growing cold, (resp. warm,) and in cold (resp. warm) weather.
Most frequently improved by warmth of bed.	Most frequently aggrav. by warmth of bed.
Better when assuming an erect position	Aggrav. oftener than improved when assuming an erect position.
Better after getting out of bed	Worse *or* better after getting out of bed.
Better or worse when rising from a seat	Worse when rising from a seat.
Better when moving the diseased part	Oftener aggrav. than improved when moving the diseased part.
Ailments from abuse of Mercury	Ailments from metallic remedies in general, from Nitric acid, Iodine, Sepia, Rhus, and Cinchona.
Predomin. **worse**	Predomin. **better**

From cold, and from being uncovered.

Predomin. **better**	Predomin. **worse**

From warmth, wrapping up, and when walking out doors*.

N.B. The oversensitiveness to pain, peculiar to Aurum, is very rarely found with Sulphur.

* Both remedies have predom. improvement from being out doors, while Sulphur-complaints are aggravated in a crowded room, the *warmth of a stove* also improves complaints of both remedies.

Baryt.	Calc.
Itching aggravated by scratching	Itching improved oftener than aggrav. by scratching.
Left side, partic. *upper left, lower right side.*	*Right* side, partic. *upper right, lower left side.*
Complaints predom. in exterior parts . .	Complaints predom. in internal parts.
Is oftener indicated with old people, partic. when they are *fat* than with children.	Is often indicated with children and young people, partic. when they are fat.
Rending pain downwards	Rending pain upwards.
Inclination for open air	Sensitiveness and aversion to open air.
When asleep, lying on the side—Apoplexia nervosa.	When asleep, lying on back with arms over the head, or on belly—Apoplexia sanguinea.
Pulse generally accelerated, but weak . .	Pulse quick and full, often trembling.
First chill, then heat	First heat, then chill.
Thirst, partic. during chill	Only during chill, sometimes want of thirst.
Sweat stinking, often only on one side . .	Sweat sticky, coloring, or bloody; sweat often confined to front side of body.

Baryt.	Calc.
Distrust — Absent-mindedness — No delirium.	Embarrassment — Amativeness — Delirium — Ailments from embarrasment, hearing bad news, and from vexation with fright, dread, or fear.
Pupils immoveable—Optical illusions generally in bright colors.	Pupils dilated — Optical illusions in black or dark colors.
Complaints oftener on *external* than inner ear.	Complains oftener in *inner* than on external ear.
Complaints on *external* nose	Complaints of the *inner* oftener than external nose.
Eruption on *upper* lip	Eruption predom. on *under* lip.
Complaints on *lower* teeth and *lower* jaw.	Complaints predom. on *upper* teeth and *upper* jaw.
Delicate taste—Generally loss of appetite .	Loss of taste—Generally hunger.
Waterbrash, improved by sweets	Waterbrash aggrav. by sweets.
Sexual desire lessened	Sexual desire increased.
Catamenia scanty and of long duration . .	Catamenia profuse and of long duration.
Voice hoarse, deep, or weak	Voice hoarse, or singing, nasal, or weak.
Cough, partic. in the evening till midnight —Expectoration chiefly during the evening.	Cough, partic. in evening, night, and morning—Expectoration, morning and during day.

Baryt.	Calc.
REMISSION *during day* and evening . . .	REMISSION before midnight.
Worse when looking sideways	Worse when looking up or down.

Predomin. worse — **Predomin. better**

In doors, when lifting the diseased limb, lying on painful side, when sitting, assuming an erect position, and from rubbing and scratching.

Predomin. better — **Predomin. worse**

Out doors, and when exercising out doors, letting the diseased limb hang down, lying on unpainful side, and from warmth of bed.

N.B. We rarely find the oversensitiveness of Baryt. to pain with Calc. On the other hand, Baryt. has not the sensation of numbness in suffering parts, not infrequent with Calc.

Baryt.	Phosphor.
Itching, aggravated by scratching	Itching, oftener lessened than aggravated by scratching.
Complaints (sensitiveness, etc.) predominant in external parts.	Complaints (sensitiveness, etc.) predominant in internal parts.
Left side; particularly *upper left, lower right side.*	*Right* side; particularly *upper right, lower left side.*
Thirst	Want of thirst.
Pulse generally accelerated, but weak . .	Pulse varying; generally quick, full, and hard; irregular; sometimes intermitting.
Sweat or chill on left side	Sweat or chill on right side.
Chill lessened in a warm room	Chill increased in a warm room.
Sweat increased while eating	Sweat abating while eating.

Baryt.	Phosphor.
Hopelessness—Distrust	Mood changing; glad or dejected; indifferent; haughty; amorous; ailments from fright, anger, (grief,) or from vexation with vehemence.
No delirium—Absent-mindedness—Mental dullness—Weak memory.	Delirium—Mental excitability—Ecstasies—Predominantly active memory.
Complaints predominant on external angle of eye.	Complaints predominant on inner angle of eye.
Optical illusions in bright colors	Optical illusions in black or prismatic colors.
Complaints on upper lip	Complaints on under lip.
Urine often and copious	Urine often, but scanty.
Sexual desire decreased	Sexual desire increased.
Expectoration predominant; evening . .	Expectoration not constant; morning and during day.

Baryt.	Phosphor.
Remission during day and evening . . .	Remission of complaints after midnight.
Worse in company, better when alone . .	Better *or* worse in company (or alone.)
Better *or* worse from light (or in the dark.)	Worse from light, better in the dark.
Worse on awaking	*Better or* worse on awaking; particularly worse after the siesta.
Predominantly worse after getting out of bed.	Better *or* worse after getting out of bed.
Predominantly worse after meals, particularly after a satisfying meal.	Worse *or* better after meals, particularly better after a satisfying meal.
Worse when swallowing food or saliva . .	Worse when swallowing food, partic. drink

Predomin. worse ——— **Predomin. better**

After a satisfying meal, but also on an empty stomach, when sitting, lifting the diseased limb, after sleep, from the touch, from rubbing and scratching.

Predomin. better ——— **Predomin. worse**

After breakfast, after stool, from warmth of bed, and letting the diseased limb hang down.

N.B. Baryt. has not the sensation of numbness in suffering parts of Phosphorus.

Baryt.	Pulsat.
Left side*—Complaints of external parts predom.	*Right* side—Complaints of internal parts predominant.
Itching, aggravated by scratching . . .	Itching, aggrav. *or* unchanged by scratch'g.
Ulcers, with scanty discharge	Ulcers, with copious discharge.
Local chill on upper part of body . . .	Local chill on lower part of body.
Chill, sweat, etc., predominant on left side .	Chill, heat, sweat, predominant on right side.
Chill increased by exercise, lessened in warm room.	Chill lessened by exercise, increased in a warm room.
Thirst, particularly during chill	Want of thirst; thirst only during heat.†

Baryt.	Pulsat.
Loquacity—Irritable mood—No delirium .	Taciturnity — Gentleness — Ailments from excessive joy, fright, grief, mortification, or vexation with fright, dread or fear.
Paralysis	Rarely paralysis . . . .
Complaints predominant on external angle of eye, external ear, upper lip, on external side of gums, and in upper part of chest.	Complaints predominant in inner angle of eye, inner ear, on lower lip, on inner side of gums, and in lower part of chest.
When asleep, lying on the side . . .	When asleep, lying on back, often with the arms over the head.
Generally loss of appetite	Generally hunger.
Urine frequent and copious.	Urine infrequent and scanty.
Sexual desire decreased	Sexual desire increased.
Catamenia scanty, of long duration . .	Catamenia scanty and of short duration.
Expectoration, particularly in evening . .	Expectoration morning and during day.

Baryt.	Pulsat.
Aggravation night and morning . . .	Aggravation from noon till midnight.
Worse on awaking	*Worse or* better on awaking.
Predominantly worse after getting out of bed.	Worse *or* better after getting out of bed.
Better after rising from a seat	*Better or* worse after rising from a seat.
Predominantly better when sitting down .	Worse *or* better when sitting down.
Worse when bending the diseased part . .	Better *or* worse when bending the diseased part.
Worse from pressure	*Better or* worse from pressure.
Worse when swallowing	*Worse or* better when swallowing.
Worse when looking sideways	Worse when looking upwards.

Predomin. worse — **Predomin. better**

From cold, from growing cold, and in cold weather, from motion, walking, stretching out, or lifting up diseased limb, washing or moistening the suffering part, lying on painful side, after getting out of bed and from pressure.

Predomin. better — **Predomin worse**

From warmth, from warmth of bed, from growing warm and in warm air, during rest, after lying down, while lying, when drawing up the diseased limb or letting it hang down, and when lying on the unpainful side.

N.B. Baryt. has not the sensation of numbness in suffering parts frequent with Pulsatilla.

---

* The formula "upper left, lower right side" applies to both remedies, but appears, as will be noticed, in a different manner in the local fever-symptoms.

† Besides this, Pulsatilla has thirst *before* and *after* chill and between heat and sweat.

Baryt.	Silicea.
Left side; particularly *upper left, lower right side.*	*Right* side; particularly *upper right, lower left side.*
Inclination for open air	Aversion to open air.
Constriction in internal parts	Constriction in external parts.
Itching, aggravated by scratching . . .	Itching, aggrav. or unchanged by scratching.
Complaints predominant on external angle of eye, on external nose, and in upper part of chest.	Complaints predominant in inner angle of eye, in inner nose, and in lower part of chest.
Pulse generally accelerated and weak . .	Pulse quick, small, but hard
Thirst, particularly during chill	Thirst, particularly during heat.
Chill lessened in warm room	Chill increased in warm room.

Baryt.	Silicea.
Mood irritable; distrustful—Unconsciousness.	Gentleness—Indifference—Very rarely unconsciousness.
Optical illusions, generally in bright colors.	Optical illusions, in black or dark colors.
Sexual desire too weak	Sexual desire too strong.
Coryza predominantly fluent	Coryza, dry oftener than fluent.
Expectoration, particularly in evening . .	Expectoration during day.

Baryt.	Silicea.
Remission during day and evening . . .	Remission of complaints before midnight.
Worse *or* better from light (or in the dark.)	Worse from light, better in the dark.
Better *or* worse from eructation	Predominantly better from eructation.
Worse when blowing nose	Worse when blowing nose, but better *afterwards.*
Worse when looking sideways	Worse when looking upwards . . . .

Predomin. worse ⏜ **Predomin. better**

In wet weather, in-doors, in company, on an empty stomach, from warm diet, when assuming an erect position, and from exercise.

Predomin better ⏜ **Predomin. worse**

In dry weather, out-doors, when alone, after breakfast, from cold diet, respiring deeply, and during rest.

N.B. Baryt. has not the sensation of numbness in suffering parts frequent with Silicea.

Baryt.	Sulphur.
Inclination for open air—Itching, aggravated by scratching.	Aversion to open air—Itching, lessened by scratching.
Pulse generally accelerated and weak . .	Pulse quick, full, and hard.
Thirst, particularly during chill	Thirst, particularly during heat; generally want of thirst during chill.
Apoplexy	Rarely apoplexy.

Baryt.	Sulphur.
Distrust—No delirium	Mood changing; gentle; indifferent—Delirium — Ailments from embarrassment, hearing bad news, from fright, mortification, or from vexation with fright, dread, or fear.
Optical illusions, in bright colors	Optical illusions, in dark colors.
Complaints generally on external ear and on upper gum.	Complaints generally in inner ear and on lower gum.
Urine frequent and copious	Urine frequent and scanty; sometimes also copious, that is, after quantitative doses.
Catamenia generally of long duration . .	Catamenia generally of short duration.
Expectoration predominant, particularly in evening.	Expectoration not constant; morning and during day; less frequent at night.

Baryt.	Sulphur.
REMISSION during day and evening . . .	REMISSION *afternoon* and before midnight.
Better *or* worse from light (resp. in the dark.)	Predominantly worse from light, better in the dark.
Worse when growing cold and in cold weather; better when growing warm and in warm air.	Better *or* worse from growing cold and in cold weather, (from growing warm and in warm air.)
Worse in-doors*, better in the open air .	Better or worse in-doors, (resp. in the open air.)
Better or worse from eructation.	Almost always improved by eructation.
Worse when looking sideways	Worse when looking down, particularly at running water.

Predomin. worse —— **Predomin. better**

From cold, from warm diet, scratching, from external pressure, and from exercise

Predomin. better —— **Predomin. worse**

From warmth, from warmth of bed, cold diet, after lying down, and during rest generally.

N.B. We rarely find the over-sensitiveness to pain peculiar to Baryt. with Sulphur; on the other hand, Baryt. lacks the sensation of numbness in suffering parts frequent with Sulphur.

---

* Yet we also find "improvement by warmth of stove" with Baryt. (as with Sulphur), while Sulphur-complaints are aggravated in a crowded room.

Belladonna.	Bryonia.
Upper left, lower right side — Dark hair	Upper right, lower left side—Light hair.
Obesity predom.	Emaciation predom.
Rending pain upwards	Rending pain downwards.
Constriction in internal parts	Constriction in external parts.
Humid eruptions — Induration of the cellular tissue	Dry eruptions—Suppuration of the cellular tissue.
Cold on diseased part	Chill *or* heat on diseased part.
Sweat lessened in doors	Sweat increased in doors.
Thirst very rare during chill	Thirst predom., but not constant.
Changeable mood — Cheerfulness *or* dejection—Indifference—Distrust—Malice.	Predom. *peevishness*; sadness.
Memory very active *or* very weak	Weak memory.
Vertigo inclining to fall sideways (left side) or backwards.	Vertigo, inclining to fall backwards.
Aversion to light, partic. candle light	Aversion to light, partic. sun light.
Eruption on *upper* lip	Eruption on *under* lip.
Drinks often, but little at a time	Drinks rarely, but a great deal at a time.
Predom. aversion to sour things	Appetite for sour things.
Nausea in throat or abdomen, rarely in stomach.	Nausea in stomach or abdomen, rarely in œsophagus.
Scentless flatus	Fetid flatus.
Diarrhœa generally painless	Diarrhœa generally painful.
Expectoration infrequent; morning, during day, evening.	Expectoration not constant; morning and evening, more rare during day.
Complaints predom. in *upper* part of chest, and on shin.	Complaints predom. in *lower* part of chest, and in calf of leg.
With Cows: Painful swelling of the udder.	With Cows: Painless swelling of the udder.
Remission of complaints after midnight and in *forenoon*.	Remission fore and afternoon.
Worse in cold weather and when growing cold.	In cold weather and when growing cold, sometimes better, sometimes worse.
Better when letting the diseased limb hang down.	When letting the diseased limb hang down, sometimes worse, sometimes better.
Oftener improved than aggrav. by bending diseased limb.	Worse when bending diseased limb.
Worse during full moon	Worse before a thunder storm.

Predomin. **worse**	Predomin. **better**

In the twilight, and when sitting erect.

Predomin. **better**	Predomin. **worse**

From stooping and sitting bent forward, bending the head back, when stretching out the diseased limb, and from change of position.

Belladonna.	Calcarea.
Upper left, lower right side — Dark hair.	*Upper right, lower left side* — Light hair.
Muscles rigid — Apoplexy more frequent than paralysis.	Muscles lax — Paralysis more frequent than apoplexy.
Complaints predom. on lower jaw, on upper arm, and on external side of thigh.	Complaints predom. on upper jaw, on fore arm, and on inner side of thigh.
Heat with aversion to uncover	Heat with inclination to uncover.
Thirst not constant, very rare during chill.	Thirst almost constant during all stages of the fever, only sometimes it is wanting, during chill.
Eruptions generally humid	Eruptions generally dry.
During sleep often lying with head on arm.	When asleep, often the arms above the head.
Generally insensibility of disposition . . .	Sensitiveness of disposition.
Satiety of life with longing for death . .	Satiety of life with fear of death.
Fear of being poisoned or of apoplexy . .	Fear of loss of reason.
Mood changing; distrustful; malicious.	
Ecstacy *or* mental dullness — Insanity *or* imbecility.	Imbecility.
Ailments from fright, anger, mortification, or from vexation with vehemence.	Ailments from hearing bad news.
Memory active *or* weak	Weak memory.
Headache, better during catamenia, from pressure, tying something tightly around it, and wrapping up; *worse* from warmth.	Headache *worse* during catamenia, from pressure, or tying something tight around it, & from wrapping up, *better* fr. warmth.
Eruption on upper lip	Eruption predom. on under lip.
Predom. aversion to sour things	Appetite for sour things.
Nausea in throat or abdomen, rarely in stomach.	Nausea in stomach.
Inguinal hernia small, recent, with spasmodic incarceration and difficulty to be reduced.	Inguinal hernia lax, apt to be incarcerated, (fr. cough, &c.,) but also easily reduceable.
Respiration predom. low	Respiration loud.
Expectoration infrequent; morning, during day, evening.	Expectoration not constant; morning and during day, rarely in evening.
Remission after midnight and in forenoon.	**Remission** of complaints before midnight.
Worse from light; better in the dark . .	Worse *or* better from light, (in the dark.)
Almost always worse when closing the eyes, better when opening them.	Better *or* worse when closing (resp. opening) the eyes.
Worse when looking sideways	Worse when looking upward or downward.
Worse *or* better from wine	Worse from spirituous liquor.
Worse *or* better when assuming an erect position.	Better when assuming an erect position.
Alm. always improved aft. gett'g out of bed.	*Worse or* better after getting out of bed.
Worse when rising from a seat	*Worse or* better when rising from a seat.
Worse from walking fast, running, &c. . .	Oftener aggrav. than improved by running, &c., partic. worse from exertion on an empty stomach.
Worse from heat of sun	Worse in snowy air.

Predomin. worse — **Predomin. better**

In dry weather, from being uncovered, from the touch, when drawing up, lifting or resting the diseased limb on something.

Predomin. better — **Predomin. worse**

In wet weather, from wrapping up in bed, from pressure, when stooping, bending the diseased part backward, when stretching out the suffering limb, or letting it hang down, and when boring with the finger in ear or nose.

N.B. We rarely find the oversensitiveness of Bellad. to pain with Calcarea,—with Bellad. rarely the sensation of numbness in suffering parts, frequent with Calc.

Belladonna.	Cantharid.
Aversion to exercise — Obesity predominant.	Inclination for exercise — Emaciation predominant.
Crawling sensation in external parts . . .	Crawling sensation in internal parts.
Rending pain upwards — Apoplexy . . .	Rending pain downwards — No apoplexy.
Ulcers, with scanty discharge	Ulcers, with copious discharge.

Belladonna.	Cantharid.
Changing mood—Cheerfulness *or* dejection; Indifference; distrust; malice.	Amativeness.
Sleeplessness *before midnight.*	Sleeplessness *after midnight.*
When the pulse grows slow, it is full and strong.	When the pulse grows slow, it is weak.
Heat descending	Heat predominantly ascending.
Thirst not constant; most rare during chill; but appears *before* the chill, and also *after* sweat.	No thirst during chill; but appears *after* chill and during heat.
Drinks often, but little at a time	Drinks seldom, but much at a time.
Nausea in throat or abdomen, rarely in stomach.	Nausea in stomach.
Coryza* predominantly dry	Coryza predominantly fluent.
Voice nasal	Voice trembling.
Expectoration from morning till evening .	Expectoration in evening.
Complaints predominant in hollow of knee, in shin, and in sole of foot.	Complaints predominant in hollow of elbow, in calf of leg, and in the instep.

Belladonna.	Cantharid.
Remission of complaints after midnight and during *forenoon.*	Remission of complaints morning and evening, till midnight.
Worse while sweating	*Better after* sweating.

Predomin. better — **Predomin. worse**

After getting out of bed, and when stooping.

*** Only during the sweating stage of fever fluent coryza is predominant with Belladonna.**

Belladonna.	China.
Right side predominant—Obesity	*Left* side—Emaciation.
Aversion to exercise*; Apoplexia sanguinea.	Inclination for exercise—Apoplexia nervosa.
Rending pain upwards	Rending pain downwards . . . . . .
Pulse generally full (large)	Pulse predominantly small . . . . . .
Sweat on front or right side of body . .	Sweat on back of body, or only on left side.
Sweat sometimes general, with exception of the head.	Sweat sometimes general, with exception of the feet.
Thirst not constant; most rare during the chill.	Thirst mostly during sweat; besides this, particularly between the several stages.
Changing mood — Fear; Distrust; Dejection *or* cheerfulness.	Sadness. ? Scheming. C.Hg.
Mental dullness oftener than mental excitability.	Rarely unconsciousness or delirium in fevers.
Consequences of fright, anger, or mortification.	Ecstasies.
Vertigo, inclining to fall sideways (left side) or backwards.	Vertigo, inclining to fall backwards.
Pupils *dilated* first, then contracted . . .	Pupils first *contracted*, then dilated.
Far-sightedness	Short-sightedness.
Eyes protruding	Eyes generally sunken.
Complaints predominant in *inner* angle of eye, on *lower* jaw, in *upper* part of chest, in the liver, and on the shin.	Complaints predominant in *external* angle of eye, on *upper* jaw, in *lower* part of chest, in spleen (oftener than in liver,) and on calf of leg.
Predominant aversion to sour things . .	Appetite for sour things.
Nausea in throat or abdomen; rarely in stomach.	Nausea in throat or stomach.
Scentless flatus	Fetid flatus.
Lochia suppressed	Lochia continue bloody too long.
Voice hoarse or raised	Voice hoarse or deep.
Respiration predominantly low	Respiration generally loud.
Expectoration infrequent; morning, during day, and evening.	Expectoration not constant; during day and evening.
Remission *forenoon* and after midnight .	Remission *afternoon* and evening.
Aggravation in the Spring	Aggravation in the Autumn.
Worse during sleep; generally also *after* sleep.	*Worse* during sleep, better *after* sleep; that is, after sufficient sleep; for awaking from sleep, when roused, is generally followed by aggravation.
Worse during sweat, predominantly better *after* it.	*Worse after* the sweat.
Ailments from abuse of Cinchona, Plumb., sting of insects, or contagious Anthrax.	Ailments from abuse of Sulphur or of Calc.

Predomin. worse — **Predomin. better**

In dry weather, when uncovering the head, sitting erect, drawing up the diseased limb, lying on left side, and after sleep.

Predomin. better — **Predomin. worse**

In wet weather, from wrapping up the head, when sitting, particularly sitting and leaning forward, stretching out the diseased limb, in bed, lying on back, when stooping, bending the head backwards, lying on the right side, and after the sweat.

* Belladonna also has inclination for constant motion in single or in the suffering parts.

Belladonna	Conium.
Dark hair—Jerking pain in external parts.	Light hair—Jerking pain in internal parts.
Painful swelling of the glands	Painless swelling of the glands.
Pulse generally quick, full, hard, and tense.	Pulse very irregular; generally slow and large; now and then with small and quick beats.
Partial sweat on upper part of body . .	Sweat on lower part of body.
Thirst most rare during chill; not constant.	Want of thirst.
Apoplexy more frequent than paralysis . .	Paralysis (painless) more frequent than apoplexy.
Silly merriness *or* sadness—Mood distrustful, irritable, malicious.	Mood sad; serious—Very rarely delirium.
Ailments from fright, anger, mortification, etc.	Ailments from grief.
Memory active *or* weak	Weak memory.
Vertigo, inclining to fall backwards or sideways.	Vertigo, inclining to fall sideways.
Desire for bread—Aversion to coffee . .	Aversion to bread—Appetite for coffee.
Catamenia too soon, profuse, and of long duration.	Catamenia too late, scanty, and of short duration.
Expectoration infrequent; morning, during day, evening.	Expectoration infrequent; is loosened only during day, and is swallowed.
Complaints predominant on upper arm . .	Complaints predominant on fore-arm.
REMISSION after midnight and in *forenoon*.	REMISSION of complaints in forenoon.
Better (resp. worse) when lying on back or side.	Better when lying on back, worse lying on side.
Worse or better when assuming an erect position.	Almost always aggravated when assuming an erect position.
Worse when getting out of bed	*Worse or* better when getting out of bed.
Worse (resp. better) when ascending or descending.	Better when ascending, worse when descending.
Oftener aggravated than improved by wine and other spirituous liquors.	Oftener improved than aggravated by wine, etc.
Worse from heat of sun	Worse in snowy air.

Predomin. worse — **Predomin. better**

In the sun, in dry weather, from warm diet, particularly when moving the diseased part, when walking, and closing the eyes.

Predomin. better — **Predomin. worse**

In wet weather, from cold diet*, during rest, when standing, sitting or lying, from change of position, bending the diseased part backwards, and when opening the eyes.

N.B. We rarely find the sensation of numbness in suffering parts of Conium with Belladonna.

---

* When *drinking cold water*, Belladonna also has aggravation, because one of its effects is that swallowing *fluids* inconveniences.

Belladonna.	Cuprum.
Right side; particularly *lower right, upper left side.*	*Left side;* particularly *lower left, upper right side.*
Dark hair—Muscles rigid	Light hair—Muscles lax.
Aversion to exercise*	Inclination for exercise.
Crawling sensation or bruised pain in external parts.	Crawling sensation or bruised pain in internal parts.
Apoplexia sanguinea—Paralysis often one-sided.	Apoplexia nervosa—Paralysis generally of both sides.
Complaints predominant in upper part of chest, on upper arm, in hollow of knee, and on shin.	Complaints predominant in lower part of chest, on fore-arm, in hollow of elbow, and on calf of leg.
Humid eruptions	Dry, cutaneous eruptions.
Pulse generally full and accelerated . . .	Pulse generally weak and slow.
Fear of being poisoned, or of apoplexy .	Fear of loss of reason.
Distrust—Cheerfulness *or* sadness . . .	Cheerfulness predominant.
Fancies—Cannot express a thought, without first saying something foolish.	Speaking words that one did not intend to say.
Ailments from anger or mortification . .	Ailments from hearing bad news.
Consequences of being very much overheated, or taking cold.	Consequences of violent exertion, with mental excitement. CHg.
Vertigo, inclining to fall backwards or sideways.	Vertigo, inclining to fall forwards.
Eyes protruding.	Eyes generally sunken.
Catamenia too soon	Catamenia too late.
Voice low	Voice low *or* stronger than usual.
Expectoration in morning, during day, evening.	Expectoration, with the cough in the morning.
Remiss. after midnight and in *forenoon* .	Remission of complaints during day.
Worse during full moon	Worse during and after new moon.
Toothache better when eating, worse *afterwards.*	Complaints improved by drinking, worse *afterwards.*
Better (or worse) when lying on back *or* side.	Worse when lying on back, better when lying on side.
Worse or better when assuming an erect position.	Worse when assuming an erect position.
Worse (or better) when ascending, *or* when descending.	Worse when ascending; better when descending.
Worse when looking sideways	Worse when looking upwards.
Ailments from abuse of Cinchona or Mercury, from Plumbum, Iodine, sting of insects, or contagious Anthrax.	Ailments from Calc.

Predomin. worse ———— **Predomin. better**

In dry weather, and while sweating.

Predomin. better ———— **Predomin worse**

In wet weather, from pressure, when stooping, when bending the diseased part backwards, and when turning in bed.

* With Belladonna there sometimes occurs inclination for exercise in single or suffering parts.

Belladonna.	Hyoscyamus.
Upp left, lower r. side—Hair gener'ly dark.	Upper right, lower left side—Light hair.
Skin and muscles rigid—Apopl. sanguinea.	Skin and muscles lax—Apoplexia nervosa.
Complaints of internal parts predom. .	*Complaints of external parts* predom.
Crawling sensation in external parts . . .	Crawling sensation in internal parts.
Paralysis generally painful — Eruptions, d°.	Paralysis generally painless—Eruptions d°.
Generally increased beats of pulse . . .	The number of puls's decreases at first. C.Hg.
When the pulse becomes slow, it is full . .	When the pulse becomes slow, it is small.
Sweat on upper part of body	Sweat on lower part of body.
Heat descending—Humid eruptions . . .	Heat ascending—Dry eruptions.
Thirst not constant, most rare during chill.	Thirst is wanting only during chill.
Dejection, Indifference, Absent-mindedness.	Haughtiness—Amativeness—Jealousy.
Ailments from mortification. (Spasms in consequence of vexation. C.Hg.) . .	Ailments from grief or jealousy.
Headache increased by exercise, partic. aggravated out doors.	Headache improved by walking. C.Hg.
The pupil of diseased eye is larger than that of the healthy one.	The pupil of the suffering eye is more contracted.
Dimsightedness more frequent than clearsightedness—Farsightedness.	Clearsightedness more frequent than dimsightedness — Shortsightedness more frequent than farsightedness.
When the pupils are dilated, staring look, eyes lusterless, dull, glazed.	When the pupils are dilated, eyes sunken, staring and lustrous. C.Hg.
Angles of the eyes painful when touched . .	Rending pain in angles of eyes, disappearing by touch. d°.
Sense of smell generally too sensitive . .	Sense of smell weak or entirely lost. d°.
More pain in lower part of belly	More complaints in upper belly. d°.
Too great irritability of the urethra . . .	Paralysis of the bladder. d°.
Indifference to sexual desire	Excessive sexual desire. d°.
Milk predom. increased	Secretion of milk decreased.
Catamenia predom. too soon	Catamenia too late.
Expectoration not often, sometimes only during day; in the morning and not in the even'g, or in the ev'g & not in the morn'g.	Expectoration not often, only sometimes in morning; on the other hand chiefly during day.
Respiration predom. low	Respiration loud.
Compl'ts predom. on upper arm & on shin.	Compl'ts pred. in fore arm & on calf of leg.
Tension and stiffness in hip and knee . .	Cramp in calf of leg and of the toes. C.Hg.
Rending pain in sole of foot, with stitches when walking.	Rending pain in sole of foot, generally during rest, disappearing when walking, appearing again when sitting down. C.Hg.
With Horses: Amaurosis with eyes reddened and constant restlessness.	With Horses: Amaurosis with winking of eyes and carrying the head high.
With Horses: Founder with dragging of the hind legs.	With Horses: Inflammation of brain with wavering on the common.
Remission *forenoon* and after midnight	Remission of complaints during day.
All compl'ts worse in afternoon 3 or 4 o'cl.	Symptoms are worst in evening. C.Hg
Worse, partic. from *candle* light	Worse, partic. from *day* light.
Better when lying, and in bed	*Worse* wh. lying, but *better* fr. warmth of bed.
Worse when getting out of bed; *better afterwards.*	*Better* when getting out of bed; *worse afterwards.*

Predomin. worse ⁀ **Predomin. better**

From external pressure, sitting bent forward, holding the diseased part bent, when lying and *after* getting out of bed.

Predomin. better ⁀ **Predomin. worse**

***When* getting out of bed, and when sitting erect.**

Belladonna.	Lachesis.
Blood coagulates easily	Blood incoagulable.
Dark hair—Muscles rigid	Light hair—Muscles lax—Very rarely paralysis.
Anxious dreams	Pleasant dreams.
Most frequently insensibility of disposition.	Sensitiveness of disposition.
Changing mood—Hopelessness—Sadness.	Haughtiness—Amativeness.
Hasty deliration—Merry talkativeness . .	Mania for relation, but one word often leads into the midst of another story. C.Hg.
Ailments from anger, vexation, mortification.	Ailments from jealousy.
Difficult comprehension; mental dullness *or* mental excitability.	Comprehends easily; mental excitability.
Memory very active *or* very weak . . .	Weak memory—Very rarely unconsciousness.
Pulse most frequently quick, full, hard and tense.	Pulse very unequal; generally quick, but small and weak, often alternating with full and hard beats.
Cold shudders or heat descending . . .	Cold shudders or heat ascending.
Thirst not constant, most rare during chill.	No thirst during chill, is not frequent during heat.
Sweat lessened when and after getting out of bed.	Sweat increased when and after getting out of bed.
Farsightedness	Shortsightedness.
Aversion to beer and to sour things . . .	Appetite for beer or sour things.
Scentless flatus	Fetid flatus.
Catamenia too profuse and of long duration.	Catamenia too scanty and of short duration.
Coryza predom.* dry	Coryza predom. fluent.
Expectoration from morning till evening .	Expectoration, which is generally swallowed, is loosened, in morning and during day.
REMISSION after midnight and in *forenoon*.	AGGRAVATION afternoon and evening till midnight.
Worse during sleep, generally also *afterwards*.	Predom. *better* during sleep, but *worse afterwards*.
Worse when swallowing and after drinking.	Quite as often improved as aggrav. when swallowing and after drinking.
Complaints predom. after meals	Complaints predom. before meals. C.Hg.
Worse in dry, cold weather; *better* in damp and warm air.	Better in dry, cold weather; *worse* in damp cold or warm air.
Worse during full moon	Worse before a thunder storm.

Predomin. worse ——— **Predomin. better**

In dry cold weather, from exercise, shaking the head, respiring deeply, drinking coffee, and when drawing up the diseased limb.

Predomin. better ——— **Predomin. worse**

In damp, warm air, during rest, when sitting and lying, when stretching out the diseased limb, when holding the suffering part bent, from change of position, from external pressure, and from eructation.

N.B. We rarely find the oversensitiveness to pain of the Balladonna-patient, with Lach.

N.B. Both remedies have great sensitiveness around the throat, even to the touch of the bed-clothes. C.Hg.

* Fluent coryza is preval. only during the sweating stage of fever with Bellad.

Belladonna.	Mercur.
Dark hair—Muscles rigid	Light hair—Muscles lax.
Rending pain upwards—Induration of cellular tissue.	Rending pain downwards—Suppuration of cellular tissue.
Complaints predominant on roof of mouth, on upper arm, in hollow of elbow, on patella, and on outer side of thigh.	Complaints predominant on soft palate, on fore-arm, on tip of elbow, and on inner side of thigh.
When the pulse becomes slow, it is full	When the pulse becomes slow, it is weak.
Thirst constant; more *before* than *during* the chill.	Thirst predominant during all stages of the fever, but not constant.
Dreams of fire, etc.	Dreams of water, etc.
Fear of being poisoned, or of apoplexy	Fear of loss of reason.
Silly merriness *or* dejection—Distrust	Seriousness.
Love of being alone	Fear of being alone.
Tries to get out of the bed	Tries to run out of the house. C.Hg.
Mental excitability *or* dullness	Mental dullness.
Ailments from fright, anger, or vexation	Ailments from emotion in general.
Memory active *or* weak	Weak memory.
Toothache, with sleepiness	Toothache, with sleeplessness.
Nausea in throat or abdomen, rarely in stomach.	Nausea in œsophagus or stomach, rarely in throat.
Catamenia too soon	Catamenia too late.
Milk most frequently increased	Milk decreased *or* spoiled.
Coryza predominantly dry	Coryza fluent oftener than dry.
Expectoration infrequent; morning, during day, evening.	Expectoration not constant; during day.
REMISSION after midnight and in *forenoon*.	REMISSION of complaints during day.*
Worse in Spring	Worse in Autumn.
Better (resp. worse) when lying on back *or* on side.	Better when lying on back; worse when lying on side.
Worse when growing cold, better when growing warm.	When growing cold, worse *or* (after warmth of bed) better.
Better from cold, worse from warm diet	Worse from cold *or* warm diet; when warm diet aggravates, cold diet improves.
Sugar lessens burning sensation in the throat, water does not.	Desire for sweets, but worse after partaking of them.
Worse *or* better from wine	Worse from drinking wine.
Almost always aggravated when swallowing.	Better *or* worse when swallowing; particularly worse when swallow'g saliva or drink.
Worse *or* better when leaning against anything; particularly better when leaning ag'st something hard (and from pressure.)	Better when leaning against anything.
Ailments from Mercurius, Plumbum, Iodine, or contagious Anthrax.	Ailments from Arsenic or Copper vapors, from Sulphur or Calc.

Predomin. worse — **Predomin. better**

In dry weather, and from smoking.

Predomin better — **Predomin. worse**

In wet weather, from pressure, when stooping, when holding the breath, and when turning in bed.

N.B. Although Mercurius has the character of increased constitutional irritability, yet we rarely find the over-sensitiveness to pain peculiar to Belladonna with this remedy.

* Except toothache, which sometimes rages all day and ceases at night. C.Hg.

Belladonna.	Mezereum.
Right side; particularly *lower right, upper left side.*	*Left* side; particularly *lower left, upper right side.*
Dark hair—Aversion to open air	Light hair—Inclination for open air.
Crawling sensation, or jerking pain in external parts.	Crawling sensation, or jerking pain in internal parts.
Apoplexy—Obesity—Swelling of suffering parts.	No apoplexy—Emaciation, particularly of suffering parts.
Ulcers, with scanty discharge	Ulcers, with copious discharge.
Complaints predominant on lower jaw, lower teeth, and in upper part of chest.	Complaints predominant on upper jaw, upper teeth, and in lower part of chest.
Sleeplessness before midnight	Sleeplessness predominant after midnight.
Pulse changed	Pulse changed very little.
Thirst not constant; most rare during chill, often after sweat and *before* the chill.	Thirst, particularly during chill.
Chill increased out-doors	Chill lessened out-doors.

Belladonna.	Mezereum.
Likes to be alone—Restlessness and haste.	Aversion to being alone—Indolence and phlegma.
Memory active *or* weak	Weak memory.
Sensation like drunkenness; worse after eating.	Sensation of drunkenness; better after meals.
Eruption on upper lip	Eruption on under lip.
Aversion to fatty food	Appetite for bacon.
Nausea in throat or abdomen; rarely in stomach.	Nausea in throat or stomach.
Voice often nasal	Voice failing or interrupted.
Expectoration infrequent; morning, during day, and evening.	Expectoration infrequent; morning.

Belladonna.	Mezereum.
REMISSION after midnight and in *forenoon*.	REMISSION after midnight and *during day*.
Better *or* worse when bending the diseased part.	Worse when bending the diseased part.
Oftener aggravated than improved when eating.	Almost always improved when eating.
Worse from warm diet; better from cold diet.	Better from warm *or* cold diet; when better from cold diet, warm diet aggravates.
Worse *or* better from wine	Worse from drinking wine.
Ailments from sting of insects, contagious Anthrax, or abuse of Cinchona, Plumb., or from Iodine.	Ailments from poisoning by Phosphor.*

Predomin. worse — **Predomin. better**

Out-doors, when growing cold†, when sucking the gums, when swallowing‡, and when drawing up the suffering limb.

Predomin. better — **Predomin. worse**

In-doors, when growing warm, after lying down, while lying, in bed, from pressure, and when stretching out or bending the diseased part backwards.

---

* Both remedies are useful against the consequences of abuse of Mercurius.

† This refers particularly to complaints already existing and caused either by disease or medicine; with both remedies cold favors the production of new complaints.

‡ Belladonna has aggravation, particularly when swallowing drink; Merzereum aggrav. when swallowing saliva.

Belladonna.	Moschus.
Plethora predom.—Apoplexia sanguinea—Paralysis.	Anæmie — Apoplexia nervosa — No paralysis of the limbs.
Trembling with convulsive shocks, or of the hands and feet, with sudden screams.	Violent trembling, shaking without chill, so that the bed is shaken; at the same time screaming she must die. C.Hg.
Fainting fits from standing	Fainting fits when rising, accompanied by vertigo and vomiting followed by headache, or itching over the whole body.
Sleeplessness with strong desire for sleep .	Sleeplessness with nervous erethism. C.Hg.
Heat or sweat with aversion to being uncovered.	Heat or sweat with inclination for being uncovered.
Thirst not constant, rare during chill; more frequent *before* chill and after sweat.	Want of thirst predom.
Delirium; seeing animals, particularly black ones, or spectres.	Delirium; supposes himself three times in bed, once again on each side. C.Hg.
Cheerfulness *or* dejection—Distrust—Irritability—Malice.	Amativeness more frequent than with Belladonna.
Hypochondriasis of women with Erethism.	Hypochondriasis with a tensive, tonic-spasmodic state—Hysterismus virilis. C.Hg.
Memory active *or* weak.	Weak memory.
Disgust for coffee	Desire for coffee without milk. C.Hg.
Nausea in throat or abdomen, rarely in stomach.	Nausea in stomach.
Sexual indifference	Excited sexual desire. C.Hg.
Complaints predom. in upper part of chest and on upper arm.	Complaints predom. in lower part of chest and on fore arm.
REMISSION after midnight and in *forenoon*.	REMISSION morning and forenoon.
Increases (in potencies) the sensibility to cold damp air.	Diminishes the insensibility to potentized medicines. C.Hg.
Better when lying down, partic. on something hard.	The part lain on, pains as though sprained or broken. C.Hg.
Better (resp. worse) when lying on painful *or* unpainful side.	Worse when lying on painful side, better when lying on unpainful side.
Great weakness, noticeable mostly when standing and moving.	Great weakness more perceptible during rest than when moving. C.Hg.

Predomin. worse — **Predomin. better**

From motion, partic. when moving diseased limb, when walking, when walking out doors *, when getting out of bed † and from being uncovered.

Predomin. better — **Predomin. worse**

During rest, after lying down, in bed ‡, when lying, sitting, and standing, when stooping, from pressure, and from wrapping up.

N.B. Moschus has not the oversensitiveness to pain of the Belladonna-patient.

N.B. Belladonna and moschus are principal remedies in the often fatal spasmus glottidis of children, (laryngismus,) the comparison given above will readily decide the choice. C.Hg.

* Here motion must decide; for both remedies have predom. aggrav. out doors.
† Both remedies have improvement of symptoms "*after* getting out of bed."
‡ The warmth of the bed also predominantly improves in moschus-complaints.

Belladonna.	Nux vom.
Upper left, lower right side—Obesity pred.	*Lower left, upper right side*—Emaciation.
Coldness of the suffering (painful) part . .	Sweat on suffering side.
Sweat on the front side of body	Sweat often confin'd to the back part of body.
Sweat increased during sleep, heat after sleep.	Sweat less during sleep—Heat less after sleep.
Thirst very rare during chill	Thirst most frequ't dur'g cold stage of fever.
Compl'ts predom. on upper arm & on shin.	Compl'ts pred. on fore arm & on calf of leg.
Sleeplessness before midnight	Sleeplessness preval. after midnight.

Most frequently insensibility of disposition.	Sensitiveness of dispos'n—Sensitive feel'gs.
Mood changing; cheerful *or* sad; distrustful.—Ecstacies—Insanity—Imbecility.	Sadness—Amativeness—Ailments fr. grief, disappointed love, jealousy, or from vexation with indignation.
Delirium tremens: Walking busily about, undertaking many things; seeing various objects, (water, glass, cats;) talks, laughs much; stammering; rush of blood to head, chill and heat, desire for beer, disgust for brandy.	Del. tr.: Tormenting fear, sees people about him that ask questions, pressure in forehead, cold face, hands and feet; heat and sweat; aversion to coffee, or it disagrees, thirst, but vomiting of drink, nausea, bitter vomiting, pain in the region of liver, cheeks and eyes yellowish *
Dimsightedness	Clearsightedness predom.
Aversion to beer	Inclination for, *or* aversion to beer.
Tobacco smoke is unbearable	Desire or disgust for tobacco. C.Hg.
Nausea in throat or abdomen, less frequently in stomach.	Nausea, partic. in stomach, less frequently in œsophagus.
Scentless flatus	Fetid flatus.
False labor pains, with headache and redness of face.	False labor pains with urging to urinate and to stool. Lippe.
Respiration low, *or* rattling	Respirat. loud, but without rattl'g of mucus.
Expectoration infrequent	Expectoration not constant.

REMISSION after midnight and in *forenoon*.	REMIS. of complaints, evening till midnight.
Worse from being overhurried	Worse when idle *or* fr. being overhurried †.
Worse from light, partic. candle light . .	Worse from light, partic. day light.
Worse when sneezing	*Worse or* better when sneezing.
Worse during sweat	*Worse or* better during sweat.
Almost always aggrav. when swallowing .	*Worse or* better when swallowing.
Worse when swallowing, partic. swallowing drink.	Worse when swallowing food, and when swallowing saliva, often better when swallowing drink.
Worse after drinking	*Worse or* better after drinking
Worse from heat of sun	Worse in snowy air.
Ailments from Mercury, sting of insects or contagious anthrax.	Ailments from Arsenic or Copper vapors, from Sulph. or Phosph.

Predomin. worse —— **Predomin. better**

From lying on the left side, after sleeping ‡, from washing and moistening the diseased part, when sitting erect, from warm diet, and when swallowing drink.

Predomin. better —— **Predomin. worse**

From lying on right side, when turning in bed, sitting bent forward, and from cold diet. §

---

* In delirium tremens both remedies have great restlessness, which does not permit the patient to remain in any one place: vertigo, trembling, bitter taste, disgust for meat, pain in the stomach, and other symptoms; therefore the one has often been given when the other should have been, and thus the cure was retarded. C. Hg.

† These symptoms are not opposites here, but are both caused by the *same* state of mind: impatience

‡ We find however with Nux vom., complaints after sleeping *too long* —The improvement of Nux vom. complaints follow only after *sufficient* sleep; when roused, the complaints are aggravated.

§ Bellad. also has aggrav. from drinking *cold water*, because it has difficulty in *swallowing drink*.

Belladonna.	Opium.
Dark hair—Heat, with aversion to being uncovered.	Light hair—Heat, with inclination for being uncovered.
Pulse generally quick, full, hard, and tense.	Pulse varying; full and slow, with snoring respiration; quick and hard, with heat and quick respiration.
Thirst not constant; most rare during chill, more frequent *before* chill.	Want of thirst; thirst almost only between heat and sweat.
Anxious dreams	Dreams predominantly pleasant . . . .
Complaints predominant on upper lip and on upper arm.	Complaints predominant on under lip and on fore-arm.
Merry or dejected and despondent . . .	Cheerfulness and boldness—Gentleness *or* rage.
Mood distrustful, peevish, irritable, malicious. H.Gr.	Imbecility of will, as though annihilated. C. Hg.
Difficult comprehension—Cannot express a thought, without first saying something foolish.	Easy *or* difficult comprehension—Says nothing but "yes."
Ailments from mortification	Ailments from excessive joy, or from shame.*
Nausea in throat or abdomen, rarely in stomach.	Very rarely nausea.
Scentless flatus predominant	Fetid flatus.
Respiration predominantly low	Respiration predominantly loud.
Expectoration infrequent; morning, during day, evening.	Expectoration infrequent; during day.
REMISSION after midnight and in *forenoon*.	REMISSION during day and evening.
Better (resp. worse) when lying on back, *or* on side.	Better when lying on back, worse when lying on side.
Worse or better when assuming an erect position.	Worse when assuming an erect position.
Ailments from Mercurius, Iodine or abuse of Cinchona, from sting of insects or contagious Anthrax.	Ailments from charcoal vapors, Strychnine, or Digitalis.

Predomin. worse —— **Predomin. better**

In the open air, from being uncovered, from cold, from growing cold, and in cold weather, from motion,† when walking, and from drinking coffee.

Predomin. better —— **Predomin. worse**

In-doors, from wrapping up, from warmth, from growing warm, and in warm air, during rest, after lying down, in bed, when lying, sitting, and standing.

N.B. Predominant painlessness characterizes the effects of Opium, and over-sensitiveness to pain Belladonna. Yet with Belladonna, whose constitutional character is rather vascillating, we also find sensation of numbness, probably only in parts that were painful at first.

* Both remedies have aggravation "*when moving the diseased part.*"

† Opium also has epileptic fits from fear or fright, or after bitter reproaches. C.Hg.

Belladonna.	Phosphor.
Upper left, lower right side—Obesity . .	Upper right, lower left side—Emaciation—Fat only in single internal parts.
Often indicat. with children a. young women.	Often indicated with old people.
Hæmorrhages—Blood coagulates easily .	Hæmorrhages — Blood uncoagulable, or coagulates slowly.
Apoplexia sanguinea—Apoplexy more frequent than paralysis.	Apoplexia nervosa — Paralysis more frequent than apoplexy.
Paralysis often only one-sided	Paralysis generally of both sides.
Humid cutaneous eruptions	Dry eruptions.
Pulse equal	Pulse unequal.
Heat or sweat, with aversion to being uncovered.	Heat or sweat, with inclination for being uncovered.
Heat descend'g; sweat on upper part of body.	H. ascend'g*; sweat on lower part of body.
Thirst not constant; rare during chill; more frequent *before* chill and *after* sweat.	Almost constant want of thirst.
Chill increased out-doors; heat and sweat lessened in-doors.	Chill lessened out-doors; heat and sweat increased in-doors.
Love of being alone	Fear of being alone.
Fear of apoplexy or of being poisoned . .	Fear of apoplexy or of loss of reason.
Distrust	Haughtiness—Amativeness (more than Bel.)
Mental excitability *or* dullness.	Mental excitability predominant.
Spasms, partic. in the side not paralysed .	Spasms, particularly in the paralysed side.
Hydrocephalus acutus	Hydrocephaloid.
Eyes protruding—Pupils most frequently dilated—Far-sightedness.	Eyes sunken—Pupils generally contracted—Short-sightedness.
Complaints predominant on upper lip . .	Complaints predominant on under lip
Tongue and pituitary membrane of the mouth red.	Tongue and pituitary membrane of mouth most frequently white.
Aversion to sour things; appetite for salt fish.	Appetite for sour things; aversion to salt fish.
Nausea in throat or abdomen, rarely stomach.	Nausea in stomach.
Voice raised or nasal	Voice trembling or hissing.
Expectoration infrequent; morning, during day, and evening.	Expectoration not constant; morning and during day.
REMISSION after midnight and in *forenoon*.	REMISSION of complaints after midnight.
Worse during full moon	Worse before a thunder-storm.
Predominantly better in bed	Worse *or* better in bed.
Better (or worse) when lying on the painful *or* on unpainful side.	Worse when lying on painful side, better when lying on unpainful side.
Worse during sleep	Worse *or* better during sleep.
Predomin. worse on awaking from sleep .	*Better or* worse on awaking, particularly worse after the siesta.
Generally improved after getting out of bed.	Worse *or* better after getting out of bed.
Worse dur'g sweat, generally better *after* it.	Dur'g sweat better *or* worse, worse *after* it.
Worse *or* better from wine	Better from drinking wine.
Ailments from Mercurius, from abuse of Cinchona, or from animal poisons.	Ailments from abuse of table-salt.

Predomin. worse — **Predomin. better**

During twilight, in dry weather, out of doors, from being uncovered, after drinking, from drinking cold water, from drinking beer, from the touch, when sitting erect, when lifting or resting the diseased limb on anything, when drawing up the diseased limb, and after sleep.

Predomin. better — **Predomin. worse**

In wet weather, in-doors, from wrapping up, from pressure, when sitting bent forward, letting the diseased limb hang down, when stretching it out, when bending the suffering part backwards, from change of position, and after sweat.

* Belladonna has chills creeping up the back and down the front of body. Phosphor has heat the same. C.Hg.

Belladonna.	Phosph. acid.
Aversion * to exercise—Obesity	Inclination for exercise—Emaciation.
Rending pain upwards—Apoplexy	Rending pain downwards—No apoplexy.
Painful swelling of glands	Painless swelling of glands.
Ulcers with scanty discharge	Ulcers with copious discharge.
Pulse generally quick, full, hard, and tense.	Pulse generally quick, small, and weak; in general irregular.
Thirst not constant, rare during chill, more frequent *before* chill and *after* sweat.	Thirst infrequent, almost only during sweat; is wanting during chill.
Sweat on front part of body	Sweat on back part of body.
Complaints predom. on lower jaw and lower teeth, on *roof of mouth* in upper part of chest, on upper arm, in hollow of elbow, and on patella.	Complaints predom. on upper jaw and upper teeth on soft palate, in lower part of chest, on fore arm and on tip of elbow.

Belladonna.	Phosph. acid.
Mood changing; distrustful	Mood very rarely irritable or malicious.
Memory active *or* weak	Weak memory.
Mental excitability—Ecstacies—Insanity.	Mental dullness—Imbecility.
Ailments from fright, anger, or from vexation with fright, fear, or vehemence.	Ailments from grief, disappointed love, and jealousy, shame, or from vexation with reserved displeasure.
Vertigo inclining to fall backwards or sideways.	Vertigo inclining to fall backwards or forwards.
Eyes protruding—Farsightedness	Eyes sunken—Shortsightedness.
Eruption on upper lip	Eruption on under lip.
Gums and mucous membrane of mouth red.	Gums & mucous membrane of mouth white.
Nausea in throat or abd'n, rarely in stom'ch.	Nausea in throat, rarely in stomach.
Milk most frequently increased	Milk decreased or spoiled.
Expectoration infrequent; morning, during day, evening.	Expectoration with the cough almost constant; morning.

Belladonna.	Phosph. acid.
REMISSION *forenoon* and after midnight.	REMISSION afternoon and before midnight.
Better (resp. worse) when lying on the painful or unpainful side.	Worse when lying on painful side, better when lying on unpainful side.
Almost always improved after getting out of bed.	Worse *or* better after getting out of bed.
Predom. worse when growing cold, better when growing warm.	Better *or* worse when growing cold, (resp. warm.)
Worse from heat of sun	Worse in snowy air.

Predomin. worse — **Predomin. better**

Out of doors, and when walking out doors, from exercise generally, when walking, moving the diseased part, when lifting the suffering limb, when eating and swallowing †.

Predomin. better — **Predomin. worse**

In doors, during rest, after lying down, in bed, and from warmth of bed, when lying, sitting, and standing, when letting the diseased limb hang down, and when stooping.

N.B. Oversensitiveness to pain is frequent with Bellad., infrequent with Phosph. ac.

---

* Bellad. sometimes has inclination for continual motion in single or suffering parts.

† Bellad. has aggrav. when swallowing drink; Phosph. ac., aggrav. when swallowing food.

Belladonna.	Pulsatilla.
Aversion to open air—Apoplexia sanguinea .	Inclination for open air—Apoplexia nervosa.
No suppuration; ulcers with scanty discharge.	Suppuration; ulcers with copious discharge.
Coldness of the painful part	Heat of the painful part.
Pulse predominantly strong	Pulse predominantly weak; sometimes imperceptible.
Sweat on front part of body	Sweat often confined to back part of body.
Sweat increased after sleep	Sweat lessened after sleep.
Sweat, sometimes only in bed	Sometimes much sweat, except in bed, when it appears only on falling asleep, and disappears on awaking.
Sweat all over body, except the head . . .	Sweat only on head.
Thirst remaining *after* the sweat	Thirst *between* the different stages, particularly between chill and heat.
The hands often under the head during sleep .	The arms often *above* the head during sleep.

Belladonna.	Pulsatilla.
Satiety of life, with longing for death . . .	Satiety of life, with fear of death.
Mood cheerful *or* sad; irritable; malicious .	Disposition good-natured, but bold; calm sadness of gentle dispositions—Amativeness—Greediness.
Consequences of anger	Consequences of grief.
Memory active *or* weak	Weak memory.
Vertigo, inclining to fall sideways (left side) or backwards.	Vertigo, inclining to fall backwards.
Growing black before the eyes when rising after lying.	Growing black before the eyes while lying.
Far-sightedness—Eyes protruding	Short-sightedness—Eyes sunken.
Pupils oftener dilated than contracted . . .	Pupils oftener contracted than dilated.
Swelling, etc., predominant on *upper* lip . .	Swelling, etc., predominant on *under* lip.
Desire for milk—Avers. to beer and sour things.	Avers. to milk—Appet. for beer or sour things.
Hiccough, with eructation at the same time .	Hicc., alternat'g with paroxysms of suffocation.
Scentless flatus—Diarrhœa predom. painless .	Fetid flatus—Diarrhœa generally painful.
Catam. too soon, profuse, of long duration . .	Catam. too late, scanty, of short duration.
Spasmodic labor-pains, with heat, rigidity and contraction of the os tincæ, or with inclusion of some parts of the child.	Deficient labor-pains, with relaxed and open os tincæ, somnolence, etc., *or* spasmodic labor-pains, with the same concomitants.
Dry coryza (except during sweating stage of fever.)	Coryza fluent (particularly right side) oftener than dry.
Respiration predominantly low	Respiration loud.
Expectoration infrequent; morning, during day and evening.	Expectoration predominant, but not constant; morning and during day.
Upper part of chest predominant	Lower part of chest predominant.
The horse has a restless eye, stares, does not allow the forefeet to be examined, refuses to be mounted, overturns himself.	The horse is sensitive to the touch, particularly on the ears, and, therefore, cannot be bridled.

Belladonna.	Pulsatilla.
Remission after midnight and in *forenoon* . .	Remission from midnight till noon.
Worse during sweat, better afterwards . . .	*Worse during and after* sweat.
Worse during full moon and from exertion. .	Worse before a thunder-storm—Oftener improved than aggravated by bodily exertion.
Worse, particularly when swallowing drink .	Worse when swallowing saliva.

Predomin. worse — **Predomin. better**

In dry weather, out-doors, from cold, from growing cold, from being uncovered, from exercise, bending the suffering part sideways, lying on painful side, from washing or moistening the diseased part, from weeping, from sour things, and when sitting erect.

Predomin. better — **Predomin. worse**

In wet weather, in-doors, from warmth, from growing warm, wrapping up, during rest, when standing, sitting, and lying, particularly when sitting bent forward, when lying on unpainful side, bending the diseased part backwards, from change of position, picking the teeth, and after sweat.

Belladonna.	Rhus.
Complaints of internal parts predominant . .	Complaints of external parts predominant.
Aversion to motion—Dark hair	Inclination for motion—Light hair.
Apoplexy more frequent than paralysis . . .	Paralysis more frequent than apoplexy.
Ulcers, with scanty discharge	Ulcers, with copious discharge; partic. on the dropsical legs spontaneous disch. of water.
Cold on painful part	Sweat on suffering side.
Pulse predominantly strong—Sweat right side.	Pulse predominantly weak—Sweat left side.
Thirst rare dur'g chill—Heat lessened in-doors.	Thirst not constant—Heat increased in-doors.

Mood cheerful *or* sad; indifferent; peevish; irritable; malicious; distrustful.	Dejection.
Satiety of life, with longing for death . . .	Satiety of life, with fear of death.
Memory active *or* weak	Weak memory.
Vertigo, inclining to fall backwards or sideways (left side.)	Vertigo, inclining to fall backwards or forwards.
Horses: Water on the brain, with a staring look.	Horses: Water on the brain, with jerk'g of head.
Complaints predomin. in upper part of chest, on upper arm, shin, and on sole of foot.	Complaints predominant in lower part of chest, on fore-arm, calf of leg, and top of foot.
Nausea in throat or abdomen, rarely in stomach.	Nausea in œsophagus or stomach, rarely in throat.
Diarrhœa predominantly painless	Diarrhœa generally painful.
Urine oftener dark than pale	Urine pale.
Coryza predominantly dry (except during the sweating stage of fever.)	Fluent coryza.
Respiration predominantly low	Respiration loud.
Expectoration infrequent; morning, during day, evening.	Expectoration not constant; morning.

REMISSION after midnight and during *forenoon.*	REMISSION of complaints during day.
Worse during full moon	Worse during increase of moon.
Better in bed and from warmth of bed . . .	Oftener improved than aggravated in bed and by warmth of bed.
Better (worse) when lying on back *or* side . .	Worse when lying on back, better lying on side.
Better (worse) when lying on painful *or* unpainful side.	Better when lying on painful side, worse when lying on unpainful side.
Worse or better when assum. an erect position.	Generally worse when assum. an erect position.
Worse when getting out of bed	Better *or* worse when getting out of bed.
Almost always impr. *after* getting out of bed.	*Worse or* better *after* getting out of bed.
Worse *or* better after sweat	*Better* after sweat.
Worse after drinking	*Worse or* better after drinking.
Worse after stool	*Better or* worse after stool.
Better when sitting down	*Worse or* better when sitting down.
Ailments from sleep'g in the sun or moonlight.	Ailments from sleeping on damp ground.
Worse when swallowing, particularly drink .	Worse when swallowing food and swall. saliva.

Predomin. worse ⏟ **Predomin. better**

In dry weather, when moving, walking, moving the diseased part, and when walking in the open air,* from warm diet, when sitting erect, and after breakfast.

Predomin. better ⏟ **Predomin. worse**

In wet weather, during rest, after lying down, when lying, sitting, and standing, from cold† diet, when sitting bent forward, when stooping, bending the diseased part backwards, from change of position, from eructation, and before breakfast.

N.B. Rhus has not the over-sensitiveness to pain of Belladonna; Belladonna has not the sensation of numbness in suffering parts.

---

* Here motion decides; for both remedies have aggrav. in the open air generally, improvement of complaints in-doors

† Belladonna also has aggrav. from drinking cold water, because of difficulty in *swallowing drink.*

Belladonna. Stramonium.

Belladonna.	Stramonium.
Right side predom.—Generally dark hair .	*Left* side—Generally light hair.
Obesity—Apoplexia sanguinea	Emaciation—Apoplexia nervosa.
Paralysis often painful, one-sided	Paralysis generally painless & of both sides
Painful eruptions	Painless eruptions.
Pulse sometimes intermittent and slow with quick respiration.	Pulse sometimes double and very quick with quiet respiration.
When the pulse becomes slow, it is full . .	When the pulse becomes slow, it is weak.
Thirst very rare during chill, often *before* chill and continues *after* sweat.	Thirst during heat and sweat and between both stages; none during chill.
Drinks often, but little at a time	Drinks seldom, but much at a time.
Inflammation of brain with aggrav. when lying down.	Inflammation of brain with improvement when lying, involuntary movements of the head and frequ't raising of middle of body.

Belladonna.	Stramonium.
Love of being alone	Fear of being alone.
Fear of being poisoned or of apoplexy—Distrust—Ailments from anger.	Fear of loss of reason — Haughtiness — Amativeness—Ailm. fr. hearing bad news.
Memory very active *or* very weak.	Weak memory.
Farsightedness	Shortsightedness.
Painful jerking of single muscles of the face.	Painless jerking of single muscles of the face.
Complaints predom. on *roof of mouth* and on *upper* arm.	Complaints predom. on *soft* palate, and on fore-arm.
Aversion to sour things	Appetite for sour things*.
Scentless flatus	Fetid flatus.
Urine oftener dark than pale—Incontinence more frequent than retention of urine.	Urine pale — Retention of urine more frequent than involuntary discharge.
Catamenia predom. too soon	Catamenia predom. too late.
Puerperal convulsions with congestions to the head.	Puerperal convulsions with copious sweating. Lippe.
Respiration predom. low	Respiration loud.
HORSES stare and have a restless look; refuse to have their fore-feet examined or to be mounted; overturn themselves.	HORSES: Uneasy with the least noise, likes to run off, bites and kicks with very quick motions.

Belladonna.	Stramonium.
REMISSION after midnight and in *forenoon.*	Aggrav. night and morning — REMISSION during day and evening.
Worse from light, partic. candle light . .	Improved quite as often as aggrav. by light; worse partic. from sun-light.
Worse in Spring	Worse in the Autumn.

Predomin. worse ——— **Predomin. better**

From sour things, lying on left side, and when lying on painful side.

Predomin. better ——— **Predomin. worse**

When stooping, from external pressure, lying on right side, and when lying on unpainful side.

N.B. Stram. has not the oversensitiveness to pain of Bellad. in accordance with the predom. characteristic of constitutional want of irritability, which is peculiar to Stramon. H.Gr. Except with paronychiæ and other suppurations where on the contrary the greatest sensitiveness to pain indicates Stramon. C.Hg.

---

* Acids are not antidotes in cases of poisoning with Bellad., but are antidotal to poisoning with Stramon. C.Hg.

Belladonna.	Sulphur.
Apoplexy more frequent than paralysis . . .	Paralysis more frequent than apoplexy.
Paralysis oftener one-sided—Rending pain upwards.	Paralysis oftener both sides—Rending pain downwards.
External parts become black	Red parts become white.
Humid eruptions	Eruptions generally dry.
Painful swelling of glands	Painless swelling of glands.
Sweat sometimes only on front part of body .	Sweat sometimes only on back part of body.
Sweat right side—Cold shudders, or heat descending.	Sweat left side—Cold shudders, or heat ascending.
Sweat often general, with exception of head .	Heat sometimes general, with except. of head.
Sweat increased after sleep	Sweat lessened after sleep.
Heat or sweat, with aversion to uncover . .	Heat or sweat, with inclination to uncover.
Generally insensibility of disposition . . .	Sensitiveness of disposition.
Silly merriness—Distrust—Malice	Seriousness.
Cannot express a thought without first saying something foolish.	Says something different from what was intended, or repeats all the words spoken to him on account of difficult comprehension.
Ecstasies—Memory active *or* weak	Ailm. from hearing bad news—Weak memory.
Periodical vertigo every morning; ceases after copious nose-bleeding.	Vertigo, with nose-bleeding C.Hg.
Hot spots on the head	A cold spot on the head.
Eyes protruding—Complaints on inner angle of eye — Pupils generally dilated — Far-sightedness.	Eyes generally sunken—Complaints predominant on external angle of eye—Pupils generally contracted—Short-sightedness.
Nausea in throat or abdom., rarely in stomach.	Nausea, partic. in stomach, rarely in throat.
Scentless flatus	Fetid flatus.
Voice hoarse or raised	Voice hoarse or deeper than usual.
Respiration predominantly low	Respiration predominantly loud.
Expectoration infrequent; morning, during day, evening.	Expectoration not constant; morning and during day, less frequently at night.
Milk generally increased	Milk decreased.
Complaints predominant on upper arm, on outer side of thigh, and on shin.	Complaints predominant on fore-arm, on inner side of thigh, and on calf of leg.
REMISSION after midnight and in *forenoon* . .	REMISSION before midnight and in *afternoon*.
Worse from heat of sun	Worse in snowy air.
Worse in the open air, better in-doors . . .	Better (resp. worse) in the open air *or* in-doors.*
Worse when growing cold and in cold weather, better when growing warm and in warm air.	Better *or* worse when growing cold and in cold weather (growing warm and in warm air.)
Almost always improv. after gett'g out of bed.	Worse *or* better after getting out of bed.
Worse when resting the diseased limb on anything.	Oftener improved than aggravated when resting the limb on anything.
Better or worse when bend'g the diseased part.	Worse when bending the suffering part.
Predom. imp. when stretch'g the diseased limb.	Mostly aggrav. when stretching out the limb.
Worse when moving the diseased part . . .	Worse *or* better when moving diseased part.
Almost always aggravated by the touch . .	*Worse or* better from the touch.
Worse when looking sideways	Worse when looking downwards.
Worse when swallowing drink	Worse when swall. dry food and on swall. saliva.
Ailments from Iodine or from animal poisons, from Ferrum, Plumbum, Cuprum, Platina, Aconitum, or Hyoscyam.	Ailments from abuse of metallic substances, from Iod., Cinchona, Rhus, Nitr. acid., or Sepia.

Predomin. worse ——— **Predomin. better**

In dry weather, from cold, being uncovered, when getting out of bed, when drawing up the diseased limb, when sitting erect, and from warm diet

Predomin. better ——— **Predomin. worse**

In wet weather, from warmth and warmth of bed†, from wrapping up, after lying down, when lying, from change of position‡, when bending the diseased part backwards, while standing, from cold diet§, when stretching out the suffering part, and when sitting bent forward.

* Sulphur complaints are improved by warmth of stove, and aggravated in a crowded room.
† "*In bed*" generally Sulphur complaints are as often improved as aggravated
‡ Sulphur-symptoms are almost as often improved as aggravated "*when turning in bed.*"
§ Belladonna also has aggravation from drinking *cold water* on account of having difficulty in *swallowing drink.*

Borax.	**Nux vom.**
Light hair—Skin and muscles lax . . .	Dark hair—Skin and muscles rigid.
Want of bodily irritability—Inclination for open air.	Increased bodily irritability—Aversion to open air.
Pulse often unchanged	Pulse generally quick, full, and hard.
Heat or sweat, with inclination to uncover .	Heat or sweat, with aversion to uncover.
Sweat increased during sleep—Heat after sleep.	Sweat lessened during sleep—Heat lessened after sleep.
Thirst not constant; is generally wanting during the chill.	Most thirst during the chill; thirst also before and after the fever, and between heat and sweat.
Skin getting callous	Skin getting sore. C.Hg
Apoplexy or paralysis not yet observed .	Apoplexy—Paralysis.
Affections of the spleen predominant . .	Affections of the liver predominant.
Painless diarrhœa	Constipation predominant; when diarrhœa occurs, it is painful and scanty.
Sexual desire too weak	Sexual desire too strong.
During pregnancy swelling, itching, and burning of the vagina, with a discharge like gonorrhœa. Bute.	During pregnancy an internal swelling of the vagina, in most cases one-sided, like a prolapsus, with burning shooting pains, worse from the touch. C.Hg.
False labor-pains or spasmodic labor, with frequent eructations.	Spasmodic labor-pains, with urging to urinate, or to stool. Lippe.
Galactorrhœa; milk coagulating	Galactorrhœa; milk spoiled. C.Hg.
Disagreeable sensation of emptiness in mammæ after suckling the child. Guernsey.	Violent, painful drawing in the nipples; worse when suckling. C.Hg.
Nipples aphthous	Nipples whitish in the centre, without suppuration. C.Hg.
Fluent coryza	Generally dry coryza, particularly in the open air; fluent coryza in-doors.
Complaints predominant on upper arm . .	Complaints predominant on fore-arm.
Remission night and forenoon	Remission evening till midnight.
Worse from light, particularly candle-light.	Worse from light, particularly daylight.
Worse after sleep	Worse on awaking, when roused from sleep; but better after sufficient and not too long sleep.
Almost always improved after getting out of bed.	Worse or better after getting out of bed.
Worse when eating	*Better or* worse when eating.
Worse when swallowing	Worse while *or* when not swallowing.
Better from eructation	Worse *or* better from eructation.
Worse when sneezing	*Worse or* better when sneezing.
Better *or* worse after stool	Worse after stool.
Worse when stooping	Better *or* worse when stooping.
Generally aggrav. by washing and moistening the diseased part.	Generally improved by washing and moistening the diseased part.

Predomin. worse — **Predomin. better**

In wet weather, in-doors, from wrapping up, after lying down, while lying, in bed, after sleep, from warm diet, on inspiration, when lifting up the diseased limb, and from washing and moistening the diseased part.

Predomin. better — **Predomin. worse**

In dry weather, out-doors, from being uncovered, when assuming an erect position, from cold diet, on expiration, and when letting the diseased limb hang down.

N.B. Borax has not the over-sensitiveness of Nux vom. to pain, which is entirely in accordance with the constitutional character of both remedies.

Brom.	Ammon. carb.
L. ⟶ R.	R. ⟶ L. C.Hg.
Pulse very much accelerated	Pulse quick, hard, and tense.
Complaints of external nose predominant .	Complaints of inner nose.
Coryza, with stoppage of right nostril . .	Coryza, with stop. of left nostr. or both. CHg.
Sexual desire too strong	Sexual desire too weak.
Catamenia too soon and generally profuse—Menstrual blood bright-red.	Catamenia predomin. too late and scanty—Menstrual blood dark.
AGGRAV. of complaints even'g till midnight.	AGGRAV. of symptoms morn'g and even'g.
Worse from cold diet.	Worse from warm diet.
Predominantly better after eating . .	Predominantly worse after eating.
Worse from external pressure	Predominantly better from pressure.
Better from exertion	Worse from bodily exertion.

N.B. Brom. seems to lack the over-sensitiveness to pain of Ammon.

Brom.	Hepar s. c.
Affections of the glands, without suppuration.	Affections of the glands, with suppuration.
Pulse very much accelerated	Pulse quick, full, and hard; sometimes intermitting.
Thirst seems to be wanting.	Thirst predominant, but not constant; most rare during chill.
No delirium	Delirium.
Involuntary seminal emissions	Efflux of succus prostat.
Sexual desire strong	Sexual desire weak.
Coryza generally fluent	Dry coryza.
Respiration with dry sound	Respiration oftener with moist than dry sound.
Expectoration infrequent	Expectoration not constant.
AGGRAVATION of complaints, particularly evening till midnight.	REMISSION afternoon—AGGRAVATIONS occur at all other times of the day or night.
Worse when swallowing *drink;* less frequently when swallowing food or saliva.	Worse when swallowing food and when swallowing saliva.

Predomin. worse ——— **Predomin. better**

In wet weather, and when bending the diseased limb.

Predomin. better ——— **Predomin. worse**

In dry weather, from bodily exertion, from riding, drinking coffee, and after eating.

Brom.	Iod.
Left side, partic. ~~*upper left, lower right*~~ *side.*	~~*Right*~~ side, partic. *upper right, lower left side.*
Blue eyes; light hair	Brown eyes; dark hair. C.Hg.
Itching lessened by scratching	Itching, unchanged by scratching.
Pulse quick	Pulse accelerated, (partic. by every movement,) at the same time oftener large and full, than weak and like a thread.
Thirst seems to be wanting	Thirst, partic. during sweat.
Respiration with dry sound	Respiration predom. with moist sound—Expiration aggravates.
Cough generally without expectoration	Cough generally with expectoration
AGGRAVATION of symptoms, evening till midnight.	REMISSION forenoon and before midnight.

Predomin. worse — **Predomin. better**

In cold weather, from being uncovered, and on inspiration.

Predomin. better — **Predomin. worse**

In warm air, from wrapping up, from running, from bodily exertion in general, and on expiration.

Brom.	Spongia.
Itching, lessened by scratching	Itching, unchanged *or* aggrav., *or* changed to another part of body by scratching.
Pulse very much accelerated	Pulse very quick, full, and hard.
Thirst seems to be wanting	Thirst predom., but not constant.
Quick comprehension	Difficult comprehension.
Saliva increased	Saliva generally decreased.
Fluent coryza	Dry coryza.
Complaints of right lung	Complaints of left lung.
AGGRAVATION of symptoms evening till midnight.	AGGRAVATION afternoon and before midnight.

Predomin. worse — **Predomin. better**

In wet weather, when lying on left side, when rising from a seat, and when swallowing.

Predomin. better — **Predomin. worse**

In dry weather, when lying on right side, from rubbing and scratching, and from bodily exertion.

N B. It seems, Brom. has not the sensation of numbness in suffering parts that we find with Spong.

Bryonia.	Lycopodium.
Sensitiveness in internal parts	Insensibility or sensation of numbness in external parts.
Complaints predom. on external ear, on underlip, in lower part of chest, on upper-arm, and on front part of thigh.	Complaints predom. in inner ear, on upper lip, in upper part of chest, on fore-arm, and on back part of thigh.
Erysipelas or œdema around the joints . .	Sweat around the joints.
Cutaneous eruptions generally dry . . .	Eruptions generally humid.
Pulse quick at night, slow during the day.	Pulse quick in the even'g, slow in the morn'g.
Heat or cold, partic. in right side of body.	Heat or chill, partic. in left side.
Burning sensation in the veins	Sensation of coldness in the veins.
Thirst predom., but not constant; drinks much at a time.	Thirst is wanting only during chill; drinks little at a time.
Irritable mood—Dejection	Gentleness—Cheerfulness *or* dejection.
Rarely sensation of numbness in the suffering parts.	Sensation of numbness in the suffering parts very frequent.
Vertigo inclining to fall backwards . . .	Vertigo inclining to fall forward.
Optical illusions in bright or prismat. colors.	Optical illusions in dark colors.
Nausea, partic. in abdomen, less frequently in stomach or œsophagus.	Nausea in stomach.
Fetid flatus	Predom. scentless flatus.
Diarrhœa generally painful	Diarrhœa painless.
Catamenia too soon *or* too late	Catamenia too late.
Oozing out of milk, secret'n gen'ly increased.	Oozing out of milk, secretion scanty.
REMISSION of complaints during day . .	REMIS. after midnight and during *forenoon*.
Worse before a thunder-storm	Worse during new moon.
Worse from light, partic. sun light . . .	Worse from light, partic. candle-light.
Almost always improved in bed and from warmth of bed.	Worse *or* better in bed and from warmth of bed.
Worse or better from change of position .	Worse from change of position.
Worse when getting out of bed or rising from a seat.	Worse *or* better when getting out of bed or rising from a seat.
Better *or* worse when opening the eyes, (or closing them.)	Worse when opening the eyes, better when closing them.
Better *or* worse after drinking	Worse after drinking.
Worse *or* better from eructation	Better from eructation.
Worse *or* better from the touch	Almost always aggrav. by the touch.
Worse *or* better when walking bent forward.	Better when walking bent forward.

Predomin. worse — **Predomin. better**

In dry weather, from cold, in the open air during continued motion, when walking, after getting out of bed or rising from a seat, when lifting up diseased limb, when ascending, when stooping, lying on the unpainful side, from needle-work, and from warm diet.

Predomin. better — **Predomin. worse**

In wet weather, from warmth * in doors, during rest, after lying down, while lying, sitting, and standing, lying on painful side, when letting the diseased limb hang down, when descending, from pressure, from cold diet, drinking cold water, and after stool.

* Both remedies have aggrav. of symptoms as often as improvement, when growing cold and in cold weather, (respect. growing warm and in warm weather.)

Bryonia.	Nux vom.
Light hair—Clonic spasms	Dark hair—Tonic spasms predominant.
Painless ulcers	Ulcers oftener painful than painless.
Sleeplessness prevalent before midnight	Sleeplessness prevalent after midnight.
Pulse quick at night, slow during day	Pulse quick in morning, slower in evening.
One-sided heat; right side	One-sided heat; left side.
Chill or heat on diseased part	Sweat on diseased side.
Chill after sleep—Heat lessened after stool.	Chill less. after sleep—Heat incr. after stool.
Thirst predominant, but not constant; drinks seldom, but much at a time.	Most thirst during chill; drinks often, but little at a time.
Greasy, sour-smelling sweat during sleep, particularly towards morn'g; worse when eating, from the least movement, in cold air, and when the other complaints are aggravated; better during rest.	Fetid sweat on one side of head and face, which feel cold, with decrease of pain, fear, aversion to being uncovered, partic. aft. midn. & towards morn'g; better from wash'g and when sitt'g still in a warm room.
Taciturnity	Loquacity—Amativeness.
Complaints from anger, in the evening	Complaints from anger, in the morning.
Vertigo, inclining to fall backwards	Vert., inclin'g to fall sideways or backwards.
Appetite for sour things—Aversion to greasy food.	Aversion to sour things predominant—Inclination for greasy food.
Nausea in abdomen	Nausea in stomach.
Desire for beer	Inclination for *or* aversion to beer.
After vomiting sensation as if the stomach were distended.	After vomiting continued stretching. [Compare Appendix.]
Urine dark; often but scanty; only exceptionally copious.	Urine generally pale; infrequent and scanty.
Expect. *morn'g* and even'g, rarely dur'g day.	Expectoration from morning till evening.
Complaints predominant on *upper* arm	Complaints predominant on *fore*-arm.
Hardness in groups of muscles affected by neuralgia.	Tetanic tension of single muscles.
Horses: Walk stiff from lameness of joints.	Horses: Walk stiff from lameness of muscles.
Remission of complaints during day	Remission evening till midnight.
Worse in the evening (but some symptoms better in the evening-*twilight.*)	*Worse* in the morning.
Worse when stretching out or bending the diseased limb; also when walking bent forward; *better* when assuming an erect position.	*Worse* when drawing up the diseased limb; *better* when stretching out the diseased limb, when walking bent forward, often also when stooping.*
Generally worse from washing with cold water, but improved by warm baths.	Oftener improved than aggravated by washing.
Sometimes worse, sometimes better from the touch, from growing cold and in cold weather.	*Worse* from the touch, growing cold and in cold weather.
Complaints after bodily exertion.	Complaints after mental exertion. C.Hg.

Predomin. worse — **Predomin. better**

After sleep†, while lying on side, particularly on unpainful side, when walking bent forward, from stretching out the diseased limb, and from warm diet.

Predomin. better — **Predomin. worse**

After stool, when lying on back or on painful side, when drawing up the diseased limb, from cold diet, and on an empty stomach.

---

* "*Aggravations, when assuming an erect position*" and "*when stooping,*" are found with both remedies.

† "*After sleeping too long,*" Nux vom. has aggravation; on awaking (when roused) from sleep, quite as often aggravation as improvement. It is evident from this that improvement only follows after sufficient, but not too long sleep.

Bryonia.	Phosphor.
Light hair — Erysipelas or œdema around the joints.	Dark hair — Vesicles around the joints.
Itching, lessened or unchanged by scratching.	Itching lessened oftener than aggrav. by scratching.
Pulse more equal than with Phosphor. . .	Pulse sometimes double.
Thirst predom.	Want of thirst predom.
Nervous fever with pain in limbs	Painless nervous fever.
Chill after sleep — Heat or chill lessened while sitting.	Chill less after sleep—Heat or chill increased while sitting.
Sweat lessened after stool	Sweat increased after stool.
Dejection—Despondency *	Cheerfulness or dejection — Indifference — Haughtiness.
Weak memory	Pred. active memory.
Optical illusions in bright or prismat. colors.	Optical illusions in black or prismatic colors.
Nausea in abdomen	Nausea in stomach.
Predom. bitter vomit	Generally *sour* vomit.
Fetid flatus—Constipation predom.; when there is diarrhœa, it is generally painful.	Scentless flatus — Generally painless diarrhœa.
Catamenia too profuse	Catamenia too profuse *or* scanty.
Voice often raised or nasal.	Voice often trembling or hissing.
Expectoration not constant; morning and evening, less frequently during day.	Expectoration not constant; *morning* and during day.
Complaints predom. on front side of thigh and on calf of leg.	Complaints predom. on back part of thigh and on shin.
REMISSION of complaints during day . .	REMISSION after midnight.
Better in bed	Worse *or* better in bed.
Most frequently worse when lying on side, better when lying on back	Generally better when lying on side, worse when lying on back.
Generally worse when lying on unpainful side, better when lying on painful side.	Generally better when lying on unpainful side, worse when lying on painful side.
Worse or better from change of position.	Worse from change of position.
Worse during sleep	Worse *or* better during sleep.
Generally aggrav. *after sleep*	Gen'ly improv. *after* sleep; but worse after the siesta, and on being roused from sleep.
Worse *or* better when assuming an erect position.	Almost always aggrav. when assuming an erect position.
Predom. worse after getting out of bed . .	Worse *or* better after getting out of bed.
Worse *or* better from touch	Almost always improved by the touch.
Generally improved by pressure	Generally aggrav. by pressure.
Better from rubbing and scratching . . .	*Better or* worse from rubbing & scratching.
Almost always aggrav. after eating, partic. after a satisfying meal.	Worse *or* better after eating, partic. better after a satisfying meal.
Worse *or* better after drinking	Almost always improved after drinking.
Ailm'ts from abuse of Mercury or Cinchona.	Ailments from Iod or table salt

Predomin. worse — **Predomin. better**

In dry weather, in the open air †, when lifting up diseased limb, and after a satisfying meal.

Predomin. better — **Predomin. worse**

In wet weather, in doors, from warmth of bed, when letting the diseased limb hang down, after perspiration, and after stool.

N.B. The sensation of numbness in suffering parts, frequent with Phosph. is rarely found with Bryonia.

* Peevish, irritable mood, is found with both remedies and is predom. with Bryonia.

† Phosph. has aggrav. (in consequence of the motion) as well as improvement "*when walking out doors.*"

Bryonia.	Pulsatilla.
Light hair	Dark hair. Bonnighansen.*
Upper right, lower left side†	Upper left, lower right side.
Aversion to open air	Inclination for open air.
Oftener indicated amongst old people . .	Oftener indicated amongst children.*
Itching, unchanged *or* lessened by scratching.	Itching, unchanged *or* aggrav. by scratching.
Predominant redness of diseased parts . .	Predominant blueness of diseased parts.*
Pressing pain, more from inside outward .	Pressing, crowding pain, more from outside inward.*
A great deal of bursting pain	A great deal of contracting, labor-like pain.*
Pain piercing, compressive; rarely jerking.	Pain as though drawn up with a jerk, then loosened.*
Spasmodic complaints; starting, twitching of the limbs.	Heaviness; numbness; sensation of emptiness or hollowness.*
Fixed, acute rheumatism, aggravated by motion — Travels slowly from joint to joint.	Wandering, acute rheumatism, worse during rest and in the beginning of motion — Pain changing suddenly from joint to joint.*
Stitches in all the serous membranes . . .	Pain dragging, jerking, twinging, and jumping from place to place.*
Inflammation; more of internal parts, with burning, dryness, avidity, heat of internal parts.	More inflammation of external parts, with festering pain, suppurating pain, bruised pain.*
Jaundice	Chlorosis.*
Pulse frequent, full, hard, and tense; frequent at night, slower during day.	Pulse generally quick, small, and weak; frequent at night, slow in the morning.
Chill increased by exercise; sweat after awaking and when walking out-doors.	Chill lessened by exercise; sweat lessened after awaking and when walking out of doors.
Chill and heat in diseased part	Heat in diseased part.
More coldness than chilliness	More chilliness than coldness.*
Chills with the heat	Chills with the pains.*
Thirst predominant, but not constant . .	Want of thirst, particularly during chill; thirst *only* during heat.
Drinks seldom, but much at a time . . .	When thirsty drinks often, but little at a time.

Bryonia.	Pulsatilla.
Peevish irritability. (Hahnemann.*) — Anxious disposition, with fear of want of subsistence. H. Hartlaub.*	Disposition gentle, but bold; chang'g mood; calm, tearful sadness, indifference, distrust, avarice, amativeness, absent-mindedness.
With nocturnal heat, restlessness, fear — Peevish, refractory.	With nocturnal heat, restlessness, fear — Lachrymose, resigned.*
Ailments from anger, or from vexation with vehemence.	Ailments from grief, from vexation with fright, from excessive joy.
Headache predominant in forehead; into the eyes, and down into face.	Headache more in the back of head; to back of neck and shoulders.*
Complaints predominant on external ear, in inner nose, and in palms of hands.	Complaints most frequent in inner ear, on external nose, and on back of hand.
Stitches, more in the hips	Stitches, more in shoulders.*
Tongue viscous, bilious	Tongue white.*
Hard swelling of spleen; rattling, from motion. H. Hartlaub.*	Stitches in the region of liver, particularly when walking.*
Nausea in abdomen	Nausea in throat and stomach, or abdomen.
Vomit, watery, bitter	Vomit, sour.*
Generally constipation	Generally diarrhœa.
Urination frequent but scanty; only exceptionally copious.	Urine infrequent and scanty.

Bryonia.	Pulsatilla.
(Continued.)	
Catamenia too profuse and of long duration.	Cat. predom. too scanty and of too short dur.
When menses do not appear, bleeding from ear and nose.	When menses do not appear, general nervous complaints.*
Milk too plentiful	Milk too scanty.*
Dry coryza	Fluent coryza (partic. right side) oftener than dry coryza.
Respiration predom. with moist sound . .	Respiration predom. with dry sound.
Expectoration brown, like liver; or, in complaints of liver, yellow.	Expectoration greenish or yellow.*
Expectoration *morning* and evening, less frequently during day.	Expectoration morning and during day.
More sleepiness during day	More sleepiness in evening.*
Children dislike to be carried	Children wish to be carried, but slowly.*
In horses: Dung in small balls (hard)—Alternate lameness and swelling of the hock-joins, especially if the feet swell while at rest.	In horses: Dung in large balls (soft)—Alternate lamen. chang'g from one foot to another at short intervals, worse when beginning to move.
During distemper, swelling and coldness of the feet, especially of the hind feet.	During distemper, swelling and coldness of the feet, especially of the fore-feet

---

Bryonia.	Pulsatilla.
Remission of complaints during day . .	Remission from midnight till noon.
Better in the evening-twilight	*Worse* in the evening-twilight.
Worse evening and night	Worse afternoon and evening.*
Some compl. better on an empty stomach .	Some complaints improved after eating.‡
A great many symptoms directly after dinner and during the first half of afternoon.	Afternoon symptoms increase toward evening.*
Nocturnal symptoms, some after nine o'clock, some *after midnight.*	Nocturnal symptoms almost all before midnight.*
Better from loosening the clothes	Predom. better from tightening the clothes.
Cabbage, potatoes, and other vegetables, partic. the nitrogenized, disagree.	Fat (pork), and particularly such animal food which is non-nitrogenized, disagree.*

Predomin. worse ——— **Predomin. better**

In dry weather, from exercise and bodily exertion, when washing and moistening the diseased limb, and when stretching it out.

Predomin better ——— **Predomin. worse**

In cloudy or wet weather, during rest, in bed, after perspiring, and from rubbing and scratching.

N.B. The sensation of numbness in suffering parts peculiar to Pulsatilla is very rarely found with Bryonia.

N.B. Both remedies meet in gastric and rheumatic affections, and in swellings of the knee; Bryonia is more effectual in gout; Pulsatilla is preferable in hæmorrhoids; Bryon. acts more on the arteries and articular synovial membranes, Pulsatilla more on the veins. (H. Hartlaub.) Bryonia more on the functions of the eye, Pulsatilla more on the organic parts of the eye; Bryonia alone has the buccal eruption. Pulsatilla the earache; Bryonia has more swelling of the feet, Pulsatilla of the face; Pulsatilla has many changes of taste, while Bryonia has only the bitter taste with liver-complaints; the inflammations of the eye are drier, more rheumatic or gouty with Bryonia, with Pulsatilla humid, catarrhal, scrofulous; on the heart, testicles, and ovaries, Pulsatilla acts almost alone.* (Bryonia more on the pericardium. J. C. Morgan.)

N.B. * added by C.Hg.

---

† Both remedies have pains in joints, in the upper right, lower left side, but these pains are very different. Bryonia has more chill right side, and more pain left side; Pulsatilla has sweat on upper right and lower left side.*

‡ "Aggravation after eating" is found with both remedies.

Bryonia.	Rhododendron.
Lower left, upper right side	Upper left, lower right side.
Complaints of internal parts predom.—Pain pressing outwards.	Complaints of external parts predom.—Pain pressing inwards.
Increased bodily irritability—Aversion to open air.	Want of bodily irritability—Inclination for open air.
Plethora—Hot swelling of glands . . .	Anæmie—Cold swelling of glands.
Apoplexy	No apoplexy.
Pulse accelerated, full, hard, and tense, sometimes intermitting.	Pulse often unchanged; generally slow and weak.
Thirst predom., but not constant	Thirst is almost always wanting.
Sleeplessness preval. before midnight . .	Sleeplessness after midnight.
Anxious dreams	Pleasant dreams.

Bryonia.	Rhododendron.
Complaints predom. in the liver	Complaints predom. in spleen.
Diarrhœa generally painful	Diarrhœa painless.
Expectoration not constant; *morning* and evening, less frequently during day.	Expectoration infrequent; *night*, less in the evening and morning.
Complaints predom. on upper arm and calf of leg.	Complaints predom. on fore-arm and shin.

Bryonia.	Rhododendron.
Remission of complaints during day . .	Remis. *during day* and before midnight.
Worse *or* better from the touch	Worse from the touch.
Worse or better from growing cold and in cold weather, (or growing warm and in warm air.)	Worse from growing cold & in cold weather; better when growing warm and in warm air.
Worse when eating	Worse *or* better when eating.
Predom. worse from warm diet, better from cold diet and drinking cold water.	Predom. worse from cold diet and drinking cold water; sometimes however worse also from warm diet.

Predomin. worse ——— **Predomin. better**

In dry weather, out doors, during continued exercise, when walking, when ascending, when moving, stretching out, washing or moistening the diseased limb, after sleep, *after* getting out of bed or rising from a seat, and after breakfast.

Predomin. better ——— **Predomin. worse**

In wet weather, in doors, during rest, after lying down, in bed,* when lying, sitting, and standing, when descending, when drawing up diseased limb, on an empty stomach, and after stool.

N.B. In accordance with the character of constitutional want of irritability, which is peculiar to Rhodod., this remedy lacks the oversensitiveness to pain of the Bryonia-patient.

---

* The painful symptoms of Rhododed. are also often improved by *warmth* of bed.

Bryonia.	Rhus.
Upper right, lower left side — Complaints (pressing, cutting pain, &c.) predom. in *internal* parts.	Upper left, lower right side — Complaints (pressing, cutting pain, &c.) predom. in *external* parts.
Itching, unchang'd *or* improv. by scratch'g.	Itching, improved by scratching.
Eruptions generally dry	Eruptions generally humid.
Erysipelas around the joints	Itching of the skin on the outer side of joints.
Eruption predom. on *under* lip . . .	Eruption predom. on *upper* lip.
Pulse quick, full, hard, and tense	Pulse generally accelerated, weak and soft.
Chill or heat on diseased part	Sweat on suffering side.
Coldness of right side	Coldness of left side.
Heat, then chill—Thirst predom. and drinks much at a time.	Chill, then heat—Thirst not constant, drinks little at a time.
Chill lessened by drinking — Chill or heat lessened when sitting.	Chill increased by drinking. Chill or heat increased when sitting.
Peevishness—Ailm. fr. anger, mortification, or of vexation with fear or vehemence.	Sadness and dejection—Ailments from vexation with fear.
Vertigo inclining to fall backwards . . .	Vertigo inclining to fall forwards or backwards.
Desire for spirituous liquors	Aversion to spirituous liquors*.
Nausea in abdomen, less frequently in stomach or œsophagus.	Nausea in œsophagus or stomach, less frequently in throat.
Incarceration of a hernia after eating cold fruit.	Incarceration of hernia from falling, overstraining, or fr. taking cold by moisture, with meteorism, paralysis, or typhoid inflammation of an intestine.
Costiveness predom.	Diarrhœa.
Urine dark; often, but scanty; only exceptionally copious.	Urine pale; often and copious.
Pred. dry coryza — Abdominal respiration.	Fluent coryza—Thoracic respiration.
Respiration pred. with moist sound . . .	Respiration with dry sound.
Expector. morn. & even., rarely during day.	Expectoration chiefly in morning.
Complaints of inner nose predom.	Complaints of external oftener than of inner nose.
Catamenia too soon *or* too late	*Catamenia* too soon.
Complaints predom. on upper arm, in palm of hand, and on *front* part of thigh.	Complaints predom. on fore-arm, on back of hand, and on *back* part of thigh.
AGGRAV. of symptoms, partic. of the fever and pain in limbs, in the *evening;* but some sympt. *better* in the even'g *twilight.*	AGGRAVATION, partic. of the fever and pain in limbs, in the *morning;* but some symptoms worse in the evening *twilight.*
Worse before a thunder storm	Worse during increase of moon.
Generally better when growing cold, worse when growing warm.	Worse when growing cold; better when growing warm.

Predomin. worse (Bryonia) — **Predomin. better** (Rhus)

In dry weather, during continued (moderate) exercise, when walking bent forward, from bending the head back, when lying on side, from warm diet, *after* breakfast, when growing warm, and when stretching out the suffering limb.

Predomin. better (Bryonia) — **Predomin. worse** (Rhus)

In cloudy and wet weather, during rest, when standing, sitting, lying, partic. lying on back, when drawing up the suffering limb, from cold diet, on an empty stomach, when growing cold, and in the evening twilight.

N.B. Rhus lacks the oversensitiveness of the Bryonia-patient to pain.—Bryonia rarely has the sensation of numbness in the suffering parts, peculiar to Rhus

N.B. Both remedies have complaints *after* bodily exertion, H.Gr.; Rhus also after moderate exercise.—Rhus has many complaints when commencing to walk, which cease after continued motion.—Bryon. has complaints *while* walking. C.Hg.

* Both have a desire for malt-liquors; particularly Bryonia; beer agrees with Bryonia, disagrees with Rhus, except in some cases when it palliates the sufferings, for inst. intolerable throbbing in the pit of stomach, but only for a very short time. C.Hg.

Bryonia.	**Sulphur.**
Right side; partic. *upper right, lower left side.*	*Left* side; partic. *upper left, lower right side.*
Increased bodily irritability—Pinching pain in internal parts.	Want of bodily irritability—Pinching pain in external parts.
External parts become black	Red parts become white.
Itching, unchang'd *or* lessen'd by scratching.	Itching, lessened by scratching.
Chill predom. right side—Thirst predom., but not constant; drinks seldom, but much at a time.	Chill predom. left side—Thirst most during heat; during chill most frequently want of thirst—Drinks often, but little at a time.
Chill increased in a warm room—Sweat after sleep.	Chill lessened in a warm room—Sweat lessened after sleep.
Erysipelas or œdema around the joints . .	Itching, erysipelas, or vesicles around the joints.
Complaints predom. on external ear, in lower part of chest, on upper arm, and on front part of thigh.	Complaints predom. in inner ear, in upper part of chest, on fore-arm, and on back part of thigh.
Mood irritable.	Mood changing; serious, solemn; indifferent; gentle *or* irritable.
Ailments from anger or from vexation with vehemence.	Ailments from shame or from vexation with fright—Absent-mindedness—Insanity—Imbecility.
Optical illusions in bright colors	Optical illusions in dark colors.
Eruption on lower lip	Eruption predom. on upper lip.
Nausea in abdomen, less frequently in stomach or in œsophagus.	Nausea in stomach, rarely in throat.
Predom. *bitter* vomit	Generally *sour* vomit.
Catamenia too profuse and of long duration.	Cat. *generally* scanty and of short duration.
Milk generally increased	Milk decreased.
Voice hoarse or raised more than usual .	Voice hoarse or deeper than usual.
Expectoration morning and evening, rarely during day.	Expectoration morning and during day, less frequently at night.
Remission of complaints during day . .	Remission evening and before midnight.
Predom. worse out doors, better in doors.	*Better or* worse * out doors, (or in doors.)
Almost always improved after stool . . .	Worse *or* better after stool.
Almost always improved after sweat . . .	Oftener aggrav. than improved after sweat.
Worse in an extended position	Better in an extended position.
Generally worse after getting out of bed .	Worse *or* better after getting out of bed.
Predom. better on an empty stomach . .	Worse *or* better on an empty stomach.
Worse *or* better after drinking	Almost always aggrav after drinking.
Worse *or* better from eructation	Almost always improved by eructation.
Worse when stooping	Worse *or* better when stooping.

Predomin. worse ——— **Predomin. better**

In dry weather, from cold, from warm diet, during continued† motion, *after* rising from seat, and in an extended position.

Predomin. better ——— **Predomin worse**

In cloudy or wet weather, from warmth‡ and warmth of bed, from cold diet, during rest, after lying down, while lying, sitting, and standing, in a contracted position, and after sweat.

---

* Sulphur-complaints are improved by warmth of stove, aggravated in a crowded room.
† Both remedies have predom. aggrav. from bodily exertion, and when moving the diseased part.
‡ When growing cold and in cold weather, (respectively when growing warm and in warm air,) both remedies have aggrav. quite as often as improvement.

Calcarea.	Causticum.
L. ⟶ R.	**R. ⟶ L.** C.Hg. *
Complaints (sensation of fullness, &c.) predom. in internal parts.	Complaints (sensation of fullness, &c.) predom. in external parts.
Light hair—Skin and muscles lax . . .	Dark hair— Muscles rigid.
Hæmorrhages bright red	Hæmorrhages dark.
Pulse full and accelerated, often trembling.	Pulse often unchanged, only towards evening somewhat irritable.
Chill increased in bed—Sweat less in doors.	Chill less in bed—Sweat increased in doors.
Thirst with fever, which is aggrav. by drinking cold water.	Want of thirst; in fevers when there is thirst, it is easily quenched by drinking water.
Cheerfulness *or* dejection—Amativeness—Imbecility more frequent than insanity—Apoplexy – Ailments from vexation with fear or fright.	Dejection — Distrust — Haughtiness — Absent-mindedness — Melancholy — Apoplexy not yet observed — Ailments from fright, mortification, grief, or from disappointed love.
Itching, lessened oftener than aggrav. by scratching.	Itching aggrav. oftener than lessened by scratching.
Vertigo inclining to fall backwards or sideways.	Vertigo, inclining to fall forwards or sideways.
Emaciation of face	Emaciation of feet.
Complaints of inner oftener than of external nose; complaints pred. on upper jaw and upper teeth, and in upper part of chest.	Complaints of external oftener than of inner nose; complaints predom. on lower jaw and lower teeth, and in lower part of chest.
Sour vomiting of food	Watery vomit.
Urine too often.	Urine often, but scanty.
Catamenia too soon and too profuse . . .	Catamenia too late and scanty.
Catamenia day and night	Catamenia only during day, intermitting at night. C.Hg.
Sexual desire increased	Sexual desire decreased.
Mild leucorrhœa	Acrid leucorrhœa.
Nasal secretion thick, often with bad odor.	Nasal secretion watery.
Expectoration partic. morning and during day.	Cough generally dry. When there is expectoration, it is loosened from evening till morning, but is generally swallowed.
Pain in chest when bending the arm back .	Pain in the back, when bend'g the arm back.
AGGRAVATION after midnight and in *morning*, also during full moon.	AGGRAVATION from evening till morning, also during new moon.
REMISSION before midnight	REMISSION during day.
Worse after a satisfying meal	Worse when hungry.
Oftener aggrav. than improved by exertion.	Oftener improved than aggrav. by exertion.

Predomin. worse ⁓ **Predomin. better**

In wet weather, from washing and drinking cold water †, from continued motion ‡, from stretching and twisting, from pressure, lying on side, and on an empty stomach, (comp. Sep. and Silic. C.Hg.)

Predomin. better ⁓ **Predomin. worse**

In dry weather, from rubbing the suffering part, during rest, from change of position, lying on back, and after breakfast.

N.B. This comparison is principally based by H.Gr. on a treatise of Bœnninghausen in A. b. Z. vol. 63, p 86, who published it to instruct some ignorant wiseacres who objected to our *Causticum*, because we do not know what it is, according to the theories of the chemistry of our day. But we can prepare it, can use it and heal the sick with it according to its symptoms, and it is one of our most valuable instruments. Twenty years ago the chemists discovered Ozon, twenty years hence they may tell us, what Hahnemann's Causticum is; why should we wait for that and let the sick suffer? C.Hg.

---

* In the chest only Calcarea acts decidedly l. to r., in mouth and teeth Calc. has more symptoms on right side; in belly and womb. Calc. l. s., Caust. r. s.; in hypochondria both r. s., in chest and limbs both more l. s. C.Hg.

† Even in epilepsy and cramp in stomach. C.Hg.

‡ When connected with exertion, the reverse is the case. C.Hg.

Calcarea.	China.
Predom. *right* side; partic. *upper right, lower left side.*	*Left* side; part. *upper left, lower right side.*
Light hair—Want of bodily irritability . .	Dark hair—Increased bodily irritability.
Hæmorrhages bright red—Apoplexia sanguinea; but paralysis more frequent than apoplexy.	Hæmorrhages dark—Apoplexia nervosa—Oftener indicated with apoplexy than paralysis.
Rending pain upwards	Rending pain downwards.
Itching, generally lessened by scratching, but often also aggrav.	Itching, lessened by scratching.
Deep ulcers predom.	Flat ulcers.
Pulse full and accelerated, often trembling.	Pulse quick, hard, but small; quieter after eating; irregular, sometimes intermitting.
Thirst almost constant	Thirst partic. before and between the different stages of fever.
Sweat often only on front part of body . .	Sweat often only on back part of body.
First heat, then chill	First chill, then heat.
Heat or sweat increased after meals . . .	Heat or sweat abating after meals.
Mood silly *or* dejected – Ailments from hearing bad news—Mental dullness.	Dejection—Very rarely unconsciousness—Mental excitability.
Vertigo, inclining to fall sideways or backwards.	Vertigo, inclining to fall backwards.
Compl. of inner oftener than of external ear.	Complaints of external ear.
Loss of smell and taste	*Acute* smell and taste.
Complaints predom. in inner nose, in liver, in upper part of chest, on fore-arm, and on back part of thigh.	Complaints predom. on external nose, in spleen, (oftener than liver,) in lower part of chest, on upper arm, and on front part of thigh.
Dislike for coffee	Appetite for coffee, also for roasted coffee beans.
Nausea in stomach	Nausea in throat or stomach.
Urine too often; sediment generally whitish.	Urine infrequent and scanty; sediment generally reddish.
Nasal secretion thick—Breath hot . . .	Nasal secretion watery—Breath cold.
Expectoration predom., but not constant; partic. in the morning and during day.	Expectoration not constant; during day and evening.
Swelling of or pain in the breasts *before* the catamenia.	Swelling of the breasts with suppressed catamenia.
REMISSION of complaints before midnight .	REMISSION afternoon and evening.
Ailments from Phosphor., Digitalis or abuse of Cinchona.	Ailments from abuse of Sulphur, from Iodine, or Calc.
Some symptoms *better* on expiration . .	Some symptoms *better* on inspiration.
Complaints from sleeping too long.	Compl'ts from having been awake at night.

Predomin. worse —— **Predomin. better**

Lying on left side, lying with head high, after sleep, on an empty stomach, and from pressure.

Predomin. better —— **Predomin. worse**

Lying on back, in a horizontal (with head low) position, in general after lying down *, lying on right side, after breakfast, and when sitting.

N.B. With Calc. we seldom find the oversensitiveness to pain of Cinchona, with Cinchona seldom the sensation of numbness in suffering parts peculiar to Calc.

* Warmth of bed often aggrav. with both remedies.

Calcarea.	Cuprum.
Predom. *right* side—Hæmorrhages bright-red—Apoplexia sanguinea.	*Left* side—Hæmorrhages dark—Apoplexia nervosa.
Bruised pain in external parts	Bruised pain in internal parts.
Itching, *lessened or* aggravated by scratching.	Itching, unchanged by scratching.
Pulse accelerated and full, often trembling .	Pulse generally slow and weak.
Clonic spasms during chill	Clonic spasms during heat or sweat.
Chill increased after meals	Chill lessened after meals.
Silly merriness *or* sadness—Peevish, irritable mood—Imbecility more frequent than insanity.	Merriness—Maliciousness—Insanity oftener than imbecility.
Vertigo, inclining to fall backwards or sideways.	Vertigo, inclining to fall forwards.
Complaints oftener in inner than on external ear.	Complaints predominant on external ear.
Complaints predominant on upper jaw and in upper part of chest.	Complaints predominant on lower jaw and in lower part of chest.
Nausea in stomach	Nausea in throat, stomach or abdomen.
Predominantly sour vomit	Bitter vomit.
Urine too often—Incontinence—Sediment generally white.	Urine infrequent and scanty—Retention of urine—Sediment reddish.
Catamenia generally too soon and profuse .	Catamenia too late; oftener too scanty than too profuse.
Breath hot—Cough generally with expectoration.	Breath cold—Cough generally without expectoration.
Expectoration in morning and during day .	Expectoration only in morning.
Remission before midnight	**Remission** during day.
Affections of stomach and intestines, worse from drinking cold water.	Affections of stomach and intestines, better from drinking cold water.
Aggrav. of symptoms during full moon . .	*Aggrav.* during new moon.
Worse from sleeping too long	Worse from having been awake at night.

Predomin. worse — **Predomin. better**

When lying on side, when letting diseased limb hang down, on inspiration, from drinking cold water, from tying the clothes tight, from warmth of bed, and during sweat.

Predomin. better — **Predomin. worse**

When lying on back, from lifting up diseased limb, on expiration, from the touch, and from loosening the clothes.

N.B. Calcarea rarely has the over-sensitiveness to pain of Cuprum, Cuprum rarely the sensation of numbness in suffering parts peculiar to Calcarea.

Calcarea.	Fluor. acid.
Muscles lax—Predom. morbid nervous irritability (in torpid constitutions.)	Muscles rigid—Predom. morbid depression of nervous system (in sensitive constitutions.)
Diseases of the bones, particularly of the end of joints.	Diseases of the bones, particularly of the cylindrical bones.
Spasms—Chill—Vertigo	No spasms—No chill—No vertigo.
Apoplexy—Pain pressing inwards	Pain pressing outwards.
Mania-a-potu	Dropsy of drunkards.
Pulse quick and full, often trembling	Pulse accelerated only by motion.
Heat increased by washing	Heat abated by washing.
Sweat increased after eating, less in-doors	Sweat less after meals, increased in-doors.

Calcarea.	Fluor. acid.
Mood is better in the evening than during day.	Mood better in morning than evening.
Fear—Silly merriness *or* dejection	Excessive hilarity.
Hopelessness—Fear of loss of reason—Fancies—Delirium.	Fear of apoplexy.
Complaints predominant in external angle of eye, on fore-arm, back of hand, and on patella.	Complaints predominant in inner angle of eye, on upper arm, in palm of hand, and on tip of elbow.
Oftener indicated with children than with old people.	Complaints of old age, also premature old age in consequence of syphilitic mercurial dyscrasy.
With Children: Large head and open sutures.	Atrophy of brain.
In the evening, in bed, when closing the eyes: Palpitation of heart, roaring in ears, jerks in the head, and fanciful imaginations. In the morning, on awaking: Feeling as though one had not had enough sleep.	In the evening, in bed: Becomes wide-awake again and cannot sleep because of thought. In the morning, on awaking from a short sleep: Feels as though he had slept all night.
Diarrhœa generally painless	Diarrhœa painful.
Urine sour	Urine alkaline.
Leucorrhœa mild	Leucorrhœa acrid.
Collection of mucus in larynx	Dryness in larynx and trachea.
Cough generally with expectoration	Cough dry.

Calcarea.	Fluor. acid.
Remission of complaints before midnight	Remission morning and before midnight.
Worse from sleeping too long	Worse from being awake at night.
Worse during and after sweat	Better while perspiring.
Ailments from Phosph., Digitalis, Mercurius, or Cinchona.	Ailments from Silicea.

Predomin. worse — **Predomin. better**

While perspiring, from washing with cold water, from tightening the clothes, and from boring with the finger (in ear or nose.)

Predomin. better — **Predomin. worse**

From loosening the clothes.

Calcarea.	Ipecacuanha.
Pain pressing inwards	Pain pressing outwards.
Paralysis more frequent than apoplexy . .	Apoplexy more frequent than paralysis.
Itching, lessened oftener than aggravated by scratching.	Itching, unchanged by scratching.
Pulse accelerated and full, often trembling .	Pulse very much accelerated, but often impercepible.
First heat, then chill	First chill, then heat.
Sweat less in-doors	Sweat increased in-doors.
Thirst during all stages of the fever . . .	Thirst not constant.
Fear—Hopelessness—Amativeness . . .	No fear, etc.
Ailments from hearing bad news — Delirium—Fancies—Imbecility.	Ailments from emotion generally — Very rarely unconsciousness.
Optical illusions, particularly in dark colors.	Optical illusions in bright colors.
Generally hunger	Loss of appetite predominant.
Vomit, sour oftener than bitter	Vomit, bitter oftener than sour.
Urine too often; Sediment generally whitish.	Urine scanty; Sediment generally reddish.
Expectoration predom. with cough, but not constant; morning and during day.	Expectoration infrequent; morning.
Remission of complaints before midnight .	**Remission** during day.
Worse or better in bed	Better in bed.
Predominantly worse on awaking and after sleep.	Better after sufficient sleep; but worse when roused from sleep.
Worse *or* better from light (resp. in the dark.)	Worse from light, better in the dark.
Worse *or* better when opening (resp. closing) the eyes.	Worse when opening the eyes; better when closing them.
Worse from sleeping too long	Worse from wakefulness at night.
Worse or better after getting out of bed .	Worse after getting out of bed.
When growing cold, worse *or* (from warmth of bed) better; likewise when growing warm.	Better when growing cold; worse when growing warm.
Worse or better from exertion	Worse from bodily exertion.
Worse or better when bending diseased part.	Worse when bending diseased part.
Worse after stool	Worse *or* better after stool.
Ailments from Phosphor, Mercurius, Sulph. acid, or Digitalis.	Ailments from Arsenic or Copper vapors, from Nux vom., Arnica, or Opium.

Predomin. worse —— **Predomin. better**

In wet weather, from cold, after perspiring, after drinking, in bed, and after sleep.

Predomin. better —— **Predomin. worse**

In dry weather, from warmth, from the touch, and when sitting down.

N.B. Ipecacuanha has not the sensation of numbness in suffering parts peculiar to Calcarea; Calcarea, on the other hand, seldom has the over-sensitiveness to pain of Ipecacuanha; still both remedies have the character of constitutional want of irritability.

Calcarea.	Kreosot.
Right side—Want of bodily irritability .	*Left* side—Increased bodily irritability.
Constriction in internal parts	Constriction in external parts.
Is often indicated with young women . .	Often indicated with old women.
Hæmorrhages, blood light-red—Paralysis.	Hæmorrhages, dark—Paralysis has not been observed.
Cutaneous eruptions generally dry . . .	Eruptions generally humid.
Pulse full and accelerated, often trembling .	Pulse small and weak, with strong ebullition of blood.
Chill (heat and sweat) with thirst . . .	Chill, without thirst; (heat, with thirst.)
Heat or sweat, with inclination to uncover .	Heat or sweat, with aversion to uncover.

Ailments from vexation with fear or fright; also from hearing bad news.	Ailments from emotion in general.
Affections of the inner oftener than the external ear.	Affections of external ear.
Eruption predominant on under lip . . .	Eruption on under lip.
Urine acid—Sediment generally white . .	Urine alkaline—Sediment generally reddish.
Sexual desire too strong	Sexual desire predominantly weak.
Leucorrhœa mild	Leucorrhœa predominantly acrid.
Expectoration not constant; morning and during day.	Expectoration not constant; morning and evening.

REMISSION of complaints before midnight .	REMISSION forenoon and evening.
Worse *or* better from cold (resp. warm) diet.	Worse from cold diet; better from warm diet.

Predomin. worse —— **Predomin. better**

From wrapping up, on awaking, and after sleep, when letting diseased limb hang down, from pressure, and after stool.

Predomin. better —— **Predomin worse**

From uncovering, when assuming an erect position, when lifting up diseased limb, from the touch, and when sitting down.

N.B. With Kreosot we seldom find the sensation of numbness in suffering parts peculiar to Calcarea. This is quite in accordance with the constitutional character of both remedies.

N.B. To spell what Reichenbach, the discoverer, named KREOSOT with a C is an old-fogyish imitation of the middle ages; to spell it Kreasot is doing violence to the spirit of the Greek language (comp. kreophagia) and copying British snobism. C.Hg.

Calcarea	Lycopodium.
Aversion to open air	Inclination for open air, oftener than aversion to it.
Hæmorrhages, blood bright red—Pain pressing inwards—Rending pain upwards.	Hœmorrhages, blood dark— Pain pressing outward—Rending pain downwards.
Dry itch	Humid itch.
Complaints of glands worse in morning. .	Complaints of glands worse in evening.
Often indicated with young women . . .	Often indicated with old women.
Pulse full and accelerated, often trembling.	Pulse accelerated somewhat only after eating and in the evening.
Burning sensation in veins	Sensation of coldness in veins.
Chill increased after getting out of bed . .	Chill less after getting out of bed.
Thirst during all the stages of the fever . .	Thirst is wanting only during chill.
Imbecility oftener than insanity	Insanity oftener than imbecility—Changing mood; gentle; distrustful; avaricious; haughty; malicious—Absent-mindedness.
Ailments from vexation with fright and from hearing bad news.	Ailments from fright, anger, mortification, or fr. vexation with reserved displeasure.
During the erethic stage of acute affections of the brain.	Diseases of brain with somnolence.
Vertigo, inclining to fall backwards or sideways.	Vertigo inclining to fall forwards.
Complaints predom. on under lip, and on patella.	Complaints predom. on upper lip, and in hollow of knee.
Appetite for bread	Aversion to bread, partic. rye bread.
Urine too often — Incontinence predom. .	Urine often, but scanty—Retention of urine oftener than incontinence.
Urinal sediment generally whitish . .	Urinal sediment red (sandy) *or* whitish.
Catamenia generally too soon	Catamenia generally too late.
Leucorrhœa mild	Leucorrhœa predom. acrid.
Milk increased*	Milk decreased.
Expectoration predom., but not constant; morning and during day.	Expectoration almost constant; morning and evening.
Remission before midnight	**Remission** after midnight and in *forenoon*.
Worse after sweat	Oftener improved than aggrav. after sweat.
Better after lying down, but the pain in joints worse from warmth of bed.	*Worse* after lying down, but the pain in joints better from warmth of bed.
Better when resting the diseased limb on something, *worse* when letting it hang down.	*Worse* when resting diseased limb on something, but sometimes also worse when letting it hang down.
Better when assuming an erect position .	Worse *or* better when assuming an erect position.
Worse when looking up or down	Worse when looking at any thing which turns.

Predomin. worse ——— **Predomin. better**

From cold, out doors, from continued (moderate) motion, (when stooping,) and on an empty stomach.

Predomin. better ——— **Predomin. worse**

From warmth, in doors, during rest, while standing, from the touch, when resting the diseased limb on any thing, and after breakfast.

N.B. We seldom find the oversensitiveness of Lycopodium to pain, with Calcarea.

* When milk is decreased, Calcarea is indicated only then, when there is no inflammability of the breast.

Calcarea.	Mercur.
Lower left, upper right side—Want of bodily irritability.	Upper left, lower right side—Increased bodily irritability.
Pain pressing inward—Rending pain upwards.	Pain pressing outward—Rending pain downwards.
Heat or sweat, with inclination to uncover.	Heat or sweat, with aversion to uncover.
Thirst constant.	Thirst predominant, but not constant.
Dreams of fire, quarrel, sickness, dead persons.	Dreams of water, falling, shooting, and misfortunes.
Silly merriness *or* sadness	Seriousness—Despondency—Malice.
Ailments from hearing bad news, mortification, or from vexation with fear or fright.	Ailments from emotion in general.
Delirium.	Rarely delirium—Absent-mindedness.
Complaints more frequent in inner than on external nose.	Complaints more frequent on external than in inner nose.
Nasal secretion thick	Nasal secretion watery.
Eruption predominant on under lip . . .	Eruption on upper lip.
Complaints predominant on upper jaw and upper teeth, and on roof of mouth.	Complaints predominant on lower jaw and lower teeth, and on soft palate
Generally hunger	Generally loss of appetite.
Appetite for spirituous liquors	Aversion to wine; but appetite for beer.
Nausea in stomach	Nausea in œsophagus or stomach.
Vomit oftener sour than bitter	Bitter vomit.
Predominant complaints after coition . .	Complaints in consequence of pollutions.
Catamenia most frequently too soon . . .	Catamenia too late.
Leucorrhœa mild	Leucorrhœa acrid.
Expectoration predominant, but not constant; morning and during day.	Expectoration not constant; during day.
Complaints predominant on patella . . .	Complaints predominant on tip of elbow, and in hollow of knee.
Sweat of feet stinking	Sweat of feet scentless.
REMISSION before midnight.	REMISSION of complaints during day.
Worse *or* better from light (resp. in the dark.)	Worse from light, better in the dark.
Better when assuming an erect position .	Worse *or* better when assum. an erect posit'n.
Worse *or* better after getting out of bed .	Better after getting out of bed.
Worse when eating, and when swallowing.	Better *or* worse when eat'g or swallow'g, partic. worse when swallow'g saliva and drink.
Oftener aggrav. than improv. by smoking .	Better from smoking.
Better *or* worse when moving the part . .	Worse when moving diseased part.
Worse or better when bending diseased part.	Worse when bending diseased part.
Better when sitting down	Worse *or* better when sitting down.
Ailments from Mercurius, Phosph., or Digitalis.	Ailments from Calc., Sulph., from Arsen. or Copper vapors, and from sting of insects.

Predomin. worse ——— **Predomin. better**

From wrapping up, when letting diseased limb hang down, lying on left side, and lying on unpainful side.

Predomin. better ——— **Predomin. worse**

From uncovering, when lifting up diseased limb, lying on right side, lying on painful side, and from the touch.

N.B. With Mercurius we seldom find the sensation of numbness in suffering parts frequent with Calc., in accordance with the constitutional character of both remedies.

Calcarea.	Natr. mur.
Eruptions generally dry	Eruptions generally humid.
Complaints predominant in internal parts .	Complaints predominant in external parts.
Light hair—Skin and muscles lax . . .	Dark hair—Skin and muscles rigid.
Lower left, upper right side	*Upper left, lower right side.*
Aversion to open air	Generally inclination for open air.
Oftener indicated with children and young women than with old people.	Often indicated with old people, particularly with old women.
Emaciation of the face	Emaciation of the feet.
Epilepsy, with unconsciousness	Epilepsy, with full consciousness.
Pulse full and accelerated	Pulse very irregular, intermitt'g; sometimes frequent and weak, somet. full and slow.
Heat, then chill	Chill, then heat.
Heat or sweat, with inclination to uncover.	Heat or sweat, with aversion to uncover.
Thirst during all stages of the fever . . .	Thirst during the fever and apyrexy.
Aversion to washing with cold water . .	Inclination for washing with cold water.

Fear—Delirium—Fancies	Changing mood; indifferent; malicious—Absent-mindedness.
Ailments from vexation with fright, and from hearing bad news.	Ailments from fright, anger, mortification, or of vexation with reserved displeasure.
Vertigo, inclination to fall backwards or sideways.	Vertigo, inclining to fall forward.
Complaints predominant in inner nose, on roof of mouth, in upper part of chest, on back of thigh, and on patella.	Compl. predom. on external nose, on soft palate, in lower part of chest, on front side of thigh, and in hollow of knee.
Generally hunger	Generally want of appetite.
Appetite for bread	Generally avers. to bread. partic. rye-bread.
Cramp in stomach, lessened by loosening the clothes.	Cramp in stomach, better from tightening the clothes.
Urine acid, generally with white sediment .	Urine alcaline, with red sediment.
Catamenia generally too soon—Leucorrhœa mild.	Catamenia too late—Leucorrhœa predominantly acrid.
Sexual desire increased or strong . . .	Sexual desire decreased or weak.
Palpitation of heart, with even, strong beats, particularly in evening, in bed.	Palpitation of heart, with irregular, intermitting beats.
Expectoration predominant, but not constant; morning and during day.	Expectoration very seldom, and then only in morning.
Paralysis prevalent in arms.	Paralysis prevalent in legs.

Remission of complaints before midnight.	Remission afternoon.
*Better** when lying in a horizontal position, or with head low.	*Better* when lying with head high.
Better when assuming an erect position . .	Worse *or* better when assum'g an erect posit

Predomin. worse — **Predomin. better**

On an empty stomach, out-doors, from washing with cold water, from wrapping up, and from tight clothes.

Predomin better — **Predomin. worse**

After breakfast, in-doors, from uncovering, from loosening the clothes and from the touch.

*** Lying down of itself improves in both remedies. Warmth of bed aggravates in both.**

Calcarea.	Nitr. acid.
Upper right, lower left side—Light hair .	Upper left, lower right side—Dark hair.
Skin and muscles lax	Skin and muscles rigid.
Hæmorrhages light red—Eruptions generally dry.	Hœmorrhages dark—Eruptions humid.
Cures warts, lipomæ, &c., by suppuration.	Causes atrophy of warts.
Emaciation of face	Emaciation of feet.
Epilepsy with unconsciousness	Epilepsy with full consciousness.
Oftener indicated with children and young women than with old people.	Often indicated with old people, partic. old women.
Pulse accelerated, full, often trembling . .	Pulse very unequal, double, intermitting.
Thirst during all stages of fever	Thirst is wanting during chill; is not constant during heat.
Hopelessness—Amativeness—Imbecility .	Malice.
Ailments from vexation with fright, dread or fear, and from hearing bad news.	Ailments from emotion in general—Very rarely apoplexy or paralysis.
Complains predom. on under lip	Complaints predom. on upper lip.
Appetite for bread	Aversion to bread.
Urine too often; acid, generally with red sediment.	Urine scanty; oftener alcaline than acid, with white *or* red sediment.
Leucorrhœa mild	Leucorrhœa acrid.
Impotence with increased sexual desire . .	Erections with less desire and potence.
Cough generally loose	Cough generally dry.
REMISSION of complaints before midnight .	REMISSION forenoon.
Better after lying down, but worse from warmth of bed.	*Worse* after lying down, but *better* from warmth of bed.
Ailments from Phosphor. or abuse of Cinchona, also from Nitr. acid.	Ailments from Calcarea.

Predomin. worse — **Predomin. better**

In cold weather, from stooping, from riding, after sweat, from use of spirituous liquors, before breakfast and from warmth of bed.

Predomin. better — **Predomin. worse**

In warm air, when assuming an erect position, from the touch, after breakfast, and after lying down.

N.B. Nitric acid lacks the sensation of numbness in suffering parts, frequent with Calc. Both remedies, however, have the character of constitutional want of irritability.

Calcarea.	Nux vomica.
Light hair—Skin and muscles lax	Dark hair—Skin and muscles rigid.
Want of bodily irritab.—Pain press'g inwards.	Increased bodily irritab. — Pain pressing outward.
Epilepsy with unconsciousness	Epilepsy with full consciousness.
Paralysis, generally of legs	Paralysis, predom of arms.
Apopl. sang. — Hæmorrhages, blood light red.	Apoplex. nervosa—Hœmorrhages, blood dark.
Heat or sweat with inclination to uncover	Heat or sweat with aversion to uncover.
Sweat, partic. on front of body — Thirst pred.	Sweat, parict. on back of body—Thirst, partic. during chill.
Chill or heat after sleep — Heat while sitting.	Chill or heat less during sleep—Heat lessened while sitting.
Sleeplessness preval. before midnight	Sleeplessness preval. after midnight.
Taciturnity — Cheerfullness *or* dejection	Loquacity—Sadness—*Malice.*
Ailments from hearing bad news, and from vexation with fright.	Ailm. from contradiction, anger, fright, mortification, grief, disappointed love, jealousy, or fr. vexation with indignation or vehemence.
Sweat on head, partic. on back part, in evening, from the least motion, increased in cold air, when having cold feet; better when sitting still in a warm room.	Fetid sweat on one side of head and face, which is cold, after midnight and in morning, with fear and abatement of pain; better from washing and when sitting still in warm room.
Optical illusions in black or dark colors	Optical illusions in bright colors.
Dimsightedness	Clear-sightedness predom.
Compl. predom. on upper jaw and upper teeth.	Compl. predom. om lower jaw and lower teeth.
Generally hunger—Appetite for bread or sour things.	Generally loss of appetite—Aversion to bread, partic. rye bread, and to sour things.
Desire for beer	Inclination for *or* aversion to beer.
Urine too often predom. dark; sediment generally white—Urinal stream small.	Urine infrequent and scanty; generally pale; sediment reddish—Urinal stream large.
Complaints predom after coition	Complaints predom. after pollutions.
Nasal secretion thick	Nasal secretion watery.
Cough generally loose — Expectoration morning and during day.	Cough generally dry—Expectoration morning, during day and evening.
Old, large inguinal hernia, easily reducible	Old, large inguin. hernia difficult to be reduced.
Complaints predom. on patella	Complaints predom. in hollow of knee.
Remission of complaints before midnight	Remission evening till midnight.
Worse *or* better from light (resp. in the dark.)	Worse from light, better in the dark.
Worse when lying on side, better when lying on back.	Generally better when lying on side, worse when lying on back.
Worse when lying on unpainful side, better when lying on painful side.	Worse (resp. better) when lying on painful *or* on unpainful side.
Predom. worse on awaking and after sleep	Better after sufficient and not too long sleep; but worse when roused from sleep.
Oftener improved than aggrav. after breakfast.	Oftener aggrav. than improved after breakfast.
Worse when eating	Oftener improv. than aggrav. when eating.
Worse *or* better from cold (resp. warm) diet	Pred. worse fr. cold diet; better fr. warm diet.
Worse when swallowing and when sneezing	*Worse or* better when swallowing or sneezing.
Worse or better when rising from a seat	Worse when rising from a seat.
Worse or better from exertion, running, &c.	Worse from exertion, running, &c.
Worse when stooping	Oftener improv. than aggrav. when stooping.
Worse *or* better when moving diseased part	Worse when moving diseased part.
Worse when bending back or stretching out diseased part.	Oftener improv. than aggrav. when bending backwards or stretching out diseased part.
Better when drawing up diseased part	Oftener aggrav. than improv. when drawing up diseased limb.
Worse after drinking	Worse *or* better after drinking.

Predomin. worse — **Predomin. better**

In wet weather, from wrapping up, in bed *, and fr. warmth of bed, lying with the head high, and lying on left side, after sweat, on inspiration, from pressure, and fr. washing or moistening diseased part.

Predomin. better — **Predomin. worse**

In dry weather, when uncovering, when assuming an erect position, in a horizontal position, lying on right side, on expiration, and from the touch.

* Both remedies have predom. improvement after lying down and while lying down generally.

Calcarea.	Phosphor.
Light hair—Skin and muscles lax . . .	Dark hair—Skin and muscles rigid.
Oftener indicated with children and young women than with old people.	Often indicated with old people.
Diseases of bones, partic. of the epiphyses.	Diseases of bones, partic. of the diaphyses.
Emaciation of face—Apoplexia sanguinea.	Emaciation of hands—Apoplexia nervosa.
Pain pressing inwards	Pain pressing outwards.
Epilepsy, with unconsciousness	Epilepsy, with full consciousness
Pulse full and accelerated, but equal . . .	Pulse varying; irregular, sometimes intermitt'g; most frequently quick, full & hard.
Heat one-sided—Left side	Heat one-sided—Right side.
Chill after sleep	Chill less after sleep.
Heat lessened after breakfast	Heat increased after breakfast.
Sweat more when eating; less in-doors . .	Sweat less when eating; increased in-doors.
First heat, then chill—Thirst constant . .	First chill, then heat—Want of thirst const't.

Calcarea.	Phosphor.
Loquacity—Hopelessness	Taciturnity—Changing mood—Indifference—Haughtiness.
Mental dullness—Imbecility	Mental excitability—Insanity.
Ailments from vexation with dread or fear, and from hearing bad news.	Ailments from anger, fright, or from vexation with vehemence.
Weak memory	Active memory.
Pupils dilated	Pupils contracted.
Complaints of inner oftener than of external ear; complaints predominant on upper jaw and on patella.	Complaints of external oftener than of inner ear; complaints predominant on lower jaw and in hollow of knee.
Appetite for bread	Aversion to bread . . . .
Urine too often; smelling sour, generally with white sediment.	Urine often, but scanty; sometimes sour, but oftener smelling like Ammoniac, with white, yellow, or reddish sediment.
Leucorrhœa mild	Leucorrhœa acrid.
Voice singing or nasal	Voice trembling or hissing.
Expectoration predom., but not constant .	Expectoration not constant.

Calcarea.	Phosphor.
REMISSION before midnight	REMISSION of complaints after midnight.
Worse in cold, wet weather	*Worse* before or during thunder-storm.
Worse *or* better from warm diet	Always aggravated by warm diet.
Worse during full or new moon	Worse before thunder-storm.
Ailments from Phosph., Mercur., Cinchona, Digitalis, or Nitr. acid.	Ailments from Iodine or from abuse of table-salt.

Predomin. worse ——— **Predomin. better**

In the open air, and when walking out-doors, when stooping, lying on side, in the evening twilight, after sleep,* on an empty stomach, but also after a satisfying meal, from sweets, coffee, wine, and drinking cold water.

Predomin. better ——— **Predomin. worse**

In warm room, from assuming an erect position, lying on back, from change of position, and after breakfast.

N.B. Calcarea rarely has the over-sensitiveness of Phosph. to pain.

*** As an exception, Phosph. has aggravation after the siesta, and likewise after being roused from sleep.**

Calcarea.	Pulsatilla.
Lower left, upper right side — Pain pressing inwards.	Upper left, lower right side — Pain pressing outward.
Want of bodily susceptibility — Aversion to open air.	Increased susceptibility—Inclination for open air.
Paralysis more frequent than apoplexy . . .	Apoplexy more frequent than paralysis.
Hæmorrhages, blood light red — Apoplexia sanguinea.	Hæmorrhages, blood dark — Apoplexia nervosa.
Itching. oftener improved than aggravated by scratching.	Itching, aggrav. *or* unchanged by scratching.
Pulse preval. full	Pulse predom. small and weak; sometimes imperceptible.
Chill with thirst—Thirst constant	Chill without thirst—Thirst only during hot [stage.
Heat l. s.—Heat first, then chill	Heat r. s.—Chill first, then heat.
Sweat, partic. on front of body	Sweat, partic. on back part of body.
Heat increased after washing; sweat when walking out doors.	Heat lessened by washing — Sweat lessened when walking out doors.
Mood silly *or* despondent; embarrassed; irritable.	Mood changeable—Calm sadness—Gentleness Boldness—Avarice—Distrust.
Ailments from hearing bad news	Ailments from excessive joy, fright, grief, mortification.
Imbecility oftener than insanity	Absent-mindedness—Melancholy.
Vertigo, inclining to fall sideways or backwards, partic. in the morning.	Vertigo, inclining to fall backwards, partic. in the evening.
Pupils generally dilated—Optical illusions in black or dark colors.	Pupils most frequently contracted — Optical illusions in bright colors.
Stye on right eye	Stye on left eye. C.Hg.
Internal nasal compl'ts oftener than external.	*External* nasal compl'ts oftener than internal.
Complaints predom. on upper jaw and upper teeth, and on outer side of gums.	Complaints predom. on lower jaw and lower teeth, and on inner side of gums.
Food tastes as though salted too little . . .	Food tastes too salty.
Appetite for bread	Aversion to bread.
Nausea in stomach	Nausea in throat, stomach, or abdomen.
Predom. sour vomit	Vomit. oftener bitter than sour.
Urine too often; sour; sediment whitish . .	Ur. seldom & scanty; alkaline; sedim. reddish.
Catamenia most frequently too soon, profuse, and of long duration.	Catamenia most frequently too late, scanty and of short duration.
Complaints predom. in upper part of chest .	Complaints predom. in lower part of chest.
Complaints predom. from coition	Complaints after pollutions.
Complaints predom. on fore-arm and patella .	Complaints predom. on upper arm and in hollow of knee.
Remission of complaints before midnight . .	Remission from midnight till noon.
Worse (resp. better) when opening the eyes, *or* when closing them.	Better when opening the eyes; worse when closing them.
Better when assuming an erect position . .	Worse *or* bett. when assum'g an erect posit'n.
Worse when getting out of bed	Impr. oftener than aggr. when gett'g out of bed.
Aggrav. oftener than improv. by exertion . .	Improv. oftener than aggrav. by exertion.
Better when sitting down	Worse *or* better when sitting down.
Worse or better from smoking	Worse from smoking.
Worse when swallowing, and after stool . .	Better *or* worse when swallow'g & after stool.
Worse or better from pressure	*Better or* worse from pressure.
Generally improved by rubbing and scratching.	Worse from rubbing and scratching.
Worse during full or new moon	Worse before a thunder-storm.

Predomin worse — **Predomin. better**

In the open air; from cold and in cold weather; from drinking cold water; during continued motion; when walking; from exertion; when stretching out; bending sideways; washing or moistening the diseased limb; on inspiration; when lying with head high; from tightening the clothes and from pressure

Predomin. better — **Predomin. worse**

In doors; from warmth and in warm air; during rest; after lying down; while lying, sitting, and standing; in a horizontal position; from change of position; from the touch; when drawing up diseased limb; on expiration; from loosening the clothes, and from rubbing and scratching.

N.B. We rarely find the oversensitiveness to pain of Pulsatilla with Calcarea.

Calcarea.	Rhus.
Upper right, lower left side	Upper left, lower right side.
Complaints predom. in internal parts . .	Complaints predom. in external parts.
Eruptions generally dry	Eruptions generally humid.
Skin and muscles lax	Skin and muscles rigid.
Pain pressing inwards, partic. also in the glands.	Pain pressing outwards, partic. also in the glands.
Cures warts, lipomæ, &c., by suppuration.	Causes atrophy of warts.
Pulse rapid and full	Pulse irregular; generally rapid, but weak, faint and soft, sometimes imperceptible and intermitting.
First heat, then chill	First chill, then heat.
Heat or sweat with inclination to uncover.	Heat or sweat with aversion to uncover.
Thirst during all stages of the fever . . .	Thirst not constant.

Calcarea.	Rhus.
Mood silly *or* sad; irritable	Dejection.
Fear of loss of reason	Fear of being poisoned.
Vertigo, inclining to fall sideways or backwards.	Vertigo, inclining to fall forwards or backwards.
Eruption predom. on underlip	Eruption on upper lip.
Internal oftener than external nasal complaints; compl. predom. on upper jaw and upper teeth, in upper part of chest; most frequently on sole of foot.	*External* oftener than internal nasal complaints; compl. predom. on lower jaw and lower teeth, in lower part of chest; most frequently on top of foot.
Generally hunger—Desire for wine . . .	Predom. loss of appetite—Aversion to wine.
Nausea in stomach	Nausea in œsophagus or stomach, less frequently in throat.
Diarrhœa generally painless	Diarrhœa generally painful.
Inguinal hernia easily reducible	Inguinal hernia difficult to reduce.
Urinal stream small; urine dark—Sediment white, less frequently reddish.	Urinal stream spread; urine pale — Sediment white.
Impotence with increased sexual desire . .	Erections (with desire to urinate. C.Hg.)
Cough generally loose — Expectoration in morning and during day.	Cough, generally dry—Expectoration, particularly in the morning.
Worse after mental exertion	Consequences of bodily exertion. C.Hg.

Calcarea.	Rhus.
REMISSION before midnight	REMISSION of complaints during day.
Worse after passing urine, and during and after sweating	*Worse before* passing urine and while sweating, *better after* the sweat.
Worse after a satisfying meal	Worse when hungry.

Predomin. **worse** ——— Predomin. **better**

When lying on side; when stretching out or when letting diseased limb hang down; during continued (moderate) motion; from wrapping up and warmth of bed*; from pressure; from boring with finger (in ear or nose) and after sweat.

Predomin. **better** ——— Predomin. **worse**

When lying on back; when drawing up, lifting or resting diseased limb on anything; during rest; after lying down, when standing and sitting; from being uncovered; change of position, and from the touch.

---

* We find aggrav. by warmth of bed rarely only with Rhus (and N. vom.).

Calcarea.	Sepia.
Light hair—Skin and muscles lax	Dark hair—Skin and muscles rigid.
Complaints of internal parts predom.	Complaints of external parts predom.
Rending pain upwards—Pain pressing inwards.	Rending pain downwards—Pain pressing outwards.
Hæmorrhages: blood light red	Hæmorrhages: blood dark.
Itching, improved oftener than aggrav. by scratching.	Itching, always aggrav. by scratching.
Pulse frequent and full	Pulse, accelerated partic. by vexation and motion; frequent and full, and then often intermitting at night, slower during day.
Chill increased after getting out of bed	Chill lessened after getting out of bed.
Thirst constant, only sometimes absent during chill.	Want of thirst; only during chill there is thirst.
Taciturnity—Fear of losing one's reason	Loquacity—Fear of apoplexy.
Silly merriness *or* dejection—Amorousness.	Seriousness—Despondency—Indifference—Absent-mindedness.
Delirium	Insanity.
Pupils dilated	Pupils contracted.
Nose-bleeding during the (too copious) menses	Nose-bleeding with suppressed or too scanty menses, or during pregnancy. C.Hg.
Generally hunger—Appetite for bread	Generally loss of appetite—Aversion to bread.
Predom. sour vomiting	Predom. bitter vomiting.
Urinary sediment generally whitish—Frequent passing of urine.	Urinary sediment *red* or whitish—Passing urine too seldom.
Catamenia generally too soon—Leucorrhœa mild.	Catamenia generally too late—Leucorrhœa acrid.
Nasal secretion thick	Nasal secretion watery.
Expectoration in the morning and during day.	Expectoration is loosened at night and in the morning; is swallowed.
Complaints predom. on patella	Complaints predom. on tip of elbow.
Remission of complaints before midnight.	Remission afternoon.
Aggrav. oftener during full moon than during new moon.	Aggravation during new moon.
Worse in cold weather, better in warm air.	Better *or* worse in cold (rsp. warm) weather.
Worse from warmth of bed	*Better or* worse from warmth of bed.
Worse *or* better fr. light (resp. in the dark.)	Worse from light; better in the dark.
Predom. worse on awaking and after sleep.	Better after sufficient sleep, but worse on awaking when roused from sleep.
Worse when getting out of bed; worse *or* better *after* getting out of bed.	Improved oftener than aggrav. *during* and *after* getting out of bed.
Aggrav. oftener than improv. by smoking.	Improved oftener than aggrav. by smoking.
Worse or better when bending the part	Worse when bending diseased part.
Aggrav. oftener than improv. by exertion.	Improved oftener than aggrav. by exertion.

Predomin. worse — **Predomin. better**

In wet weather; when walking in the open air; from walking and exercise in general; from bodily exertion; on inspiration; from warmth of bed; from wrapping up; lying on side; after sleep; when getting out of bed; from drinking cold water, (and from smoking.)

Predomin. better — **Predomin. worse**

In dry weather; during rest; when lying, sitting, and standing; on expiration; from uncovering, lying on back, and from scratching.

N.B. We very rarely find the oversensitiveness of Sepia to pain with Calcarea; with Sepia rarely the sensation of numbness in suffering parts peculiar to Calc.

Calcarea.	Silicea.
Apoplexia sanguinea	Apoplexia nervosa.
Complaints (constriction, etc.) predominant in internal parts—Want of irritability.	Compl. (constriction, etc.) predom. in external parts—Increased bodily irritability.
Obesity *or* emaciation	Emaciation.
Rending pain upwards	Rending pain downwards.
Pain pressing inwards	Pain pressing outwards.
Itching, *improved or* aggrav. by scratch'g.	Itching, unchanged *or* aggrav. by scratch'g.
Pulse frequent and full, often trembling . .	Pulse frequent, hard, but small; often irregular.
Sweat on front of body	Sweat often confined to back part of body.
Heat, with inclination for uncovering . .	Heat, with aversion to uncovering.
Dreams of dead people, fire, quarrel, dispute, etc.	Dreams of thieves, water, business, etc.
Sleeplessness prevalent before midnight . .	Sleeplessness prevalent after midnight.

Calcarea.	Silicea.
Fear—Cheerfulness *or* dejection—Irritable mood—Delirium.	Indifference—Gentleness—Dejection—Absent-mindedness.
Vertigo, inclining to fall backwards or sideways.	Vertigo, inclining to fall forwards.
Pupils dilated—Complaints predominant on external angle of eye.	Pupils contracted—Complaints predom. on inner angle of eye.
Complaints generally in inner ear	Complaints generally on external ear.
Eruption predominant on under lip . . .	Eruption on upper lip.
Complaints predominant on upper jaw, on upper teeth, and in upper part of chest.	Complaints predominant on lower jaw, on lower teeth, and in lower part of chest.
Generally hunger	Loss of appetite predominant.
Vomit oftener sour than bitter	Bitter vomit.
Stool generally like diarrhœa	Stool generally costive.
Urinary sediment generally whitish, seldom reddish.	Urinary sediment reddish or yellow.
Catamenia generally too soon	Catamenia generally too late.
Leucorrhœa mild	Leucorrhœa acrid.
Expectoration predominant, but not constant: morning and during day.	Expectoration rather constant; only during day.
Numbnesss of fingers	Heat in fingers.

Calcarea.	Silicea.
Worse in wet, cold weather	*Worse* in cold, dry air.
Worse from cold *or* warm diet	*Worse* from cold diet, *better* from warm diet.
Worse when blowing the nose	*Better after* blowing the nose.
Ailments from Phosph., Digitalis, or abuse of Cinchona, also from Nitric acid.	Ailments from sting of insects, or from abuse of Sulphur.

Predomin. worse ——— **Predomin. better**

In wet weather, when lying on side, when letting suffering limb hang down, from wrapping up, in bed, during continued moderate motion, and on an empty stomach.

Predomin. better ——— **Predomin. worse**

In dry weather, when lying on back, when lifting up or resting suffering limb on anything, from uncovering, from the touch, during rest, after breakfast, and from scratching.

N.B. Over-sensitiveness to pain is very rarely found with Calc., but more frequently with Silicea.

Calcarea.	Sulphur.
Right side; partic. *upper right, lower left side.*	*Left* side; partic. *upper left, lower right side* *.
Rending pain upwards — Pain pressing inwards.	Rending pain downwards—Pain pressing outwards.
Hæmorrhages, blood light red—Apoplexy	Hæmorrhages, blood dark—Rarely apoplexy.
Itching, improved oftener than aggravated by scratching.	Itching, almost always improved by scratching.
Eruptions better in the open air	Eruptions worse in the open air. C.Hg.
Cures warts &c. by suppuration	Causes atrophy of warts, &c.
Pulse sometimes trembling	Pulse semetimes intermitting.
Sweat, partic. anteriorly	Sweat, partic. posteriorly.
Thirst constant during all stages of the fever.	Thirst mostly during heat; generally absence of thirst during chill.
Silly merriness *or* despondency — Amorousness.	Mood changing; serious, solemn, sad, gentle indifferent.
Consequences of hearing bad news—Imbecility predom.	Consequences of shame or mortification—Insanity predom.
Pupils generally dilated	Pupils generally contracted.
Complaints predom. on lower eye-lids	Complaints predom. on upper eye-lids.
Eruption predom. on under-lip	Eruption predom. on upper lip.
Complaints predom. on upper gum	Complaints predom. on lower gum.
Generally hunger	Generally loss of appetite.
Appetite for bread and for spirituous liquors.	Aversion to bread, partic. rye bread—Inclination *or* aversion to beer and spirit. liquors.
Catamenia generally too soon, profuse and long.	Catamenia generally too late, scanty, and of short duration.
Leucorrhœa mild	Leucorrhœa acrid.
Nasal secretion thick	Nasal secretion watery.
Expectoration predom., but not constant	Expectoration not constant.
Remission of complaints before midnight	Remission *evening* and before midnight.
Worse during *full moon or* new moon	Worse during full moon, or before a thunderstorm.
Predom. worse out doors; better in doors	Better (resp. worse) out doors *or* in doors †.
Worse when growing cold and in cold weather; better when growing warm and in warm air.	Worse *or* better when growing cold and in cold weather, resp. growing warm or in warm air.
Better (resp worse) from warm *or* cold diet	Predom. worse from cold diet, better from warm diet.
Worse or better after eating	Worse after eating.
Worse or better from smoking	Worse from smoking.
Worse when stooping	Worse *or* better when stooping.
Better when assuming an erect position	Aggrav. oftener than improved when assuming an erect position.
Better when sitting down	*Better or* worse when sitting down.
Aggrav. oftener than improved when rising from a seat.	Worse when rising from a seat.
Worse, after mental exertion, than aft. bodily.	Worse after bodily exertion more than after mental exertion. C.Hg.
Better from being touched	Aggrav. oftener than improved by the touch.
Worse or better when bending the part	Worse when bending diseased part.
Ailments from Phosphor. or Digitalis	Ailments from abuse of metallic medicines, &c.
Worse when looking up or down	Worse when looking down.

Predomin. worse —— **Predomin. better**

During continued motion; when getting out of bed; lying with head high; when letting diseased limb hang down; from pressure; after stool, and from boring with finger (in ear or nose).

Predomin. better —— **Predomin. worse**

During rest; when standing, sitting, and lying; in horizontal position, or with head low; when lifting up diseased limb; from change of position; when assuming an erect position, and from being touched.

---

* In rare single cases, the formula "upper right, lower left side" can also be applied to Sulphur.

† Sulphur-complaints are improved by warmth of stove; aggrav. in a crowded room.

Calcarea.	Zincum.
Right side—Light hair	*Left* side—Dark hair.
Complaints (constriction, etc.) predominant in internal parts.	Complaints (constriction, etc.) predominant in external parts.
Rending pain upwards—Apoplexy . . .	Rending pain downwards—No apoplexy.
Hydrocephalus	Hydrocephaloid. C.Hg.
Itching, lessened oftener than aggravated by scratching.	Itching, generally lessened by scratching, but often also unchanged, or appearing in another place.
Pulse frequent and full, often trembling .	Pulse small and frequent in evening; slower in morning and during day; sometimes intermitting.
Thirst constant	Thirst not constant.
Sweat increased while eating	Sweat lessened while eating.

Calcarea.	Zincum.
Silly merriness *or* fear and despondency	Mood changing; cheerful; indifferent.
Ailments from hearing bad news	Ailments from fright.
Solicitude concerning bodily welfare . . .	Solicitude concern'g spiritual welfare. CHg.
Unconsciousness—Fancies—Imbecility . .	Absent-mindedness.
Vertigo, inclining to fall backwards or sideways.	Vertigo, inclining to fall sideways (left side.)
Optical illusions in black or in dark colors .	Optical illusions in bright colors.
Eruption predominant on under lip . . .	Eruption on upper lip.
Urine generally dark; sediment white, less frequently red.	Urine predominantly pale; sediment yellow.
Catam. too profuse and generally too soon.	Catam. predom. scanty and gener'y too late.
Larynx and trachea filled with mucus . .	Larynx and trachea dry.
Expectoration predominant, but not constant; morning and during day.	Expectoration almost constant; morning.
Complaints predominantly in upper part of chest, on inner side of thigh, and on sole of foot.	Complaints predominant in lower part of chest, on outer side of thigh, and on top of foot.

Calcarea.	Zincum.
REMISSION of complaints before midnight .	AGGRAVATION afternoon and *evening*, less frequently at night.
Worse when looking up or down	Worse when looking upwards.
Worse or better when bend'g diseased limb.	Worse when bending diseased limb
Aggrav. oftener than improved by exertion, (particularly mental exertion.) C.Hg.	Worse from bodily exertion.
Ailments from Phosph., Mercurius, Nitr. acid, Cinchona, or Digitalis.	Ailments from Baryta.

Predomin. worse —— **Predomin. better**

Out-doors, when getting out of bed, when stretching out diseased limb, from pressure, when swallowing and eating, from tight clothes, from boring with finger (in ear or nose), and before breakfast.

Predomin. better —— **Predomin. worse**

In-doors, after lying down, when drawing up diseased limb, when assuming an erect position, from loosening the clothes, and after breakfast.

N.B. Although both remedies have the predominant character of constitutional irritability, yet we often find with Zinc (very rarely with Calcarea) over-sensitiveness to pain; on the other hand, the sensation of numbness in suffering parts peculiar to Calcarea is very rarely found with Zinc.

Camphora.	Apis.
Complaints (burning, pressing, etc.) predominant in internal parts.	Complaints (burning, pressing, etc.) in external parts.
Want of irritability—Muscles lax . . .	Increased irritability—Muscles rigid.
Aversion to open air—Apoplexia nervosa .	Inclination for open air—Apoplexia sanguinea.
No paralysis of limbs	Paralysis of limbs.
Pulse predominantly slow, small, and weak.	Pulse accelerated and predominantly large.
Congestion of blood to ears	Congestion of blood to eyes.
Want of thirst predominant	Thirst seems to be wanting only during sweat.
Chill lessened in warm room	Chill increased in warm room.
Heat, without thirst, with aversion to uncover.	Heat, with thirst and inclination to uncover.

Camphora.	Apis.
Mental excitability	Eccentric merriness—Fickleness—Ailments from hearing bad news, from vexation, anger or jealousy.
Predominant insanity	Absent-mindedness—Mental dullness—Predominant imbecility.
Pupils contracted—Clear-sightedness . .	Pupils generally dilated—Dim-sightedness.
Very rarely nausea	Nausea.
Predominantly *sour* vomit	Bitter vomit.
Urine infrequent and scanty	Urine often, and at the same time generally less than usual.
Palpitation of heart, with regular, but generally slow beats.	Beating of heart and pulse often intermitting.
Complaints predominant on patella . . .	Complaints predominant in hollow of knee.

Camphora.	Apis.
AGGRAVATION afternoon and *night* . . .	AGGRAVATION from evening till morning.
Ailments, partic. from abuse of Cantharides, from Copper vapors, or Squilla.	Ailments from sting of musquitoes, from contagious Anthrax, Iodine, or from abuse of Cinchona.

Predomin. worse —— **Predomin. better**

In the open air, from cold,* from uncovering, and from drinking wine.

Predomin. better —— **Predomin worse**

In-doors, from warmth, from wrapping up, after lying down, in bed, and from warmth of bed, from drinking beer, and from drinking cold water.

---

* Both remedies have aggravation in cold weather.

Camph.	Cantharid.
Want of bodily irritability—Apoplexy . .	Increased irritability—Paralysis.
In afebrile diseases dryness of skin . . .	Inclination to sweat and perspiring easily.
Predom. want of thirst	Thirst is wanting during chill, but appears *after* chill and in heat.

Camph.	Cantharid.
Mental excitability	Amorousness—Fancies.
Eyes sunken	Eyes protruding.
Acute taste	Loss of taste.
Very rarely Nausea	Nausea, partic. in stomach.
Stream of urine thin	Stream of urine spread.
Urine seldom and scanty	Urine seldom and scanty, but with paralytic affections copious and often.
Complaints predom. on fore-arm, on inner side of thigh, and on foot.	Complaints predom. on upper arm, on outer side of thigh, and on hand.

Camph.	Cantharid.
Aggravation afternoon and *night* . . .	Aggrav. after midnight and *during day*.
Better from rubbing and scratching . . .	Better *or* worse from scratching, &c.
Worse when lying on side; better when lying on back.	Better (resp. worse) when lying on side *or* on back.
Worse after stool	Better *or* worse after stool.

Predomin. worse ⁀ **Predomin. better**

When closing the eyes; from pressure, and from drinking wine.

Predomin. better ⁀ **Predomin. worse**

When opening eyes, and from drinking cold water.

Camphora.	Opium.
Trembling sensation in internal parts—Apoplexia nervosa predominant.	Trembling of external parts—Apoplexia sanguinea.
No paralysis of the limbs	Paralysis of the limbs.
Pulse slow, small, weak, often imperceptible.	Pulse variable; full and slow with snoring respiration; quick and hard, with heat and quick, anxious respiration.
Coldness predominant—Heat or sweat, with aversion to uncover	Heat predominant—Heat or sweat, with inclination to uncover.

Camphora.	Opium.
Sadness—Mental excitability—Insanity .	Cheerfulness—Ecstasies *or* mental dullness—Gentleness—Boldness—Fancies—Ailments from shame, fright, anger, vexation, or joy—Imbecility more frequent than insanity.
Eyes sunken—Pupils contracted	Eyes protruding—Pupils dilated.
Clear-sightedness	Dim-sightedness.
Saliva increased—Acute taste	Saliva decreased—Loss of taste.
Predominantly *sour* vomit	Predominantly bitter vomit.
Cholera asiatica, first stage; sudden coldness, etc.	Cholera asiatica, second typhoid stage, or after too much camphor.
Very rarely costiveness—Diarrhœa predominantly painless.	Predominant costiveness; when there is diarrhœa, it is also painless.*
Urine seldom and scanty	Urine seldom and scanty, but sometimes (with paralysis) copious.

Camphora.	Opium.
AGGRAVATION afternoon and *night* . . .	AGGRAVATION night and morning.
Worse from sunlight	Worse from candle-light.
Worse after sleep	Generally worse, rarely better after sleep.
Worse from drinking wine	*Worse or* better from wine.
Better *or* worse from smoking	Worse from smoking.
Ailments from Cantharides, Scilla, or Copper vapors.	Ailments from Charcoal vapor, Digitalis, Strychnine, or Plumb.

Predomin. worse —— **Predomin. better**

From cold, growing cold and in cold weather, out-doors†, from uncovering, when moving‡, when sitting bent forward, from pressure, and from drinking coffee.

Predomin. better —— **Predomin worse**

From warmth, from growing warm, and in warm air, in-doors, from wrapping up, during rest, after lying down, in bed and from warmth of bed, when lying, standing, and sitting, particularly sitting erect, and when assuming an erect position.

N.B. Camph. has over-sensitiveness to pain, Opium predominant painlessness. Camph. sometimes has sensation of numbness, but less frequently than Opium.

---

* Both remedies have costiveness a great deal, and with retention of urine or infrequent, scanty discharge of urine With Camph. it seems to be more the inactivity of the kidneys, with Opium of the rectum. C Hg.

† With Camphor, as with most other remedies, as in nearly all other cases, congestive compl. are improv. out of doors

‡ Both remedies have aggravation "when moving painful part."

Camph.	Veratr. alb.
Want of bodily irritability—Trembling sensation in internal parts.	Increased irritability — Trembling of external parts.
Pulse more regular	Pulse not so regular.
Heat or sweat, with aversion to uncover .	Heat or sweat, with inclination to uncover.
Predominant want of thirst — Desire for drink without thirst.	Thirst more frequent than want of thirst—Thirst with aversion to drink.
No paralysis of the limbs	Paralysis of limbs.
Sadness — Rarely rage — Mental excitability—Insanity not so frequent as with Veratrum.	Cheerfulness *or* dejection—Fear—Haughtiness—Ailments from grief, anger, or from vexation with fear—Absentmindedness—Fancies—*Ecstasies or* mental dullness—Insanity more frequent than imbecility.
Saliva predominantly increased — Acute taste.	Saliva generally decreased—Loss of taste.
Very rarely nausea	Nausea in stomach, which, however, is often wanting when vomiting.
Sour vomit	Predominantly bitter vomit.
Urine seldom and scanty	Urine seldom and scanty, *or* copious.
Labor-pains weak or ceasing	Spasmodic labor-pains.
Cough, without expectoration	Cough, generally with expectoration.
Complaints predominant on fore-arm . .	Complaints predominant on upper arm.
AGGRAVATION afternoon and *night* . . .	AGGRAVATION night and morning.
Generally aggravated by pressure	Generally improved by pressure.
Predominantly better in bed	*Worse or* better in bed.
Worse when growing cold, better when growing warm.	Worse *or* better when growing cold (resp. growing warm.)
Worse after meals	Better *or* worse after meals.
Worse after stool	Worse *or* better after stool.
Ailments from Cantharides, Scilla, or Copper vapors.	Ailments from abuse of Cinchona, Iron, or Arsenic.

Predomin. worse 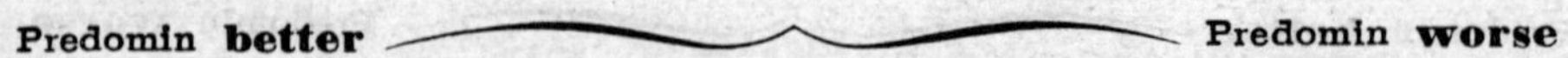 **Predomin. better**

Out of doors, from uncovering, when moving, when walking, from sitting bent forward, and from pressure.

Predomin better — **Predomin worse**

In-doors, from wrapping up, during rest, after lying down, when lying, standing, and sitting, partic. sitting erect, when assuming an erect position, from warmth of bed, from drinking cold water and beer.

N.B. Camph. has not the sensation of numbness in suffering parts frequent with Veratrum; on the other hand, Veratrum rarely has the over-sensitiveness to pain which Camph has. This seems in contradiction to the constitutional character of each remedy; but compare preface.

Cannabis.	Cantharides.
Complaints (quivering, tension, sore pain, etc.) predominant in internal parts.	Complaints (quivering, tension, sore pain, etc.) predominant in external parts.
Complaints predominant on upper eyelids, in lower part of chest, on feet, on the thighs, particularly on front part of thighs.	Complaints predominant on lower eyelids, in upper part of chest, on hands, on legs, and on back part of thighs.
In diseases without fever, dryness of skin; with fever, dry heat.	In afebrile states, easy perspiration; in febrile diseases, sweat.
Pulse slow and weak, (small and soft) . .	Pulse variable; generally quick, full, and hard.
Thirst, particularly during chill	Thirst is wanting during chill, but appears *fter* chill and during heat.
Seriousness — Cheerfulness — Irritability— Absentmindedness—Mental excitability— Ecstasies—Clairvoyance.	Mood irritable—Amativeness—Raving delirium—Insanity.
Heart-diseases	Spasms—Paralysis of the nervous system.
Diseases of the mucous membranes of the sexual and respiratory organs.	Diseases of the mucous membranes, of the uropoetic and digestive organs.
Urine often, but scanty	Urine infrequent and scanty; only exceptionally copious.
Incontinence oftener than retention of urine.	Retention of urine oftener than incontinence.
Changeable sexual desire	Increased (violent) sexual desire.
Dry coryza — Stoppage of nose—Respiration loud.	Fluent coryza—Running of nose—Respiration low.
Cough generally with expectoration . .	Cough generally dry.
AGGRAVATION forenoon and night . . .	REMISSION of symptoms morning and evening, till midnight.

Predomin. worse — **Predomin. better**

From warmth, on expiration, from eructation, and by external pressure.

Predomin. better — **Predomin. worse**

From cold, washing with cold water, on inspiration, and from stooping.

Cannabis.	Euphrasia.
Right side — Pinching pain in internal parts.	*Left* side — Pinching pain in external parts.
Pulse changed; small, weak, slow, intermitting, etc.	Pulse unchanged.
Awaking too early	Awaking too late.
Paralysis	No paralysis observed as yet.

Cannabis.	Euphrasia.
Seriousness *or* cheerfulness — Madness — Ecstasies — Absent-mindedness — Delirium.	Indifference.
Optical illusions in bright colors	Optical illusions in black or in dark colors.
Urine often, but scanty	Urine often and copious.
Dry coryza	Fluent coryza . . . .
Expectoration predominant; evening; is generally swallowed.	Expectoration predominant; morning.
Complaints predominant in lower part of chest.	Complaints predominant in upper part of chest.

Cannabis.	Euphrasia.
REMISSION morning, afternoon, evening .	REMISSION of complaints during day.
Worse or better out-doors; *better* or worse in-doors.	Better out-doors; worse in-doors.
Worse when awaking from sleep	Aggravated oftener than improved after sleep.
Almost always improved after meals . .	Worse *or* better after meals.
Worse from the touch	Better *or* worse from the touch.

Predomin. worse ⏞ **Predomin. better**

Out-doors, from exercise, when walking, on expiration, and from eructation.

Predomin. better ⏞ **Predomin. worse**

In-doors, during rest, after lying down, while lying, in bed, while sitting and standing, on inspiration, and when stooping.

N.B. Euphrasia has not the over-sensitiveness to pain which is found with Cannabis.

Cannabis.	Opium.
Lower left, upper right side — Dark hair.	Upper left, lower right side—Light hair.
Inclination for open air	Aversion to open air.
Sensation of heaviness in external parts .	Sensation of heaviness in internal parts.
Pulse slow and weak	Pulse variable; full and slow with snoring respiration; quick and hard, with heat and quick anxious respiration.
Thirst, partic. during cold stage	Want of thirst predom.
Sleeplessness predom., partic. after midnight.	Somnolence predom.—When there is sleeplessness, it appears before midnight.
No apoplexy observed yet	Apoplexy more frequent than paralysis.

Cannabis.	Opium.
Cheerfulness *or* peevishness — Ecstacies — Rarely insensibility.	Gentleness — Boldness — Hilarity — Indifference—Ecstacies *or* mental dullness.
Pupils generally contracted	Pupils generally dilated.
Nausea in stomach, rarely in throat . . .	Very rarely nausea.
Urine often, but scanty	Urine infrequent and scanty, *or* (with paralysis) copious.
Stream of urine spread	Stream of urine retarded and interrupted on acc. of spasm of neck of bladder.
Incontinence more frequent than retention of urine.	Retention of urine more frequent than incontinence.
Sexual desire changing	Sexual desire strong.
Respiration predom. with dry sound . .	Respiration generally with moist sound.
Cough generally with expectoration — Expectoration in evening; is generally swallowed.	Cough generally dry — Expectoration during day.

Cannabis.	Opium.
REMISSION morning, afternoon, and evening.	REMISSION of complaints during day and evening.
Aggrav. oftener than improved in the open air.	Improved oftener than aggrav. in the open air.
Improved oftener than aggrav. in doors	Aggrav. oftener than improved in doors.
Worse or better when assuming an erect position.	Worse when assuming erect position.
Worse *or* better after getting out of bed .	Better after getting out of bed.
Almost always improved after meals . .	Worse after meals.

Predomin. worse — **Predomin. better**

In the open air; from motion*; when walking, on expiration; from eructation, and from pressure.

Predomin. better — **Predomin. worse**

In doors; during rest; after lying down; in bed; when lying, sitting and standing; on inspiration; after meals, and when stooping.

N.B. Opium has predom. painlessness; therefore it lacks the oversensitiveness to pain, which we find with Cannabis.

---

* Both remedies have aggrav. when moving diseased part.

Cannabis.	Pulsatilla.
Upper right, lower left side — Inclination for motion.	*Upper left, lower right side*—Aversion to motion.
Quivering sensation in internal parts—Paralysis.	Quivering sensation in external parts — Apoplexy more frequent than paralysis.
Sleeplessness after midnight; awaking too early.	Sleeplessness before midnight — Awaking too late.
Chill with thirst—Pulse preval. slow	Chill without thirst; thirst only during heat — Pulse accelerated.
Chill increased in the open air	Chill lessened in the open air.

Want of reserve — Cheerfulness — Madness —Ecstacies—Clairvoyances—Rarely unconsciousness.	Taciturnity—Calm sadness of gentle dispositions —Anxiousness — Distrust—Avarice—Boldness—Indifference.
Complaints predom. on external ear	Oral complaints internal oftener than external.
Nausea in stomach, less frequently in throat.	Nausea in throat, stomach, or abdomen.
First vomiting, then hunger	First ravenous hunger, eating greedily,—afterwards vomiting.
Complaints of spleen predom.	Liver complaint predom.
Costiveness predom.	Diarrhœa predom.
Stream of urine spread	Stream of urine thin.
Urine often, but scanty	Urine infrequent and scanty.
Sexual desire changing	Sexual desire increased
Scrotum contracted	Scrotum relaxed. C.Hg.
Dry coryza	Fluent coryza more frequ. than dry coryza.
Expectoration predom.; evening.	Expectoration predom., but not constant; morning and during day.
Complaints predom. on patella	Complaints predom. in hollow of knee.

Aggravation night and forenoon	Aggravation from noon till midnight.
Worse from pressure	*Better or* worse from pressure.
Worse when moving diseased part	*Better or* worse when moving diseased part.
Better when bending diseased limb	Worse *or* better when bending the limb.
Worse (resp. better) when lying on painful *or* on unpainful side.	Better when lying on painful side; worse when lying on unpainful side.
Worse before breakfast	Better *or* worse before breakfast.
Almost always improved after meals	*Worse or* better after meals.
Worse from eructation	Aggrav. oftener than improv. by eructation.

Predomin. worse ⁀ **Predomin. better**

Out of doors; from motion; when walking, running, and from bodily exertion; when stretching out diseased limb; from pressure, and from sour things.

Predomin. better ⁀ **Predomin. worse**

In doors; during rest; after lying down; in bed; when lying, sitting and standing; when drawing up diseased limb; when stooping, and after meals.

F.B. With Cannabis we rarely find the sensation of numbness in suffering parts peculiar to Pulsatilla.

Cannabis.	Thuya.
Right side; particularly ***upper right, lower left side.***	*Left* side; particularly ***upper left, lower right side.***
Dark hair—Inclination for exercise and open air.	Light hair—Aversion to exercise and open air.
Tension or sore pain in internal parts . .	Tension or sore pain in external parts.
Thirst, particularly during chill	Thirst is wanting during chill; generally appears during heat; is not constant during sweat.
Chill, with thirst—No apoplexy	Chill, generally without thirst—Apoplexy.
Pulse slow and weak	Pulse slow and weak in morning; quick and full in evening.

Cannabis.	Thuya.
Want of reserve—Fear of apoplexy . .	Taciturnity—Fear of loss of reason.
Cheerfulness *or* peevishness—Rarely mental dullness—Delirium.	Peevishness and dejection—Haughtiness—Mental dullness—Rarely delirium.
Complaints predominant on external ear, in lower part of chest, and on patella.	Complaints predominant in inner ear, in upper part of chest, and in hollow of knee.
Urine often, but scanty	Urine often and copious.

Cannabis.	Thuya.
AGGRAVATION forenoon and night . .	REMISSION forenoon and before midnight.
Worse when turning in bed . .	Worse *or* better when turning in bed.
Worse when awaking from sleep . . .	*Worse or* better after sleep.
Worse when moving diseased part . . .	Better *or* worse when moving the diseased part.
Worse *or* better from scratching	Better from scratching.

Predomin. worse — **Predomin. better**

From motion, when walking, from touch and from pressure, on an empty stomach, and from eructation.

Predomin. better — **Predomin worse**

During rest, in bed, when lying, sitting, and standing, from washing, after breakfast, after meals, and when stooping.

Cantharides. — Lycopodium.

Cantharides.	Lycopodium.
Sensitiveness in internal parts	Numbness in internal parts.
Lancinating pain from without inwardly—Stitches upwards.	Lancinating pain from within outwardly—Stitches downwards.
Sleeplessness prevalent after midnight . .	Sleeplessness prevalent before midnight.
Pulse generally quick, full, and hard . . .	Pulse somewhat accelerated only in the evening and after meals.
Heat, with aversion to uncover	Heat, with inclination to uncover.
Chill increased after getting out of bed . .	Chill lessened after getting out of bed.
Predom. external chill, with internal heat .	Predom. internal chill, with external heat.
Thirst; drinking much at a time . . .	Thirst; drinking little at a time.
Apoplexy not observed as yet	Apoplexy.
Loquacity	Taciturnity.
Solicitude concerning bodily welfare . . .	Solicitude concerning spiritual welfare. CHg.
Complaints predominant on lower eyelids, on upper lip, on upper arm, and on outer side of thigh.	Complaints predominant on upper eyelids, on under lip, on fore-arm, and on inner side of thigh.
Eyes protruding	Eyes sunken.
Styes, right side	Styes, left side. C.Hg.
Pain in belly abating after stool	Pain in belly worse after stool.
Urine infrequent and scanty, but sometimes (with paralysis) copious—Sediment red.	Urine frequent, but scanty—Sediment red (sandy) *or* whitish.
Catamenia too soon	Catamenia too late.
Expectoration infrequent; evening . . .	Expector. almost constant; morn'g & even'g.
AGGRAVATION night, particularly after midnight and during day.	REMISSION after midnight and in *forenoon.*
Better in bed and from warmth of bed.	Worse *or* better in bed & fr. warmth of bed.
Better (resp. worse) lying on side *or* back.	Worse lying on side, better lying on back
Better when assuming an erect position. .	Worse *or* better when assum'g an erect posit.
Better when sitting down	Worse *or* better when sitting down.
Better after sweat	Worse *or* better after sweat.
Worse from growing cold, better from growing warm.	Better *or* worse from growing cold (resp. growing warm.)
Worse when uncovering; better when wrapping up.	*Generally* better from uncovering*; worse from wrapping up.
Worse from weeping	*Better or* worse from weeping.
Better *or* worse after stool	Worse after stool.

Predomin worse — **Predomin. better**

In the open air and when walking out-doors, from cold, from motion, from walking, after getting out of bed, when stooping, when closing the eyes, and from weeping.

Predomin. better — **Predomin worse**

In-doors, from warmth, during rest, after lying down, while lying, sitting, and standing, from pressure, when opening the eyes, and from drinking wine and other spirituous liquors.

N.B. In accordance with the character of increased susceptibility, which is peculiar to Cantharides, this remedy lacks the sensation of numbness in suffering parts peculiar to Lycop.

N.B. Dr. LUDLAM, on diphtheria, calls our attention to Cantharides in cases where the patient has urinary difficulties, too copious or difficult micturition, the urine containing shreds or casts of the uriniferous tubuli, shows extreme prostration, sinking, death-like turns, particularly if there appears a rash upon the skin or under (shining through) the epidermis. As Lycop. also has the urinary difficulty and according to Dr. Raue (Lecture on Diphtheria), the latter is indicated when the fauces have a darkish hue, worse on the right side, which is not unsimilar to Cantharides, we may be able to decide by Ludlam's other characteristics, or by the following of Dr. Raue, for Lycop. (worse from swallowing warm drinks, has to breathe through the mouth, or dilates the nostrils with every inspiration, the child is naughty, cross, kicks, awaking from a nap); but in cases where such symptoms are not given, we may use the differential comparison with advantage. Also look to Lachesis or Apis. C.Hg.

* Deviations can be explained by the various influences which warmth of bed has on the Lycopod. complaints. The same can be said of the varied influences which growing cold has on Lycopod. symptoms.

Capsicum.	**Nux vomica.**
Preval. *left* side—*Upper left, lower right side.*	*Right* side—*Upper right, lower left* **side.**
Light hair—Want of bodily irritability . .	Dark hair—Increased irritability.
Phlegmatic temperament—Obesity . . .	Sanguine, choleric temperament—Emaciation.
Skin and muscles lax	Skin and muscles rigid.
Inclination for open air	Aversion to open air.
Pulse often unchanged; very irregular . .	Pulse generally hard, full and accelerated, partic. during heat.
Thirst is wanting only during sweat . . .	Thirst most frequent during chill, also *before* and *after* the fever, and between heat and sweat.
Changing mood—Gentleness—Phlegma—Apoplexy or paralysis not observed as yet.	Dejection—Irritable mood—Amorousness—Absent-mindedness—Fancies.
Bursting headache, in evening, better from lying with head high.	Bursting headache, in morning, partic. with mental exertion, better when sitting still in warm room.
Dim-sightedness	Predom. clear-sightedness.
Pupils most frequently contracted, partic. during cold stage.	Pupils almost always dilated.
Chill or sweat lessened when walking out of doors.	Chill or sweat increased when walking out of doors.
Heat or sweat lessened by motion . . .	Heat or sweat increased by motion.
Complaints predom. on external ear . . .	Complaints predom. in inner ear.
Appetite for coffee—Diarrhœa . . .	Aversion to coffee—Predom. costiveness.
Sexual desire weak	Sexual desire strong.
Respiration slow	Respirat'n more frequently quick than slow.
Expectoration infrequent; partic. in morning.	Expectoration not constant; from morning till evening.
REMISSION *during day* and before midnight.	REMISSION evening till midnight.
Improved quite as often as aggrav. after stool.	Worse after stool.

Predomin. worse — **Predomin. better**

During rest; in bed; after lying down; while lying, sitting, standing; lying on left side and from pressure.

Predomin. better — **Predomin worse**

During continued motion; when walking out doors *; when stepping heavily; after rising from seat, and when lying on right side.

N.B. In accordance with the constitutional character of each remedy, we very rarely find the over-sensitiveness to pain of the Nux vom. patient with Capsicum.

* The improvement of the Capsicum-symptoms, when walking out doors, must be attributed more to motion than to open air.

Capsicum.	Pulsatilla.
Preval. *left side*—Want of irritability . .	*Right* side—Increased bodily irritability.
Skin lax—Pulse unchanged	Skin rigid—Pulse changed, intermitting, &c.
Itching lessened *or* aggrav. by scratching.	Itching unchanged *or* aggr. by scratching.
Sleeplessness after midnight; awaking too early.	Sleeplessness before midnight; therefore awaking too late.
Pulse often unchanged; very irregular . .	Pulse generally accelerated, small and weak, sometimes imperceptible.
First sweat, then heat	First heat, then sweat.
Thirst predom., but not constant; is wanting during sweat.	Predom. want of thirst, partic. during chill; thirst appears more *before* and *between* the different stages of the fever

---

Capsicum.	Pulsatilla.
Phlegma—Indolence—Malice.—Apoplexy and paralysis not observed as yet.	Sanguine temperament—Disposition gentle, but bold – Good-naturedness – Indifference – Distrust—Avarice - Calm sadness —Amorousness – Absent-mindedness—Fancies.
Home-sickness with redness of cheeks and sleepiness.	Sits sleepily in a place and refuses to move from it, (face pale.) C.Hg.
Complaints predom. on external ear; on fore-arm, and on thigh.	Ear-complaints internal oftener than external; complaints predom on upper arm and on leg.
Nausea in stomach	Nausea in throat, stomach, or abdomen.
Retention of urine predom.	Incontinence oftener than retention of urine.
Sexual desire weak	Sexual desire strong.
Respiration slow	Respiration quick.
Expectoration infrequent; partic. in the morning.	Expectoration predom., but not constant; in morning and during day.

Capsicum.	Pulsatilla.
REMISSION *during day* and before midnight.	REMISSION from midnight till noon.
Better while eating; worse *afterwards*. .	Better while drinking, worse *afterwards*.

Predomin. worse — **Predomin. better**

Out doors; from cold, and in cold weather; when lying on unpainful side; from tightening the clothes*, and from pressure.

Predomin. better — **Predomin. worse**

In doors; from warmth, and in warm air; when lying on unpainful side; while eating, and from walking heavily.

N.B. Capsicum lacks the sensation of numbness in suffering parts, peculiar to Pulsatilla; on the other hand Caps. very rarely has the oversensitiveness to pain of Pulsat.

*** Yet we also find "Sensation of clothes being unbearable" with Pulsatilla.**

Carbo animal.	Arsenic.
Tension in external parts, bruised pain in internal parts.	Tension in internal parts, bruised pain in external parts.
Paralysis not yet observed	Paralysis of limbs.
Disposition to sweat and perspiring easily.	In sickness without fever, dryness of skin.
Humid eruptions	Eruptions generally dry.
Stinging pain in scars	Burning pain in scars. C.Hg.
Hot swelling of glands	Cold swelling of glands.
Pulse accelerated and irritable, partic. towards evening; slower in morn'g, quicker in evening.	Pulse very quick, small and weak, or intermitting; quicker in morning, slower in evening.
Chill while eating or after the meals . . .	Chills lessen after eating With the chill more hunger than thirst. C.Hg.
Thirst partic. during heat	Least thirst during chill, most during sweat.
Sweat increased after sleep, during motion, and when walking out doors.	Sweat abating after sleep, during motion, and when walking out doors.
Sleeplessness before midnight	Sleeplessness preval. after midnight.

Carbo animal.	Arsenic.
Mood changing — Cheerfulness predom.— Ailments from mortification.	Mood despondent; indifferent; peevish; irritable; malicious; greedy — Ailments from grief, fright, or from vexation with dread, fear, reserved displeasure or vehemence.
Urine copious	Urine scanty (with diarrhœa) *or* copious.
Predom. dry coryza	Predom. fluent coryza.
Complaints predom. on fore-arm, on top of foot, and on thigh.	Complaints predom. on upper arm, on sole of foot, and on leg.
Worse (rsp. better) in wet *or* in dry weather.	Predom. worse in dry weather, better in wet weather.
Worse on awaking	Better after sufficient sleep; but worse on awaking when roused.
Worse on assuming an erect position . .	*Better or* worse when assuming an erect position.
Improved oftener than aggr. when stooping.	Aggrav. oftener than improved by stooping.
Better after getting out of bed	Better *or* worse after getting out of bed.
Better *or* worse from scratching	Worse from scratching.

Predomin. worse — **Predomin. better**

From motion; when walking; when getting out of bed; lying on side; after sleep; before breakfast; in company; from pressure. and when drawing up diseased limb.

Predomin. better — **Predomin. worse**

During rest; after lying down; while lying and sitting; lying on back; after breakfast; when alone; after drinking, and when stretching out diseased limb.

N.B. Although both remedies have the character of constitutional want of irritability, yet we find oversensitiveness to pain frequently with Arsenic, very rarely with Carbo animal.

N.B. The characteristic appearance of symptoms with Carbo anim. *after shaving*, particularly in the region of the nervus trigeminus, is an oversensitiveness not very rare. C.Hg.

Carb. anim.	Bellad.
Bruised pain in internal parts	Bruised pain in external parts
Apoplexy or paralysis not yet observed . .	Apoplexy—Paralysis.
Complaints predominant on fore-arm, on tip of elbow, on inner side of thigh, and on top of foot.	Complaints predominant on upper arm, in hollow of elbow, on patella, on outer side of thigh, and on sole of foot.
Thirst, particularly during heat	Thirst not constant; most rare during chill; thirst *before* and *after* the fever.
Cheerfulness.	Mood cheerful *or* sad; indifferent; peevish; irritable; malicious; distrustful.
Ailments from grief	Ailments from anger, fright, mortification, or from vexation with dread, fear, fright, or vehemence – Absentmindedness—Fancies— Unconsciousness — Delirium—Ecstasies *or* mental dullness—Insanity.
Sensitive disposition	Generally insensitiveness of disposition.
Expectoration not constant; during day .	Expectoration infrequent; morning, during day, evening.
REMISSION *during day* and before midnight.	REMISSION after midnight and in *forenoon*.
Worse (resp. better) in dry *or* in wet weather.	Worse in dry weather; predominantly better in wet weather.
Worse when lying on side, better when lying on back.	Better (resp. worse) when lying on side *or* on back.
Worse when lying on painful side, better when lying on unpainful side.	Better (resp. worse) when lying on painful *or* on unpainful side.
Worse when assuming an erect position .	*Worse or* better when assuming an erect position.
Generally aggravated *before* breakfast . .	Better before breakfast.
Worse from spirituous liquors	Worse *or* better from spirituous liquors.

Predomin. worse —————— **Predomin. better**

In the dark, in bed, from external pressure, and on an empty stomach.

Predomin. better —————— **Predomin. worse**

From light, after drinking, and after breakfast.

N.B. With Carb. anim., whose predominant characteristic is want of susceptibility, we rarely find the over-sensitiveness to pain peculiar to Belladonna. On the other hand, Belladonna rarely has the sensation of numbness in suffering parts of Carb. anim.

Carb. anim.	Calc.
Bruised pain in internal parts	Bruised pain in external parts.
Apoplexia or paralysis not yet observed .	Apoplexy—Paralysis.
Humid eruptions	Eruptions generally dry.
Chill while eating, or after the meals . .	With the chill more thirst than hunger. CHg.
Complaints predominant on tip of elbow and on thigh.	Complaints predominant on patella and on leg.
Mood changing; cheerful	Silly merriness *or* sadness—Mood despondent; peevish; irritable; amorous.
Ailments from grief or mortification. . .	Ailments from hearing bad news, or from vexation with dread, fear, or fright—Delirium – Fancies—Mental dullness.
Urine copious—Sexual desire too weak. .	Urine too frequent—Sexual desire generally too strong.
Complaints after pollutions	Predominant complaints after coition.
Nasal secretion watery	Nasal secretion thick . . . .
Expectoration not constant; during day .	Expectoration predominant, but not constant; morning and evening.
Remission *during day* and before midnight.	Remission of complaints before midnight.
Worse (resp. better) in dry *or* in wet weather.	Better in dry weather, worse in wet weather.
Worse when closing the eyes; better when opening them.	Worse (resp. better) when closing the eyes, *or* when opening them.
Predominantly worse in the dark; better from light.	Worse *or* better from light (resp. in the dark.)
Almost always improved after getting out of bed.	Worse *or* better after getting out of bed.*
Worse when rising from a seat	*Worse or* better when rising from a seat.
Worse from smoking	*Worse or* better from smoking.

Predomin. worse — **Predomin. better**

When lying on painful side, from uncovering, when drawing up diseased limb, when assuming an erect position, and from the touch.

Predomin better — **Predomin. worse**

When lying on unpainful side, from wrapping up, when stretching out diseased limb, when stooping, and after drinking.

* This may be traced back to the different influences which rest and warmth of bed have on Calcarea-complaints; the first improves, the latter aggravates.

Carb. anim.	Carb. veg.
Tension or piercing pain in external parts.	Tension or piercing pain in internal parts.
Apoplexy or paralysis not yet observed. .	Apoplexy—Paralysis.
Stinging in the scars.	Scars burn, pain when weather changes; break open. C.Hg.
Pulse irritated and accelerated, particularly towards evening.	Pulse, weak, faint, unequal, or intermitting
Heat, with aversion to uncover	Heat, with inclination to uncover.
Thirst, particularly during heat	Want of thirst predominant; thirst prevalent only during chill.

Carb. anim.	Carb. veg.
Mood changing; cheerful—Ailments from grief or mortification.	Mood irritable—Excited imagination—Unconsciousness—Delirium.
Far-sightedness	Short-sightedness.
Painless diarrhœa.	Painful diarrhœa
Secretion of urine profuse	Urine scanty.
Sexual desire weak, decreased	Sexual desire strong, increased.
Expectoration not constant; during day .	Expectoration not constant; morning.
Complaints predominant on fore-arm and on top of foot.	Complaints predominant on upper arm and on sole of foot.

Carb. anim.	Carb. veg.
REMISSION *during day* and before midnight.	REMISSION afternoon and after midnight.
Almost always improved after getting out of bed.	Worse *or* better after getting out of bed.
Worse from growing cold; better from growing warm.	*Better or* worse* from growing cold (warm.)
Worse after stool	*Worse or* better after stool
Worse from drinking cold water	Better from cold diet; worse from warm diet.

Predomin. worse ⁀ **Predomin. better**

When uncovered, when assuming an erect position, when drawing up diseased limb. and on an empty stomach.

Predomin. better ⁀ **Predomin worse**

From wrapping up, when stooping, stretching out diseased limb, when lying, after breakfast, and after drinking.

---

* The lessening of Carb. veg. symptoms, when growing cold, are without doubt attributable to the aggravation by warmth of bed and hot rooms.

Carb. anim.	Graphit.
Complaints (ulcerative pain, bruised pain, etc.) predominant in internal parts.	Complaints (ulcerative pain, bruised pain, etc.) predominant in internal parts.
Painful tension in external parts	Tensive pain in internal parts.
Paralysis not yet observed	Paralysis of limbs.
Stinging in scars	Burning of scars, break open. C.Hg.
Pulse irritated and accelerated, particularly towards evening.	Pulse full and hard, but not perceptibly accelerated.
Thirst, particularly during heat	Want of thirst, particularly during heat.
Chill increases after drinking	Chill lessens after drinking. C.Hg.

Carb. anim.	Graphit.
Mood predominantly cheerful — Ailments from mortification.	**Mood sad; despondent; peevish; amorous; Absent-mindedness—**
Secretion of urine copious	Urine scanty.
Complaints after pollutions.	Complaints after coition.
Catamenia too soon and too profuse . .	Catamenia too late and too scanty.
Respiration with moist sound	Respiration with dry sound.
Expectoration not constant; during day .	Expectoration predominant; during day and evening.
Complaints predominant on top of foot .	Complaints predominant on sole of foot.

Carb. anim.	Graphit.
Remission *during day* and before midnight.	Remission of complaints during day.
Almost always improved after getting out of bed.	Worse *or* better after getting out of bed.
Predominantly worse from growing cold; better from growing warm.	Worse or better* from growing cold (warm.)
Almost always aggravated after eating . .	Worse *or* better after eating.

Predomin. worse — **Predomin. better**

Out-doors,† in the dark, when drawing up diseased limb, before breakfast, when swallowing, from drinking wine, and from pressure.

Predomin. better — **Predomin. worse**

In-doors, from light, when stretching out diseased limb, after breakfast, and when stooping.

N.B. We very rarely find the over-sensitiveness to pain with Carb. anim. which belongs to Graphit, whose constitutional character, on the whole, is undecided.

---

* Graphit-complaints are sometimes improved, sometimes aggravated by warmth of bed also.

† Both remedies have predominant aggravation when "walking out-doors; therefore the influence of open air is not decisive here, but the effect of motion.

Carb. anim.	Phosphor.
Ulcerative pain in internal parts . .	Ulcerative pain in external parts.
Apoplexy or paralysis *not* observed as yet .	Apoplexy—*Paralysis.*
Stinging in scars	Pinching, contraction in scars; they break open and bleed. C.Hg.
Humid eruptions	Dry eruptions.
Disposition to sweat	Dryness of skin predom.
Chill lessened in warm room	Chill increased in warm room.
Chill while eating or after meals	Chill lessened after eating; with the chill more hunger than thirst. C.Hg.
Sweat increased when eating	Sweat lessened when eating.
Pulse irritated & accelerated, part. in evening.	Pulse different, irregular; sometimes intermitting.
Thirst, partic. during heat	Want of thirst almost constant.

Cheerfulness	Mood cheerful *or* dejected; indifferent, irritable; amorous.
Ailments from mortification (or grief.) . . .	Ailments from anger, fright, or from vexation with vehemence, (or from grief)—Unconsciousness—Delirium—Ecstacies—Fancies—Insanity.
Pupils dilated—Far-sightedness	Pupils generally contracted—Short-sightedness.
Urine copious	Urine often, but scanty.
Sexual desire decreased, weak	Sexual desire increased, strong.
Catamenia predom. profuse	Catamenia profuse *or* weak.
Nasal secretion watery	Nasal secretion thick or viscid.
Expectoration not constant; during day . .	Expectoration not constant; morning and during day.
Complaints predom. on tip of elbow, on thigh and on top of foot.	Complaints predom. in hollow of elbow, on leg and on sole of foot.

Remission *during day* and before midnight .	Remission of complaints after midnight.
Worse in cold weather, better in warm air. .	Worse (resp. better) in cold *or* in warm air
Worse (resp. better) in dry *or* wet weather .	Predom. better in dry weather, worse in wet weather.
Worse in company; better when alone . . .	Better (resp. worse) in company *or* when alone.
Worse when closing eyes; better when opening them.	Better (resp. worse) when closing eyes, *or* when opening them.
Worse lying on side, better when lying on back.	Generally better when lying on side, worse when lying on back.
Worse from uncovering; better when wrapping up.	Generally better from uncovering, worse from wrapping up.
Worse on awaking	Better after sufficient sleep; but worse on awaking when roused and after the siesta.
Almost always better after getting out of bed.	Worse *or* better * after getting out of bed.
Almost always aggrav. after meals, partic. worse after eating bread.	Worse *or* better after meals, partic. after eating bread.
Worse from pressure	Aggrav. oftener than improved by pressure.

Predomin. worse —— **Predomin. better**

In the open air†, in the dark, when lying on side, from uncovering, from touch, when drawing up diseased limb, on an empty stomach, from drinking wine, drinking cold water, and after sleep.

Predomin. better —— **Predomin. worse**

In doors, from light, lying on back, wrapping up, when stretching out diseased limb, and after breakfast.

N.B. We very rarely find the oversensitiveness of Phosphor. to pain with Carbo anim.

---

* This difference can be traced to the predominantly different influence which rest and warmth of bed have on Phosphor-complaints.

† "*While walking out doors*" Phosph. complaints are quite as often improved as aggravated: — if the latter is the case, motion, and not the open air, decides.

Carb. anim.	Pulsatilla.
Want of bodily susceptibility—Aversion to open air.	Increased susceptibility — Inclination for open air.
Paralysis or apoplexy not yet observed . .	Apoplexy more frequent than paralysis.
Disposition to sweat and slight perspiration.	Dryness of skin in sickness without fever.
Chill while eating or after the meals . . .	With the chill hunger and thirst. C.Hg.
Chill lessened in warm room	Chill increased in warm room.
Thirst partic. during heat	Want of thirst predom., partic. during chill; thirst *before & between* the differ. stages.
Sweat increased after sleep and when walking out doors.	Sweat less after sleep; abating when walking out doors.
Mood predom. cheerful	Mood lachrymose, sad; gentle; indifferent; bold; avaricious; distrustful—Amorousness—Ailments fr. excessive joy, fr. fright, or fr. vexation with dread, fear, or fright.
No unconsciousness or delirium	Absent-mindedn.—Fancies—Unconsciousn.
Pupils dilated—Far-sightedness	Pup. gen'ly contracted—Short-sightedness.
Diarrhœa predom. painless	Diarrhœa generally painful.
Urine copious	Urine infrequent and scanty.
Sexual desire decreased, weak	Sexual desire increased, strong.
Catamenia too soon and profuse	Catamenia too late and generally scanty.
Dry coryza	Fluent coryza (partic. r. s.) more frequent than dry coryza.
Respiration with moist sound	Respiration predom. with dry sound.
Expectoration not constant; during day .	Expectoration predom., but not constant; morning and during day.
Complaints predom. on fore-arm, on tip of elbow, on thigh and top of foot.	Complaints predom. on upper arm, in hollow of elbow, on leg and on sole of foot.
REMISSION *during day* and before midnight.	REMISSION from midnight till noon.
Generally worse in the dark, better from light.	Generally better in the dark, worse from light.
Worse when lying on side; better when lying on back.	Worse (resp. better) when lying on side *or* on back.
Worse on awaking	*Worse or* better after sleep.
Worse when assuming an erect position .	Worse *or* better when assuming an erect position.
Aggrav. oftener than improved when getting out of bed.	Improved oftener than aggrav. when getting out of bed.
Almost alw. improv. *after* gett'g out of bed.	*Better or* worse *after* getting out of bed.
Better when sitting down	Worse *or* better when sitting down.
Worse when rising from seat	*Worse or* better when rising from seat.
Worse from pressure	*Better or* worse from pressure.
Better *or* worse from scratching . . .	Worse from scratching.
Almost always aggrav. after meals . . .	*Worse or* better after meals.
Worse when swallowing; also after stool .	Better *or* worse wh. swallow'g, & after stool.
Worse when drawing a deep breath . . .	Better *or* worse when drawing a deep breath.
Worse (resp. better) in wet *or* dry weather	Worse in wet weather, better in dry weather.

Predomin. worse —— **Predomin. better**

In the open air, and when walking out doors; from cold, from growing cold, and in cold weather; from uncovering, from motion, while walking, on inspiration; when lying on painful side, drinking cold water; from pressure, and when getting out of bed.

Predomin. better —— **Predomin. worse**

In doors; from warmth, from growing warm, and in warm air; from wrapping up; during rest; when lying, sitting, and standing; on expiration; when lying on unpainful side; after drinking, and when stooping.

N.B. The oversensitiveness of Pulsat. to pain is rarely found with Carbo anim.

Carb. anim.	Sepia.
Complaints (ulcerative pain, etc.) predom. in internal parts.	Complaints (ulcerative pain, etc.) predom. in external parts.
Hot swelling of glands	Painless swelling of glands.
Apoplexy or paralysis not yet observed .	Apoplexy—Paralysis of limbs.
Pulse irritated and accelerated in evening, slow in morning.	Pulse quick and full at night, slower during day.
Thirst, particularly during heat	Predominant want of thirst; thirst constant only during chill.

Mood changing; predominantly cheerful.	Mood sad; despondent; serious; indifferent; peevish; irritable; greedy.
Ailments from grief or mortification—No unconsciousness.	Ailments from vexation with fear—Absent-mindedness—Fancies—Mental dullness—Insanity.
Pupils dilated	Pupils contracted.
Sexual desire weak	Sexual desire changing.
Catamenia too soon	Catamenia oftener too late than too soon.
Respiration with moist sound	Respiration predom. with dry sound.
Expectoration not constant; during day .	Expectoration predominant, but not constant; is loosened night and morning, and is generally swallowed.

Remission *during day* and before midnight.	**Remission** of complaints in afternoon.
Worse (resp. better) in wet or dry weather.	Generally better in wet weather, worse in dry weather.
Worse in cold weather; better in warm air.	Worse *or* better in cold (resp. warm) air.
Worse when walking out-doors	Better *or* worse when walking out-doors.
Worse when closing eyes, better when opening them.	Predominantly better when closing eyes, worse when opening them.
Almost always aggravated in bed . . .	*Better or* worse in bed and from warmth of bed.
Worse on awaking	Better after sufficient sleep; but worse on awaking when roused.
Generally aggrav. when getting out of bed.	Geenerally improv. when getting out of bed.
Worse when rising from seat	Better *or* worse when rising from seat.
Better *or* worse from scratching	Worse from scratching.
Almost always aggravated after meals . .	*Worse or* better after meals.

Predomin. worse — **Predomin. better**

From motion, when walking, when assuming an erect position, when drawing up diseased limb, when lying on side, lying on painful side, from drinking cold water, in the dark, after sleep, and after getting out of bed.

Predomin. better — **Predomin. worse**

During rest, when lying, sitting and standing, when stooping, when stretching out diseased limb, when lying on back, lying on unpainful side, after drinking, and from light.

N.B. With Carb. anim. we rarely find the over-sensitiveness of Sepia to pain; rarely with Sepia the sensation of numbness in suffering parts which belongs to Carb. anim Both remedies have mere sensitiveness (to the touch, etc.) The first is caused by the character of constitutional want of irritability, which is predominant with Carb. anim.

Carb. anim.	Sulphur.
Pinching pain in internal parts	Pinching pain in external parts.
Apoplexy or paralysis not yet observed . .	Paralysis more frequent than apoplexy.
Humid eruption	Eruptions generally dry.
Pulse irritated and accelerated, particularly towards evening; slower in the morning.	Pulse frequent night and morning; slower during day and evening.
Sweat increased after sleep	Sweat lessened after sleep.
Heat, particularly on upper part of body .	Heat on lower part of body, or general, with exception of head.
Mood cheerful	Mood serious; solemn; gentle; sad and dejected; indifferent; peevish; irritable.
Ailments from grief	Ailments from shame, or from vexation with dread, fear, or fright—Absent-mindedness—Fancies—Delirium—Mental dullness—Insanity.
Pupils dilated—Far-sightedness	Pupils generally contracted—Predom. short-sightedness.
Urine increased	Urine often, but scanty; sometimes copious.
Catamenia too soon and profuse	Catamenia generally too late and scanty.
Expectoration not constant; during day	Expectoration not constant; morning and during day; less frequent at night.
Complaints predominant on tip of elbow and on top of foot.	Complaints predominant in hollow of elbow, on patella, and on sole of foot.
Remission *dur'g day* and before midnight.	**Remission** afternoon and before midnight.
Worse (resp better) in wet *or* dry weather.	Predom. worse in wet weather, better in dry weather.
Worse from grow'g cold and in cold weather, better when grow'g warm and in warm air.	Better (resp. worse) when grow'g cold and in cold air, *or* when growing warm and in warm air.
Worse in the open air, better in-doors . .	Better *or* worse* out-doors (resp. in-doors).
Worse in bed	*Worse or* better in bed.
Generally improved after gett'g out of bed.	Worse *or* better after getting out of bed.
Worse when assuming an erect position .	Aggravated oftener than improved when assuming an erect position.
Better when stretching out diseased limb .	Aggravated oftener than improved when stretching out diseased limb.
Worse from the touch	Aggrav. oftener than improv. by the touch.
Predominantly worse *before* breakfast, better *afterwards*.	Better *or* worse before breakfast; better *or* worse *after* breakfast.
Worse from drinking cold water	Aggravated oftener than improved by drinking cold water.
Worse after stool	Better *or* worse after stool.

Predomin. worse — **Predomin. better**

In the dark. from cold, from uncovering, from motion, when drawing up diseased limb, and from pressure.

Predomin. better — **Predomin worse**

From light, from warmth, wrapping up, during rest, when lying and standing,† when stretching out diseased limb, and after drinking.

Sulphur-complaints are improved by warmth of stove, and aggravated in a crowded room.
Sulphur-complaints are aggravated by continued standing; but are improved by standing still after motion.

Carb. veg.	Bellad.
Predominant want of bodily irritability . .	*Increased irritability or* want of irritabil
Often indicated with old people	Often indic. with child'n and young women.
Rending or lancinating pain downwards .	Rending or lancinating pain upwards.
Paralysis more frequent than apoplexy . .	Apoplexy more frequent than paralysis
Suppuration or gangrene of cellular tissue.	Scleroma neonatorum.
Emaciation of diseased part	Swelling of diseased part.
Pulse weak	Pulse predominantly strong.
Heat or sweat, with inclination to uncover.	Heat or sweat, with aversion to uncover.
Predominant want of thirst; thirst preval. only during chill.	Thirst not constant; most rare during chill
Sweat more when and after gett'g out of bed.	Sweat less. when and after gett'g out of bed.
Sensitive disposition	Predominant insensibility of disposition.
Silly behavior	Mood changing; cheerful *or* sad; indifferent; peevish; distrustful; malicious.
Excited imagination	Absent-mindedness—Mental excitability *or* dullness.
Weakness of memory	Memory active *or* weak.
Short-sightedness	Far-sightedness.
Frequent complaints on upper jaw . . .	Frequent complaints on lower jaw.
Appetite for sour things	Aversion to sour things.
Fetid, humid warm flatus	Scentless flatus.
Costiveness predominant; when diarrhœa occurs, it is generally painful.	Painless diarrhœa.
Expectoration not constant; morning.	Expectoration infrequent; morning, during day, evening.
Complaints predominant in lower part of chest, in shoulder-joint, on inner side of thigh, and on calf of leg.	Complaints predominant in upper part of chest, in hip-joint, on outer side of thigh, and on shin.
Remission after midnight and in afternoon.	Remission after midnight and in *forenoon.*
Worse (resp. better) in wet *or* dry weather.	Predominantly better in wet weather, worse in dry weather.
Worse (resp. better) in cold *or* warm air .	Worse in cold air, better in warm air.
Worse when lying on side, better when lying on back.	Better (resp. worse) when lying on side *or* on back.
Worse or better after getting out of bed .	Mostly improved after getting out of bed.
Worse when looking upwards	Worse when looking sideways.
Better when assuming an erect position .	*Worse or* better when assum'g an erect pos.
Worse when stooping	*Better or* worse when stooping.
Better when leaning against anything . .	When leaning against anything worse *or* (if it is hard) better.
Worse from spirituous liquors	Worse *or* better from spirituous liquors.
Improved by eructation	Worse *or* better from eructation.
Worse when swallowing food	Worse, particularly when swallowing drink.

Predomin. worse ⁓ **Predomin. better**

In the dark, in bed and from warmth of bed, from wrapping up, from change of position, when lying or standing, when bending diseased part backwards, when stretching out suffering limb, and from pressure.

Predomin. better ⁓ **Predomin. worse**

From light, when growing cold, from uncovering, and when drawing up diseased limb.

N.B. The over-sensitiveness of Belladonna to pain is very rarely found with Carb. veg.; the sensation of numbness in suffering parts, belonging to Carb. veg., rarely with Belladonna. Yet mere sensitiveness (to the touch) is found with both remedies; also sensation of numbness generally with Belladonna, (particularly in parts painful before.)

Carb. veg.	Calc.
Often indicated with old people	Indicated oftener with children than old people.
Dark hair—Muscles rigid	Light hair—Muscles lax.
Rending pain downwards	Rending pain upwards.
Very rarely apoplexy—Humid itch . . .	Apoplexy—Dry itch.
Pulse weak, unequal, intermitting . . .	Pulse full and accelerated, often trembling.
Chill while eating, or after meals . . .	Hunger with the chill. C.Hg
Heat of only one side; right side . . .	Heat of only one side; left side.
First chill, then heat	First heat, then chill.
Thirst only during cold stage	Thirst constant dur'g all stages of the fever, only sometimes wanting during chill.

Carb. veg.	Calc.
Fear of apoplexy—Silly behavior . . .	Fear of loss of reason—Silly merriness or despondency—Peevishness—Amorousness.
Excited imagination	Imbecility
Nasal complaints external	Nasal compl. internal oftener than external.
Eruption on upper lip	Eruption predominant on under lip.
Predominant aversion to salt things . .	Appetite for salt things.
Diarrhœa generally painful	Diarrhœa generally painless.
Urine infrequent and scanty; alkaline . .	Urine too often; acid.
Complaints after pollutions . . .	Predominant complaints after coition.
Leucorrhœa acrid	Leucorrhœa mild.
Breath cold—Cough generally dry . .	Breath hot—Cough generally with expector.
Expectoration in morning	Expectoration morning and during day.
Complaints predominant in lower part of chest, on upper arm, and on thigh.	Complaints predominant in upper part of chest, on fore-arm, and on leg.

Carb. veg.	Calc.
Remission after midnight and in afternoon.	Remission of complaints before midnight.
Better (resp. worse) in wet *or* dry weather.	Worse in damp air, better in dry air.
Worse *or* bett.r in cold (resp. warm) air	Worse in cold weather, better in warm air.
Worse in the evening air	Worse from exertion on an empty stomach.
Worse in the dark, better from light . . .	Worse *or* better from light (resp. in the dark.)
Worse when looking upwards	Worse when looking up or downwards.
Worse after breakfast	Aggravated more frequently *before* breakfast than *after* it.
Worse after meals	Better *or* worse after meals.
Better from cold diet, worse from warm .	Worse from drinking cold water.
Worse or better after stool	Worse after stool.
Worse when rising from seat	*Worse or* better when rising from seat.
Ailments from (Mercurius, Cinchona, Alcohol, or) Lachesis.	Ailments from (Mercurius, Cinchona, Alcohol) Nitr acid., Phosph., or Digitalis.

Predomin. worse — **Predomin. better**

When growing warm, after rising from a seat, from the touch, and after breakfast.

Predomin. better — **Predomin. worse**

When growing cold, and on an empty stomach.

Carb. veg.	China.
Aversion to exercise	Inclination for exercise.
Want of bodily irritability—Hæmorrhages, bright-red blood.	Increased irritability—Hœmorrhages, dark blood.
Paralysis more frequent than apoplexy	Apoplexy more frequent than paralysis.
Stitches downwards	Stitches upwards.
Deep ulcers wiih scanty discharge	Shallow ulcers, with copious, ichorous discharge.
Distention of veins of feet	Distention of veins of hands.
Predom. internal chill with external heat	Predom. external chill with internal heat.
Chill while eating and after the meals	More hunger than thirst with the chill. C.Hg.
Thirst only during cold stage	Thirst constant only during sweat, appears partic. *before* and *between* the different stages.
Pulse weak, unequal	Pulse small, but hard and quick; more quiet after meals; irregular.
Sweat increased after meals	Sweat lessened after meals.

Carb. veg.	China.
Sensitive disposition Fear—Silly merriness.	Predom. insensibility of disposition—Mood sad; indifferent; peevish; amorous.
Ailments from fright or fear	Ailments from vexation — Absent-mindedness—Rarely unconsciousness.
Complaints predom. in inner angle of eye.	Complaints predom. in external angle of eye.
Costiveness predom.—Diarrhœa generally painful.	Diarrhœa predom., generally painless.
Expectoration not constant; morning	Expectoration not constant; during day and evening.
Complaints predom. on shoulder joint, on wrist, and on back part of thigh.	Complaints predom. in hip joint, in ankle, and on front side of thigh.

Carb. veg.	China.
REMIS. after midnight and in the afternoon.	REMISSION *afternoon* and evening.
Better (resp. worse) in wet *or* dry weather.	Worse in wet weather; bett. in dry weather.
Worse (resp. better) in cold *or* warm air	Worse in cold air; better in warm air.
Worse from wrapping up; better from uncovering.	Worse (resp. better) from wrapping up, *or* from uncovering.
Worse from lying on side, better when lying on back.	Aggrav. oftener than improved when lying on back.
Worse after sleep	Better after sufficient sleep; worse on awaking when roused.
Worse when getting out of bed	Worse *or* better when getting out of bed.
Worse *or* better *after* getting out of bed	Better *after* getting out of bed.
Worse when rising from seat	Worse *or* better when rising from a seat.
Worse after meals	Worse *or* better after meals.
Worse *or* better after stool	Worse after stool.
Worse in the Spring	Worse in the Autumn.

Predomin worse — **Predomin. better**

In the dark, when growing warm, when sitting erect, when bending diseased part backwards, *after* rising from a seat, from pressure, and when eating.

Predomin. better — **Predomin. worse**

From light, when growing cold; when sitting, partic. bent forwards; when leaning against something, and from eructation.

N.B. In accordance with the constitutional character of each remedy, we very rarely find with Carb. veg. the oversensitiveness of Cinchona to pain,—rarely with Cinchona the sensation of numbness in suffering parts, which belongs to Carb. veg. However, mere sensitiveness (to the touch. &c.) is found with both remedies,—and with Cinchona also general numb sensation, (partic. in parts which were *before* painful.)

Carb. veg.	Ferrum.
Want of bodily irritability—Muscles rigid.	Increased irritability—Muscles lax.
External parts become black	Red parts become white.
Paralysis more frequent than apoplexy . .	Apoplexy more frequent than paralysis.
Pulse weak, unequal	Pulse full and hard.
Thirst *only* during chill	Thirst, partic during chill.
Chill while eating or after the meals . .	Chill better after eating. C.Hg.
Sweat increased after meals	Sweat lessened after meals.

Carb. veg.	Ferrum.
Mood anxious	Changeable mood; also alternating cheerful one evening, sad the next—Haughtiness.
Excited imagination — Unconsciousness — Fancies.	Rarely delirium.
Predom. hunger	Generally loss of appetite.
Appetite for sour things	Aversion to sour things.
Costiveness predom. — Diarrhœa generally painful.	Diarrhœa predom.; painless.
Catamenia too soon	Catamenia preval. too late.
Labor pains weak or ceasing	Spasmodic labor pains.
Respiration with moist sound	Respiration predom. with dry sound.
Breath cold — Expectoration not constant.	Breath hot — Expectoration predom. with the cough.
Complaints predom. in wrist and on thigh.	Complaints predom. on ankle and on leg.

Carb. veg.	Ferrum.
Remission afternoon and after midnight .	Remission *during day* and before midnight.
Better (resp. worse) in wet *or* dry weather.	Worse in wet weather, better in dry weather.
Better (resp. worse) in cold *or* warm air .	Worse in cold air, better in warm air.
Worse *or* better after getting out of bed .	Better after getting out of bed.
Worse *or* better when swallowing . . .	Worse when swallowing.

Predomin. worse — **Predomin. better**

When getting out of bed, after breakfast, from drinking wine *, when ascending, from exerting the mind or the eyes, after rising from a seat, when sitting erect, and from exercise.

Predomin. better — **Predomin. worse**

After lying down, when growing cold, when descending; when sitting, partic. sitting bent forward; on an empty stomach, and during rest.

N.B. In accordance with the constitutional character of each remedy, we very rarely find the over-sensitiveness of Ferrum to pain, with Carb. veg. — Both remedies sometimes have mere sensitiveness. (to the touch, &c.)

---

* Wine improves Ferrum-complaints only, when it is not acid; on the other hand we find aggrav. with Ferrum from drinking beer. In corresponding cases Ferrum cures mania-a-potu; however this is rarely caused by wine, most frequently by beer and brandy. Comp. note Ars. and Ferr.

Carb. veg.	Graphit.
Lancinating pain in internal parts . . .	Lancinating pain in external parts.
Consequences of being overheated—Palpitation of heart, without anxiety.	Consequences of taking cold—Palpitation of heart, with anxiety.
Pulse weak, unequal, intermitting . . .	Pulse often unchanged; generally full and hard, but not perceptibly accelerated.
Thirst only during chill	Want of thirst, particularly during heat.
Heat, with inclination to uncover	Heat, with aversion to uncover.
Loosing the hair, particularly on back part of head.	Loosing the hair, particularly on top and sides of head, and from the whiskers.

Carb. veg.	Graphit.
Mood irritable—Rarely amorousness—Unconsciousness—Fancies—Excited imagination.	Mood changing; peevish; sad; dejected—Absent-mindedness – No delirium.
External nasal complaints — Complaints predominant on upper jaw and on upper arm.	Nasal complaints internal oftener than external—Complaints predominant on lower jaw and on fore-arm.
Painful diarrhœa	Painless diarrhœa.
Urine alkaline	Urine generally acid.
Complaints from pollutions	Complaints from coition.
Catamenia too soon and too profuse . .	Catamenia too late and too scanty.
Leucorrhœa thick	Leucorrhœa watery.
Rattling of mucus	Respiration with dry sound.
Expectoration not constant; morning . .	Expectoration predominant; during day and evening.

Carb. veg.	Graphit.
REMISSION afternoon and after midnight .	REMISSION of complaints during day.
Worse from riding	*Better* while riding, *worse afterwards*.
Worse after a satisfying meal	Worse when hungry.

Predomin. worse —— **Predomin. better**

Out-doors, from wrapping up, from warm diet, from riding, from pressure, in the dark, when lying, after rising from a seat, after sweat, and from drinking wine.

Predomin. better —— **Predomin. worse**

In-doors,* from uncovering, from cold diet, after vomiting, from light, and while sitting.

N.B. In accordance with the character of want of irritability belonging to Carb veg. we very rarely find over-sensitiveness to pain, which is peculiar to Graphit. with this remedy.

---

* We also find aggravation in-doors with Carb. veg., that is when the room is too warm.

Carb. veg.	Lycopod.
Hæmorrhages; blood light-red	Hæmorrhages; blood dark.
Dark hair—Muscles rigid	Light hair—Muscles lax.
Lancinating pain in internal parts . . .	Lancinating pain in external parts.
Reaction ceases after fruitless efforts . .	Exhaustion after acute fevers.
Sensitiveness* in internal parts	Sensation of numbness in internal parts.
Silly merriness - Rarely amorousness—Very rarely delirium - Excited imagination—Very rarely apoplexy	Seriousness — Gentleness—Cheerfulness *or* dejection—Peevishness—Dejection—Distrust — Malice — Greediness — Haughtiness—Change of moods—Absentmindedness—Mental dullness—Insanity.
Pulse weak, unequal, intermitting - Heat right side.	Pulse somewhat accelerated only in evening and after meals -Heat left side †
Thirst only during cold stage of fever . .	Thirst is wanting only during chill.
Sweat increased when and after getting out of bed.	Sweat lessened when and after getting out of bed,
Flatus predominantly fetid, humid, warm .	Flatus predominantly scentless.
Diarrhœa, when it appears, painful . . .	Diarrhœa, when it appears, painless.
Urine infrequent and scanty . . .	Urine often, but scanty.
Incontinentia urinæ predominant . . .	Retention of urine more frequent than incontinence.
Catamenia too soon	Catamenia too late.
Cough generall dry — Expectoration in morning.	Cough generally with expectoration, which is loosened, particularly in morning and evening.
Complaints predominant in lower part of chest, on upper arm, on wrist, and on thigh.	Complaints predominant in upper part of chest, on fore-arm, on ankle, and on leg.
REMISSION after midnight and in the afternoon.	REMISSION after midnight and in the *forenoon.*
Worse sometimes in wet, sometimes in dry weather.	*Worse* in wet weather, *better* in dry air.
Worse from warmth of bed	Better *or* worse from warmth of bed.

Predomin. worse —— **Predomin. better**

In the open air, from cold, from warm diet, after rising from a seat, when sitting bent forward, when stooping, after sweat, during exercise, and in the dark.

Predomin. better —— **Predomin. worse**

In-doors, from warmth and rest‡, from cold diet, when sitting, particularly sitting erect, after lying down, and from light.

---

* Carb. veg. also has sensitiveness predominant in external parts, Lycopodium generally has sensation of numbness; yet we find oversensitiveness to pain much more prominant with Lycopodium than with Carb. veg., in accordance with the prevailing characteristic of want of irritability peculiar to Carb. veg.; the sensation of numbness generally appears in the painful parts, predominantly after paroxysms of acute pain.—Both remedies have sensitiveness to the touch.

† Lycopodium has chill as well as heat on one side only—the left side—thus deviating in this from the predominant side of its other symptoms.

‡ Yet we also find aggrav. *after* exercise, and improvement during continued moderate exercise, with Carb. veg

Carb. veg.	Mercur.
Dark hair	Light hair.
Want of bodily irritability—Muscles rigid.	Increased irritability—Muscles lax.
Often indicated with old people — Very rarely apoplexy.	Often indicated with children—Very rarely paralysis.
Humid itch—Thirst only during chill	Dry itch—Thirst during all stages.
Pulse weak, unequal	Pulse irregular, gen'ly full and accelerated.
Heat of only one side, r. s.	One-sided heat, left side.
Chill lessened in warm room — Sweat increased when or after getting out of bed.	Chill increased in warm room — Sweat abates while and after getting out of bed.
Silly merriness — Fear of apoplexy - Excited imagination.	Seriousness—Fear of loss of reason.—Despondency — Peevishness — Malice — Absent-mindedness—Imbecility.
Complaints predom. on upper jaw	Complaints predom. on lower jaw.
Hunger predom.	Generally loss of appetite.
Aversion to milk	Appetite for milk.
Costiveness more frequent than diarrhœa	Diarrhœa more frequent than costiveness.
Urine infrequent and scanty; smelling like ammoniacum.	Urine often and copious; smelling acid.
Catamenia too soon	Catamenia too late.
Expectoration in morning	Expectoration during day.
Complaints predom. in lower part of chest, on upper arm and on calf of leg.	Complaints predom. in upper part of chest, on fore-arm and shin.
REMISSION after midnight and in the afternoon.	REMISSION of complaints during day.
Better (resp. worse) in wet *or* dry weather.	Worse in wet weather; better in dry weather.
Better (resp. worse) in cold *or* warm air	Worse in cold air; better in warm air *.
Worse from wrapping up; better from uncovering.	From wrapping up, (resp. uncovering;) better *or* worse †.
Worse *or* better after getting out of bed	Better after getting out of bed.
Almost always aggrav. when eating	Better *or* worse when eating.
Worse from warm diet; better from cold diet.	Worse from cold *or* warm diet.
Worse or better after stool	Worse after stool.
Worse in the Spring	Worse in the Autumn.
Ailments from abuse of Mercury	Ailments from sting of insects, Arsenic or Copper vapors, Sulph. or Calc.

Predomin. worse — **Predomin. better**

In the dark, while lying ‡, after rising from a seat, and after breakfast.

Predomin. better — **Predomin. worse**

From light, and on an empty stomach.

N.B. The sensation of numbness in suffering parts belonging to Carb. veg. is rarely found with Mercur.

---

* Both remedies undecided as regards "growing cold" and "growing warm."

† This difference can be traced back to the different influence which warmth of bed and other warmth has on Mercurial-complaints

‡ We also find improvement of complaints with Carb. veg "*after lying down.*"

Carb. veg.	Nux vom.
Want of bodily irritability—Hæmorrhages, bright-red blood.	Increase of irritability — Hæmorrhages, blood dark.
Clonic spasms—Very rarely apoplexy . .	Tonic spasms predom.—Apoplexy.
Sleeplessness preval. before midnight . .	Sleeplessness preval. after midnight.
One-sided chill predom. l. s.; heat pred. r. s.	One-sided chill predom. r. s.; heat pred. l. s.
Distention of veins of feet	Distention of veins of hands.
Thirst only during cold stage—Pulse weak, unequal.	Thirst mostly during cold stage — Pulse generally full, hard, and accelerated.
Chill while eating and after the meals . .	Hunger with the chill. C.Hg.

Carb. veg.	Nux vom.
Very rarely amorousness	Dejection—Peevishness—Malice.
Excited imagination	Absent-mindedn.—Weak reasoning powers.
Short-sightedness	Far-sightedness.
Complaints predom. on upper jaw . . .	Complaints predom. on lower jaw.
Hunger predom.	Generally loss of appetite.
Appetite for sour things—Aversion to fat things.	Predom. aversion to sour things—Appetite for rich (fat) dishes.
Urine generally dark	Urine generally pale.
Respiration with moist sound—Breath cold.	Respiration with dry sound—Breath hot.
Expectoration in morning	Expectoration in morning, during day, and evening.
Complaints predom. in upper arm and on wrist.	Complaints predom. on fore-arm and on ankle.

Carb. veg.	Nux vom.
Remis. after midnight and in the afternoon.	Remission evening till midnight.
Better (resp. worse) in wet *or* dry weather.	Predom. better in wet weather, worse in dry weather.
Worse from washing and moistening . .	Improv. oftener than aggr. by washing, &c.
Better (resp. worse) in cold *or* warm air .	Worse in cold weather; better in warm air.
Worse in the evening air	Better in the night air (congestion to head.)
Worse when lying on side; better when lying on back.	*Generally* better when lying on side, worse when lying on back.
Worse after sleep	Better after sufficient and not too long sleep; worse on awaking when roused.
Worse from pressure	*Better or* worse from pressure.
Worse when stooping	Better *or* worse when stooping.
Worse when sneezing	*Worse or* better when sneezing.
Better from eructation	Worse *or* better from eructation.
Worse or better after stool	Worse after stool.
Ailments from abuse of Mercur.	Ailm. from Arsenic or Copper vapors, from Sulph., Calc., Phosph., Iodine, or Plumb.
Bad effects fr. stale fish, decayed vegetables.	Bad effects fr. spices, ginger, onions. C.Hg.

Predomin. worse — **Predomin. better**

In the dark, when growing warm, from warmth of bed, from wrapping up, from warm diet, when eating, when sitting erect, when lying, after sweat, when stretching out suffering limb, when bending diseased part backwards, when lying on side, after sleep, from washing and moistening diseased part, and from pressure.

Predomin. better — **Predomin. worse**

From light, when growing cold, from uncovering, from cold diet, when sitting bent forward, when drawing up diseased limb, when lying on back, and when assuming an erect position.

N.B. In accordance with the constitutional character of each remedy, we very rarely find the over-sensitiveness of Nux vom. to pain with Carb. veg., — rarely with Nux vom. the sensation of numbness in suffering parts, which belongs to Carb. veg. Mere sensitiveness (to touch, &c.) however, we find with both remedies.

Carb. veg.	Phosph.
Eruptions generally humid — Scars burn, painful with change of weather, break open	Eruptions generally dry — In scars pinching contraction, break open and bleed. C. Hg.
One-sided chill, predominantly left side . .	One-sided chill, predominantly right side.
Local sweat on upper part of body . . .	Partial sweat on lower part of body.
Distention of veins of feet	Distention of veins of hands.
Chill or sweat lessened in (warm) room	Chill or sweat increased in (warm) room.
Chill while eating or after meals	Chill with hunger, and lessened by eating something. C. Hg.
Sweat increased when eating	Sweat abating when eating.
Thirst only during cold stage of fever — Pulse weak.	Want of thirst — Pulse most frequently quick, full, and hard; unequal.
Want of bodily irritability	*Increased irritability or* want of irritabil.
Sensitive disposition	Disposition *insensible or* sensitive.
Fear of apoplexy — Very rarely amorousness.	Fear of apoplexy or of loss of reason — Mood changing, cheerful *or* sad and dejected; indifferent; peevish; haughty.
Weak memory	Active memory — Insanity.
Complaints predominant on upper jaw and upper lip.	Complaints predominant on lower jaw and lower lip.
Fetid flatus	Hot, scentless flatus.
Costiveness predominant; when diarrhœa occurs, it is generally painful.	Diarrhœa predominant; generally painless.
Urine infrequent and scanty	Urine often, but scanty.
Leucorrhœa greenish	Leucorrh. (or nasal secretion) ochre-yellow.
Labor-pains weak or ceasing	Labor too painful.
Breath cold — Expectoration in the morning.	Breath hot — Expect. morn'g and dur'g day.
Compl. predom. on thigh and calf of leg .	Complaints predominant on leg and shin.
REMISSION after midnight and in afternoon.	REMISSION of complaints after midnight.
Worse in the evening air	Worse in the evening twilight.
Better (resp. worse) in wet *or* dry weather.	Predominantly worse in wet weather, better in dry weather.
Worse in bed	Worse *or* better in bed.
Worse when lying on side, better when lying on back.	Generally better when lying on side, worse when lying on back.
Worse after sleep	Better after sufficient sleep, but worse on awak'g when roused, and after the siesta.
Worse from pressure	*Worse or* better from pressure.
Worse after meals	Worse *or* better after meals.
Better from eructation	Worse *or* better from eructation.
Worse or better after stool.	Worse after stool.

Predomin. worse — **Predomin. better**

When growing warm, out-doors,* in the dark, when sitting erect, after rising from a seat, from the touch, after a satisfying meal, after drinking, when lying on side, and after sleep.

Predomin. better — **Predomin. worse**

When growing cold, in-doors, from light, when sitting bent forward, and when lying on back.

N.B. The over-sensitiveness of Phosph. to pain is very rarely found with Carb. veg.

* "When walking out-doors," Phosphor-complaints are aggravated quite as often as improved. In the first case it is exercise, and not open air, which aggravates.

Carb. veg.	Pulsat.
Want of bodily irritability — Often indicated with old people.	Increased irritability — Often indicated with children.
Hæmorrhages, bright-red blood — Ulcers with scanty discharge of pus.	Hæmorrhages, dark blood—Ulc'rs with copious suppuration.
Thirst only during cold stage — Pulse weak, unequal.	Thirst is wanting during chill — Pulse generally quick, small, and weak.
Paralysis more frequent than apoplexy . . .	Apoplexy more frequent than paralysis.
Complaints predom. on upper jaw, on upper lip, and on thigh.	Complains predom. on lower jaw, on lower lip, and on leg.
Mood irritable; silly, merry; rarely dejected or peevish; rarely amorous.	Mood changing; — gentle; sad; indifferent; bold; greedy; distrustful; amorous. — Ailments from excessive joy, grief, fright, or vexation.
Excited imagination	Absent-mindedness.
Costiveness predom.	Diarrhœa predom
Catamenia too soon and profuse	Catamenia generally too late and scanty.
Coryza dry oftener than fluent	Coryza fluent oftener than dry.
Cough generally dry—Expectoration in morning—Rattling of mucus.	Expectoration predom., but not constant; morning and during day — Respiration generally with dry sound.
Remission after midnight and in the afternoon.	Remission from midnight till noon.
Better (resp. worse) in wet *or* dry weather. .	Worse in wet weather, better in dry weather.
Worse or better in cold weather; *better or* worse in warm air.	Better in cold weather; worse in warm air.
Worse in the dark, better from light . . .	*Generally* better in the dark, worse in the light.
Worse after sleep	Worse or better after sleep.
Worse when getting out of bed	Improved oftener than aggrav. when getting out of bed.
Better when sitting down	Worse *or* better when sitting down.
Worse when sitting erect; better when sitting bent forward.	*Generally* better when sitting erect, worse when bending forward.
Worse when rising from a seat	*Worse or* better when rising from a seat.
Predom. worse *after* rising from a seat . . .	*Generally* better *after* rising from a seat.
Better when assuming an erect position . .	Worse *or* better when assuming an erect position.
Worse from pressure	*Better or* worse from pressure.
Worse after meals	*Worse or* better after meals.
Predom. worse after stool	Improved oftener than aggrav. after stool.
Better from loosening the clothes	Predom. better from tying clothes tight.

Predomin. worse — **Predomin. better**

In cold weather, from cold*, out doors and when walking out doors; from washing, moistening, or stretching out diseased part; from weeping, from pressure, tightening the clothes, from exercise; when getting out of bed, when sitting erect; after rising from a seat, after stool, and in the dark.

Predomin. better — **Predomin. worse**

In warm air, from warmth, in doors, when sitting, after † lying down, when drawing up diseased limb, from eructation, during rest ‡, from loosening the clothes, when sitting bent forward, and from light.

N.B. We rarely find the oversensitiveness of Pulsat. to pain with Carb. veg. — Mere sensitiveness (to touch, &c.) is found with both remedies.

---

* Both remedies have predom. improvement "*when growing cold,*" and aggrav. of compl. "*when growing warm.*"
† When lying, in bed, from warmth of bed, and from wrapping up, both remedies have predom. aggrav. of symptoms.
‡ Yet we also find with Carb. veg. (as with Pulsat.) aggrav. *after* exercise, and improvement during continued, moderate exercise.

Carb. veg.	Sepia.
Hæmorrhages, bright-red blood — Rarely apoplexy.	Hœmorrhages, dark blood — Apoplexy.
Eruptions generally humid	Eruptions generally dry.
Pulse weak	Pulse frequent and full at night, slow during day; accelerated by vexation and exercise.
Chill first. then heat	Heat first, then chill.
Mood silly; rarely dejected or peevish . .	Mood serious; sad; indifferent — Greediness — Ailments from vexation with fear — Absent-mindedness.
Delirium—Excited imagination	Insanity—Imbecility.
Short-sightedness	Far-sightedness.
Eruption on upper lip	Eruption on under-lip.
Hunger predom.	Generally loss of appetite.
Predom. aversion to salt things	Appetite for salt things.
Catamenia too soon	Catamenia oftener too late than too soon.
Leucorrhœa,—thick	Leucorrhœa watery.
Rattling of mucus	Respiration predom. with dry sound.
Cough generally dry; expector in morning.	Cough generally with expectoration, which is loosened at night and in the morning, and is generally swallowed.
Complaints predom. on upper arm . . .	Complaints predom. on fore-arm.
Remis. after midnight and in the afternoon.	**Remission** of complaints in the afternoon.
Better (resp. worse) in dry *or* wet weather.	Predom. better in wet weather, worse in dry weather.
Worse when walking out doors; but also worse in overheated rooms.	Better *or* worse when walking out doors; worse in a crowded room.
Predom. better after lying down	*Worse or* better after lying down.
Almost always aggrav. in bed	Better *or* worse in bed.
Worse after sleep	Better after sufficient sleep; worse on awaking when roused from sleep.
Worse when getting out of bed	Improv. oftener than aggrav. when getting out of bed.
Aggrav. oftener than improv. *after* getting out of bed.	Improv. oftener than aggrav. *after* getting out of bed.
Worse after meals*	*Worse or* better after meals.
Worse when rising from a seat	Worse *or* better when rising from a seat.

Predomin. **worse** — Predomin. **better**

In the dark, when growing warm, from wrapping up, from warmth of bed, lying on side, when turning in bed, after sleep, when and after getting out of bed, from exercise, after breakfast, when sitting erect, and after rising from a seat.

Predomin. **better** — Predomin. **worse**

From light, when growing cold †, from uncovering, lying on back; when sitting, part. when sitting bent forward; when leaning against something, from eructation, during rest ‡, and on an empty stomach.

N B. With Carb. veg. we rarely find the oversensitiveness of Sepia to pain, and with Sepia rarely the sensation of numbness in suffering parts, belonging to Carb. veg.—Mere sensitiveness (to touch) is found with both remedies.

---

* Both remedies have aggrav. after a satisfying meal.
† Both remedies have predom. aggrav. form cold, improv. from warmth — in cold (resp. warm) weather improv. quite as often as aggrav. of symptoms.
‡ Yet we also find aggrav. with Carb. veg. after exercise, and improvement during continued moderate exercise.

Carb. veg.	Sulphur.
Hæmorrhages, bright-red blood—Pinching pain in internal parts.	Hæmorrhages, dark blood—Pinching pain in external parts.
External parts grow black	Red parts become white.
Eruptions generally humid	Eruptions generally dry.
Pulse weak and unequal	Pulse full, hard, and accelerated.
Thirst only during cold stage of fever . .	Generally want of thirst during chill—Most during heat.
Yellow fever	Asiatic cholera. C.Hg.
Mood foolishly merry; rarely depressed or peevish.*	Mood serious, solemn; changing; sad; gentle; indifferent—Absentmindedness—Insanity – Imbecility.
Hot spots on the head	Cold spot on the head.
Complaints predom. in inner angle of eye.	Complaints predom. in external angle of eye.
Saliva predominantly increased	Saliva generally decreased.
Hunger predominant	Generally loss of appetite.
Urine infrequent and scanty; with odor-like ammoniac.	Urine often, but scanty; but sometimes (only after strong doses of Sulph.) copious; acid.
Catamenia too soon and profuse	Catamenia generally too late and scanty.
Expectoration in the morning	Expectoration in the morning and during day; less frequent at night.
Complaints predominant in lower part of chest and on upper arm.	Complaints predominant in upper part of chest and on fore-arm.
REMISSION afternoon and after midnight .	REMISSION afternoon and before midnight.
Better (resp. worse) in wet *or* dry weather.	Worse in wet weather, better in dry weather.
Worse out-doors, better in-doors; but worse in overheated rooms.	Better *or* worse out-doors (resp. in-doors), particularly worse in crowded rooms.
Worse when turning in bed	*Worse or* better when turning in bed.
Predominantly worse *after* breakfast . .	Improved quite as often as aggravated *after* breakfast.
Worse when stooping	Better *or* worse when stooping.
Better when assuming an erect position .	Aggravated oftener than improved when assuming an erect position.
Worse when looking upwards	Worse when looking down.
Worse from touch	Aggravated oftener than improved by the touch.
Aggravation oftener than improvement after stool.	Aggravated quite as often as improved after stool.

Predomin. worse —— **Predomin. better**

In the dark, from cold, from warm diet, when getting out of bed, when sitting erect, after rising from a seat, from pressure, and from exercise.

Predomin. better —— **Predomin. worse**

From light, warmth, cold diet, after lying down,† during rest, when sitting bent forward, and when assuming an erect position.

N.B. Of all our medicines Carbo vegetabilis is, according to its symptoms, the most similar to the characteristic symptoms of yellow fever, as much so as Sulphur corresponds to the characteristics of Asiatic cholera. Hence each remedy respectively, when it can be given in time, is best given in the first symptoms of these epidemics, in order to reduce each case at least to a milder form—an immense advantage. It is worthy of note that charcoal would put an end to the spreading of yellow fever, if the excrements of each patient, and every corpse, were covered by coarse charcoal powder; but whether the internal use of it will prevent the disease with individuals has not yet been ascertained. Sulphur prevents Chol. asiat. with individuals, if the finest powder, called milk of Sulphur, is put into the stockings, so as to come in contact with the soles of the feet; a pinch a day is sufficient to cause a gentle pouring out of sulphurated hydrogen through the pores of the skin, all over the body, blackening bright silver. But whether the substance which carries the disease is destroyed by it, has not been ascertained yet. C.Hg.

* Irritable mood occurs with both remedies.
† We find aggravation predominant with both remedies "while lying."

Causticum.	Clematis.
Right side—Dark hair—Skin and muscles rigid.	*Left* side—Light hair—Skin and muscles lax.
Paralysis of limbs	Paralysis not yet observed.
Itching, relieved *or* aggravated by scratching.	Itching, unchanged by scratching.
Pulse somewhat irritated only towards evening, on account of ebullition of blood.	Pulse excited, with throbbing in the veins.
Thirstlessness	Thirst.
Chill lessened in a warm room	Chill increased in a warm room.
Dejection — Distrust — Haughtiness — Ailments from fright, mortification, grief, or disappointed love.	Irritable mood—Contrit'n of spirit —Homesickness — Ailments from home-sickness or contrition of spirit.
Absent-mindedn. — Fancies — Unconsciousness.	Difficulty in thinking.
Catamenia too late	Catamenia too soon.
Expectoration not constant; is loosened in the evening, night, and morning; is generally swallowed.	Expectoration quite seldom
Complaints generally on top of foot. . .	Complaints on sole of foot.
AGGRAVATION *evening*, night, morning . .	AGGRAVATION night and morning.
REMISSION during the day	REMISSION during day and evening.
Better or worse from warmth of bed . .	Worse from warmth of bed, yet often better in bed.
Worse when closing the eyes, better when opening them.	Better (resp. worse) when closing *or* when opening the eyes.
Improved oftener than aggravated by washing and moistening diseased part.	Worse from washing and moistening diseased part.
Improved oftener than aggravated by eating bread.	Worse from eating bread.
Worse after stool	Better *or* worse after stool.
Ailments from Plumbum or abuse of Cinchona, from Asa fœt., Euphrasia or Colocynthis.	Ailments from abuse of Mercury.

Predomin. worse ⁀ **Predomin. better**

In dry weather, during rest, when standing,* and after breakfast.

Predomin. better ⁀ **Predomin. worse**

In wet weather, from motion, when walking, but also when lying, from touch, on an empty stomach, from eating bread, and from washing and moistening diseased part.

N.B. Clematis lacks the sensation of numbness in suffering parts peculiar to Causticum.

---

* The symptoms of Clematis are improved by standing still after motion, but are aggravated when standing "for any length of time." Compare Sulphur.

Causticum.	Lachesis.
Upper right, lower left side— Dark hair . .	*Upper left, lower right side*— Light hair.
Muscles rigid	Muscles lax.
Complaints (heaviness, &c.) predom. in external parts.	Complaints (heaviness, &c.) predom. in internal parts.
Eruptions dry *or* humid	Eruption predom. humid.
Apoplexy not yet observed	Apoplexy.
Paralysis, often of both sides (paraplegie) . .	Paralysis generally only one-sided.
Pulse generally unchanged, only towards evening somewhat accelerated on account of orgasm of blood.	Pulse changed in strength and quality, generally small, weak, accelerated, and irregular, sometimes intermitting or trembling.
Heat descending	Heat ascending.
External chill with internal heat predom. . .	Internal chill with external heat predom.
Want of thirst	No thirst during chill, but *before* chill ; is not constant during the hot stage.
Sweat increased while eating, lessened when getting out of bed.	Sweat lessened while eating, increased when getting out of bed.
Lying on the side dur'g sleep—Anx's dreams.	Lying on back during sleep—Pleasant dreams.
Mood depressed ; taciturn ; peevish	Mood serene ; loquacious ; irritable ; amorous.
Ailments from fright, mortification, grief, or disappointed love.	Ailments from fright or jealousy.
Cloudiness of mind—Melancholy	Comprehending easily (quickly) ; mental excitement—Ecstasies.
Very rarely delirium or insanity	Very rarely absent-mindedness or unconsciousness.
Far-sightedness	Short-sightedness.
Nasal-complaints predom. external	Nasal complaint predom. internal.
Urine often, but scanty	Urine too often.
Sexual desire too weak	Sexual desire too strong.
Catamenia of too long duration and generally too late.	Catamenia of too short duration ; at the same time too soon *or* too late.
Expectoration not constant ; is loosened evening, night and morning ; must generally be swallowed.	Expectoration infrequent ; is loosened morning and during day, and in some cases is swallowed.
Aggravation *evening*, night, morning ; remission during day.	*Worse* from noon till midnight ; better from midnigt till noon, (except in the morning on awaking.) C.Hg.
Worse during new moon, less frequently during a thunderstorm.	*Worse* before a thunder-storm.
Worse in snowy air	Worse from heat of sun (sun-stroke).
Worse on inspiration and on expiration . .	Better on inspiration.
Worse after sleep	*Worse or* better after sleep.
Worse when eating and swallowing	When eating and swallowing improved oftener than aggravated.
Almost always aggravated after meals . . .	Better *or* worse after meals.
Worse after drinking	Better *or* worse after drinking.
Worse from spirituous liquors	Better *or* worse from spirituous liquors.
Generally better when lying on painful side, worse when lying on unpainful side.	Worse when lying on painful side, better when lying on unpainful side.

Predomin. **worse** — Predomin. **better**

In dry, cold weather ; in doors, when lying on back, when letting diseased limb hang down, when bending suffering part backwards, after breakfast, after pollutions, from shaking the head, when lying on unpainful side, on inspiration, and when swallowing and eating.

Predomin. **better** — Predomin. **worse**

In damp and warm air, out doors *, while lying †, lying on side, when lifting up diseased limb, from bodily exertion, on an empty stomach, from the touch, and from pressure.

N.B. Lachesis lacks the sensation of numbness in suffering parts which is often found with Caust.; — on the other hand, sensitiveness (to touch, &c.) is predom. with Lachesis—oversensitiveness to pain it has less frequently.

---

* Both remedies have predom. aggrav. when *walking* out doors.
† Both remedies have predom. improv. in bed.

Causticum.	Phosphor.
Complaints (pinching pain, &c.) predom. in external parts.	Complaints (pinching pain, &c.) predom. in internal parts.
Gnawing sensation in internal parts—Hæmorrhages &c., dark blood.	Gnawing pain in external parts — Hæmorrhages, bright-red blood.
Emaciation of feet; distention of veins of feet.	Emaciation of hands; distent. of veins of hands.
Numbness, partic. in suffering parts	Sensation of numbness in suffering parts, *or* in distant parts.
Itching, aggravated oftener than lessened by scratching.	Itching, lessened oftener than aggravated by scratching.
Eruptions humid *or* dry	Eruptions almost always dry.
Ailments from abuse of Plumb. or Cinchona, from Asa fœtida, Euphrasia or Colocynth.	Ailments from Iodine or Natr. mur.
Ulcers, also fistulous ones, or after burns, with throbbing and burning pain and watery pus.	Ulcers painless, or with piercing, festering pain, with viscous pus.
Diseases of bones, partic. of Epiphyses . . .	Diseases of bones, partic. of Diaphyses.
Pulse often unchanged—Varicosities . . .	Pulse accelerated, irregular, often intermitting.
Chill lessened in bed and in warm room, increased out doors.	Chill increased in bed, and in warm room, lessened out doors.
Sweat increased when eating	Sweat lessened when eating.
Net-like appearance of capillaries—Chill predom. l. s.	Chill r. s. — Throbbing in veins; distention of veins.—Congestions.
Heat descending	Heat ascending.
Epilepsy with loss of consciousness	Epilepsy with full consciousness.
Painful paralysis	Painless paralysis.
Phlegmatic temperament	Sanguine choleric temperament.
Sensitive disposition—Mood despondent, very rarely irritable—Very rarely delirium—Absent-mindedness — *Weak memory* — Melancholy — Ailments from mortification or disappointed love.	Insensibility *or* sensitiveness of disposition — Chang'g mood; indifferent; irritable; cheerful; despondent. — Very rarely distrust — Amativeness—Irritable excitability—Ecstacies — Predom. *active memory*—Insanity— Ailments from anger or from vexation with fright or vehemence.
Far-sightedness	Short-sightedness.
Appetite for beer	Aversion to beer.
Thirst with disgust for drink	Desire for drink without thirst.
Sexual desire weak—Catamenia scanty. . .	Sexual desire strong—Catamenia increased *or* scanty.
Nasal secretion watery	Nasal secretion thick.
Expectoration with putrid or greasy taste, is generally swallowed, loosened at *night*, morning and evening.	Expectoration with salty, sour or sweetish (and putrid) taste, loosened morning and during day.
Complaints most frequent in inner ear and on instep.	Complaints most frequent on external ear, and on sole of foot.
Remission of complaints during day	Remission after midnight.
Worse in dry weather, better in damp air . .	Aggrav. more frequ. in wet than dry weather.
Washing improves in most cases	Washing aggravates in most cases.
Worse during new moon, less frequently during thunder-storm.	Worse before thunder-storm.
Improved oftener than aggrav. by exertion .	Worse from bodily exertion.

Predomin. worse — **Predomin. better**

In dry weather; during rest when standing and sitting, particularly when sitting erect; from rubbing, and after sleep*.

Predomin. better — **Predomin. worse**

In wet weather, from continued moderate motion †, from sitting bent forward, from pressure, and from washing and moistening suffering part.

N.B. Caust. has not the oversensitiveness of Phosph. to pain.

---

* Exceptionally Phosph. has aggrav. after sleeping in the afternoon; on awaking (when roused) from sleep, it has aggrav. quite as often as improvement, therefore the latter follows only after *sufficient* sleep.

† Both remedies have aggrav. when beginning to move; an "improvement during motion" which occurs with Phosphor. seems to refer exclusively to pain in joints, therefore to suffering part when moved.

Causticum.	Pulsatilla.
Upper right, lower left side.	Upper left, lower right side.
Complaints (pinching pain, etc.) predominant in external parts; sensitiveness predominant in internal parts.	Complaints (pinching pain, etc.) predominant in internal parts; sensitiveness to touch in external parts.
Apoplexy not yet observed	Apoplexy.
Paralysis, generally painful	Paralysis of rare occurrence and painless.
Itching, lessened *or* aggravated by scratching.	Itching, aggravat'd *or* unchang'd by scratch'g.
When asleep lying on side	When asleep lying on back, often with arms thrown over the head.
Pulse generally unchanged	Pulse changed, sometimes intermitting; generally quick, small, weak.
Chill or sweat on suffering part — Chill predominantly left side.	Heat on suffering part—Chill predominantly right side.
Chill lessened in bed and in warm room; increased out-doors.	Chill increased in bed and in warm room; lessened out-doors.
Sweat increased when walking out-doors	Sweat lessened when walking out-doors.
Want of thirst	Thirst very rarely during chill.

Causticum.	Pulsatilla.
Hopelessness	Mood changing; indifferent; bold; greedy; amorous—Calm sadness of gentle disposit's.
Ailments from disappointed love	Ailments from vexation or excessive joy—Delirium.
Vertigo, inclining to fall forwards or sideways.	Vertigo, inclining to fall backwards.
Far-sightedness — Optical illusions in dark colors.	Short-sightedness—Optical illusions in bright colors.
Sour vomit	Vomit bitter oftener than sour.
Urine often, but scanty	Urine infrequent and scanty.
Sexual desire decreased	Sexual desire increased.
Catamenia of long duration	Catamenia of short duration.
Respiration with moist sound	Respiration prevalent with dry sound.
Cough generally dry—Expectorat. is loosened even'g, night & morn'g, & is mostly swallow.	Cough generally with expectoration—Expectoration morning and during day.
Complaints predominant on fore-arm & instep.	Compl. predom. on upper arm and sole of foot.

Causticum.	Pulsatilla.
Aggravation from *evening* till morning	Aggravation from noon till midnight.
Worse dur'g new moon, less frequently dur'g thunder-storm.	Worse before thunder-storm.
Better in bed	Generally aggravated in bed.
Better or worse from warmth of bed	Worse from warmth of bed.
Worse after sleep	*Worse or* better after sleep.
Worse after meals	Worse *or* better after meals.
Worse when swallowing	Worse *or* better when swallowing.
Generally improved by eating bread	Worse from bread.
Worse after stool	*Better or* worse after stool.
Worse after bodily exertion	Aggravated by mental oftener than by bodily exertion. C.Hg.
Worse when moving diseased limb	*Better or* worse when moving diseased limb.
Almost always improved when sitting down	*Worse or* better when sitting down.
Almost always aggrav. when ris'g from a seat.	Worse *or* better when rising from a seat.
Better *after* rising from a seat	Better *or* worse *after* rising from a seat.
Worse on inspiration and expiration	Worse on expiration; better on inspiration.

Predomin. worse — **Predomin. better**

In dry weather, from cold, from growing cold and in cold weather, when walking out-doors*, lying on back, lying on left side, when stretching out diseased limb, from vinegar and sour things, from tying clothes tight, after stool, and when moving suffering part.

Predomin. better — **Predomin worse**

In wet weather, from warmth, from growing warm and in warm air, lying on (right) side, when lying generally, drawing up diseased limb, from the touch, loosening the clothes, and from eating bread.

N.B. Causticum has not the over-sensitiveness of Pulsatilla.

---

* Both remedies have improvement of complaints out-doors generally.

Causticum.	Rhus.
Upper right, lower left side—Dark hair . .	Upper left, lower right side—Light hair.
Gnawing pain, or sensitiveness in intern. parts.	Gnawing pain or sensitiveness in extern. parts.
Apoplexy not yet observed	Apoplexy.
Itching aggrav. *or* lessened by scratching . .	Itching, lessened by scratching.
Hæmorrhages, dark blood— Painful ulcers . .	Hæmor., bright-red blood—Painless ulcers.
Cures moles, varices, and cystic tumors by suppuration—Eruptions dry *or* humid . .	Causes atrophy of warts—Eruptions generally humid.
When asleep lying on side	When asleep lying on back, sometimes on belly.
Pulse often unchanged	Pulse quick, small, soft, sometimes trembling, irregular or intermitting.
Chill, coldness, &c., chiefly on left side . . .	Coldness of right side predom *.
Heat on back part of body	Heat on front part, coldness on back part of body.
Distention of veins of feet	Distention of veins of hands.
Congestion to ears	Congestion to eyes.
Chill lessened by drinking	Chill increased by drinking.
Heat abated by drinking water	Heat increased by drinking water.
Chill on diseased part—Want of thirst predom.	Sweat on diseased part—Thirst not constant.

Causticum.	Rhus.
Peevishness—Distrust—Absent-mindedness .	Sadness and despondency—Delirium.
Ailments from fright, mortification, grief, disappointed love.	Ailments from vexation with fear.
Vertigo inclining to fall forwards or sideways.	Vert., inclining to fall forewards or backwards.
Appetite for beer—Aversion to sweets . . .	Aversion to spirituous liquors— Appetite for sweets.
Urine often, but scanty	Urine often and copious.
Sexual desire and potency diminished . . .	Erections.
Catamenia too late and scanty	Catamenia too soon and profuse.
Nasal secretion watery—Respirat. with moist sound.	Nasal secretion thick— Respiration with dry sound.
Expectoration is loosened from evening till morning; is swallowed.	Expectoration in the morning.

Causticum.	Rhus.
Worse during new moon	Worse during increase of moon.
Almost always improved † in bed	Worse *or better* in bed.
Almost always aggrav. after meals	Worse *or* better after meals.
Improved oftener than aggrav. by exertion .	Worse from bodily exertion.
Worse when moving diseased part	Improved oftener than aggrav. by moving the part.
Almost always improved when sitting down .	Worse *or* better when sitting down.
Almost always aggrav. when rising from a seat.	*Worse or* better when rising from a seat.
Better *after* rising from a seat	Worse *or* better *after* rising from a seat.
Worse on in- and expiration	Worse on inspiration; better on expiration.
Worse after stool	Improved oftener than aggrav. after stool.
Worse when looking upwards	Worse when looking down.

Predomin. **worse** — Predomin. **better**

In dry weather, in doors, but also when *walking* out doors, when stretching out diseased limb, when letting it hang down, from warm diet, *after* breakfast, after stool, and when moving suffering part.

Predomin. **better** — Predomin. **worse**

In wet weather, out doors, when drawing up diseased limb, when lifting it up or resting it on anything, when washing or moistening suffering part, from cold diet, and drinking cold water, from eating bread, when lying, from touch‡, and on an empty stomach.

---

* All other one-sided complaints Rhus as well as Caust. has predom. on r. s. On the other hand **we find—going to** sleep of the whole *left* side with *Caust.*, while with *Rhus* the same symptom appears on r. s.

† With both remedies we find improvement oftener than aggrav. from warmth of bed.

‡ The complaints of both remedies are predom. improved by pressure.

Causticum.	Sepia.
Sensitiveness predominant in internal parts.	Sensitiveness predom. in external parts.*
Rending pain upwards—Lancinating pain from without inwards.	Rending pain downwards — Lancinating pain from within outwards.
Itching, lessened *or* aggravated by scratching.	Itching, always aggravated by scratching.
After the itch transparent blisters, which leave a clean, sore spot on skin, after they burst, on which new blisters soon appear.	*After itch* corroding blisters full of discolored matter, confluent, generally humid, and with bad odor; when these blisters burst, they leave an impure ulcer.
Warts disappear by suppuration	Warts become atrophic.
Pulse irritated and accelerated in evening, slow in morning.	Pulse quick and full at night, slow during day.
Heat descending	Heat ascending.
Want of thirst	Thirst constant only during chill.

Causticum.	Sepia.
Taciturnity—Mood distrustful—very rarely irritable.	Loquacity — Seriousness — Indifference—Greediness—Insanity—Imbecility.
Ailments from fright, grief, or mortification.	Ailments from vexation with fear.
Apoplexy not yet observed	Apoplexy.
Discharge of moisture or fetid pus from the ears.	Discharge chiefly of blood from the ears.
Sour vomit	Predominantly bitter vomit.
Discharge of urine too often and scanty .	Discharge of urine too seldom.
Sexual desire weak	Sexual desire changing, with diminished potency.
Catamenia too scanty	Catamenia too profuse *or* too scanty.
Respiration with moist sound	Respiration predominant with dry sound.
Cough, particularly evening till midnight; most frequently dry; expectoration is loosened from evening till morning, and is generally swallowed.	Cough, particularly forenoon and evening, till midnight; generally with expectoration, which is loosened night and morning and generally swallowed.

Causticum.	Sepia.
Remission of complaints during day . .	Remission of complaints afternoon.
Worse when hungry	Worse after a satisfying meal.
Complaints predominant on patella . . .	Complaints predominant on tip of elbow.
Ailments from Plumbum, Asa fœt., Eupras. or Colocynth.	Ailments from Sulphur or from sting of insects.

Predomin. worse — **Predomin. better**

From moving suffering parts, and after breakfast.

Predomin. better — **Predomin worse**

From touch or external pressure, from washing, on an empty stomach, and after eating bread.

---

* This corresponds to the twofold influence of touch and external pressure. On the other hand, Causticum lacks the over-sensitiveness of Sepia to pain, and Sepia generally the sensation of numbness in suffering parts belonging to Caust

Causticum.	Sulphur.
Right side; particularly *upper right, lower left side.*	*Left* side; particularly *upper left, lower right side.*
Rending pain upwards—Lancinating pain from without inwards.	Rending pain downwards — Lancinating pain from within outwards.
Itching, aggravated *or* lessened by scratching; seldom unchanged.	Itching, almost always lessened by scratching.
Painful ulcers	Painless ulcers.
Pulse often unchanged; only towards evening somewhat irritated and accelerated; slow in morning.	Pulse generally quick, full, and hard; accelerated, particularly night and morn'g; slower during day and evening.
Descending heat	Ascending heat.
Heat on painful part	Coldness on painful parts.
Predom. external chill, with internal heat.*	Predom. internal chill, with external heat.
Chill lessened in bed	Chill increased in bed.
Want of thirst predominant	Thirst, mostly during heat.
Cures moles, cystic tumors, etc., by suppuration and forming scabs.	Causes atrophy of warts.
Distrust—Rarely irritable mood	Mood changing; serious; solemn; gentle; indifferent.
Ailments from fright, grief, disappointed love.	Ailm. fr. shame or vexation with fright, dread or fear—Delirium—Imbecility—Insanity.
Complaints predominant on inner angle of eye—Far-sightedness.	Complaints predominant on external angle of eye—Short-sightedness.
Saliva generally increased	Saliva generally decreased.
Desire for beer	Des. for *or* avers. to beer & spirituous liquor.
Urine often, but scanty	Urine often and scanty, sometimes (after strong doses) copious.
Catamenia of too long duration	Catamenia generally of short duration.
Spasmodic labor-pains	Labor-pains weak or ceasing.
Expectoration is loosened evening, night, and morning; it is generally swallowed.	Expectoration morning and during day; less frequently at night.
REMISSION of complaints during day . .	REMISSION afternoon and before midnight.
Worse during new moon	Worse during full moon.
Almost always improved in bed	*Worse or* better in bed.
Generally improved by warmth of bed .	Generally aggravated by warmth of bed.
Predominantly worse when lying on back, better when lying on side.	Worse (resp. better) when lying on side or on back.
Worse when turning in bed	*Worse or* better when turning in bed.
Better *before* breakfast, worse *afterwards.*	W. *or* b. on empty stom. (resp. after breakf't).
Worse when hungry	Worse after a satisfying meal.
Worse after stool	Better *or* worse after stool.
Almost always improved by the touch .	Aggravated oftener than improved by touch.
Improved oftener than aggrav. by washing.	Almost always aggravated by washing.
Worse from moving diseased part . . .	*Worse or* better from mov'g diseased part.
Improv'd oftener than aggravat'd by exert'n.	Worse from bodily exertion.
Worse when looking upwards	Worse when looking down.
Worse from grow'g cold & in cold air, better when grow'g warm and in warm air.	Better *or* worse from grow'g cold & in cold weather (resp. grow'g warm & in warm air).

Predomin. **worse** — Predomin. **better**

In dry weather, from cold, from warm diet, lying on right side, and when letting diseased limb hang down.

Predomin. **better** — Predomin. **worse**

In wet weather, from warmth, from cold diet and from drinking cold water, from eating bread, when lying, lying on left side, when lifting up diseased limb, in bed and from warmth of bed, from touch, and from bodily exertion.

* This relation corresponds exactly to the influence of cold, and of warm diet, on the one hand, and that of warmth and of cold diet on the other hand.

Chamomilla.	Belladonna.
Left side—Light hair—Skin & muscles lax.	*Right* side—Dark hair—Skin & muscl. rigid.
Inclination for motion—No apoplexy . .	Aversion to motion * — Apoplexy.
Very rarely paralysis	Paralysis.
Pulse accelerated and tense, but small . .	Pulse generally quick, tense, full, and hard
Sweat only on head	Sweat general, except on head.
Sweat increased when and after getting out of bed.	Sweat lessened, when and after getting out of bed.
Thirst constant	Thirst not constant; most rarely dur'g chill.
Sensitive disposition	Generally insensibility of disposition.
Seriousness—Sadness—Rarely distrust . .	Mood changing; foolishly merry *or* sad; malicious.
Mental dullness—Very rarely delirium . .	Mental excitability *or* dullness—Fancies—Insanity.
Pupils contracted, (first contracted, then dilated.)	Pupils generally dilated, (first *dilated*, then contracted.)
Complaints predom. on under-lip	Complaints predom. on upper lip.
Appetite for sour things—Nausea in stomach.	Aversion to sour things—Nausea in throat, or abdomen, less frequently in stomach.
Hot, fetid flatus	Scentless flatus.
Respiration loud—Voice hoarse or deep .	Respiration predom. low—Voice hoarse or raised.
Expectoration during day	Expectoration never at night.
The milk runs from the breast; it is diminished or spoiled.	The milk runs from the breast and is generally increased.
Inguinal hernia easily reducible . . .	Inguinal hernia, small, recent, difficult to reduce.
Complaints predom. on calf of leg . . .	Complaints predom. on shin.
Aggrav. evening & night, partic. bef. midn.	Remis. after midnight and in the forenoon.
Better or worse when growing cold (resp. growing warm.)	Worse from growing cold, better from growing warm.
Better or worse from uncovering (resp. wrapping up.)	Worse from uncovering, better from wrapping up.
Better after sweat	Worse *or* better after sweat.
Worse when lying on back, better when lying on side.	Better (resp. worse) when lying on back or side.
Better when lying on painful side, worse when lying on unpainful side.	Worse (resp. better) when lying on painful or on unpainful side.
Worse *or* better after getting out of bed .	Almost always improved after getting out of bed.
Better *or* worse from coffee	Worse from drinking coffee.
Worse when swallowing food	Worse, partic. when swallowing drink.
Worse *or* better from pressure	Predom. better from pressure.
Worse from eructation	Improved oftener than aggr. by eructation.
Worse or better when moving diseased part.	Worse when moving diseased part.
Almost always improved when bending diseased part.	*Better or* worse when bending diseased part.
Ailments from Coffea, Colocynth., Ignat., Nux vom., Pulsat., Valeriana.	Ailments from animal poisons, Cinchona, Iodine, Mercur., or Plumb.

Predomin. worse ——— **Predomin. better**

From warmth, during rest, when standing, after lying down, while lying, in bed, and from warmth of bed, when stooping, when stretching out diseased limb, and from eructation.

Predomin. better ——— **Predomin. worse**

From cold, from exercise, when walking, when drawing up diseased limb, from drinking cold water † and after stool.

* We also find inclination for motion in single or suffering parts with Belladonna.

† From cold diet in general, both remedies have predom. improvement of complaints; — from warm diet predom. aggravation. Comp. complaints concomitant to swallowing.

Chamomilla.	Cocculus.
Left side—Inclination for exercise—Gnawing sensation in external parts.	*Right* side—Aversion to exercise—Gnawing sensation in internal parts.
Very rarely paralysis—No apoplexy . . .	Paralysis—Apoplexy.
Congestion to head	Congestion to feet.
Chill lessened in warm room	Chill increased in warm room.
Heat increased in bed	Heat lessened in bed.
Thirst constant in fevers	Predom. want of thirst—Thirst only sometimes during hot stage.
Pulse often unequal	Pulse often imperceptible.

Taciturnity—Irritable mood	Loquacity—Gentleness.
Ailments from anger, mortification, or from vexation with vehemence.	Ailments from vexation with reserved displeasure.
Delirium	Fancies—Insanity.
Appetite for sour things—Aversion to beer.	Aversion to sour things—Desire for *or* aversion to beer.

AGGRAVATION evening and night, partic. before midnight.	REMISSION night and forenoon.
Worse from warmth of bed	*Worse or* better from warmth of bed.
Worse (resp. better) from wrapping up, *or* from uncovering	Worse from uncovering; better from wrapping up.
Better *or* worse from drinking coffee . .	Worse from drinking coffee.
Worse from eructation	Better *or* worse from eructation.
Better *or* worse when assuming an erect position.	Worse when assuming an erect position.
Worse or better when moving diseased part.	Worse when moving diseased part.
Worse *or* better from pressure	Better from pressure.

Predomin. worse — **Predomin. better**

During rest, while lying, in bed, from warmth, and from warm diet.

Predomin. better — **Predomin. worse**

From exercise, when walking, when bending suffering part, from cold*, from drinking cold water, after stool, and from change of position.

N.B. With Chamomilla we rarely find the sensation of numbness in suffering parts, peculiar to Cocculus.

* Both remedies have predom. aggravation when growing cold, and in cold weather,—improvement of symptoms when growing warm, and in warm air.

Chamomilla.	Ignatia.
Inclination for exercise – Gnawing sensation in external parts.	Aversion to exercise—Gnawing sensation in internal parts.
Itching (aggravated or) unch'd by scratching.	Itching, lessened *or* changed to another place by scratching.
Painful ulcers, also with proud flesh . . .	Painless ulcers.
No apoplexy—Very rarely paralysis . .	Apoplexy—Paralysis.
Pulse quick and tense, but small	Pulse generally accelerated, full, and hard, with throbbing in veins.
Chill or sweat, increased after getting out of bed.	Chill or sweat, lessened after getting out of bed.
Chill often confined to front part of body .	Chill often only on back part of body.
Thirst during all stages of the fever . .	**Thirst only during chill and after sweat.**
Seriousness — Dejection — Vexation, with paroxysms of rage.	**Mood changing; cheerful *or* sad and despondent—Reserved mortification—Gentleness—Amativeness—Boldness.**
Ailments from anger, or from vexation with vehemence.	**Ailments from hearing bad news, from shame, grief, disappointed love, and jealousy, or from vexation with reserved displeasure.**
Unconsciousness	Fancies—Insanity.
Catamenia increased	Catamenia too scanty.
Inspiration quick; expiration slow . . .	Inspiration slow; expiration quick.
Expectoration during day	Expectoration in the evening, rarely in the morning.
AGGRAVATION evening and night, particularly before midnight.	REMISSION of complaints before midnight.
When growing cold (resp. growing warm) better *or* worse.	Predominantly worse when growing cold, better when growing warm
Worse (resp. better) from uncovering *or* wrapping up.	*Generally* better from uncovering, worse from wrapping up.
Worse when lying on back, better when lying on side.	*Generally* better when lying on back, worse when lying on side.
Worse when getting out of bed	Better *or* worse when getting out of bed.
Better *or* worse from drinking coffee . .	Worse from drinking coffee.
Almost always aggravated when eating .	Improv. oftener than aggrav. when eating.
Worse when swallowing food	Worse when swallowing drink.

Predomin. worse —— **Predomin. better**

From warmth, from warm diet, when swallowing, after breakfast, during and after meals, from eructation, on inspiration, when taking a deep breath, from weeping, when rising from a seat, when lifting up or stretching out diseased limb, and when closing the eyes.

Predomin. better —— **Predomin. worse**

From cold,* from cold diet, from drinking cold water, on an empty stomach, after stool, on expiration, after sweat, when letting diseased limb hang down or when drawing it up, when bending suffering part, particularly when bending it backwards, and when opening the eyes.

* Both remedies have predominant aggravation in *cold weather*, improvement in warm air.

Chamomilla.	Mercurius.
Inclination for exercise — Hæmorrhages; blood dark.	Aversion to exercise—Hæmorrhages; blood bright-red.
Apoplexy not yet observed	Apoplexy.
Itching, (aggrav. or) unchang'd by scratch'g.	Itching, aggravat'd *or* improv'd by scratch'g.
Pulse accelerated, small and tense	Pulse generally full and accelerated.
One-sided heat, right side	One-sided heat, left side.
Partial sweat on head	Sweat general, except head.
Congestion to eyes	Congestion to ears.
Chill lessened in warm room	Chill increased in warm room.
Sweat increased when and after getting out of bed.	Sweat lessened when and after getting out of bed.

Chamomilla.	Mercurius.
Irascibility	Malice—Amorousness—Very rarely delir'm.
Ailm's from anger or vexat'n with vehemence.	Ailments from insults—Fancies.
Pupils contracted	Pupils dilated.
Nasal complaints predominantly internal	Nasal compl. external oftener than internal.
Toothache during sweating stage	Sweat with toothache; chill after it. C.Hg.
Complaints on under lip	Complaints on upper lip.
Nausea in stomach	Nausea in œsophagus or stomach.
Catamenia too soon and profuse	C. too late; at the same time scanty *or* profuse.
Expectoration infrequent	Expectoration not constant.
Complaints predominant on calf of leg	Complaints predominant on shin.

Chamomilla.	Mercurius.
AGGRAVATION evening and night, particularly before midnight.	AGGRAVATION from evening till morning.
Generally worse in dry weather, better in wet weather.	Better in dry weather, worse in wet weather.
Better (resp. worse) from uncovering *or* wrapping up.	*Generally* worse from uncovering, better from wrapping up.
Worse when lying on back, better when lying on side.	*Generally* better when lying on back, worse when lying on side.
Worse *or* better after getting out of bed.	Better after getting out of bed.
Worse when eating and swallowing, particularly when swallowing food.	Better *or* worse when eat'g & swallow'g, partic. worse when swallow'g saliva & drink.
Predominantly worse from warm diet, better from cold diet.	Worse from cold *or* warm diet; in the latter case bettered by cold diet.*
Better *or* worse from coffee	Worse from drinking coffee.
Worse when blowing nose	Worse when blowing nose, better *afterw.*
Better *or* worse from pressure	Predominantly worse from pressure.
Worse or better when moving the part	Worse when moving diseased part.
Ailments from Coffea, Colocynth., Ignatia, Nux vomica, Pulsatilla, or Valeriana.	Ailments from sting of insects, Arsenic or Copper vapors, from Sulphur, Calcarea, or abuse of Cinchona.

Predomin. worse —— **Predomin. better**

In dry weather, during rest, when standing and lying†, lying on unpainful side, and after breakfast.

Predomin. better —— **Predomin. worse**

In wet weather, from exercise, when walking, when lying on painful side, before breakfast, from drinking cold water, after sweat, after stool, when bending diseased part, and from change of position.

N.B. We rarely find the over-sensitiveness of Chamom. to pain with Mercurius, although the character of increased constitutional irritability belongs to both.

---

* The improvement sometimes found with Mercurius, by cold diet, refers exclusively to food, as cold drinks always aggravate the symptoms of this remedy, (in consequence of characteristic aggravation *when swallowing drink.*

† We find the complaints of both remedies predominantly aggravated when in bed and from warmth of bed.

Chamom.	Nux vom.
Predom. *left* side — Skin and muscles lax.	*Right* side—Skin and muscles rigid.
Hair light—Inclination for exercise—Child desires to be carried.	Hair dark — Aversion to exercise; inclination to lie down.
Epilepsy with loss of consciousness . . .	Epilepsy with full consciousness.
Secretions predom. increased*.	Secretions pred. diminished or suppressed.
Pulse quick and tense, but small, often very unequal.	Pulse generally frequent, full and hard, sometimes intermitting.
Thirst constant	Thirst, mostly during chill, but also before and after the attack of fever, and between heat and sweat.
Sweat increased during sleep	Sweat lessened during sleep.
Sleep after sweat	Sleep between chill and heat.
One-sided chill predom. l. s., heat pred. r. s.	One-sided chill predom. r. s., heat pred.
No apoplexy—Rarely paralysis	Apoplexy—Paralysis.
Taciturnity—Seriousness—Indifference . .	Loquacity—Amorousness—Maliciousness.
Very rarely delirium	Delirium—Fancies.
Complaints after vexation with anger in evening.	After vexation with anger in the morning. C.Hg.
Sensitiveness of internal parts	Generally sensitiveness of external parts.
Throbbing, generally one-sided headache, worse from night air, better from warm applications and from walking about in the room.	Hæmorrhoidal congestion to head worse from motion, bettered by night air and cold applications.
Pupils contracted	Pupils dilated.
Appetite for sour things—Cramp in stomach, generally improved by coffee.	Predom. aversion to sour things — Cramp in stomach, which is aggrav. by coffee.
Aversion to beer	Desire for *or* aversion to beer.
Inguinal hernia, easily reduced	Inguinal hernia difficult to reduce.
Diarrhœa—Sediment of urine yellow . . .	Constipation—Sediment of urine reddish.
Expectoration during day	Expector. morning, during day and evening.
Milk decreased	Milk increased.
AGGRAVATION evening and night, partic. before midnight.	REMISSION of complaints evening till midnight.
Worse from eructation and from warmth of bed.	Generally improv. by eructation and warmth of bed.
Worse after sleep	*Better* after sleep, when it is not of too long duration, but yet sufficient — On awaking, when roused, aggrav.

Predomin. worse ——— **Predomin. better**

From warmth and warmth of bed, from warm diet, when sitting erect, when lying, partic. when lying on unpainful side, during rest in general, after sleep, from washing or moistening diseased part†, and when lifting up or stretching out suffering limb.

Predomin. better ——— **Predomin. worse**

From cold ‡ and cold diet, from sitting bent forward, when lying on painful side, when letting diseased limb hang down, bending or drawing it up, when walking, from motion generally,§ also on expiration *after* stool, after sweat, and from change of position.

* Excepting the secretion of milk, — with N. vom. it is true, we also find the secretions of the mucous membrane sometimes increased, but then they are always not "ripened," no deciding crisis.

† Chamomilla has aggrav. by wet cold applications, improv. by warm ditto.

‡ Both remedies have aggrav. in cold *weather*, the same *while* sweating.

§ Yet Chamom. has aggrav. oftener than improv. *while moving the diseased part.*

Chamom.	Pulsat.
Chill and other complaints predom. *left* side.	Chill and other compl'ts predom. *right* side.
Aversion to open air—Inclination for exercise.	Inclination for open air—Aversion to exercise.
Chill lessened in warm room	Chill increased in warm room.
Pulse quick, small, but tense; very often unequal.	Pulse frequent, small, and weak; sometimes intermitting or imperceptible.
Thirst constant	Predom. lack of thirst, partic. during chill — Thirst especially *before* and *between* the different stages.
Chill increased out doors; sweat when and after getting out of bed.	Chill less out doors; sweat abating when and after getting out of bed.
Fixed, acute rheumatism without swelling .	Peregrinating acute rheumatism in joints with swelling.
Pain, partic. at night, during sweat, better *after* sweat.	Pain at night, either exclusively during sweat, or during and after sweat.
Sensitiveness of internal parts	*Generally* sensitiveness of external parts.

Chamom.	Pulsat.
Quarrelsome peevishness	Lachrymose mood and calm sadness of gentle dispositions — Changing mood; greediness; distrust; boldness; amorousness—Fancies.
Ailments from anger, or from vexation with vehemence.	Ailments from joy, grief, or from vexation with reserved displeasure.
Children easier when carried about . . .	Childr. want to be carried about, but slowly.
Nasal complaints internal; complaints predom. in palm of hand.	Nasal complaints external oftener than internal complaints; predom. on back of hand.
Acute smell	Loss of smell, or weak smell predom.
Loss of appetite predom.	Generally hunger.
Nausea in stomach	Nausea in throat, stomach or abdomen.
Sediment of urine yellow	Sediment of urine reddish.
Catamenia too soon and too profuse . .	Catam. too late, and generally too scanty
Milk decreased	Milk generally increased.
Expectoration during day	Expectoration in morning and during day.

Chamom.	Pulsat.
Aggravation evening and night, partic. before midnight; after sunrise, and in dry cold weather.	Aggravation from noon until midnight; after sunset, and in wet cold weather.
Some compl'ts better on an empty stomach.	Some complaints better after eating.
Ailments from Coffea, Colocynth., Ignatia, N. vom.	Ailments from Copper-vapors, Mercury, Sulphur, or abuse of Cinchona.

Predomin. worse ——————— **Predomin. better**

In dry weather, while walking out doors, from wet cold applications, from weeping, and when lifting up diseased limb.

Predomin. better ——————— **Predomin. worse**

In wet weather, in warm room, (from warm applications.) from change of position, from bending the head back, when letting diseased limb hang down, and *after* sweat.

N.B. We rarely find the sensation of numbness in suffering parts, peculiar to Pulsat., with Chamom.

China.	Cina.
Upper left, lower right side	Upper right, lower left side.
Complaints predominant in internal parts .	Complaints predominant in external parts.
Itching in external parts	Itching in internal parts.
Itching, lessened by scratching	Itching, unchanged *or* lessened by scratching.
Stitches from within outwards	Stitches from without inwards.
Pulse unequal, intermitting	Pulse often unchanged.
Thirst not constant; it is most conspicuous *before* and *between* the different stages, also during and after sweat.	Thirst predominant before and during chill, not constant during heat.
Chill lessened in warm room	Chill increased in warm room.

China.	Cina.
Apoplexy or paralysis	Neither apoplexy nor paralysis has yet been observed.
Ulcers with copious discharge	Ulcers with scanty discharge.
Complaints predominant on upper jaw and in lower part of chest.	Complaints predominant on lower jaw and in upper part of chest.
Optical illusions in black or dark colors .	Optical illusions in bright colors.
Acute taste	Loss of taste.
Expectoration during day and evening . .	Expectoration in evening.

China.	Cina.
REMISSION *afternoon* and evening . . .	REMISSION during day and evening.
Pressure improves; touch aggravates . .	*Worse* from touch and pressure.
Worse when swallowing food	Worse when swallowing drink.
Worse or better from shaking head . . .	*Bettered* by shaking head.
Worse from light, particularly sunlight . .	Worse from light, particularly candle-light.
Ailments from Iodine, Mercurius, Sulph., Calcarea, or Veratrum.	Ailments from Capsicum or abuse of Mercury.

Predomin. worse ——— **Predomin. better**

From cold, lying on back, after lying down, in bed, after breakfast, after stool, and while moving.

Predomin. better ——— **Predomin. worse**

From warmth, lying on side, after sleep*, after getting out of bed, on an empty stomach, from deep respiration, during rest, and from pressure.

*** The improvement of Cinchona-complaints follows exclusively after sufficient sleep; for on awaking, when roused from sleep, we find these complaints aggravated quite as often as improved.**

China.	Ferrum.
Upper left, lower right side—Piercing pain upwards.	Upper right, lower left side—Piercing pain downwards.
Hæmorrhages, blood dark, coagulates neither easily nor entirely. (Comp. Apis.)	Hæmorrhages; blood light-colored; coagulates easily.
External parts grow black	Red parts grow white.
Ulcers very ichorous, also somewhat inflammatory (and very sensitive).	Ulcers impure, pale, œdematous.
Pulse small, quick, and hard; more quiet after meals; irregular.	Pulse full and hard.
Sweat on upper part of body	Sweat often confined to lower part of body.
Sweat increased while speaking	Sweat lessened while speaking.
Distention of veins of hands	Distention of veins of feet.
Mood indifferent; peevish; sad; hopeless—Amorousness—Absent-mindedness.	Cheerfulness *or* dejection; particularly also alternating cheerful one evening, sad the next.
Mental excitement—Fancies	Changing mood—Rarely delirium.
Ailments from vexation—Apoplexia nervosa.	Ailments from anger—Apoplexia sanguinea.
Nocturnal blindness	At night, capability to see in the dark, with hysteric persons.
Aversion to warm food	Inclination for warm food.
Appetite for sour things	Aversion to sour things.
Impotence	Sterility.
Catamenia too soon and too profuse . .	Catamenia generally too late, but profuse.
Predominant labor-pains weak or ceasing .	Spasmodic labor-pains.
Breath cold—Expectoration not constant; during day and evening.	Breath hot—Expectoration rather constant; in the morning.
Pituitous consumption of drunkards . . .	Consumption in consequence of erethic chlorosis.
Moving suffering part aggravates *or* improves.	Always *improved* by moving suffer'g part.
Better *or* worse from eating meat . . .	*Worse* from eating meat.
Worse *or* better from letting diseased limb hang down.	*Better* from letting diseased limb hang down.
Worse after vomiting	Better *or* worse after vomiting.
REMISSION *afternoon* and evening . . .	REMISSION *during day* and before midnight.
Ailments from Sulphur, Calcarea, Mercurius, Veratrum or Coffea.	Ailments from abuse of Cinchona or Arsenic.

Predomin. **worse** ——— Predomin **better**

After breakfast, from mental and bodily exertion, when leaning against anything, lying on back, from drinking wine*, and while moving

Predomin. **better** ——— Predomin. **worse**

After sleep, on an empty stomach, from bending diseased part backwards, and during rest.

N.B. The aggravation of Cinchona-complaints, when lying on back, is apparently contradicted by two recent cures (one of prolaps. uteri, and the other of Empyema). However, we cannot attach great importance to these cases, as lying on belly became unbearable on account of mechanical conditions. Neither can we attach importance to another cure with Cinchona, where bending the head back (when lying on belly) relieved relatively, because only in this way the patient could avoid lying on back, and also avoid the aggrav. caused by enveloping the head (with the bedding).

* Wine improves Ferrum-complaints only when it is not acid.

China.	Helleb.
Suppurative pain in external parts . . .	Suppurative pain in internal parts.
Increased irritability	Want of bodily (constitutional) irritability.
Apoplexy—Paralysis, painful	Very rarely paralysis, and then painless.
Itching, lessened by scratching — Painful ulcers.	Itching, unchanged by scratching — Painless ulcers.
Pulse frequent, small and hard; more quiet after meals; irregular, sometimes intermitting.	Pulse generally slow, small and weak.
Chill first, then heat	Heat first, then chill.
Thirst most prominent during sweat, and before and between the different stages.	Want of thirst constant.
Chill increased out doors	Chill lessened out doors.
Sleeplessness, part. before midnight . . .	Somnolence predom.

Mood peevish; irritable — Amorousness — Ailments from vexation.	Mood gentle — Distrust — Ailments from grief, mortification, or from vexation with reserved displeasure.
Ment. excitability—Rarely unconsciousness.	Mental dullness—Imbecility
External parts become black	Red parts become white.
Compl'ts predom. on external angle of eye.	Complaints predom. on inner angle of eye.
Tootache during the sweat	Toothache during the chill. C.Hg.
Nausea in throat or stomach	Nausea in stomach.
Spleen affected oftener than liver	Liver complaint, partic. after abuse of Cinchona.
Urine infrequent and scanty	Urine often, but scanty.
Expectoration not constant.	Cough without expectoration.

Remission *afternoon* and evening . . .	Remission of complaints during day.
Better (resp. worse) from uncovering *or* wrapping up.	Worse from uncovering; bettered by wrapping up.
Better after sufficient sleep; but worse on awaking when roused.	Predom. *better* after sleep.
Worse (resp. better) when opening *or* when closing the eyes.	Better when opening eyes; worse when closing them.
Better after getting out of bed	Worse *or* better after getting out of bed.
Generally worse on expiration, better when inspiring.	Better on expiration, worse on inspiration.
Better or worse when respiring deeply . .	Worse when respiring deeply.
Ailments from Helleborus, Iodine, Sulphur, Calcar., or abuse of Mercurius.	Ailments from abuse of Cinchona.

Predomin. worse — **Predomin. better**

Out doors *, while sitting, and after the sweat.

Predomin. better — **Predomin worse**

In doors, when sitting down, and when bending diseased part backwards.

N.B. We very rarely find the oversensitiveness of Cinchona to pain with Helleborus.

---

* We find Helleborus-complaints (like those of Cinchona) also aggrav. "*when walking out doors*." In this case there fore the influence of motion must decide and not that of the open air.

China	Ipecac.
Left side predom. — Increased bodily irritability.	*Right* side - Want of irritability.
Dark hair—Hæmorrhages—Blood dark .	Light hair—Hæmor., blood bright-red.
Generally Anæmie.	Plethora.
Itching lessened by scratching	Itching, unchanged by scratching.
Pulse frequent, small and hard, more quiet after meals; irregular, sometimes intermitting.	Pulse very much accelerated, but often imperceptible.
Thirst most prominent *before, between* and *after* the different stages of fever.	Thirst not constant.
Chill increased out doors, lessened in a warm room.	Chill lessened out doors, increased in a warm room.
Sweat lessened in doors	Sweat increased in doors.
Chill increased by drinking	Chill lessened by drinking.
External chill with internal heat	Internal chill with external heat.
Sweat on upper part of body, (which however is sometimes also confined to lower part of body.)	Coldness of upper part of body.
Amorousness — Absent-mindedness — Mental excitement — Fancies — Delirium — Ailments from vexation.	Rarely sadness or dejection—Ailments from anger, mortification, or from vexation with indignation.
Paralysis	Very rarely paralysis.
Ailments from Mercurial vapors	Ailments from Copper or Arsenic vapors.
Complaints from light, partic. sun-light . .	Complaints from light, partic. candle-light
Optical illusions, partic. in black or in dark colors.	Optical illusions in bright colors.
Acute, sensitive smell	Loss of smell.
Acute taste	Loss of taste.
Nausea in throat or stomach	Nausea in stomach, rarely in abdomen.
Vomit is sour oftener than bitter	Vomit is bitter, oftener than sour.
Labor-pains predom. weak or ceasing . .	Spasmodic labor-pains.
Expectoration not constant; during day and evening.	Expectoration infrequent; morning and during day.
REMISSION *afternoon* and evening . . .	REMISSION of complaints during day.
Worse in the Autumn; in wet cold weather.	*Worse* in winter, and in dry weather.
Worse, partic. *after* sweat	*Worse during* sweat.
Better in doors.	Better in doors, but worse if the room is too warm.
Better when sitting down, but *worse* whlie sitting.	*Worse* when sitting down, but *better* while sitting.
Ailments from Mercury, Iodine, Sulphur. Calc., Helleborus, or Coffea.	Ailments from Copper vapors, Arnica, or Opium.

Predomin. worse ——— **Predomin. better**

In wet weather, from cold, lying on back, lying on right side, while sitting, and after drinking.

Predomin. better ——— **Predomin. worse**

In dry weather; from warmth; lying on side, partic. on left side, and when sitting down.

China.	Lachesis.
Left side predominant—Dark hair - Inclination for exercise.	*Right* side – Light hair—Predominant aversion to exercise.
Ulcerative pain in external parts—Apoplexia nervosa.	Ulcerative pain in internal parts—Apoplexia sanguinea.
Itching in external parts—Blood coagulates easily.	Itching in internal parts — Blood uncoagulable.
Ulcers with copious discharge	Ulcers with scanty discharge.
Predominant external chill, with internal heat.	Predom. internal chill, with external heat.
Pulse frequent, small, but hard; more quiet after meals.	Pulse frequent, small and weak; often alternating with full and strong beats.
Sweat less when and after getting out of bed.	Sweat incr. when & after gett'g out of bed.
Thirst most prominent *before, between* and *after* the different stages.	Thirst not during, but *before* chill; not frequent during heat.
Dreams predominantly unpleasant . . .	Dreams generally pleasant.

China.	Lachesis.
Taciturnity	Loquacity.
Mood indifferent; peevish; sad; despondent.	Cheerfulness—Distrust.
Difficulty in comprehend'g—Rarely delirium.	Easy comprehension—Insanity.
Ailments from vexation	Ailments from fright or jealousy.
Nasal affections predominantly external .	Nasal affections predominantly internal.
Spleen is affected oftener than liver . . .	Liver complaints predominant.
Urine infrequent and scanty	Urine too often.
Catamenia too strong and of long duration.	Catamenia generally scanty and of short duration.
Expectoration not constant; during day and evening.	Expectoration infrequent; is loosened in the morn'g and dur'g day; is swallowed

---

China.	Lachesis.
REMISSION of complaints *afternoon* and evening.	**AGGRAVATION afternoon and evening till midnight.**
Worse in the Fall, in wet and foggy weather, and also during increase of moon.	Worse in the Spring, in wet weather, and before thunder-storm.
Worse after drinking	Better *or* worse after drinking.
Aggravated oftener than improved by shaking head.	Bettered by shaking head.
Ailments from Iodine, Sulph., Calcarea, Veratrum or Coffea.	Ailments from abuse of Cinchona, or from sting of insects.

Predomin. worse ——— **Predomin. better**

From motion, in bed, during sleep, after breakfast, and from wrapping up the head.

Predomin. better ——— **Predomin. worse**

During rest, after sleep*, after getting out of bed, on an empty stomach, from uncovering the head, and from external pressure.

N.B. With Lachesis we rarely find the over-sensitiveness to pain of Cinchona. Mere sensitiveness to touch is found with both remedies.

*** The improvement of Cinchona-symptoms follows exclusively after sufficient sleep; for on awaking (when roused) from sleep, we find these symptoms aggravated at least quite as often.**

China.	Mercur.
Dark hair—Inclination for exercise . . .	Light hair—Aversion to exercise.
Itching, lessened by scratching	Iching, lessened *or* aggrav. by scratching.
Ailments from Mercurial vapors	Ailments from Copper or Arsenic vapors.
Pulse small, hard, and accelerated; more quiet after meals.	Pulse generally full and accelerated.
Chill lessened in warm room	Chill increased in warm room.
Sweat sometimes general, with excep. of feet.	Sw. somet's general, with except'n of head
Sweat often only on back part of body . .	Sweat often only on front part of body.
Thirst is often wanting*	Thirst predom. during all stages of fever.
Hæmorrhages, blood dark—When asleep lying on back.	Hæmorrhages, blood bright-red — When asleep lying on side.

China.	Mercur.
Mental excitability—Ailments from vexation.	Mental dullness — Seriousness — Ailments from offences.
Delirium	Very rarely delirium.
Paralysis	Very rarely paralysis.
Eyes predom. sunken, rarely protruding .	Eyes protruding.
Complaints generally on upper jaw . . .	Complaints predominant on lower jaw.
Toothache during sweating stage of fever .	T. dur. chill; with the toothache sweat. CHg.
Acute taste	Loss of taste.
Inclination for sweets	Aversion to sweets.
Desire for spirituous liquors	Aversion to wine; but appetite for beer.
Nausea in throat or stomach	N. in œsophagus or stomach, rarely in throat.
Vomit is sour oftener than bitter . . .	Bitter vomit.
Spleen is affected oftener than liver . .	Liver-complaints predominant.
Diarrhœa generally painless	Diarrhœa predominantly painful.
Urine infrequent and scanty	Urine often and copious.
Catamenia too soon and profuse . . .	C. too late, at the same time scanty *or* prof.
Expectoration during day and evening .	Expectoration during day.
Complaints predominant in lower part of chest, on upper arm, on patella, and on front part of thigh.	Complaints predominant in upper part of chest, on fore-arm, on tip of elbow, and on back part of thigh.

China.	Mercur.
Remission *afternoon* and evening . . .	Remission of complaints during day.
Generally better on inspirat'n, worse on exp.	Worse on inspiration, better on expiration.
Better or worse when respiring deeply .	Worse when respiring deeply.
Generally worse when lying on back, better when lying on side.	Predominantly better when lying on back, worse when lying on side.
Better (resp. worse) from uncovering *or* wrapping up.	*Generally* worse from uncovering, bettered by wrapping up.
Predominantly worse from growing cold; improved when growing warm.	Worse *or* better from growing cold (resp. growing warm).
Better *or* worse when moving the part .	Worse when moving diseased part.

Predomin. worse ——— **Predomin. better**

When standing, when sitting, particularly sitting bent forward, and from smoking.

Predomin. better ——— **Predomin. worse**

When sitting erect, and from pressure.

N.B. With Mercurius we rarely find the over-sensitiveness of Cinchona to pain. But mere sensitiveness (to touch, etc.) is found with both remedies, as both also have the character of increased constitutional irritability.

---

* Compare diagnosis of Cinchona : Lachesis.

China.	Natr. mur.
Left side predominant—Muscles oftener lax than rigid.	*Right* side—Muscles rigid.
Complaints predominant in internal parts.	Complaints predominant in external parts.
Inclination for exercise; aversion to open air.	Aversion to exercise—Inclination for open air.
Apoplexy oftener than paralysis	Paralysis oftener than apoplexy.
Pulse frequent, small, but hard; more quiet after meals.	Pulse sometimes frequent and weak, sometimes full and slow.
Distention of veins of hands	Distention of veins of feet.
Sweat lessened after getting out of bed and after meals.	Sweat increased after getting out of bed and after meals.
External chill, with internal heat	Internal chill, with external heat.
Thirst is often wanting*	Thirst during and between the attacks of fever.

China.	Natr. mur.
Dejection — Rarely malice — Mental excitability — Fancies — Rarely unconsciousness—Ailments from vexation.	Changing mood—Cheerfulness or dejection —Mental dullness—Ailments from anger, fright, mortification, or from vexation with reserved displeasure.
Vertigo, inclining to fall backwards	Vertigo, inclining to fall forwards.
Complaints oftener on external than in inner ear.	Complaints oftener in inner than on external ear.
Acute, sensitive smell and taste	Loss of smell—Loss of taste.
Appetite for coffee, or roasted coffee-beans.	Disgust for coffee.
Nausea in throat or stomach	Nausea in stomach.
Urine infrequent and scanty	Urine too often.
Catamenia too soon and too profuse	Catamenia too late, at the same time scanty *or* profuse.
Nasal secretion watery—Breath cold	Nasal secretion thick—Breath hot.
Expectoration not constant; during day and evening.	Expectoration infrequent; in morning.

China.	Natr. mur.
AGGRAVATION in the Fall	AGGRAVATION in the Spring.

Predomin. worse — **Predomin. better**

Out-doors, from cold, after lying down, while standing and sitting, in bed, particularly when lying on back, when stretching out diseased limb, after sweat, from tying clothes tight, and lying on right side.

Predomin. better — **Predomin. worse**

In-doors, from warmth, **when respiring deeply, from external pressure, lying on side, particularly left side, and from loosening the clothes.**

N.B. Natr. mur. lacks the over-sensitiveness of Cinchona to pain. On the other hand, we but rarely find the sensation of numbness in suffering parts peculiar to Natr. mur. with Cinchona. Mere sensitiveness (to the touch, etc.) is met with in both remedies.

---

* With Cinchona thirst is most prominent in the transition from chill to heat, and from heat to sweat, also *after* the sweat-stage of the fever and *before* the chill.

China.	Nux vom.
Left side predominant, particularly *upper left, lower right side.*	*Right* side, particularly *upper right, lower left side.*
Muscles frequently lax—Lancinating pain outwards.	Muscles rigid—Lancinating pain from without inwards.
Pulse frequent, hard, but small; more quiet after meals; irregular.	Pulse quick, hard, and full, particularly during hot stage of fever.
Cold or sweat of left side	Cold or sweat of right side.
Thirst appears mostly during sweat . . .	Thirst appears mostly during chill.
More sweat during sleep—Heat or sweat lessened after meals.	Sweat lessened during sleep—Heat or sweat increased after meals.
Sleeplessness before midnight	Sleeplessness prevalent after midnight.
Inclination for exercise	Aversion to exercise.
Insensibility of disposition predominant .	Great sensibility.
Rarely fear—Rarely malice—Rarely unconsciousness or delirium—*Ecstasies.*	*Mental dullness.*
Ailments from vexation	Ailments from fright, anger, mortification, grief, disappointed love or jealousy, and from vexation with fright, dread, fear, indignation or vehemence.
Vertigo, inclining to fall backwards . . .	Vertigo, inclining to fall sideways or backw.
Headache better when opening eyes . . .	Headache worse when opening the eyes.
Dim-sightedness—Short-sightedness . . .	Predom. clear-sightedness - Far-sightedn's.
Optical illusions in black or in dark colors.	Optical illusions in bright colors.
Complaints generally on upper jaw . . .	Complaints predominant on lower jaw.
Spleen affected oftener than liver	Liver diseased oftener than spleen.
Complaints predominant on upper arm . .	Complaints predominant on fore-arm.
Acute taste predominant	Loss of taste predominant.
Appetite for coffee or for sour things . .	Predom. aversion to coffee or sour things.
Aversion to fat things	Appetite for fat things.
Nausea in throat or stomach	Nausea in stomach, rarely in œsophagus.
Diarrhœa predominant; generally painless.	Costiveness—When diarrhœa occurs, it is painful.
Urinal stream small Breath cold . . .	Urinal stream large—Breath hot.
Expectoration during day and evening . .	Expector. morn'g, during day and evening.
Swelling of breasts instead of catamenia .	Swelling of the breasts with each attack of neuralgia uteri.
Ailments from Mercurial vapors	Ailm. from Arsen., Lead or Copper vapors.
Ulcers with copious discharge	Ulcers with scanty discharge.
Remission *afternoon* and evening	Remission of compl. evening till midnight.
Better on an empty stomach	Worse *or* better on an empty stomach.
Predominantly *better* from external pressure.	Generally improved by pressure.
Better *or* worse from bend'g diseased limb.	Worse when bending diseased limb.
Worse after the sweat	*Worse during* sweat, predom. *better after* it.
Worse in wet cold weather	*Worse* in dry cold weather.
Better from warm applications	Better from cold applications.

Predomin. worse ——— **Predomin. better**

In wet weather, from wrapping up head, from stretching out suffering limb, from washing it with cold water or moistening it, after lying down, in bed, when standing and sitting, and after sweat.

Predomin. better ——— **Predomin. worse**

In dry weather, from uncovering the head, from drawing up diseased limb, and from deep respiration.

China.	Phosph. acid.
Increased irritability—Hot, painful swelling of glands.	Want of bodily irritability—Painless swelling of glands.
Pulse frequent, small, but hard; more quiet after meals.	Pulse generally frequent, small and weak; more rarely full and strong.
Coldness left side	One-sided coldness, predominant right side.
Thirst most frequent dur'g sweat, also *before*, *between* and *after* the different stages.	Want of thirst predominant; almost constant during chill.
Sweat lessened after meals	Sweat increased after meals.
Apoplexy	No apoplexy.
Mood irritable—Amorousness.	Mood very rarely irritable.
Ecstasies—Rarely unconsiousness (except in fainting spells).	Mental dullness.
Vertigo, inclining to fall backwards . . .	Vertigo, inclin'g to fall forwards or backw.
Compl. predom. on external corner of eye.	Compl. predom. on inner corner of eye.
Saliva increased Aversion to warm food. .	Sal. generally decr.—Desire for warm food.
Urine infrequent and scanty	Urine often and copious; sometimes scanty.
Sexual desire predominantly strong . . .	Sexual desire diminished, weak.
Expectoration not constant; during day and evening.	Expectoration rather constant; morning.
Complaints predominant on upper arm, on patella, on front part of thigh, and on calf of leg.	Complaints predominant on fore-arm, on tip of elbow, on back part of thigh, and on shin.
REMISSION *afternoon* and evening . . .	REMISSION afternoon and before midnight.
Predominantly worse from growing cold, better from growing warm.	Better (resp. worse) from growing cold *or* warm.
Better (resp. worse) from uncovering *or* wrapping up.	Worse from uncovering, better from wrapping up
Worse *or* better when getting out of bed .	Worse when getting out of bed.
Better after getting out of bed	*After* getting out of bed worse *or* better.
Worse *or* better when rising from a seat .	Worse when rising from a seat.
Worse *or* better when moving diseased part.	Better when moving diseased part.
Worse *or* better after meals	Worse after meals.
Ailments from Veratrum, Iodine, Calcarea, Sulph., or Coffea.	Ailments from Lachesis.

Predomin. worse ——— **Predomin. better**

In wet weather, in the open air, when walking out-doors, from exercise, when swallowing, and from change of position.

Predomin. better ——— **Predomin. worse**

In dry weather, in-doors, and during rest.

N.B. Over-sensitiveness to pain is frequent with Cinchona, infrequent with Phosph. acid.

China.	Pulsat.
Complaints (cold, heat, sweat, &c.) predom. *left* side.	Complaints (cold, heat, sweat, &c.) predom. *right* side.
Inclination for exercise—Painful paralysis .	Aversion to exercise—Painless paralysis.
Itching, lessened by scratching	Itching, unchanged or aggrav. by scratching.
Pulse frequent, small, but hard; irregular . .	Pulse generally accelerated, small and weak, sometimes imperceptible.
Chill increased by exercise and in the open air, lessened in warm room.	Chill lessened by exercise and in the open air, increased in warm room.
Heat or sweat, increased when walking out doors.	Heat or sweat lessened when walking out doors.
Sweat sometimes general, with exception of feet.	Coldness sometimes general, with exception of feet.
Thirst is often wanting *	Thirst only during hot stage of fever; is always wanting during chill.

China.	Pulsat.
Generally insensibility of disposition . . .	Sensitive disposition—Changing moods.
Bashfulness—Rarely fear	*Boldness*—Distrust—Greediness—Rarely irritability.
Rarely unconsciousness—*Mental excitability.*	*Mental dullness.*
Ailments from vexation	Ailments from fright, excessive joy, grief, mortification, or from vexation with fright, dread or fear.
Optical illusions in black or in dark colors .	Optical illusions in bright colors.
Complaints pred. in external corner of eye, on external ear, on upper jaw, and of *the spleen.*	Complaints predom. in inner corner of eye, in inner ear, on lower jaw, and of liver.
Acute smell	Predom. loss of smell.
Subjective cadaverous smell	Objective stench from nose; subjective fragrant odors, or smell of inveterate catarrh.
Acute taste.	Loss of taste.
Appetite for sweets	Appetite for sour and refreshing things.
Nausea in throat or stomach	Nausea in throat, stomach, or abdomen.
Vomit is sour oftener than bitter.	Vomit is bitter oftener than sour.
Diarrhœa generally painless	Diarrhœa generally painful.
Catamenia too soon, profuse and of long duration.	Catamenia too late, of short duration and predom. scanty.
Lochial discharge remains bloody too long .	Lochiæ suppressed.
Expectoration during day and evening . . .	Expectoration morning and during day.

China.	Pulsat.
Remission *afternoon* and evening	Aggrav. afternoon and evening till midnight.
Worse from washing.	Generally bettered by washing and moistening.
Worse *or* better from uncovering	*Better* from uncovering; *worse* from wrapping up.
Worse during increase of moon	Worse before thunder-storm.

Predomin. worse —— **Predomin. better**

Out doors, by cold, when lying on painful side, from tying the clothes tight, when bending the head sideways, from exertion (bodily); from partaking of sour things, from exercise, lying on right side, when stretching out diseased limb, and from washing and moistening suffering part.

Predomin. better —— **Predomin. worse**

In warm room, from warmth in general, when lying on unpainful side, or on a cold pillow, when drawing up diseased limb, when eating, during rest, lying on left side, from loosening the clothes, and from rubbing and scratching.

N.B. With Cinchona we very rarely find the sensation of numbness in suffering parts peculiar to Pulsatilla.

* Thirst is most prominent during transition from chill to heat, from heat to sweat, also *after* the sweating stage of fever; Pulsat. also has thirst during the intervals, partic. between chill and hot stage, but not *after* sweat.

China.	Sulphur.
Increased irritability — Ulcerative pain in external parts.	Want of bodily irritability—Ulcerative pain in internal parts.
Apoplexy more frequent than paralysis . .	Paralysis more frequent than apoplexy.
Paralysis, eruptions and ulcers *painful* . .	Paralysis, eruptions and ulcers *painless.*
External parts become black	Red parts become white.
Pulse frequent, hard, but small; irregular .	Pulse quick, hard and full.
External chill with internal heat	Internal chill with external heat.
Sweat lessened after meals	Sweat increased after meals.
Thirst is wanting only sometimes during chill*.	Thirst mostly during heat; during chill want of thirst is predom.
Toothache during the sweat	Toothache during the chill. C. Hg.
Generally insensibility of disposition — Rarely fear.	Sensitiveness of disposition—Changing mood—Gentleness—Amorousness rarely observed.
Ailments from vexation	Ailments from shame, mortification, or vexation with fright, dread or fear.
Mental excitability—Rarely delirium . . .	Mental dullness—Imbecility—Insanity.
Complaints predom. on external ear, in lower part of chest, on upper arm, and on front part of thigh.	Complaints predom. in inner ear, in upper part of chest, on fore-arm, and on back part of thigh.
Diseases of the periosteum predom.	Diseases of bones predom.
Subjective cadaverous smell	Objective stench from nose predom.
Secretion of saliva predom. increased . . .	Saliva generally diminished.
Delicate taste	Loss of taste.
Urine infrequent and scanty — Sediment generally red.	Urine often, but scanty; yet sometimes copious —Sediment oftener white than red.
Catamenia too soon, profuse and of long duration.	Catamenia *generally* too late, scanty and of short duration.
Expectoration during day and evening . . .	Expectoration morning and during day, less frequently at night.
REMISSION *afternoon* and evening	REMISSION *afternoon* and before midnight.
Worse dur'g increase of moon; in the Autumn.	Worse during full moon; in the Spring.
Pred. worse fr. growing cold & in cold weather; better from growing warm and in warm air.	Better or worse from growing cold and in cold air, (resp. growing warm and in warm air.)
Worse in the open air, better in doors . . .	Bett. (resp. worse) in the open air *or* in doors†.
Worse (resp. better) from uncovering *or* wrapping up.	Predom. better from uncovering, worse from wrapping up.
Generally worse when lying on back; better when lying on side.	*Generally* better when lying on back, worse when lying on side.
Better when lying with head high; worse when lying low.	Oftener improved when lying with head high, than low.
Better after sufficient sleep; worse on awaking when roused from sleep.	Worse after sleep.
Better after getting out of bed	Worse *or* better after getting out of bed.
Pred. better *before* breakf.; worse afterwards.	Worse *or* better before (resp. after) breakfast.
Worse *or* better after meals	Worse after meals.
Worse after stool	Better *or* worse after stool.
Better or worse from biting	Worse from biting.
Worse from touch	Aggrav. oftener than improved by touch.
Worse *or* better when bending the part . .	Worse when bending diseased part.
Worse *or* better when rising from a seat . .	Worse when rising from a seat.
Worse from being awake at night	Worse from sleeping too long.

Predomin. worse — **Predomin. better**

From cold, when moving, from eructation, and when lying on right side.

Predomin. better — **Predomin worse**

From warmth, during rest, when bending diseased part backwards, when lying on left side, after sleep, and when clenching the teeth.

N.B. We very rarely find the oversensitiveness of Cinchona to pain with Sulph., rarely with Cinchona the sensation of numbness in the suffering parts peculiar to Sulphur.—*Both* remedies have sensitiveness to touch.

* Thirst is most prominent *after* the different stages of the fever.
† Sulphur-symptoms are improved by warmth of stove, aggravated in crowded rooms, (when among many people.)

China.	Veratrum.
Left side—Dark hair	*Right* side—Light hair.
Ulcerative pain in external parts	Ulcerative pain in internal parts.
Apoplexy more frequent than paralysis . .	Paralysis more frequent than apoplexy.
Paralysis painful	Paralysis painless.
Ulcers with copious discharge	Ulcers with scanty discharge.
Pulse frequent, small, and hard; more quiet after meals.	Pulse generally slow, small, and weak; sometimes slower than beating of heart.
Thirst often wanting *	Thirst not constant.
Sadness and dejection — Embarrassment — Indifference — Rarely fear — Malice — Haughtiness—Ailments from vexation—Wrapt in thought.	Cheerfulness *or* dejection—Boldness—Distrust—Ailments from fright, anger, grief, or from vexation with dread or fear—Being beside one's self.
Mental excitability — Rarely unconsciousness—Rarely delirium.	Ecstasies or mental dullness—Insanity.
Optical illusions in black or in dark colors.	Optical illusions in bright colors.
Acute, sensitive sense of smell	Loss of smell.
Complaints predom. on outside of nose, on upper jaw, and on upper teeth.	Complaints predom. on inside of nose, on lower jaw, and lower teeth.
With the sweat toothache	With the toothache sweat. C.Hg.
Secretion of saliva predom. increased . .	Saliva *generally* diminished.
Acute taste	Loss of taste.
Vomit sour oftener than bitter	Vomit predom. bitter.
Spleen is affected oftener than liver . . .	Liver complaints predom.
Catamenia too soon—Labor pains weak or ceasing.	Catamenia too soon *or* too late — Spasmodic labor pains.
Lochial discharge bloody too long . . .	Lochial discharge suppressed.
Expectoration during day and evening . .	Expectoration during day.
Complaints predom. in lower part of chest, and on front part of thigh.	Complaints predom. in upper part of chest, and on back part of thigh.
REMISSION *afternoon* and evening . . .	REMISSION during day and evening.
Worse from growing cold; better from growing warm.	From growing cold (resp. growing warm) better *or* worse.
Worse (resp. better) from uncovering *or* wrapping up.	Bettered by uncovering; worse from wrapping up.
Worse in bed †	Worse *or* better in bed.
Generally worse when lying on back, better when lying on side.	Better when lying on back, worse when lying on side.
Better after sufficient sleep; but worse on awaking when roused from sleep.	Worse after sleep.
Better after getting out of bed	Worse *or* better after getting out of bed.
Bett. or worse wh. assum'g an erect position.	Worse when assuming an erect position.
Generally improved when eating . .	Worse when eating.
Worse after stool	Worse *or* better after stool.
Worse from being awake at night . . .	Worse from sleeping too long.

Predomin. **worse** ⏞ Predomin. **better**

Out doors, during motion, [illegible]nding, when sitting bent forward, when bending back the head, [illegible]om eructation, and after sweat.

Predomin. **better** ⏞ Predomin. **worse**

In doors, during rest, when descending, wh. sitting down, wh. sitting erect, after sleep, and while eating.

N.B. Although both remedies have the predom. character of increased irritability, yet with Veratrum we rarely find the oversensitiveness of Cinchona to pain, — rarely with Cinchona the sensation of numbness in suffering parts, which belongs to Veratr. Mere sensitiveness (to touch, &c.) is found with *both* remedies.

---

* The thirst is most intense *after* each stage of the fever, and also *before* the chill and during sweat.
† Both remedies have predom. aggrav. of complaints from *warmth* of bed.

Cicuta.	Belladonna.
Apoplexy or paralysis not yet observed .	Apoplexy—Paralysis.
Skin hardening, callous	Skin chafed; sore. C.Hg.
Ulcers with copious discharge	Ulcers with scanty discharge. C.Hg.
Pulse slow, weak, trembling	Pulse generally quick, full and hard.
Thirst	Thirst not constant; most rare during chill; appears also *before* and *after* the attack of fever.

Cicuta.	Belladonna.
Sensitive disposition—Gentleness—Impulsive (sanguine) temperament—Predom. cheerfulness—Anxious feeling in head.	Insensibility of disposition predom—Mood irritable; changeable; cheerful or dejected—Anxious feeling around the heart.
Rarely delirium	Mental excitability *or* dullness.
Ailments from hearing bad news	Ailments from fright, anger, mortification, or from vexation with fright, dread, fear, or vehemence.
Vertigo, inclining to fall forwards . . .	Vertigo inclining to fall backwards or sideways (left side).
Pupils generally contracted	Pupils generally dilated.
Eyes generally sunken	Eyes protruding.
Catamenia too late and scanty	Catamenia too soon and profuse.
Eclampsia parturentium with a cold face; eyes half closed.	Eclampsia parturentium with congestion to the head, red face, and wild look. C.Hg.
Fluent coryza predom.	Dry coryza predom.
Cough predom. with expectoration . . .	Cough generally without expectoration.
Complaints predom. in lower part of chest, and on fore-arm.	Complaints predom. in upper part of chest, and on upper arm.
With HORSES: Lockjaw, carries the head high and straightened out.	With HORSES: Lockjaw, carrying the neck very high, keeping the head more in.

Cicuta.	Belladonna.
REMISSION forenoon and evening	REMISSION after midnight and *forenoon.*
Worse when bending diseased part . . .	*Better or* worse when bending diseased part.
Worse when eating	*Worse or* better when eating.
Worse in the Fall	Worse in the Spring.

Predomin. worse ——— **Predomin. better**

In doors *, when opening the eyes, when stooping, when sitting bent forward, and when bending back the head.

Predomin. better ——— **Predomin. worse**

Out doors, when closing the eyes, and when sitting erect.

N.B. Cicuta lacks the oversensitiveness of Bellad. to pain—Mere sensitiveness (to touch, &c) is found with Bellad. oftenest in external parts, with Cicuta exclusively in internal parts.

---

* Yet we also find complaints improved by warmth of stove, with Cicuta.

Cicuta.	Ignatia.
Itching, lessened by scratching	Itching, lessened *or* changed to another place by scratching.
Skin hardening, callous	Skin chafed, sore. C. Hg.
Discharge of ulcers copious	Discharge of ulcers scanty. C. Hg.
Apoplexy or paralysis have not yet been observed.	Apoplexy—Paralysis.
Pulse slow and weak	Pulse generally accelerated, full and hard.
Heat or sweat, with aversion to uncover .	Heat or sweat, with inclination to uncover.
Thirst.	Thirst only during chill and after sweat.

Cicuta.	Ignatia.
Predominant cheerfulness—Gentleness, but impulsive (sanguine) temperament —Rage - Distrust.	Predominant sadness—Gentle disposition—Indifference—Mood changing; bold; irritable—Amorousness—Consequences of shame, reserved mortification, grief, or disappointed love.
Anxious feeling in head—Unconsciousness.	Anxious feeling in prœcordia.
Complaints predominant on external ear, on upper lip, and on fore-arm.	Complaints predominant on inner ear, under lip, and upper arm.
Desire for wine or brandy . . .	Aversion to wine or brandy.
Urine infrequent, but copious	Urine often and copious.
Retention of urine *or* incontinence . . .	Incontinence.
Catamenia too late and scanty.	Catamenia predom. too soon, but scanty.
Cough generally with expectoration . . .	Cough generally without expectoration.
Spine-disease, with gressus vaccinus . . .	Spine-disease, with gressus gallinaceus.

Cicuta.	Ignatia.
REMISSION forenoon and evening . . .	REMISSION of complaints before midnight.
Worse from bodily exertion	Improved much oftener than aggravated by exertion.
Worse when stooping	Better *or* worse when stooping.
Almost always aggravated when assuming an erect position.	Better *or* worse when assuming an erect position.
Worse on inspiration and expiration . .	Better on inspiration; worse on expiration.
Worse when eating	Improved oftener than aggravated when eating.
Worse from uncovering; better from wrapping up.	*Generally* better from uncovering; worse from wrapping up.
Ailments from Opium	Ailments from Coffea, Chamomilla, Nux vom., Pulsatilla, or Zink.

Predomin. worse ——— **Predomin. better**

In-doors*, when sitting bent forward, when rising from a seat, when lifting or resting diseased limb on anything, when swallowing, while and after eating, and from uncovering.

Predomin. better ——— **Predomin. worse**

Out-doors, when sitting erect, when standing, after lying down, while lying, in bed, from warmth of bed, when letting diseased limb hang down, and from wrapping up.

N.B. Cicuta lacks the over-sensitiveness to pain of Ignat.

---

* Yet we also find improvement from warmth of stove with Cicuta; with Ignat. also aggravation in hot room.

Cicuta.	Nux vomica.
Want of irritability	Increased irritability.
Epilepsy with unconsciousness—Thirst after the spasms; not in all the stages of the fever observed yet.	Epilepsy with full consciousness — Thirst mostly during chill.
Pulse slow and weak; tremulous	Pulse generally accelerated, full and hard, particularly during heat.
Sweat increased during sleep—Skin hardening, callous—Pus copious.	Sweat lessened during sleep—Skin chafed, getting sore—Pus scanty. C.Hg.
Apoplexy or paralysis has not yet been observed.	Apoplexy—Paralysis.

Predominant cheerfulness — Gentleness — Distrust — In rare cases malice—Anxious feeling in head — Solicitude concerning the future.	Mood anxious; sad; peevish; irritable; irascible; malicious — Amorousness — Precipitation — Anxious feeling in præcordia—Solicitude concerning the present. C.Hg.
Ailments from hearing bad news	Consequences of fright, anger, mortification, grief, disappointed love, jealousy, or from vexation with fright, fear, indignation, or vehemence.
Vertigo, inclining to fall forwards . . .	Vertigo, inclining to fall backwards or sideways.
Urine infrequent, but copious	Urine infrequent and scanty.
Catamenia too late and scanty.	Catamenia too soon and profuse.
Fluent coryza	Dry coryza most frequent, particularly in the open air; on the other hand, fluent coryza in-doors.
Respiration prevalently slow	Respiration is oftener quick than slow.
Cough generally with expectoration . . .	Cough generally without expectoration.

Remission forenoon and evening	Remission evening till midnight.
Improved by warmth of bed	Improved oftener than aggrav. by warmth of bed.
Worse after drinking	*Worse or* better after drinking.
Worse when stooping	*Better or* worse when stooping.

Predomin. worse ——— **Predomin. better**

In-doors*, when eating, and when lifting up diseased limb, or resting it on anything.

Predomin. better ——— **Predomin. worse**

Out-doors, and when letting diseased limb hang down.

N.B. Cicuta lacks the over-sensitiveness to pain of Nux vom. Mere sensitiveness (to touch, etc.) is most frequent in external parts with Nux vom.; with Cicuta it is exclusively in internal parts.

---

* Yet we also find with Cicuta (as with Nux vom.) improvement by warmth of stove.

Cicuta.	Pulsatilla.
Want of irritability	Increased irritability.
Itching, lessened by scratching	Itching, aggrav. *or* unchanged by scratch'g.
Skin hard, callous	Skin chafed, sore. C. Hg.
Thirst not yet observed with the fever—Pulse slow, weak, and trembling.	Thirst only during hot stage of fever*—Pulse generally quick, small, and weak.
Chill lessened in warm room	Chill increased in warm room.
Heat lessened in bed	Heat increased in bed.
Cheerfulness—Gentleness—Impulsive (sanguine) temperament—Rage.	Lacrymose sadness of gentle dispositions—Mood changing; anxious; ready to take offence; indifferent; peevish; bold—Amorousness—Avarice—Precipitation
Anxious feeling in head	Feeling of anxiety in præcordia.
Ailments from hearing bad news	Consequences of excessive joy, of fright, grief, mortification, or from vexation with fright, dread, or fear.
Insanity	Melancholy.
Vertigo, inclining to fall forwards	Vertigo, inclining to fall backwards.
Complaints predominant on external ear, on inside of nose, on upper lip, on fore-arm, and on thigh.	Complaints predominant in inner ear, on outside of nose, on lower lip, on upper arm, and on leg.
Generally loss of appetite	Generally hunger.
Urine infrequent, but copious	Urine infrequent and scanty.
Respiration prevalently slow	Respiration quick.
Expectoration predominant with the cough.	Expectoration predom., but not constant.
Remission forenoon and evening	Remission from midnight till noon.
Predominantly better in bed	Much oftener aggrav. than improved in bed.
Worse on awaking	*Worse or* better after sleep.
Worse on expiration and inspiration	Predom. better on inspir., worse on expirat.
Worse from bodily exertion	Improved oftener than aggrav. by exertion.
Worse from moving or bending diseased part.	Better *or* worse from moving or bending diseased part.
Better when sitting down	Worse *or* better when sitting down.
Worse when rising from a seat; better *afterwards.*	Worse *or* better *when* and *after* rising from a seat.
Almost always aggravated when assuming an erect position.	Worse *or* better when assuming an erect position.
Worse when swallowing	Worse *or* better when swallowing.
Worse after meals	*Worse or* better after meals.

Predomin. **worse** — Predomin. **better**

From cold, from growing cold and in cold weather, from uncovering, from motion, while walking, from exertion, when lifting up diseased limb or resting it on anything, and when opening the eyes.

Predomin. **better** — Predomin. **worse**

From warmth, from growing warm and in warm air, from wrapping up, during rest, after lying down, while lying, sitting and standing, from warmth of bed, when letting diseased limb hang down, when closing eyes, and from rubbing and scratching.

N.B. Cicuta lacks the over-sensitiveness of Pulsatilla to pain, generally also the sensation of numbness in suffering parts belonging to Pulsatilla. Mere sensitiveness (to touch, etc.) is found, with Pulsatilla, predominantly in external parts, with Cicuta exclusively in internal parts.

* Besides this, Pulsatilla has thirst before and after chill, also between heat and sweat.

Cina.	Calcarea.
Left side predominant—Dark hair . . .	*Right* side—Light hair.
Complaints predominant in external parts .	Complaints predominant in internal parts.
Rending pain downwards	Rending pain upwards.
Epilepsy, with rigidity and full consciousness.	Epilepsy, with unconsciousness.
Pulse often unchanged; generally quick and hard, but small.	Pulse changed, sometimes trembling; generally frequent and full.
First chill, then heat	First heat, then chill.
Thirst during and *before* chill; not constant during heat.	Thirst almost constant; during chill it is sometimes wanting.

Cina.	Calcarea.
Optical illusions in bright colors	Optical illusions in black.
Complaints predominant on lower jaw . .	Complaints predominant on upper jaw.
Cough generally dry — Expectoration in evening.	Cough generally with expectoration—Expectoration morning and during day.

Cina.	Calcarea.
Remission *during day* and evening . . .	Remission of complaints before midnight.
Worse from pressure	Better *or* worse from pressure.
Worse from resting diseased limb on anything.	*Better* from lifting up, or resting diseased limb on anything; *worse* when letting it hang down.
Ailments from Capsicum (or Cinchona). .	Ailments from Mercurius, Phosph., Digitalis, Nitric acid, (or Cinchona).

Predomin. worse — **Predomin. better**

From warmth, during rest, when standing and sitting, from the touch, and when resting diseased limb on anything.

Predomin. better — **Predomin. worse**

From cold, from motion, shaking the head, in bed, and after stool.

N.B. With Calcarea we very rarely find the over-sensitiveness to pain belonging to Cina, with Cina rarely the sensation of numbness in suffering parts frequent with Calcarea.

Cina.	Ignatia.
Complaints (pinching pain, &c.) predom. in external parts.	Complaints (pinching pain, &c.) predom. in internal parts.
Epilepsy with full consciousness	Epilepsy with unconsciousness.
Apoplexy or paralysis has not yet been observed.	Apoplexy — Paralysis —
Pulse often unchanged; generally quick, hard, but small.	Pulse generally accelerated, large, hard; very changeable.
Thirst during and *before* chill; not constant during heat.	Thirst only during chill and after sweat.
Chill increased in warm room	Chill abating in warm room.
Itching, lessened *or* unchanged by scratching.	Itching lessened *or* changed to another place by scratching.
Hunger predom.	Generally loss of appetite.
Catamenia too soon and profuse	Catamenia too soon, but scanty
Expectoration not constant	Expectoration infrequent.
Complaints predom. on the hand	Complaints predom. on foot.

REMISSION *during day* and evening . . .	REMISSION of complaints before midnight.
Worse from bodily exertion	Improved oftener than aggrav. by exertion.
Worse when assuming an erect position .	Better *or* worse when assuming an erect position.
Worse when and after getting out of bed .	Better *or* worse when and after getting out of bed.
Predom. worse on in- and expiration . .	Better on inspiration, worse on expiration.
Worse from acid wine	Better from partaking of sour things.
Ailments from Capsicum or abuse of Cinchona.	Ailments from Coffea, Chamom., N. vom., Pulsat., or Zinc.

Predomin. worse ——— **Predomin. better**

From warmth, growing warm, and in warm room, when lying on painful side, when resting upon anything, or stretching out diseased limb, from pressure, when respiring deeply, when swallowing, after meals, and from change of position.

Predomin. better ——— **Predomin. worse**

From cold*, and from growing cold, after lying down, while lying, in bed, lying on unpainful side, when drawing up diseased limb, when moving suffering part, and after stool.

*** Both remedies have predom. aggravation *in cold weather*, — improvement in warm air.**

Cina.	N. vomica.
Left side—Complaints (pinching pain, &c.) predom. in external parts.	*Right* side—Complaints (pinching pain, &c.) predom. in internal parts.
Apoplexy or paralysis has not yet been observed.	Apoplexy—Paralysis.
Pulse often unchanged; generally quick, hard, but small.	Pulse changed in quality and strength, generally hard, full and quick; sometimes intermitting.
Chill on upper part of body	Coldness on lower part of body.
Thirst during and *before* chill; not constant during heat.	Most thirst during chill, but also *before* and *after* the attack of fever, and between heat and sweat.
Heat increased after sleep	Heat lessened after sleep.

Cina.	N. vomica.
Dim-sightedness	Clear-sightedness predom.
Hunger predom.	Generally loss of appetite.
Appetite for bread	Aversion to bread, partic. rye-bread.
Fluent coryza	Coryza dry oftener than fluent, partic. out doors, — on the other hand fluent coryza in doors.
Expectoration with the cough in evening .	Expector. morning, during day, evening.

Cina.	N. vomica.
REMISSION during day and evening . . .	REMISSION evening till midnight.
Worse from light, partic. candle-light. . .	Worse from light, partic. day-light.
Worse after sleep	Better after sufficient and not too long sleep; but worse on awaking when roused from sleep.
Worse when swallowing, partic. drink . .	*Worse or* better when swallowing, partic. food and saliva; often better when swallowing drink.
Worse from acid wine	Worse from spirits, partic. from wine containing lead.
Worse when sneezing	*Worse or* better from sneezing.
Worse from pressure	Improv. oftener than aggrav. by pressure.
Predom. worse after getting out of bed . .	Better *or* worse after getting out of bed.
Ailments from Capsicum	Ailments from Arsenic or Copper vapors, from Sulph., Calc., Iodine, or Plumbum.

Predomin. **worse** —— Predomin. **better**

From warmth, and growing warm, from warmth of bed, and warmth of stove*, during rest; when sitting, partic. sitting erect; when lying on side, when resting suffering part on anything, when stretching it out, or bending it backwards; after sleep, and when swallowing drink.

Predomin. **better** —— Predomin **worse**

From cold †, and from growing cold; from motion, walking; when moving suffering part, when sitting bent forward, lying on back, when drawing up diseased limb, when shaking the head, and after stool.

---

* Both remedies have predom. improvement *in doors*, and generally aggrav. *in the open air.*
† *In cold weather* both remedies have predom. aggrav., *in warm air* improv.

Cina.	Pulsatilla.
Left side; partic. *lower l., upper r. s.* . .	*Right* side; partic. *lower r., upper l. s.*
Complaints (pinching pain, &c.) predom. in external parts.	Complaints (pinching pain, &c.) predom. in internal parts.
Aversion to open air	Inclination for open air.
Itching lessen'd *or* unchang'd by scratching.	Itching, aggr. *or* unchanged by scratching.
Pulse often unchanged; generally quick, small, but hard.	Pulse changed, sometimes intermitting; generally quick, small, weak.
Chill on upper part of body	Chill on lower part of body, heat on upper part.
Thirst during and *before* chill; not constant during heat.	Want of thirst predom., partic. during chill; — thirst, partic. *before* and *between* the different stages.
Apoplexy or paralysis not yet observed. .	Apoplexy—Paralysis.
Pupils generally dilated	Pupils generally contracted.
Appetite for bread	Aversion to bread.
Catamenia too soon and profuse	Catamenia too late and generally scanty.
Cough generally dry; expectoration in evening.	Cough generally loose; expectoration morning and during day.
Complaints predom. in upper part of chest.	Complaints predom. in lower part of chest.

Cina.	Pulsatilla.
Aggravation night and morning . . .	Aggravation from noon till midnight.
Worse after sleep	*Worse or* better after sleep.
Worse when and after getting out of bed .	*Better or* worse when and after getting out of bed.
Better after rising from a seat	*Better or* worse after rising from a seat.
Children want to be carried about . . .	Childr. want to be carried, but slowly. C.Hg.
Worse when assuming an erect position. .	Worse *or* better when assuming an erect position.
Better when moving diseased part . . .	*Better or* worse when moving diseased part.
Almost always aggravated by pressure . .	*Better or* worse from pressure.
Worse on in- and expiration	Better on inspiration; worse on expiration.
Worse when respiring deeply	Better *or* worse when respiring deeply.
Worse when swallowing, partic. worse when swallowing drink.	*Worse or* better when swallowing, partic. worse when swallowing saliva.
Worse from drinking quickly	Worse from eating quickly.
Worse from acid wine	Better from eating sour things.
Better after stool	*Better or* worse after stool.
Ailments from Capsicum	Ailments from Copper vapors, Iron, Platina, Strannum, Tartar. emet., Mercurius, Sulphur, Sulphuric acid, Chamom., Ignatia. or Sabadilla.

Predomin. worse — **Predomin. better**

In cold weather, out doors, lying on right side, or lying on painful side, when sitting erect, when resting diseased limb on anything, or when stretching it out; from bodily exertion, from shaking the head, and from pressure.

Predomin. better — **Predomin. worse**

In warm air, in doors*, lying on left side, or lying on unpainful side, when sitting bent forward, when drawing up diseased limb, after lying down, while lying, in bed, and from rubbing and scratching.

N.B. With Cina we rarely find the sensation of numbness in suffering parts, peculiar to Pulsatilla.

---

* *In warm room* both remedies have aggrav., when *walking out doors* both predom. improvement of complaints; — in the latter case, not the influence of the open air, but that of motion decides for Cina.

Clematis.	Mercur.
Itching unchanged (or lessened) by scratching.	Itching, aggrav. *or* lessened by scratching.
Eruptions generally humid	Eruptions generally dry.
Skin hardened, callous	Skin chafed, sore. C.Hg.
Apoplexy not yet observed	Apoplexy.
Pulse unchanged; excited	Pulse changed in quality and strength, generally full and accelerated; sometimes irregular or imperceptible.
One-sided heat, right side	One-sided heat, left side.
Thirst, partic. during hot stage	Thirst during all stages.

Clematis.	Mercur.
Cheerfulness *or* sadness—Home-sickness—Gentleness.	Seriousness—Dejection—Home-sickness *or* desire to travel—Malice—Amorousness.
Easy *or* difficult comprehension	Difficult comprehension — Absent-mindedness—Mental dullness—Unconsciousness.
Complaints predom. on lower lip	Complaints predom. on upper lip.
With the toothache anxiety and sweat . .	With the toothache sweat and chill after it. C.Hg.
Urine often, but scanty	Urine frequent and copious.
Sexual desire predom. weak	Sexual desire strong.
Catamenia too soon	Catamenia too late.
Complaints predom. in hollow of elbow . .	Complaints predom. on tip of elbow and in hollow of knee.

Clematis.	Mercur.
AGGRAVATION night and morning . . .	AGGRAVATION from evening till morning.
Generally worse in doors, bett. out doors*.	*Generally* better in doors, worse out doors.
Worse during continued standing; but better when standing still after motion.	Predom. better while standing.
Better *or* worse from drinking cold water .	Worse from drinking cold water.
Ailments from abuse of Mercur.	Ailments from Arsenic or Copper vapors, from Sulph., Calc., abuse of Cinchona, or from sting of insects.

Predomin. worse ——— **Predomin. better**

While lying down, and from smoking

Predomin. better ——— **Predomin. worse**

During and after sweat, and from pressure.

---

* Both remedies have aggrav. *when walking out doors;* with Clematis therefore the influence of the open air does not decide, but that of motion.

Clematis.	Sulphur.
Cutting pain predominant in external parts.	Cutting pain predominant in internal parts.
Paralysis not yet observed	Paralysis of limbs.
Itching, unchanged by scratching	Itching, lessened by scratching.
Skin hardened, callous	Skin chafed, sore. C.Hg
Painful eruptions and ulcers	Painless eruptions and ulcers.
Pulse often unchanged; excited	Pulse changed; generally full, hard, and accelerated, sometimes imperceptible or intermitting.
Heat, with aversion to uncover	Heat, with inclination to uncover.
Thirst, particularly during heat	Thirst mostly during heat, most rare during chill; sometimes appears *before* the chill.
Chill increased in warm room	Chill abating in warm room.

Mood cheerful *or* sad—Home-sickness . .	Mood changing; serious, solemn, dejected; Delirium — Fancies — Insanity — Imbecility.
Complaints predominant in inner angle of eye, and on under lip.	Complaints predominant on external angle of eye, and on upper lip.
With the toothache anxious sweat . . .	With the toothache chill. C.Hg.
Catamenia too soon	Catamenia generally too late.
Expectoration infrequent	Expectoration not constant.

Remission during day and evening . . .	Remission *afternoon* and before midnight.
Predominantly worse out-doors; better in-doors.	Better (worse) out-doors *or* in-doors; particularly better from warmth of stove, worse in crowded room.
Worse in cold weather, better in warm air .	In cold (resp. warm) air better *or* worse.
Better after sweat	*Worse or* better after sweat.
Worse from warmth of bed	Aggravated oftener than improved by warmth of bed.
Better when lying with head high . . .	Oftener improved in an elevated than in a low position.
Worse when stooping	Better *or* worse when stooping.
Worse when moving diseased part . . .	*Worse or* better when moving the part.
Worse from touch	*Worse or* better from touch.

Predomin. worse ⏞ **Predomin. better**

From cold, from uncovering, and from exercise.

Predomin. better ⏞ **Predomin. worse**

From warmth, from wrapping up, during rest*, and during and after the sweat.

---

* Both remedies have predominant aggravation while lying down.

Clematis.	Thuya.
Itching, unchanged by scratching, rarely lessened by it.	Itching, lessened by scratching.
Hot, painful swelling of glands	Cold, painless swelling of glands
Pus scanty	Pus copious. C.Hg.
Apoplexy or paralysis not yet observed .	Paralysis – Apoplexy.
Awaking too late	Awaking too early.
Pulse often unchanged; excited	Pulse changed, sometimes irregular; slow and weak in morning, accelerated and full in evening.
Heat, with aversion to uncover	Heat, with inclination to uncover.
Thirst, particularly during heat	Thirst is wanting during chill, is constant during hot stage, not constant during sweat.

Contrition of spirit—Home-sickness . .	Seriousness – Haughtiness—Excited imagination—Imbecility.
Complaints predominant on lower lip and sole of foot.	Complaints predominant on upper lip and on instep.
Urine frequent, but scanty	Urine frequent and copious.
Sexual desire prevalently weak	Sexual desire prevalently strong.
Cough predominantly dry	Cough predominantly with expectoration.

REMISSION during day and evening . . .	REMISSION forenoon and before midnight.
Complaints from the sunshine	Complaints from the moonlight.
Better during and after sweat	Worse while perspiring, better *afterwards*.
Worse on awaking	*Worse or* better after sleep.
Worse before breakfast	*Generally* better before breakfast.
Worse *or* better from drinking cold water .	Better from drinking cold water.
Worse when moving diseased part . . .	Better *or* worse from moving diseased part.
Worse during continued standing; but better when standing still after motion.	Predominantly worse while standing.

Predomin. worse —— **Predomin. better**

From cold, from uncovering, but also in-doors*, from motion, when walking, bending the head back, lying on right side, from touch, and after stool.

Predomin. better —— **Predomin. worse**

From warmth, wrapping up, out-doors, during rest, in bed†, lying on left side, and during sweat.

---

* On the other hand, Thuya-symptoms are aggravated in rooms that are too warm.

† Both remedies have aggravation while lying and from warmth of bed.

Cocculus.	Ignatia.
Right side—Inflammation of internal parts.	*Left* side—Inflammation of external parts.
Pain piercing outwards; in glands pressing inwards.	Pain piercing inwards; in glands pressing outwards.
Itching, unchanged by scratching. . . .	Itching lessened *or* place changed by scratching.
Pulse small and spasmodic often imperceptible.	Pulse generally quick, full, hard, with throbbing in veins; very changeable.
While eating chilly	Chill better after eating. C.Hg.
Predom. want of thirst, partic during chill.	Thirst *only* during chill, and after sweat.
Chill increased in warm room	Chill lessened in warm room.
Heat or sweat with aversion to uncover .	Heat or sweat with inclination to uncover.

Loquacity — Seriousness – Sadness — Gentleness.	Taciturnity — Cheerfulness *or* sadness — Mood changing; gentle *or* irritable — Amorousness.
Ailments from want of sleep. from care, mental or bodily excitement. C.Hg. .	Ailments from hearing bad news, fr. shame, mortification, disap love or jealousy.
Unconsciousness	Delirium.
Saliva predom. decreased	Saliva predom. increased
Aversion to sour things	Appetite for sour things.
Vomit predom. sour	Vomit is bitter oftener than sour.
Complaints predom. in liver	Spleen affected oftener than liver.
Complaints predom. in kidneys	Complaints predom. in bladder.
Urine frequent, but scanty	Urine often and copious.
Catamenia too late *or* too soon	Catamenia too soon.

Remission *night*, and forenoon	Remission of complaints before midnight.
Worse *or* better from growing cold, and in cold air. (resp growing warm, and in warm air.)	Predom. worse from growing cold, and in cold weather; better from growing warm, and in warm air.
Worse or better from warmth of bed . .	Worse from warmth of bed.
Worse when getting out of bed	Better *or* worse when getting out of bed.
Better *after* getting out of bed	Better *or* worse *after* getting out of bed.
Worse from bodily exertion	Improv. oftener than aggrav. by exertion.
Worse when stooping and when assuming an erect position.	Better *or* worse when assuming an erect position, and when stooping.
Almost always aggrav while eating . . .	*Better or* worse while eating.
Worse *or* better from eructation	Better from eructation.
Ailments from Ignatia or Cuprum . . .	Ailments from Coffea, Pulsatilla, or Zinc.

Predomin. worse ⁓ **Predomin. better**

From uncovering, when lying on back, when rising from a seat, when lifting up diseased limb, when swallowing *, during and after meals, and from change of position.

Predomin. better ⁓ **Predomin. worse**

From wrapping up, when lying on side, while lying, in bed, when standing, when letting diseased limb hang down, *before* breakfast, and after sweat.

N.B. With Ignatia we rarely find the sensation of numbness in suffering parts belonging to Cocculus.

---

* Cocculus, worse when swallowing saliva, and Ignatia, worse when swallowing drink.

Cocculus.	Nux vom.
Light hair—Skin and muscles lax . . .	Dark hair—Skin and muscles rigid
Crawling sensation in internal parts—Pain pressing inwards.	Crawling sensation in external parts—Pain pressing outwards.
Painless cutaneous eruptions	Painful eruptions.
Pulse small and spasmodic	Pulse generally quick, full, and hard; sometimes intermitting.
Partial sweat on front part of body . . .	Partial sweat on back part of body.
While eating chilly	During chill hunger. C.Hg.
Want of thirst predom.; partic. during chill.	Thirst predom; most during cold stage *
Desire for drink without thirst	Thirst with aversion to drink.
Gentleness—Indifference	Mood irritable; irascible; malicious—Amorousness.
Ailments from vexation with reserved displeasure.	Ailm. from disappointed love and jealousy from mortification, anger, or from vexation with indignation or vehemence.
No delirium	Delirium with the chill, with the fever or sweat.
Pupils generally contracted—Optical illusions in black or in dark colors.	Pupils generally dilated—Optical illusions in bright colors.
Saliva predom. decreased	Saliva generally increased.
Urine frequent, but scanty	Urine infrequent and scanty.
When diarrhœa appears, it is painless . .	When diarrhœa appears, it is painful.
Catamenia scanty, at the same time too late *or* too soon.	Catamenia too soon and profuse.
Expectoration tolerably infrequent . . .	Expectoration not constant.
Complaints predom. on upper arm . . .	Complains predom. on fore-arm.
REMISSION *night* and forenoon	REMISSION evening till midnight.
From growing cold, and in cold weather, (resp. growing warm, and in warm air,) worse *or* better.	Worse from growing cold, and in cold weather; better from growing warm, and in warm air.
Aggrav. oftener than improv. by warmth of bed.	Improved much oftener than aggrav. by warmth of bed.
Predom. worse after sleep	Better after sufficien sleep; but worse on awaking when roused.
Worse after drinking	*Worse or* better after drinking.
Worse when stooping	Better *or* worse when stooping.
Better from pressure	*Better or* worse from pressure.
Ailments from Nux vom. or Ignatia . . .	Ailments from Cocculus, Arsenic vapors, Iodine, Phosphor, Sulphur, Calcar., Cinchona, Coffea, Pulsat. Stramon., Plumbum, or Colchicum

Predomin. worse —— **Predomin. better**

When sitting erect, when lifting diseased limb, while eating, and after sleep.

Predomin. better —— **Predomin. worse**

When sitting bent forward, and when letting diseased limb hang down.

N.B. With N. vom. we rarely find the sensation of numbness of suffering parts, peculiar to Cocculus —Sensitiveness (to touch,) N. vom. has predom. in external parts, Cocculus exclusively in internal parts.

* N. vom. also has thirst before the chill, between heat and sweat, and *after* sweat stage.

Cocculus.	Phosphor.
Light hair—Skin and muscles lax	Dark hair—Skin and muscles rigid.
Often indicated with children and women . .	Often indicated with old people.
Pain pressing inwards—Gnawing pain in internal parts.	Pain pressing outwards—Gnawing pain in external parts.
Painless cutaneous eruptions	Painful eruptions.
Pulse small and spasmodic, often imperceptible.	Pulse generally quick, full & hard; irregular; often intermitting.
While eating chilly	During chill hunger. C.Hg
Heat with aversion to uncover	Heat with inclination to uncover.
Want of thirst predom., partic. during chill .	Want of thirst constant during all stages.
Heat or chill lessened in bed; chill increased out-doors and by drinking.	Heat or chill increased in bed; chill lessened out doors and by drinking.
Loquacity—Gentleness—Sadness—Hopelessness.	Taciturnity—Mood changing; cheerful *or* sad; irritable; haughty—Amorousness.
Ailments from vexation with fear or reserved displeasure.	Ailments from anger, or from vexation with fright or vehemence.
Weakness of memory—Absent-mindedness—Mental dullness.	Active memory pred.—Ecstacies—Delirium.
Eyes protruding	Eyes generally sunken.
Aversion to sour things—Desire for *or* aversion to beer.	Appetite for sour things—Aversion to beer.
Fetid flatus	Scentless flatus.
Costiveness most frequent	Diarrhœa most frequent. (Disposition to soft stools. C.Hg.)
Catamenia scanty	Catamenia profuse *or* scanty.
Cough generally dry	Cough either with expectoration *or* dry.
Complaints predom. on thigh	Complaints predom. on leg.
Remission night and forenoon	Remission of complaints after midnight.
Worse while perspiring	*Worse or* better while perspiring.
Worse *or* better when growing cold, (resp. growing warm.)	Predom. worse when growing cold; better when growing warm.
Predom. better in bed*	*Worse or* better in bed.
Worse from uncovering; better from wrapping up.	*Generally* better from uncovering; worse from wrapping up.
Predom. worse after sleep	Better after sufficient sleep; but worse after the siesta, and on awaking when roused from sleep.
Worse after meals	*Worse or* better after meals.
Worse when stooping	Better *or* worse when stooping.
Worse when swallowing saliva	Worse when swallowing food, and partic. when swallowing drink.
Better from pressure	Aggravated oftener than improv. by pressure.
Ailments from Chamom., Ignatia, Nux vom., or Copper.	Ailm. from Iodine or from abuse of table-salt.

Predomin. worse — **Predomin. better**

Out-doors, when sitting erect, when lifting diseased limb, from the touch, after drinking, from cold diet, and from drinking cold water; from spirituous liquors, after sleep, and from uncovering.

Predomin. better — **Predomin. worse**

In-doors*, when sitting bent forward, when letting diseased limb hang down, *after* the sweat, from warm diet, in bed, and from wrapping up.

N.B. From the decided aggravation in rooms filled with people, it is evident that the open air alone effects the improv. with the Phosph. patient; the improvement in-doors and the improvement out-doors is partly an alternating effect,—partly the improved symptoms differ essentially in kind. C.Hg.

* Both remedies have predom. aggravation from *warmth* of bed.

† Phosph. also has aggrav., partic. in *crowded* rooms. *When walking* out-doors, this remedy has improv. of complaints quite as often as aggrav., by which we see that in the latter case motion decides and not the influence of the open air.

Cocculus.	Pulsatilla.
Aversion to open air—Pain pressing inwards.	Inclinat. for open air—Pain pressing outwards.
Sensitiveness of internal parts	*Generally* sensitiveness of external parts.
Paralysis—Painless eruptions	Rarely paralysis—Painful eruptions.
Sweat or coldness on suffering side	Heat on suffering part.
Pulse small and spasmodic	Pulse generally quick, small, and weak.
Chill predom. on back part of body; sweat on front part.	Chill on front part of body; sweat on back part of body.
While eating chilly	During chill hunger. C.Hg.
Heat or chill less'd in bed; chill incr. out-doors.	Heat or chill worse in bed; chill less. out-doors.
Loquacity — Gentleness — Seriousness — No delirium.	Taciturnity—Mood changing; gentle, but bold —Avarice—Distrust—Amorousness.
Ailments from vexation with reserved displeasure.	Ailments from excessive joy, mortification, or from vexation with fright.
Optical illusions in black or in dark colors	Optical illusions in bright colors.
Eyes protruding	Eyes sunken.
Nasal complaints predominantly internal	Nasal compl. external, oftener than internal.
Nose-bleeding during pregnancy or with hemorrhoidal disposition.	Nose-bleeding with suppressed or scanty catamenia. C.Hg.
Saliva predom. decreased	Saliva generally increased.
Generally loss of appetite	Generally hunger.
Aversion to sour things — Desire for *or* aversion to beer.	Appetite for sour things and beer.
Food tastes as though salted too little	Food tastes too salty.
Vomit sour, oftener than bitter	Vomit bitter oftener than sour.
Generally constipation — When diarrhœa appears, it is painless.	Generally diarrhœa which is oftenest painful.
Cough generally dry	Cough generally with expectoration.
Urine frequent, but scanty	Urine infrequent and scanty.
Catamenia too late *or* too soon	Catamenia too late.
Complaints predom. in kidneys, and on thigh.	Complaints predom. in bladder, and on leg.
AGGRAVATION morning, afternoon, evening.	AGGRAVATION from noon till midnight.
Worse (resp. better) from growing cold and in cold air, *or* when grow'g warm & in warm air.	Better from growing cold and in cold weather; worse when growing warm and in warm air.
Worse from uncovering; better from wrapping up.	*Generally* better from uncovering, worse from wrapping up.
Better after the sweat	Almost always aggrav. after the sweat.
Predom. better in bed	*Generally* worse in bed.
From warmth of bed *worse or* better	Worse from warmth of bed.
Worse when lying on back; better when lying on side.	*Generally* better when lying on back, worse when lying on side.
Worse when getting out of bed	*Better or* worse when getting out of bed.
Better *after* getting out of bed	*Better or* worse *after* getting out of bed.
Worse when rising from a seat	*Worse or* better when rising from a seat.
Better *after* rising from a seat	*Better or* worse *after* rising from a seat.
Worse when stooping and when assuming an erect position.	*Worse or* better when stooping, and when assuming an erect position.
Better when sitting down	Worse *or* better when sitting down.
Worse when sitting erect; better when sitting bent forward.	*Generally* better when sitting erect; worse when sitting bent forward.
Worse when moving or bending diseased part.	Better *or* worse when moving or bending diseased part.
Better from pressure	Worse *or better* from pressure.
Better *before* breakfast	*Worse or* better before breakfast.
Worse after meals	*Worse or* better after meals.
Worse after stool	*Better or* worse after stool.

Predomin. worse — **Predomin. better**

Out-doors, and when walking out-doors; from cold, from cold diet, and drinking cold water; from uncovering, when getting out of bed, lying on back, when sitting erect, when bending diseased limb sideways, when lifting suffering limb, from exercise, when walking, walking fast, running; from bodily exertion generally, and after stool.

Predomin. better — **Predomin worse**

In-doors, from warmth, and warm diet; from wrapping up, when lying on side, sitting bent forward, when letting suffering limb hang down, during rest, standing & lying, in bed, and after the sweat.

Cocculus.	Rhus.
Skin and muscles lax—Aversion to exercise.	Skin and muscles rigid—Inclin. for exercise.
Complaints (sensitiveness, gnawing, pressing pain) predominantly internal.	Complaints (sensitiveness, etc.) predominant in external parts.
Pain pressing inwards—Anæmie	Pain press'g outwards—Generally plethora.
Itching, unchanged by scratching. . .	Itch.'g, less. by scratch'g, rarely unchanged.
Dry eruptions	Eruptions generally humid.
Paralysis, particularly after spasms . . .	Par., partic. after apoplexy or pain in joints.
Pulse small and spasmodic	Pulse irregular; generally accelerated, weak, faint, and soft.
Chills while eating	Chills lessened after eating C.Hg.
Heat lessened in bed	Heat increased in bed.
Want of thirst predominant	Thirst not constant.
Mood indifferent—Absent-mindedness—Insanity.	Dejection of spirits more predominant than with Cocculus.
Conseq. of vexat'n with reserv'd displeasure.	Delirium.
Pupils generally contracted	Pupils dilated.
Nasal complaints predominantly internal; nose-bleeding with hemorrhoids.	Nas. compl. extern. oftener than intern.; nose-bleed'g in place of hemorrhoid. disch. CHg.
Saliva predominantly decreased	Saliva generally increased.
Aversion to beer or desire for it	Desire for beer.
Nausea in stom., rarely in throat or abdomen.	Naus. in œsoph. or stom., rarely in throat.
Costiveness predom.—Diarrhœa painless .	Diarrhœa predominant; generally painful.
Urine frequent, but scanty	Urine frequent and copious.
Catamenia too scanty; at the same time too late *or* too soon.	Catamenia profuse and generally too soon.
Expectoration rather infrequent	Expectoration not constant.
Complaints predominant on upper arm . .	Complaints predominant on fore-arm.
REMISSION *night* and forenoon	REMISSION of complaints during day.
Worse when getting out of bed	Better *or* worse when getting out of bed.
Better *after* getting out of bed	*Worse or* better *after* getting out of bed.
Better when sitting down	Worse *or* better when sitting down.
Worse when rising from a seat	*Worse or* better when rising from a seat.
Better *after* rising from a seat	*Worse or* better *after* rising from a seat.
Worse from moving or bending diseased part.	Better *or* worse from moving or bending diseased part.
Worse when walking out-doors	Better *or* worse* when exercis'g out-doors.
Worse (resp. better) from grow'g cold and in cold weather, *or* from growing warm and in warm air.	Worse when growing cold und in cold weather; better from growing warm and in warm air.
Worse after eating or drinking	*Worse or* better after eat'g, also aft'r drink'g.
Better *or* worse from eructation	Worse from eructation.
Worse after stool	*Better or* worse after stool.
Worse when swallowing saliva	Worse when swallow'g saliva & swall. food.

Predomin. worse —— **Predomin. better**

From exercise, when walking, when sitting erect, after breakfast, and after stool.

Predomin. better —— **Predomin. worse**

During rest, when standing and lying, when sitting bent forward, from biting (clenching the teeth), and on an empty stomach.

N.B. Rhus lacks the over-sensitiveness of Cocculus to pain.

* Here the influence of motion, and not that of open air, decides in the first case; for out-doors generally both remedies have predom. aggravation, in-doors predom. improvement.

Coffea.	Belladonna
From up downwards—Inclination for motion.	*From down upwards*—Aversion to motion.*
Bruised pain in internal parts	Bruised pain in external parts.
Ischias (rending. shooting.) or neuralgia cruralis, increased by walking, relieved by pressure, except on foramen; worse afternoon and night.	Ischias in the hip joint, violent at night, compels to change position; sensitive to touch, even of the clothing, or in thigh, bearable only when the limb is hanging down. C. Hg.
Sleepless before and about mid-night; from over-excitement, feeling wide awake, with the fever, partic. during the sweat.	Sleepless before midnight, with great desire to sleep, imagines that something is entrusted to his care; fear, fright. C. Hg.
Pulse, if changed, more frequent, but less vigorous, even small and infirm. Grauvogl.	Pulse changed in frequency, strength and quality, sometimes trembling or irregular.
Thirst rather infrequent during heat, almost constant *after* heat and during sweat.	Thirst not constant, most rare during chill, often *before* the chill, and *after* the sweat.
Measles: frequent short and dry cough, hoarse when crying; skin and all senses over-sensitive; spasmodic motions, trembling; with heat and sweat in the face.	*Measles*: Dry cough, with weeping; thirst; difficult swallowing; hoarse crying on account of pain in throat; hot burning skin, violent contraction of fingers & toes. C. Hg.
Ailments from excessive joy, or from disappointed love.	Mood changing; indifferent, peevish, distrustful, malicious† — Ailments fr. mortification.
Sensitive disposition	Generally insensibility of disposition.
Memory very active — Easy comprehension — Mental excitability.	Memory active *or* weak—Difficult comprehension—Mental excitability *or* dullness.
Delirium tremens: unsteady running about, imagines that he is not at home, with trembling of hands; small, frequent pulse. (120) .	*Delirium tremens:* walking busily about, undertaking many things, rush of blood to head, chill & heat. Cmp. Bell.—Nux. C. Hg.
Threatening of apoplexy: over-excited, exalted, talkative, full of fear, pangs of conscience, aversion to open air, sleepless, convulsive grinding of teeth.	Threat of apoplexy, disposition irritable, shuns motion, inclined to sleep, fulness in the head, giddiness, reddened eyes, sensible to light, noise and touch. C. Hg.
Nose-bleeding with heaviness of the head, and ill-humor.	Vertigo in the morning ends with bleeding of nose. C. Hg.
Compl. predom. on soft palate—Fetid flatus .	Compl. pred. on roof of mouth—Scentl. flatus.
Metrorhagia, large black lumps, worse from every motion, violent pain in the groins, fever, bright-red face; in the greatest despair, believes herself dying.	Metrorhagia, blood coagulated, dark or red or changing, with bearing-down, restless, dislikes to lie on back, bruised pain in small of back, sacrum as if broken, face pale, suffer'g, thirst and chilliness, part. in the back. C. Hg.
Threatening abortion or labor-pains, excessively painful, with fear of death.	Threatening abortion or false labor-pains with headache and redness of face. C. Hg.
Childbed-fever with great excitability, trembling of hands.	Childbed-fever with gr. anxiety, despair of recovery; or mov'g the hands in the air. C. Hg.
Spasmus glottidis, starts from sleep with short inhalation, or gasping with wheezing, cold sweat, blue face, worse when put into the bath.	Spasmus glottidis, with convulsions or a croup-like cough; wheezing inspiration, without expiration, or imperceptible respiration, and apparently no pulse. C. Hg.
REMISSION forenoon and evening till midnight.	REMISSION *forenoon* and after midnight.
Worse (resp. better) from uncovering *or* wrapping up.	Worse from uncovering; better from wrapping up.
Worse from spirituous liquors	Worse *or* better from spirituous liquors.
Worse when bending diseased part	*Better or* worse when bending diseased part.
Worse when bending diseased part backwards or forwards.	Worse when bending diseased part sideways better when bending it backwards.

Predomin. worse — **Predomin. better**

When growing warm, in bed, when opening the eyes, when sitting down, when stooping, when holding diseased part bent, when bending it backwards, and from scratching.

Predomin. better — **Predomin worse**

When growing cold,‡ when closing the eyes, and after stool.

* *Belladonna* sometimes also has *inclination for motion* in single or suffering parts.
† "*Cheerfulness*" is found with both remedies.
‡ Both remedies have predom. aggrav. from *cold* generally, improvement from warmth.

Coffea.	Chamomilla.
Muscles rigid—Dark hair.	Muscles lax—Light hair.
Sensitiveness in external parts.	Sensitiveness in internal parts.
With the pain—the patient seems beside himself.	Pain seems to be unbearable. C.Hg.
Ischias or neuralgia cruralis increased by walking; is worse afternoon and night; relieved by pressure, except on foramen.	Ischias nervosa,—left side. drawing pain from hip to knee, or from tuber ischii to soles of feet, worse at night. in bed; screaming aloud even when slightly moved; sensation of numbness after the pain. C.Hg.
Apoplexy—Paralysis	Very rarely paralysis—No apoplexy.
Threatenings of apoplexy; over-excited, exalted, talkative, full of fear, pangs of conscience, discouraged, complaining, aversion to the open air, sleepless, convulsive grinding of teeth.	Threatenings of apoplexy with women in childbed; heaviness and beating; tearing pain in head, one-sided from the head into the jaws; hot sweat on the head, partic. the scalp; with fainting spells or convulsions C.Hg.
Convulsions of teething children with grinding of teeth. &c.	Convulsions of teething children; one cheek red, the other pale; smiling in sleep. C.Hg.
Pulse, if changed, more frequent, less vigorous, even small and infirm. Grauvogl.	Pulse quick, small and tense; unequal.
Thirst only before and during sweat	Thirst constant in fevers.
Measles with frequent, short, and dry cough.	*After* measles: short, dry cough. C.Hg.
Sleepless more before midnight, with awaking; with the hot, partic. the sweating stage.	Sleepless all night, anxiety drives him out of bed; sleepless dur. all stages of fever C.Hg.
Loquacity—*Cheerfulness or* dejection—Being beside one's self.	Taciturnity — Mood sad; peevish; serious — Wrapt in thought.
Ailments from excessive joy or from disappointed love.	Consequences of mortification.
Easy comprehension—Mental excitability	Difficult comprehension — Mental dullness — Unconsciousness.
Congestions to head while talking	Vertigo while talking. C.Hg.
Pupils dilated	Pupils contracted.
Hunger predom.	Loss of appetite predom.
Diarrhœa from too much thought and care about domestic affairs; watery, painless, very weakening with over-sensibility and great irritability.	Diarrhœa from vexation, from taking cold, during dentition, bilious, slimy, smelling sour, or like rotten eggs, yellowish, greenish curdled; with cutting pain; great sensibility, restlessness, crying; peevishness. C.Hg.
Metrorrhagie: large black lumps worse from every motion, with violent pain in groins and fear of death.	Metrorrhagie, dark coagulated, in sudden attacks, coldness of limbs, partic. feet; thirst; worse when lying on back, violent, contracting labor-like pains from the sacrum into abdomen. C.Hg.
Intermitting palpitation of heart	Palpitation of heart in uniform beats.
Cough without expectoration	Cough dry, rarely with expectoration.
Complaints predom. on shin	Complaints predom. on calf of leg.
AGGRAVATION afternoon, night, (partic. after midnight,) and morning.	AGGRAVATION evening and night, partic. before midnight.
Better after getting out of bed	Worse *or* better after getting out of bed.
Childr. at times cannot bear to be carried about.	Children feel better when carried about. C.Hg.
Worse when moving diseased part	*Worse or* better when moving diseased part.

Predomin. worse — **Predomin. better**

From cold, when opening the eyes, from motion, when walking, when sitting down, when bending the suffering part, when drawing up diseased limb, and on expiration.

Predomin. better — **Predomin worse**

From warmth; when closing the eyes, during rest, when standing, when lying*, and when stretching out diseased limb.

* Both remedies have predom. aggrav. *in bed*.

Coffea.	Colocynthis.
Sensitiveness of external parts—Over-sensitiveness.	Sensitiveness in internal parts—Sensation of numbness.*
Dryness of skin, but not in febrile diseases .	Disposition to sweat and perspiring easily.
Apoplexy	Apoplexy not yet observed.
Pulse, if changed, more frequent, but less vigorous, even small and infirm. Grauvogl.	Pulse changed in frequency and strength; generally hard, full, and quick.
No thirst until before and during the sweating stage.	Predominant want of thirst.
Sleeplessn. fr. overexcitement of body or mind.	Sleeplessness after vexation. C.Hg.
Loquacity — Predomin. cheerfulness—Rarely amorousness — Sanguine choleric temparament—Ailments from excessive joy, fright, disappointed love, and from vexation with fright or vehemence.	Mood taciturn; hypochondriacal; averse—Choleric temperament—Affected by misfortune, even that of others—Ailments from shame, grief, mortification, and from vexation with indignation.
Easy comprehension—Mental excitability . .	Distaste for mental labor—Heaviness in the head.
Complaints predominant on soft palate, on back part of thigh, and on shin.	Complaints predominant on roof of mouth, on front part of thigh, and on calf of leg.
Aversion to coffee	Appetite for coffee.
Diarrhœa predominantly painless	Diarrhœa predominantly painful.
Chronic disposit'n to watery, painless diarrhœa, from too much care with household affairs.	Chronic diarrhœa, watery, with pain inside of abdomen; in the morning. C.Hg.
Urine too frequent (and copious)	Urine decreased *or* increased.
Expectoration not yet observed	Expectoration rather infrequent.
Ischias or neuralgia cruralis, in attacks; rending, shooting increased by walking, relieved by pressure, except on foramen; worse afternoon and night; restless and sleepless at night.	Ischias postica, right side; shooting pain in sacral region; must lie in one position; aggravated by every motion; stitching, cutting pain from hip to knee or ankles, or like a flash of lightning from sacrum to heel, with thirst for water, worse in the evening and at night; numb and as if dead during remission. C.Hg.
Remission forenoon and evening, till midnight.	Remission night and morning.
Better after getting out of bed	*Better or* worse after getting out of bed.
Worse from cold; better from warmth . . .	Better (resp. worse) from cold *or* warmth.
Worse when walking out-doors	Worse *or* better† when walking out-doors.
Worse when stooping	*Worse or* better when stooping.
Ailments from Chamom., Colocynthis, Ignatia, or Nux vomica.	Ailments from Causticum.

Predomin. worse — **Predomin. better**

From exercise, when walking, when holding diseased part bent, and from scratching.

Predomin. better — **Predomin. worse**

During rest, while standing,‡ and while lying down.§

* Colocynthis lacks the over-sensitiveness of Coffea to pain.

† In the latter case the motion, and not the influence of the open air, decides for Colocynthis; for, in general, both remedies have aggravation out-doors.

‡ Yet we also find "improvement" with Colocynthis "when standing still after exercise."

§ Both remedies have predominant aggravation "in bed."

Coffea.	Ignatia.
Inclination for exercise	Aversion to exercise.
Sleepless more before and soon after midnight; wide awake; during the hot stage, partic. during the sweat; also *after typhoid fevers.*	Sleeplessness during the evening and before midnight; from ebullition of blood; with starting when falling asleep; inward restlessness, thirst, fever with anxiety from 2 to 5 A. M., sleep with the heat so light that he hears very distant noises.
Threatenings of apoplexy, with congestion to head. Comp. Acon. — Coffea.	Threatenings of apoplexy; head feels empty, face is pale.*
Convulsions of teething children with grinding of teeth, &c., after over-excitement.	Convulsion during dentition with frothing at the mouth, kicking with the legs; or with children after having been punished; after fear or fright.
Pulse is changed, more frequent, less vigorous, even small and infirm. Grauvogl.	Pulse changed, generally accelerated, large and hard; unequal.
Generally dislikes to be uncovered	Likes to be uncovered during the hot or sweating stage. C.Hg.
Thirst only *before* and during sweat. . . .	Thirst only during chill and *after* sweat.
Being beside one's self—Predom. cheerfulness Loquacity — Mood irritable — Rarely amorousness.	Wrapt in thought — Predom. sadness — Mood changing; gentle, indifferent, peevish, bold. — Taciturnity.
Ailments from excessive joy, anger, or from vexation with vehemence.†	Ailments from shame, grief, jealousy, mortification, hearing bad news, or from vexation with fear or reserved displeasure.
Memory active—Easy comprehension—Mental excitement—Rarely fancies.	Memory weak—Diffic. comprehension—Mental dullness—Absent-mindedness—Insanity.
Congestion to head while talking.	Congestion to head fr. being spoken to. C.Hg.
Predom. acute and sensitive hearing. . . .	Difficulty of hearing or deafness.
Complaints predom. on soft palate	Complaints predom. on roof of mouth.
Hunger predom.	Generally loss of appetite.
Eat hastily	Drink hastily—before spasms of childr. C.Hg.
Diarrhœa painless, all day, from too much care about domestic affairs.	Diarrh. painless, with rumbling noise of wind, — worse in the night and from fright with great timidity. C.Hg.
Catamenia too profuse and of long duration .	Catamenia scanty but of long duration.
Metrorhagia; — comp. Coffea — Bellad. . .	Metrorhagia from chamomile-tea. C.Hg.
Expectoration not yet observed	Expectoration infrequent.
Complaints predom. on shin	Complaints generally on calf of leg.
Ischias in attacks, rending and shooting; worse afternoon and night. Comp. Coffea—Acon., etc.	Ischias,—intermitting, chronic; better in Summer, worse in Winter, — beating as though it would burst the hip joint, accompanied by chilliness with thirst, flushes of heat, particularly in the face, without thirst. C.Hg.
REMISSION forenoon and evening till midnight.	REMISSION of complaints before midnight.
Worse during and after meals.	Impr. oftener than aggr. during & after meals.
Worse from bodily exertion	Improv. oftener than aggr. by bodily exertion.
Worse after sleep.	*Worse or* better after sleep.
Better after getting out of bed	Worse *or* better after getting out of bed.
Ailments from Nux vom., Colocynth., &c. . .	Ailments from Tabacum, Digitalis, or Zinc.

Predomin. **worse** — Predomin. **better**

When lifting up diseased limb, from uncovering the head, from rubbing and scratching, when swallowing, and during and after meals.

Predomin. **better** — Predomin. **worse**

When letting diseased limb hang down, from wrapping up the head, when standing and lying‡, and after stool.

N.B. In spite of the great similarity of many symptoms, these remedies are rarely antidotes to each other, they even act injuriously when given the one after the other; the head symptoms of both follow the same direction, — from right to left. — Comp. Acon. — Coffea.

* Consequences of disappointed love appear with both remedies.

† Both remedies have predom. aggrav. *in bed.*

‡ Both remedies may prevent apoplexy with nervous persons, with the same sensibility to noise, the same aggravation from spirituous liquors, &c., and the cases may only be distinguished by the peculiarities of the mind, of the pulse, or the fever, or others mentioned above. C.Hg.

Coffea.	Nux vom.
From up, downwards—Inclinat'n fer exercise.	From down, upwards—Aversion to exercise.
Sensitiveness of skin	Sensitiveness, but sometimes insensibility of skin. C.Hg.
Sleepless until midnight or after midnight with feeling wide awake during the heat, particularly the sweat.	Sleepless before and partic. after midnight, fidgety; restlessness in lower limbs during heat, sometimes with sweat. C.Hg.
Pulse, if changed, more frequent, but less vigorous, even small and infirm. Grauvogl.	Pulse changed in frequency and strength, generally hard, full and quick.
Thirst is mostly before and during sweat . .	Thirst mostly during chill, also *before* chill, and *before* and *after* sweat.

Coffea.	Nux vom.
Cheerfullness more frequent than sadness*—Rarely amorousness.	Mood sad, anxious, peevish; malicious.
Consequences of excessive joy	Ailments from grief, jealousy, or mortification.
Easy comprehension — Mental excitability — Rarely fancies.	Difficult comprehension — Mental dullness — Absent-mindedness—Unconsciousness.
Delirium tremens, unsteady running about, imagines that he is not at home, trembling of hands. Comp. Aconit. — Coffea.	Delirium tremens, fear, sees people, heat and sweat, vomiting. Comp. Bellad. — N. vom. C.Hg.
Threatenings of apoplexy; talkativeness; convulsive grinding of teeth.	Threatenings of apoplexy, biting together of jaws, tongue heavy. C.Hg.
Headache aggrav. after sleep	Headache better after sleep.
Toothache with lachrymose mood	Toothache with desperate mood. C.Hg.
Complaints predom. on soft palate	Complaints predom. on roof of mouth.
Acute taste	Predom. loss of taste.
Hunger predom.	Generally loss of appetite.
Diarrhœa predom. painless	Constipation pred.—When diarrhœa occurs, it is painful and scanty.
Diarrhœa, watery, painless, very weakening, with over-sensibility; from too much care.	Diarrhœa lumpy, with slime and blood, violent belly ache, with freq. urging to stool. C.Hg.
Urine predom. too often and copious . . .	Urine predom. too infrequent and scanty.
Metrorrhagia, large black lumps, worse from motion; with violent pains in groin and fear of death.	Metrorrhagia, dark, coagulated; worse from motion, bearing down in abdomen; as if the navel were drawn in — weeps about every thing. C.Hg.
Cough *without* expectoration	Expectoration not constant.
Complaints predom. on shin	Complaints generally on calf of leg.
Ischias or neuralgia cruralis, rending, shooting pains and attacks, increased by walking, relieved by pressure, except on foramen; worse afternoon and night.	Ischias, from toes to hip upwards, or from the trochanter to hollow of knee, worse at night, aggrav. very much by every motion or when lifted; much worse when pressing to stool†. C.Hg.

Coffea.	Nux vom.
Remission forenoon and evening till midnight.	Remission evening till midnight.
Worse when overhurried	Worse when idle *or* when overhurried.‡
Worse after sleep	Better after sufficient and not too long sleep; but worse on awaking when roused fr. sleep
Better after getting out of bed	Worse *or* better after getting out of bed.
Worse when stooping	Better *or* worse when stooping.
Worse when swallowing	*Worse or* better when swallowing.
Ailments from Nux vom., or Colocynthis . .	Ailments from Arsenic or Copper vapors, from Sulph., Calc., Phosph., Iodine, Plumb., or abuse of Cinchona.

Predomin. worse —— **Predomin. better**

When lifting up or bending diseased limb backwards, from rubbing and scratching, in bed, when sitting down, when eating, and after sleep.

Predomin. better —— **Predomin. worse**

When letting diseased limb hang down, and after stool.

---

* Tellurium (156) has the same extending from the sacrum downwards to the thigh, according to symptoms of Drs. Kitchen and Rau, and Dr. Bauer's cure, (243.) C.Hg

† "*Irritable mood*" is found with both remedies.

‡ These are only apparently opposites, and both arise from the mutual source of the *same* impatient disposition.

Coffea.	Pulsat.
Shunning open air	Longing for open air.
Inclination for exercise	Aversion to exercise.
With the pain, the patient seems beside himself.	With the pain, chilliness, difficult breathing, pale face. C.Hg.
Sleeplessness more after midnight; without any complaint during the fever, partic. during the sweat.	Sleeplessness more before midnight, with anxiety as if he had committed a crime, ebullition of blood, rush of ideas or one single idea; a melody, &c., occupies the mind; — during all stages of the fever. C.Hg.
Awaking too early	Awaking too late.
Pulse, if changed, more frequent, less vigorous, even small and infirm. Grauvogl.	Pulse changed, generally frequent, small, and weak.
Chill increased by exercise	Chill lessened by exercise.
Thirst, partic. during sweat*	Want of thirst predom.
With the measles, frequent, short, and dry cough, over-sensitiveness and spasmodic motions.	With the measles frequent, short, dry cough with piercing pain in chest, dry mouth; no thirst; ears aching. C.Hg.

Coffea.	Pulsat.
Cheerfulness more frequent than sadness .	Calm, lachrymose sadness.
Being beside one's self	Being wrapt in thought.
Loquacity	Taciturnity.
Mood irritable—Rarely amorousness . .	Mood gentle, but bold; changing, indifferent, peevish, greedy; distrustful.
Ailments from disappointed love, anger, or from vexation with vehemence.†	Ailments from mortification borne without complaint, sorrow, or from vexation with fear.
Memory active	Weakness of memory—Absent-mindedness.
Rarely fancies	Delirium.
Crackling noise in the head, synchronous with the pulse, in one side of the head, partic. in the morning and in the open air, better within doors.	Crackling noise in the head, synchronous with the pulse, when moving the head, or while walking; worse in the evening, and better in the open air; worse within doors.
Pupils dilated	Pupils generally contracted.
Acute and sensitive hearing predom. . .	Hardness of hearing; deafness.
Nasal complaints predom, internal . . .	Nasal complaints external, oftener than internal.
Acute, sensitive smell and taste	Predom. loss of smell; loss of taste.
Nose bleeding with heaviness of the head, and ill-humor.	Nose bleeding with suppressed catamenia. C.Hg.
Complaints predom. on soft palate . . .	Complaints predom. on hard palate.
Painless diarrhæa	Diarrhœa generally painful.
Diarrhœa from too much care	Diarrhœa, after getting the feet wet, slimy, whitish.
Urine frequent and copious	Urine infrequent and scanty.
Catamenia too profuse and of long duration.	Catamenia too scanty and of short duration.
Catamenia only during the evening . . .	Catamenia only during the day, while walking. C.Hg.

---

* Coffea has much thirst between heat and sweat, Pulsat. still more between chill and heat.

† Ailments from excessive joy occur with both remedies.

Coffea.	Pulsat.
(Continued.)	
Metrorhagia, large black lumps, worse from every motion; violent pain in groins; fear of death.	Metrorhagia, blood coagulated; ceasing and returning; worse during the evening and night with labor-like pains, sudden outcries, fainting. C.Hg.
Labor-pains ceasing with complaining loquacity and fear of death.	Labor-pains ceasing, with coldness and somnolence.
Cough without expectoration	Cough generally with expectoration.
Ischias, neuralgia cruralis in attacks; worse from motion, relieved by pressure, except on foramen.	Ischias, left side, along the nerve, forces to change position; every motion aggrav.; anxiousness even to weeping; *the greater the pain, the greater the chilliness;* — no thirst with it; worse at night. C.Hg.

REMISSION forenoon and evening till midnight.	AGGRAVATION afternoon and evening till midnight.
Worse after sleep	*Worse or* better after sleep.
Better after getting out of bed	*Better or* worse after getting out of bed.
Worse when sitting down	Better *or* worse when sitting down.
Worse when moving diseased limb . . .	*Better or* worse when moving the limb.
Worse when bending diseased part, partic. when bending it backwards or forwards.	Better when bending diseased part (sideways) *or* (backwards) worse.
Worse when swallowing	*Worse or* better when swallowing.
Better after stool	*Better or* worse after stool.
Children, at times cannot bear to be carried about.	Children desire to be carried about, but slowly. C.Hg.

Predomin. worse — **Predomin. better**

From cold, out-doors and when walking out-doors, from exercise, when walking, from bodily exertion; when lifting, or holding diseased limb bent; when opening the eyes, and from tying the clothes tight.

Predomin. better — **Predomin worse**

From warmth, in-doors, during rest; while standing, sitting, and lying;* when letting diseased limb hang down, when closing eyes, and from loosening the clothes.

N.B. With Coffea we very rarely find the sensation of numbness in suffering parts peculiar to Pulsat.

---

* Both remedies have predom. aggrav. *in bed.*

Colchicum.	Apis.
Right side—Complaints (burning, heat, etc.) predominant in internal parts.	*Left* side—Complaints (burning, heat, etc.) predominant in external parts.
Pulse sometimes trembling	Pulse sometimes intermitting.
Heat, with aversion to uncover	Heat, with inclination to uncover.
Thirst seems to be wanting only during chill.	Thirst seems to be wanting only during sweat.
Rarely despondency*	Mood hopeless; indifferent; irritable.
Ailments from grief or the misbehavior of others.	Ailments from fright, jealousy, anger, from hearing bad news, or from vexation with fright.
Anxious feeling in præcordia	Anxious feeling in head.
Rarely absent-mindedness — Rarely delirium.	Absent-mindedness – Delirium.
Paralysis — No apoplexy	Apoplexy—Rarely paralysis.
Complaints predominant on lower eyelids, and on inner ear.	Complaints predominant on upper eyelids, and on external ear.
Acute hearing predominant	Hardness of hearing; deafness.
Diarrhœa prevalently painful	Diarrhœa (except dysentery) prevalently painless.
Catamenia too scanty	Catamenia too profuse *or* too scanty.
Expectoration rather infrequent; morning and during day.	Cough, wakens before midnight and ceases as soon as anything is loosened, which is swallowed.
Remission morning and forenoon . . .	**Remission** of complaints during day.
Better (resp. worse) in cold *or* warm air .	Worse in cold weather; better in warm air.
Worse from getting wet through	Worse from getting wet through; but prevalently better from washing with cold water and moistening suffering part.

Predomin. worse —— **Predomin. better**

From uncovering, when assuming an erect position, and when sitting erect.

Predomin. better —— **Predomin. worse**

From wrapping up, when stooping and sitting bent forward, in bed, after sleep, after getting out of bed, and on inspiration.

N.B. In gouty complaints and erysipelas these remedies concur: Colchicum acts on the healthy, principally, from right to left, and was given, in many cases, with most decidedly good effect, when the gout commenced on the left and extended or threatened to extend to the right side; Apis, which acts in the opposite direction, (L. to R. Erysipelas of the face, complaints in ovaries, etc.) may have a more curative influence in gout, if the pain commenced and predominates on the right side, going from there to the left; this has been proved in diseases of the ovaries, but in gout it has not yet been ascertained. C.Hg.

* "Cheerfulness" is found with both remedies.

Colchicum.	Belladonna.
Upper right, lower left side—Paralysis . .	Upper left, lower right side — Apoplexy more frequent than paralysis.
Often indicated with old people	Often indicated with children and young women.
Cold shudders or heat ascending	Cold shudder or heat descending.
Thirst seems to be wanting only during chill.	Thirst not constant; most rare during chill; appears also before and after the attack of fever.
Sensitiveness of disposition	Generally insensibility of disposition.
Mood rarely peevish or despondent . . .	Mood changing; indifferent; irritable; malicious; distrustful.
Ailments from grief or from misbehavior of others.	Ailments from fright, anger, mortification, or from vexation with fright, dread, fear, or vehemence.
Rarely absent-mindedness, unconsciousness, or delirium.	Fancies—Insanity.
Weakness of memory	Memory active *or* very weak.
Painful diarrhœa	Painless diarrhœa.
Catamenia too soon, but scanty	Catamenia too soon and profuse.
During delivery incarceration of placenta .	During delivery inclusion of some parts of the child. C.Hg.
Fluent coryza	Predom. dry coryza.
Voice hoarse or deeper than usual . . .	Voice hoarse or raised.
Expectoration infrequent; morning and during day.	Expectoration infrequent; morning, during day and evening.
Remission morning and forenoon . . .	Remission after midnight and *forenoon*.
Better (resp. worse) in cold weather *or* in warm air.	Worse in cold weather; better in warm air.
Worse when lying on painful side, better when lying on unpainful side.	Better (resp. worse) when lying on painful *or* on unpainful side.
Worse when assuming an erect position .	*Worse or* better when assuming an erect position.
Worse when looking upwards	Worse when looking sideways.
Improv. oftener than aggrav when respiring deeply.	Worse when respiring deeply.
Worse when eating	*Worse or* better when eating.
Worse in the Fall	Worse in the Spring.

Predomin. worse — **Predomin. better**

In wet weather, from warmth, when growing warm, in-doors, when opening the eyes, when bending the head back, and from pressure.

Predomin. better — **Predomin. worse**

In dry weather, from cold, when growing cold, out-doors*, after sleep, after stool, and when closing the eyes.

N.B. With Bellad. we very rarely find the sensation of numbness in suffering parts belonging to Colch.

---

* Both remedies have predom. aggrav. when *walking out-doors;* therefore the influence of motion, and not that of the open air, here decides for Colch.

Colchicum.	Nux vom.
Pulse sometimes trembling; beating of heart the same.	Pulse sometimes intermitting the 4 to 5th beat.
Intermitting of retarded pulse	Intermitting of small, accelerated pulse.
Thirst seems to be wanting only during chill.	Most thirst during chill.
Apoplexy not yet observed	Apoplexy.
Mood cheerful *or* sad	Mood sad, irritable,—malicious—Amorousness.
Ailments from the misbehavior of others *.	Consequences of fright, anger, mortification, disappointed love, jealousy, or from vexation with fright, dread, fear, indignation, or vehemence.
Rarely absent-mindedness — Rarely unconsciousness or delirium.	Fancies.
Cataracta	Amaurosis.
Appetite for coffee—Aversion to fat food—Generally diarrhœa	Aversion to coffee—Appetite for fat food—Generally constipation.
Sediment of urine whitish	Sediment of urine reddish.
Catamenia too soon and scanty	Catamenia too soon and profuse.
Fluent coryza	Coryza generally dry, partic. out-doors; indoors; on the other hand it is fluent.
Breath cold	Breath hot.
Respiration with moist sound	Respiration with dry sound.
Expectoration infrequent; morning and during day.	Expectoration not constant; morning, during day, and evening.
REMISSION morning and forenoon . . .	REMISSION evening till midnight.
Better (resp. worse) in cold *or* warm air .	Worse in cold weather; better in warm air.
Better or worse when respiring deeply . .	Worse when respiring deeply.
Worse from getting wet through	Generally improved by washing and moistening.
Worse when swallowing	*Worse or* better when swallowing.
Better from eructation	*Better or* worse from eructation.
Worse when assuming an erect position . .	*Worse or* better when assuming an erect position.
Better when stooping	*Better or* worse when stooping.
Predom. worse when lying on side; better when lying on back.	*Generally* better when lying on side, worse when lying on back.

Predomin. worse —————— **Predomin. better**

In wet weather, from warmth, and when growing warm, in-doors, and from warmth of stove, when lying on left side, when sitting erect, when lifting diseased limb, from pressure, and while eating.

Predomin. better —————— **Predomin. worse**

In dry weather, from cold, and when growing cold, out-doors,† when lying on right side, when sitting bent forward, when letting diseased limb hang down, after stool, and when respiring deeply.

N.B. With N. vom. we rarely find the sensation of numbness in suffering parts peculiar to Colchicum.

---

* *Ailments from grief* are found with both remedies.

† Both remedies have predom. aggrav. *when walking out-doors;* therefore the influence of motion and not that of the open air, here decides for Colchicum.

Colchicum.	Pulsat.
Upper right, lower left side—**Paralysis** . .	Upper left, lower right side — **Apoplexy** more frequent than paralysis.
Often indicated with old people	Often indicated with children.
During sleep lying on side	When asleep, lying on back, often the hands above the head.
Pulse generally frequent, full, and hard . .	Pulse generally frequent, but small & weak, sometimes imperceptible.
Chill increased by exercise, lessened when sitting and after sleep.	Chill lessened by exercise, increased when sitting and after sleep.
Thirst seems to be wanting only during chill.	Thirst only during hot stage.

Mood cheerful *or* dejected	Mood changing; anxious; sad; gentle; indifferent; peevish; greedy; distrustful; bold—Amorousness.
Ailments from the misbehavior of others .	Ailments from excessive joy, fright, mortification, or from vexation with fright, dread or fear.
Rarely absent-mindedness; rarely delirium.	Fancies.
Pupils predom. dilated	Pupils generally contracted.
Predom. acute or sensitive hearing . . .	Hardness of hearing; deafness.
Acute sensitive sense of smell	Predom. loss of smell.
Nasal complaints predom. internal . .	Nasal compl. external, oftener than internal.
Complaints predom. on upper lip	Complaints predom. on under lip.
Predom. loss of appetite.	Generally hunger.
Sediment of urine whitish	Sediment red.
Catamenia too soon	Catamenia too late.
Respiration with moist sound	Respiration prevalent with dry sound.
Cough generally without expectoration . .	Cough generally with expectoration.
Complaints generally on instep	Complaints generally on sole of foot.

REMISSION morning and forenoon . . .	REMISSION from midnight till noon.
Worse from getting wet through	Better from washing and moistening; but worse after getting the feet wet.
Better (resp. worse) in cold *or* warm air .	Better in cold weather; worse in warm air.
Improved oftener than aggrav. after sleep .	Aggrav. oftener than improv. after sleep.
Worse when swallowing.	*Worse or* better when swallowing.
Better after stool	*Better or* worse after stool.
Worse when assuming an erect position .	*Worse or* better when assuming an erect position.
Worse fr. moving or bending diseased part.	*Better or* worse from bending the diseased part.

Predomin. **worse** — Predomin. **better**

When walking in the open air,* from uncovering, when lying on painful side, when sitting erect, from exercise; from walking, running, and bodily exertion; when lifting diseased limb, when opening the eyes, when bending the head sideways, and from pressure.

Predomin. **better** — Predomin. **worse**

From wrapping up, when lying on unpainful side, when sitting bent forward, when stooping, during rest; when standing, sitting, and lying; in bed, when letting diseased limb hang down, when closing the eyes, from eructation, and after sleep.

---

* Here the influence of motion decides for Colch., and not the influence of the open air; — for out of doors generally both remedies have predom. improvement.

Colchicum.	Rhus.
Upper right, lower left side—Over-sensitiveness.	Upper left, lower right side — Predom. sensation of numbness.*
Complaints predom. in internal parts	Complaints predom. in external parts.
Itching, unchanged by scratching	Itching improved by scratching.
Itching or pinkish redness around the joints.	Itching around the joints.
During sleep lying on side	During sleep lying on back.
Apoplexy not yet observed	Apoplexy.
Pulse generally frequent, full, and hard	Pulse irregular; generally accelerated, weak and soft.
Chill lessened while sitting	Chill increased while sitting.

Colchicum.	Rhus.
Mood cheerful, or sad	Mood anxious, dejected.
Ailments from grief or fr. the misdemeanor of others.	Ailments from vexation with fear.
Rarely unconsciousness	Fancies.
Predom. acute or sensitive hearing	Hardness of hearing; deafness.
Acute, sensitive smell	Loss of smell.
Nasal complaints predom. internal	Nasal compl. external oftener than internal.
Urine dark, oftener than pale; scanty	Urine pale; often and copious.
Catamenia too soon and scanty	Catamenia too soon and profuse.
Respiration with moist sound	Respiration with dry sound.
Expectoration rather infrequent; morning and during day.	Expectoration not constant; partic. in the morning.
Complaints generally on sole of foot	Complaints generally on instep.

Colchicum.	Rhus.
REMISSION morning and forenoon	REMISSION of complaints during day.
Better (resp. worse) in cold *or* warm weather.	Worse in cold weather; better in warm air.
Almost always improv. in bed	*Better or* worse in bed.
Worse when moving diseased part, and when bending it.	*Better or* worse from moving or bending diseased part.
Better *or* worse from change of position	Worse from change of position when lying or standing.
Worse when looking upwards	Worse when looking down.
Better or worse when respiring deeply	Worse when respiring deeply.
Worse after drinking	*Worse or* better after drinking.
Better after stool	*Better or* worse after stool.
Aggravation very often, after mental exertion.	Decidedly worse after bodily exertion.

C.Hg.

Predomin. worse ⏜ **Predomin. better**

From warmth and growing warm, in doors, from warmth of stove, when lying on side, lying on painful side, from exercise; when walking, partic. walking in the open air;† when bending the head back, on expiration, from pressure, and when sitting erect.

Predomin. better ⏜ **Predomin. worse**

From cold, and from growing cold, in the open air, when lying on back, lying on unpainful side, during rest; when lying, standing, and sitting, partic. when sitting bent forward; when stooping, on inspiration, when respiring deeply, and after sleep.

---

* Yet we also find with Rhus "sensitiveness of external parts," and with both remedies sensation of numbness in suffering parts; — but Rhus lacks the over-sensitiveness of Colch. to pain.

† Here the influence of motion, and not that of the open air, decides for both remedies.

Colchicum.	Sepia.
Complaints predom. in internal parts—Rending pain upwards.	Complaints predom. in external parts—Rending pain downwards.
Apoplexy not yet observed—Erysipelas, smooth.	Apoplexy—Erysipelas generally pustulous
Itching, unchanged by scratching, rarely lessened.	Itching, aggrav. by scratching.
Intermitting of retarded pulse	Intermitting of accelerated pulse.
Pulse generally frequent, full, and hard . .	Pulse frequent and full, at night, slower during day; accelerated by vexation and motion.
Heat with thirst	Heat without thirst.
Thirst seems to be wanting only during chill.	Predom. want of thirst; thirst is constant only during chill.

Mood cheerful or sad; rarely irritable . .	Mood serious, dejected, anxious, indifferent, peevish—Avarice.
Ailments from grief or from the misbehavior of others.	Consequences of fright, anger, and partic. of vexation with fear.
Rarely absent-mindedness	Fancies—Mental dullness—Insanity.
Pupils generally dilated	Pupils contracted.
Predom acute, sensitive hearing	Hardness of hearing; deafness.
Complaints predom. on upper lip	Complaints predom. on under lip.
Sediment of urine white	Sediment *red* or whitish.
Catamenia too soon and scanty	Catamenia generally too late and profuse.
Respiration with moist sound	Respiration preval. with dry sound.
Expectoration infrequent; morning and during day.	Expectoration predom., but not constant; is loosened night and morning, and is generally swallowed.

Remission morning and forenoon . . .	Remission of complaints in afternoon.
Predom. better in bed	Worse *or* better in bed.
Worse from bodily exertion	Improv. oftener than aggrav. by exertion.
Better on inspiration *	Worse *or* better on inspiration.
Worse in the Fall.	Worse in the Spring.

Predomin. worse —— **Predomin. better**

In wet weather, from warmth, and when growing warm; lying on side, partic. lying on painful side; from motion, when walking, when moving diseased part, when sitting erect, when assuming an erect position, when bending the head sideways, and while smoking.

Predomin. better —— **Predomin. worse**

In dry weather, from cold, and when growing cold, † when lying on back, lying on unpainful side, during rest; when lying, standing, and sitting, partic. when sitting bent forward; when stooping, from eructation, and after stool.

N.B. We rarely find the sensation of numbness in suffering parts, peculiar to Colch., with Sepia.

---

* Both remedies have predom. aggrav. on expiration.
† In cold (resp. warm) weather, both remedies have aggrav. quite as often as improvement.

Colocynth.	Bellad.
Upper right, lower left side — Inclination for motion.	Upper left, lower right side — Aversion to motion. *
Very rarely paralysis—Epilepsy with rigidity.	Paralysis—Apoplexy—Epilepsy with convulsions.
Sweat, which disappears when moving . .	Sweat, increased by motion.
Partial sweat on lower part of body . . .	Sweat on upper part of body.
Want of thirst predom.	Thirst not constant; rarely during chill; appears often *before* chill, and *after* sweat.
Desire for drink without thirst	Thirst with aversion to drink.
Sensitiveness of disposition — Hypochondriacal mood.	Generally insensibility of disposition—Mood changing; cheerful *or* dejected; indifferent; distrustful.
Ailments from shame, grief, and from vexation with indignation or reserved displeasure.	Ailments from fright, or from vexation with fright, dread, fear, or vehemence.
Very rarely delirium or insanity	Absent-mindedness — Unconsciousness — Fancies — Mental excitability (ecstasies) *or* dullness.
Eyes sunken.	Eyes protruding.
With the toothache pain in eyes	With the toothache pain in the ear. C.Hg.
Appetite for coffee	Aversion to coffee.
Painful diarrhœa	Painless diarrhœa.
False labor-pains extending into the thighs.	False labor-pains with headache and red face. Lippe.
Coxarthrocace, in the 2d or 3d stage . .	Coxarthrocace in the 1st stage.† C.Hg.
Complaints predom. on calf of leg and on instep.	Compl. predom. on shin and sole of foot.
REMISSION night and morning	REMISSION after midnight and *forenoon.*
Worse when lying on back, better when lying on side.	Better (resp. worse) when lying on back *or* on side.
Better when lying on painful side . . .	Better (resp. worse) when lying on painful *or* on unpainful side.
Worse when lying on unpainful side . . .	
Worse from drinking wine	Worse *or* better from wine.
Generally improved by coffee	Worse from drinking coffee.
Ailments from Causticum	Ailm. from Acon., Hyosc., Mercur., Plumb., Cinchona, from sting of insects, or from contagious anthrax.

Predomin. worse — **Predomin. better**

During rest, after lying down, while lying, in bed, while standing,† when stooping, and from cold diet.‡

Predomin. better — **Predomin. worse**

From motion, when walking, and running; § from warm diet, but also from drinking cold water;** from coffee, and from smoking.

N.B. Coloc. has not the over-sensitiveness to pain of Bellad. H.Gr. But the neuralgies of Coloc. are of a much more violent kind; with Bellad. there is more a general over-sensitiveness to all pain, which almost always appears in frequent, short attacks. C.Hg.

---

* We also find inclination for motion in single or suffering parts with Bellad.

† Both right side, partic. Coloc., while Stramon., according to Dr. Jeanes, cures it only on the left side. Silicea and Calcarea seem also to have a more curative effect on the left side in this complaint. C.Hg.

‡ Yet we also find improv. when standing still after moving, with Colocynth.

§ Bellad. has aggrav. from *drinking cold water*, because one of its effects is to render the swallowing of drink difficult.

** We also find aggrav. through physical exertion, with Colocynth.

Colocynthis.	Nux vomica.
Inclination for exercise—Throbbing sensation predominant in external parts.	Aversion to exercise—Throbbing sensation in internal parts.
Very rarely paralysis—No apoplexy . . .	Apoplexy—Paralysis.
Distention of veins of feet	Distention of veins of hands.
One-sided heat, right side	One-sided heat, left side.
Sweat on lower part of body	Sweat on upper part of body.
Sweat, which disappears when moving . .	Sweat, increased by the least movement.
Predominant want of thirst — Desire for drink without thirst.	Most thirst during chill—Thirst with aversion to drink.
Being affected by misfortune, even that of others*—Taciturnity.	Fear—Loquacity.
Ailments from shame or from vexation with reserved displeasure.	Consequences of fright, disappointed love or jealousy, and from vexation with fright, dread, fear or vehemence.
Very rarely delirium	Absent-mindedness — Unconsciousness — Fancies.
Complaints predominant on external ear .	Complaints predominant on inner ear.
Toothache with feverish heat	Toothache with break'g out of sweat. CHg.
Toothache extends to the eye	Toothache extends to the ear. CHg.
Appetite for coffee	Aversion to coffee.
Bellyache better after stool	Bellyache worse after stool.
Urine scanty *or* copious – Sediment *white* or reddish.	Urine infrequent and scanty — Sediment reddish.
Expectoration infrequent	Expectoration not constant.
Complaints predominant on patella . . .	Complaints predominant in hollow of knee.
REMISSION night and morning	REMISSION evening till midnight.
Better (resp. worse) from cold and growing cold, *or* from warmth and growing warm.	Worse from cold and growing cold, better from warmth and growing warm.
Worse when lying on back, better when lying on side.	*Generally* aggravated when lying on back, better when lying on side.
Better when lying on painful side, worse when lying on unpainful side.	*Generally* worse when lying on painful side, better when lying on unpainful side.
Better *or* worse from exertion	Worse from bodily exertion.
Predominantly worse when stooping . . .	Better *or* worse when stooping.
Generally improved by coffee	Worse from drinking coffee.
Worse or better after stool	Worse after stool.

Predomin. worse ——— **Predomin. better**

During rest, when standing, after lying down, while lying, in bed, from warmth of stove,† when sitting erect, when lifting diseased limb.

Predomin. better ——— **Predomin. worse**

From exercise, when walking, when sitting bent forward, when letting diseased limb hang down, from coffee, drinking cold water, and smoking.

N.B. Colocynthis lacks the over-sensitiveness to pain which Nux vomica seems to have.

* Hypochondriacal (despondent or irritable) mood is found with both remedies.
† In-doors generally both remedies have predominant improvement; aggravation out-doors.

Colocynthis.	Pulsatilla.
Upper right, lower left side—No apoplexy.	Upper left, lower right side—Apoplexy.
Inclination for exercise—Aversion to open air.	Aversion to exercise—Inclination for open air.
Idiopathic neuralgia	Symptomatic neuralgia.
Pulse generally full and hard.	Pulse generally accelerated, but small and weak; sometimes imperceptible.
Choleric temperament	Sanguine phlegmatic temperament—Mood changing; anxious; gentle; indifferent; bold; distrustful - Greediness.
Ailments from anger, shame, or from vexation with indignation or reserved displeasure.	Ailments from fright, excessive joy, or from vexation with fright, dread, or fear.
Rarely unconsciousness or delirium . . .	Absent-mindedness — Unconsciousness — Fancies.
Complaints predominant on external ear .	Complaints generally of inner ear.
Want of thirst	Thirst only during hot stage.
Bellyache better after stool	Bellyache after stool.
Urine diminished *or* increased—Sediment *white* or red—Predom. retention of urine.	Urine infrequent and scanty—Sediment red —Incontinence more freq. than retent'n.
Catamenia prevalently too soon and profuse.	Catam. too late and generally too scanty.
Cough generally dry	Cough generally with expectoration.
Complaints predominant on patella and instep.	Complaints generally in hollow of knee and on sole of foot.
Remission night and morning	**Remission** from midnight till noon.
Ailments from lead vapors	Ailments from Copper or Mercurial vapors.
Worse when lying on back, better when lying on side.	*Generally* better when lying on back, worse when lying on side.
Worse (resp. better) from cold and growing cold, or from warmth and growing warm.	Better from cold and growing cold, worse from warmth and growing warm.
Worse or better after stool	*Better or* worse after stool.
Ailments from Causticum or Plumbum . .	Ailments from Copper vapors, Sulph., Nitric acid, Ferrum, Merc., Platina, Chamom., Cinchona, Colch., Ignatia, or Canthar.

Predomin. worse —— **Predomin. better**

In the open air, in cold weather, from cold* diet, sour things, when sitting erect, when lifting diseased limb, when lying on back, and after stool.

Predomin. better —— **Predomin. worse**

In-doors, in warm air, from warm diet, from coffee and smoking, when sitting, when sitting bent forward, when letting diseased limb hang down, when lying on side, after sweat, from rubbing and scratching.

N.B. Colocynthis lacks the over-sensitiveness of Pulsatilla to pain, generally also the sensation of numbness in suffering parts peculiar to Pulsatilla. On the other hand, we find mere sensitiveness (to touch, etc.) with both remedies, with Pulsat. predom. in external and with Coloc. in internal parts.

* At the same time we also find with Colocynthis (as with Pulsatilla) improvement from drinking cold water.

Conium.	Nux vomica.
Upper left, lower right side—Light hair . .	Upper right, lower left side—Dark hair.
Want of bodily irritability—Pinching pain in external parts.	Increased irritability—Pinching pain in internal parts.
Coniine paralyses the motoric nerves by the intermediation of the blood.	Strychnine paralyses the motoric nerves directly, without the intermediation of the blood.
Painless ulcers and swelling of glands . . .	Painful ulcers and swelling of glands.
Pulse generally large and slow, with now and then small and quick beats.	Pulse generally accelerated, full, and hard, particularly during hot stage.
Partial sweat on lower part of body . . .	Sweat on upper part of body.
Sweat increased during sleep; heat after sleep.	Sweat lessened during sleep; heat lessened after sleep.
Want of thirst	Thirst particularly during cold stage.

Insensibility of disposition	Sensitiveness.
Mood serious; indifferent—Rarely delirium .	Mood irritable; malicious—Absentmindedness.
Solicitude concerning the future	Solicitude concerning the present. C.Hg.
Vertigo, inclining to fall sideways	Vert., inclin'g to fall backwards or sideways.
Dim-sightedness predominant	Clear-sightedness predominant.
Optical illusions in dark or prismatic colors .	Optical illusions in bright colors.
Appetite for coffee	Aversion to coffee.
When diarrhœa occurs, it is painless . . .	When diarrhœa occurs, it is painful.
Urine oftener diminished than increased . .	Urine infrequent and scanty.
Sediment white or grey	Sediment reddish.
Catamenia predominantly too late, scanty and of short duration.	Catamenia too soon, profuse, and of long duration.
Expectoration infrequent; during day; is generally swallowed.	Expectoration not constant; morning, during day, evening.
Palpitation after drinking	Palpitation after dinner. C.Hg.
Complaints predominant on patella	Complaints predominant in hollow of knee.

REMISSION of complaints forenoon.	REMISSION evening till midnight.
Worse when lying on side, better when lying on back.	*Generally* better when lying on side, worse lying on back.
Worse after sleep	Better after sufficient and not too long sleep; but worse on awaking when roused.
Worse or better when getting out of bed . .	Worse when getting out of bed.
Worse when swallowing	*Worse or* better when swallowing.
Worse after drinking.	*Worse or* better after drinking.
Better or worse after stool	Worse after stool.
Worse when sneezing	*Worse or* better when sneezing.
Better *or* worse from touch	Worse from touch.
Better from pressure	*Better or* worse from pressure.
Worse *or* better* when walking out-doors . .	Worse when walking out-doors.

Predomin. worse — **Predomin. better**

In wet weather, from washing, moistening, lifting, resting against anything, or stretching out diseased limb, when bending suffering part backwards, from scratching and rubbing, when sitting erect, when descending, during rest, when standing, sitting and lying,† after sweat, after sleep, and while eating.

Predomin. better — **Predomin. worse**

In dry weather, when letting diseased limb hang down or when drawing it up, when sitting bent forward, when ascending, from motion, partic. moving diseased part, when walking, and in the sunshine.

N.B. With Nux vom. we rarely find the sensation of numbness in suffering parts peculiar to Con.

---

* In the latter case the influence of motion, and not of the open air, here decides for Con.; for out-doors generally both remedies have predominant aggravation; improvement in-doors.

† Both remedies have predominant improvement of complaints *in bed*.

Conium.	Pulsat.
Want of bodily irritability—Often indicated with old people.	Increased irritability—Often indicated with children.
Aversion to open air—Pinching pain in external parts.	Inclination for open air—Pinching pain in internal parts.
Itching increased by scratching	Itching, aggrav. *or* unchanged by scratching.
Wounds, partic. with injury of glands . . .	Wounds, partic. with injury of bones.
Cold, painless swelling of glands	Hot, painful swelling of glands.
Pulse generally large and slow, with now and then small and quick beats.	Pulse predom. weak, small and accelerated; sometimes intermitting.
Want of thirst constant	Want of thirst, constant during chill.
Chill increased by exercise, and out-doors, better in warm room.	Chill lessened by exercise and out-doors, increased in warm room.
Heat lessened in-doors—Sweat lessened in bed.	Heat increased in-doors—Sweat increased *or* disappearing, in bed.
Insensibility of disposition	Sensitiveness of disposition.
Mood serious—Very rarely delirium	Gentleness—Distrust—Absent-mindedness.
Vertigo, inclining to fall sideways	Vertigo, inclining to fall backwards.
Staggering when walking out-doors	Stagger'g, disappears when walking out-doors.
Pupils dilated	Pupils generally contracted.
Optic. illusions pred. in dark or prismat. colors.	Optical illusions in bright colors.
Complaints predom. on upper lip	Complaints predom. on under lip.
Predom. loss of appetite—Cold (scentl.) flatus.	Generally hunger—Hot, fetid flatus.
When diarrhœa occurs, it is predom. painless.	Diarrhœa generally painful.
Urine diminished oftener than increased—Sediment white or grey.	Urine infrequent and scanty—Sediment reddish.
Expectoration infrequent; during day;—is swallowed.	Expectoration predom., but not constant; morning and during day.
Palpitations after drinking	Palpitations after dinner. C.Hg.
Compl. pred. in upper part of chest, on forearm, in the palm of hand, and on patella.	Compl. pred. in lower part of chest, on upper arm, on back of hand, and in hollow of knee.
Remission of complaints forenoon	Remission from midnight till noon.
Worse *or* better * when walking out-doors .	Better when walking out-doors.
Worse *or* better during sleep	Worse during sleep.
Worse *after* sleep	*Worse or* better *after* sleep.
Aggrav. oftener than improv. when getting out of bed.	Improv. oftener than aggrav. when getting out of bed.
Better when sitting down	Worse *or* better when sitting down.
Worse when sitting erect; better when sitting bent forward.	*Generally* better when sitting erect; worse when sitting bent forward.
Worse when rising from a seat	*Worse or* better when getting out of bed.
Better *after* rising from a seat	*Better or* worse *after* rising from a seat.
Almost always aggrav. when assuming an erect position.	Better *or* worse when assuming an erect position.
Almost alw's improv. by moving diseased part.	*Better or* worse when moving diseased part,
Worse when bending diseased part	Better *or* worse when bending diseased part.
Better *or* worse from touch	Worse from the touch.
Better from pressure	*Better or* worse from pressure.
Worse when looking sideways	Worse when looking upwards.
Worse when swallowing	Worse *or* better when swallowing.
Almost always aggrav. after meals	*Worse or* better after meals.
Generally better after spirituous liquors . .	Worse from spirituous liquors.

Predomin. **worse** — Predomin. **better**

In cold weather, from cold, from growing cold, and from cold diet; out-doors, from uncovering, from washing, moistening, lifting, resting on anything, or stretching out diseased limb; from bodily exertion, when opening the eyes, when getting out of bed, and when sitting erect.

Predomin. **better** — Predomin. **worse**

In warm air, from warmth, warmth of stove, from growing warm, and from warm diet; in-doors, † from wrapping up, when letting diseased limb hang down, or when drawing it up, when closing the eyes, when stooping and sitting bent forward, in the sun shine, in bed, and from warmth of bed, and from spirituous liquors.

* In the latter case the influence of exercise, and not that of the open air, decides for Con.

† We find aggravation in *crowded rooms*, with both remedies.

Conium.	Sulphur.
Right side—External parts become black.	*Left* side—Red parts become white.
Itching, aggrav. by scratching	Itching, improved by scratching.
Humid eruptions	Eruptions generally dry.
Cold, painless swelling of glands	Hot, but generally painless swelling of glands.
Pulse unaltered with affections of head and sensorium.	Pulse altered with every disturbance. C.Hg.
Pulse generally large and slow, with now and then small and quick beats.	Pulse full, hard, and accelerated.
Partial sweat on lower part of body	Sweat on upper part of body.
Sweat lessened by exercise	Sweat increased by exercise.
Heat or sweat with aversion to uncover	Heat or sweat with inclination to uncover.
Want of thirst	Thirst mostly during hot stage, often already *before* chill.
Insensibility of disposition	Sensitive disposition.
Solicitude concerning the future	Solicitude concerning the present. C.Hg.
Rarely delirium — Imbecility more frequent than insanity.	Gentleness *or* irritability — Rarely amorousness — Absent-mindedness — Insanity more frequent than imbecility.
Vertigo, pressure in the head w. unalt'd pulse.	Vertigo with palpitation of the heart. C.Hg.
Complaints predom. on inner angle of eye	Complaints predom. on external angle of eye.
Pupils dilated	Pupils contracted.
Predom. bitter vomit	Predom. sour vomit.
Sediment of urine white or grey	Sediment of urine white *or red*.
Milk increased	Milk diminished.*
Expectoration infrequent; during day; — is swallowed.	Expectoration not constant; morning and during day, rarely at night.
Remission of complaints in forenoon	Remission *afternoon* and before midnight.
Worse when idle	Worse from being overhurried.
Worse from growing cold and in cold weather; better from growing warm and in warm air.	Better (resp. worse) from growing cold, and in cold weather, *or* from growing warm, and in warm air.
Almost always improv.† in bed	Worse *or* better in bed.
Worse when lying on side; better when lying on back.	*Generally* worse when lying on side, better when lying on back.
Worse when turning in bed, and from change of position.	*Worse or* better when turning in bed, or from change of position.
Worse *or* better during sleep	Worse during sleep.
Worse after sweat	*Worse or* better after sweat.
Worse or better when getting out of bed	Better when getting out of bed.
Generally improv. by spirituous liquors	Generally aggrav. by spirituous liquors.
Worse in the open air; better in-doors ‡	Better (resp. worse) in the open air *or* in-doors.
Worse when sneezing	*Worse or* better when sneezing.
Almost always improv. when stooping	*Better or* worse when stooping.
Almost always aggrav. when assuming an erect position	*Worse or* better when assuming an erect position.
Generally improv. when moving diseased part.	Generally aggrav. when moving diseased part.
Worse when looking sideways	Worse when looking down, partic. at running water.

Predomin. worse — **Predomin. better**

From cold, from uncovering, when sitting erect, when resting diseased limb on anything, when descending, when getting out of bed, on expiration, and from scratching.

Predomin. better — **Predomin. worse**

From warmth and warmth of bed, from wrapping up, when sitting bent forward, when ascending, on inspiration, in the sunshine, from spirituous liquors, and when moving the suffering part.

N.B. With Sulph. we very rarely find the over-sensitiveness of Con. to pain.

---

* Sulphur acts principally on the nipples, (itching, soreness, bleeding,) it affects the mammary glands inflammatorily, and in consequence may diminish the secretion; conium causes atrophia of mammæ and diminishes the milk even in cows, it often removes hardenings in the mammæ, even of a scirrhous kind, and in some cases has afterwards brought on galactorrhœa. C.Hg.

† In general *when lying* both remedies have predom. aggravation.

‡ The symptoms of both remedies are improved by warmth of stove, aggrav. in crowded rooms.

Cuprum.	Arsenic.
Predom. *left* side; particularly *lower left, upper right side.*	*Right* side; particularly *lower right, upper left side.*
Hæmorrhages, blood dark—Muscles lax . .	Hæmorrhag., blood bright-red—Muscles rigid.
Nervous paralysis — Apoplexy	Paralysis, with atrophy of muscles—Rarely apoplexy.
Bruised pain in internal parts	Bruised pain in external parts.
Itching, unchanged by scratching . . .	Itching, aggravated by scratching.
Ulcers, with scanty discharge.	Ulcers, with copious discharge.
Predominant somnolence	Predominant sleeplessness.
Pulse generally slow and weak	Pulse generally accelerated and weak; sometimes intermitting; quick in morning, slower in evening.
Clonic spasms during heat or sweat. . . .	Clonic spasms during chill.
Thirst during hot and sweating stage, which cold water relieves.	Least thirst during chill, most during sweat; at the same time, drink'g cold water aggrav.

Mood predominantly cheerful	Mood depressed; peevish; indifferent; greedy.
Ailments from hearing bad news.	Ailments from grief, or from vexation with vehemence.
Rarely mental dullness	Unconsciousness more rare than with Cuprum.
Insanity more frequent than imbecility . . .	Imbecility more frequent than insanity.
Complaints predominant on external ear . .	Complaints predom. of inner ear.
Saliva preval. increased	Saliva predominantly diminished.
Hunger predominant.	Generally loss of appetite.
Nausea in throat, stomach, or abdomen . .	Nausea, particularly in throat.
Urine infrequent and scanty	Urine scanty (with diarrhœa) *or* copious.
Retention of urine	Incontinence more frequent than retention.
Catamenia too late	Catamenia preval. too soon.
Predom. dry coryza	Fluent coryza.
Slow inspiration, and quick expiration . . .	Deep, quick inspiration, and difficult, interrupted expiration.
Expectoration infrequent; morning	Expectoration predominant, but not constant; during day.
Complaints predominant on fore-arm and in hollow of elbow.	Complaints predominant on upper arm.
Vesicles filled with water on tips of fingers .	Vesicles filled with blood on tips of fingers; ulcers and scabs under nails.

Remission of complaints during day . . .	Remission *during day* and before midnight.
Worse from light, better in the dark . . .	Worse (better) from light *or* in the dark.
Better in bed*	In bed (rest) worse *or* (warmth) better.
Worse when stooping and when rising . . .	Better *or* worse when stoop'g and when ris'g.
Worse when bending diseased part	Better when bend'g the part or hold'g it bent.
Consequences of the greatest mental exertions and emotions.	Consequences of much bodily exertion, long marches, partic. going up hill. C.Hg.
Ailments from Aurum or Mercurius	Ailments from contagious Anthrax, Iodine, Plumb., Cinchona, Strychn., Ipec., Veratr., Lachesis, Carb. veg., Graphit., Phosphor.

Predomin. worse —— **Predomin. better**

In wet weather, from exercise, when walking, when sitting erect, from warm diet, from pressure, and when bending suffering part.

Predomin. better —— **Predomin. worse**

In dry weather, during rest, after lying down, while lying, when sitting bent forward, from cold diet, from drinking coffee, after meals, when respiring deeply, from tightening the clothes, and when perspiring.

N.B. With Cuprum we rarely find the sensation of numbness in suffering parts belonging to Arsenic.

---

* The complaints of both remedies are improved by *warmth* of bed.

Cuprum.	Cocculus.
Left side — Inclination for exercise . . .	*Right* side – Aversion to exercise.
Inflammation of external parts; insensibility of internal parts.*	Inflammation or sensitiveness of internal parts; insensibility of external parts.
Painful cutaneous eruptions	Painless eruptions.
Warts	Corns. C.Hg.
Pulse generally slow and weak	Pulse generally small and spasmodic, often imperceptible.
Chill lessened by drinking	Chill increased by drinking.
Thirst	Want of thirst predominating.
Joking — Cheerfulness — Malice	Seriousness — Dejection — Peevishness — Indifference – Gentleness.
Ailments from hearing bad news	Ailments from grief, or from vexation with reserved displeasure.
Delirium — Rarely fancies	Absent-mindedness.
Eyes generally sunken	Eyes protruding.
Pupils dilated – Cataracta	Pupils generally contracted — Amaurosis.
Saliva generally increased	Saliva predom. diminished.
Bitter vomit	Predom. sour vomit.
Predominant diarrhœa	Generally constipation.
Urine infrequent and scanty — Retention of urine.	Urine often, but scanty — Involuntary discharge of urine.
Catamenia too late	Catamenia too soon *or* too late.
Respiration with moist sound	Respiration preval. with dry sound.
Complaints predominant on fore-arm and leg.	Complaints predominant on upper arm and on thigh.
Remission of complaints during day . .	**Remission** night and forenoon.
Better from warmth of bed	Worse *or* better from warmth of bed.
Ailments from Aurum or Mercurius	Ailments from Cuprum, Nux vom., Ignatia, or Chamom.

Predomin. worse ——— **Predomin. better**

From pressure, and from warm diet.

Predomin. better ——— **Predomin. worse**

While perspiring, from cold diet, and after meals.

* Over-sensitiveness to pain is found with both remedies, on the other hand "sensation of numbness in suffering parts" chiefly with Cocculus.

Cuprum.	Ferrum.
R. → L.	**L. → R.***
Light hair	Dark hair.
Congestion to internal parts; feels as if the blood was stagnated.	Congestion to external parts; as if the blood was agitated.*
Petechiæ	Varices.*
Hæmorrhages, dark	Hæmorrhages, light blood.
Apoplexia nervosa	Apoplexia sanguinea.
Paralysis of central origin; generally on both sides.	Consecutive paralysis; generally one-sided.
Reactive spasms more frequent than paralysis.	Paralysis more frequent than spasms.
Great mobility	Nervous excitability.*
Involuntary or convulsive motions	Desire to move.*
Sudden attacks of neuralgia in the involuntary muscles, with active congestions.	Gradually increasing neuralgia in the voluntary muscles; worst during rest or on beginning to move; *without or* with passive congestion.
In the bones soreness, pressure, tearing, rending, as if broken.	In the bones less hardness, disposed to soften, to bend; fractures slowly uniting.*
Glands swollen, aching, and as if bruised	Glands swollen, with rending, tearing pains.*
Bruised pain internally	Bruised pain in external parts.
External parts grow black	Red parts become white.
Dropsy in consequence of organic diseases.	Dropsy in consequence of oligæmia.
Skin dough-like, soft or without elasticity	Over-sensitiveness of skin.*
Torpid (nervous) chlorosis, particularly during hot weather, or after abuse of iron.	Erethic chlorosis, particularly during cold weather.
Skin bluish or shrunken	Skin pale, yellowish, sallow, dirty, withered, flabby, or viscous.*
Eruptions squamous, shilfery or itch-like, or pimply.	No eruptions, only yellow or brown spots, sore to the touch.*
Pulse predominantly slow, small, and weak.	Pulse full and hard.
Thirst, particularly during heat and sweat.	Thirst, particularly during chill.
Fear of loss of reason—Anxiousness—Maliciousness.	Fear of apoplexy—Mood changing; irritable; alternating; cheerful one evening, sad the next.
Ailments from hearing bad news, from fright, or from fear with vexation.	Ailments from anger.
Insensibility—Insanity	Delirium more infrequent than with Cuprum.
Pupils predominantly dilated—Cataract.	Pupils predominantly contracted—Amaurosis.
Inclination for cold dishes	Inclination for warm dishes.
Nausea in throat, stomach, and abdomen	Seldom nausea.*
Vomiting; bilious, or slimy, or watery, or fetid.*	Vomiting; sour, or bloody, or of worms.*
Diarrhœa with pains, seldom painless, often green, frothy, streaked with blood.	Painless diarrhœa, often after the meals; of undigested food; sometimes acrid.*
Hæmorrhoids, with moderate, but long-lasting bleeding.	Hæmorrhoids, with copious bleeding, or oozing of ichor.*
Anus very sensitive to touch; tickling as of ascarides.	Anus itching; tearing pains with itching and gnawing; prolapsus.*
Urine generally dark (with acid.)	Urine alkaline.
Retention of urine	Involuntary urination.
Inflammation of glans penis	Painfulness of vagina.*

(Continued.)

Cuprum.	Ferrum.
Catamenia oftener too scanty, than profuse.	Catamenia preval. profuse.
With the catamenia asthma; the blood is viscous.	Before the catamenia, laborlike pains, the blood watery or in lumps.*
Sexual desire excited in women, lessened in men*—Impotence.	Sexual desire excited in men, lessened in women*—Sterility.
Promoting conception; produces abortion in large doses.	Impeding conception; insensibility during coition; prevents abortion in potencies.*
Scrofulous and scirrhous swelling in the uterus or the mammæ, with pains.	Pains below the uterus, dryness of vagina, pains in os tincæ on lying; bear'g down.*
Leucorrhœa not observed even with uterine diseases.	Leucorrhœa mild, milky; or itching, sharp, with soreness.*
Cold in the head fluent or stopped up, with sleepy gaping.	Cold in the head, with bloody, puruloid, greenish, whey-like, slimy, sharp disch.*
Breath cold—Respiration with moist sound.	Breath hot—Respir'n pred. with dry sound.
Respiration unequal, slow or frequent panting, or quick with rattling in the chest.	Respiration anxious, loud without rattling, except in children.*
Congestive asthma, improved when lying down.	Asthma after loss of fluids, or after itch, partic. in winter and at night, worse when lying on back and in horizontal position, bettered by moderate exertion of the body, and by uncovering the chest.
Cough generally without expectoration, (or with sputa of a metallic taste, or tough dark blood.*)	C'gh gener'y with expector., (of sweetish or putrid taste, or streaked with blood, sourish, bilious, or of bright blood coagul'd.*)
Cough better from drinking cold water, worse from eating.	Cough excited by drinking, often improved by eating.
Inflammation of lungs with redness of roof of mouth, cold, moist skin, sour sweats, simultaneous bronchitis or pleuritis, and sudden attacks of suffocation.	Inflammation of lungs with roof of mouth white; dry skin and gradually increasing oppression.
Idiopathic heart disease, acute or chronic .	Consecutive heart disease with characteristics of chlorosis.
Predom. compl. on fore arm and hand, (also in elbow, finger, point of finger, hollow of knee, ankle joint, instep, sole of foot.)	Predom. complaints on upper arm and foot, (also in shoulders, shoulder joint, hip joint, knee, and toes.*)
Remission of complaints during day . .	Remis. *during day* and before midnight †.
Worse from exerting the eyes	*Generally* better fr. exerting the eye-sight.
Ailments from Aurum	Ailments from Arsenic., Iodine, or China.
Worse from spirituous liquors	Better from wine, when not acid, but worse from drinking beer. ‡

Predomin. **worse**	Predomin. **better**

From continued motion, partic. of the suffering part; or in the head, by sudden exertion of the mind, or the body, § when walking fast and running; when ascending; when sitting erect; when lying on back; and from uncovering.

Predomin. **better**	Predomin. **worse**

During rest; when standing; after lying down; when lying; in bed; when descending; when sitting bent forward; when lying on side; from wrapping up; and during sweat.

N.B. All that is marked * has been added by C.Hg.

† With *Cuprum* the symptoms occurring between midnight and noon are more numerous than those occurring between noon and midnight, in the proportion of two to one: with *Ferrum* the inverse proportion obtains.*

‡ In suitable cases Ferrum cures delirium tremens; however the latter is generally caused by beer or brandy; rarely by wine. Compare note * to Ars. and Ferr.

§ Cuprum relieves the effects of violent mental exertion, or emotion, with bodily exertion and want of sleep; while Ferrum cures a great many effects of continued bodily exertion, (similar to Arsen.) At the same time Ferrum has improv. from mental exertion.*

Cuprum.	Mercur.
Upper right, lower left side—Hæmorrhages, blood dark.	Upper left, lower right side—Hæmorrhages, blood light-red.
Gnawing pain, sensation of crawling and numbness in internal parts.*	Sensation of gnawing, crawling, and numbness in external parts.
Itching, unchanged by scratching	Itching, improv. *or* aggrav. by scratching.
Inclination for motion—Paralysis . . .	Aversion to motion—Very rarely paralysis.
Pulse generally slow, small, and weak . .	Pulse irregular, generally full & accelerated.
Thirst, particularly during heat and sweat .	Thirst almost constant during all stages.
Clonic spasms during heat and sweat . .	Clonic spasms during chill.
Somnolence predominant	Sleeplessness predominant.
Joking — Mood generally cheerful; rarely peevish.	Seriousness — Dejection — Amorousness — Absent-mindedness—Rarely delirium.
Ailments from fright or hearing bad news .	Ailments from mortification.
Insanity oftener than imbecility	Imbecility oftener than insanity.
Eyes generally sunken	Eyes protruding.
Complaints predominant on roof of mouth.	Complaints predominant on soft palate.
Nausea in throat, stomach, or abdomen . .	Nausea in œsophagus or in stomach, more rarely in throat.
Diarrhœa generally painless	Diarrhœa preval. painful.
Urine infrequent and scanty—Retention of urine.	Urine too often and copious—Incontinence.
Dry coryza	Coryza fluent oftener than dry.
Expectoration infrequent; morning . . .	Expectoration not constant; during day.
Complaints predominant in lower part of chest, in hollow of elbow, and on calf of leg.	Complaints predominant in upper part of chest, on tip of elbow, in hollow of knee, and on shin.
Worse when swallowing	Better *or* worse when swallowing, partic worse when swallowing saliva or drink.
Better from cold diet, worse from warm diet.	Worse *or* better from cold diet, worse from warm diet.
Worse from growing cold, better from growing warm.	Better (resp. worse) from growing cold *or* warm.
Worse when lying on back, better when lying on side.	*Generally* better when lying on back, worse when lying on side.
Sugar acts as an antidote to poisonous doses.	Aversion to sugar and aggravation from it.

C.Hg.

Predomin. worse — **Predomin. better**

While sitting, and when lying on back.

Predomin. better — **Predomin. worse**

When lying on side, in bed and from warmth of bed, while sweating, on inspiration, when taking a deep breath, and from drinking cold water.

* Although Mercur. has the constitutional character of increased irritability, it seems to lack the over-sensitiveness of Cuprum to pain. Mere sensitiveness (to touch, etc.) is found with both remedies.

Cuprum.	Pulsat.
Left side; partic. *lower l., upper r. s.*	*Right* side; partic. *lower r., upper l. s.*
Inclination for motion – Paralysis generally of both sides.	Aversion to motion — Paralysis generally one-sided.
Itching, unchanged by scratching	Itching, aggr. *or* unchanged by scratching
Warts	Corns. C.Hg
Ulcers with scanty discharge	Ulcers with copious discharge.
Pulse predom. small, weak and slow	Pulse generally small, weak, but accelerated; sometimes intermitting.
Chill lessened after meals	Chill increased after meals.
Thirst	Want of thirst; thirst only during hot stage.

Cuprum.	Pulsat.
Mood cheerful; malicious; rarely peevish	Calm, lachrymose sadness of gentle dispositions—Mood good-natured; changing; indifferent; bold—Amorousness.
Ailments from hearing bad news	Ailments from reserved mortification, grief, or fr. excessive joy—Distrust—Avarice.
Insanity	Absent-mindedness – Melancholy.
Vertigo, inclining to fall forwards	Vertigo, inclining to fall backwards.
Pupils dilated	Pupils generally contracted.
Complaints predom. on external ear	Complaints generally of inner ear.
Diarrhœa generally painless	Diarrhœa generally painful.
Retention of urine	Incontinence more frequent than retention.
Catamenia of too long duration	Catamenia of too short duration.
Dry coryza	Coryza fluent oftener than dry.
Voice stronger than usual *or* low	Voice low.
Respiration with moist sound	Respiration predom. with dry sound.
Expectoration infrequent; morning	Expectoration predom., but not constant; morning and during day.
Complaints predom. on fore-arm	Complaints predom. on upper arm.

Cuprum.	Pulsat.
AGGRAVATION from evening till morning	AGGRAVATION from noon till midnight.
Worse during and after new moon	Worse before a thunder-storm.
Worse when lying on back, better when lying on side.	*Generally* better when lying on back; worse when lying on side.
Worse from uncovering, better from wrapping up.	*Generally* better from uncovering; worse from wrapping up.
Worse when stooping and when rising	*Worse or* better when stooping and when rising.
Better after rising from a seat	*Better or* worse after rising from a seat.
Worse when bending diseased part	Worse *or* better when bending diseased part, partic. better when bending it sideways or holding it bent.
Better when taking a deep breath	Better *or* worse when taking a deep breath.
Worse when swallowing	Worse *or* better when swallowing.
Worse after stool	*Better or* worse after stool.

Predomin. worse —— **Predomin. better**

From uncovering, when growing cold, from motion, when walking, walking fast, running; from bodily exertion generally; when lifting diseased limb, when sitting erect, when lying on painful side, or on back; from pressure, and from weeping.

Predomin. better —— **Predomin. worse**

From wrapping up, when growing warm, during rest, while standing, after lying down, while lying, in bed, and from warmth of bed; when letting diseased limb hang down, when sitting bent forward, when lying on unpainful side, and lying on side generally, and during sweat.

N.B. With Cuprum we rarely find the sensation of numbness in suffering parts, peculiar to Pulsatilla.

Cuprum.	Sulphur.
Upper right, lower left side	Upper left, lower right side.
Insensibility of internal parts *	Insensibility of external parts predom.
Painful eruptions and ulcers	Painless eruptions and ulcers.
Dry eruptions	Eruptions dry oftener than humid.
External parts grow black	Red parts grow white.
Itching, unchanged by scratching (rarely aggr.)	Itching, lessened (rarely aggr.) by scratching.
Pulse predom. small, weak and slow	Pulse generally quick, full, and hard; sometimes intermitting.
Chill lessened after meals	Chill increased after meals.
Somnolence predom.	Sleeplessness predom., partic. before midnight.
Jesting—Mood cheerful; haughty; malicious.	Mood serious, solemn; gentle, depressed, and sad; indifferent; peevish; irritable.
Unconsciousness more freq't than with Sulph.	Absent-mindedness—Weak memory.
Speaking words, that one did not intend to say.	Repeating every thing said to him, on account of difficult comprehension.
Pupils dilated	Pupils generally contracted.
Complaints predom. on external ear	Complaints of inner ear predom.
Saliva predom. increased	Saliva generally diminished.
Hunger predom.	Generally loss of appetite.
Vomit, bitter	Vomit, sour, oftener than bitter.
Nausea in throat, stomach or abdomen	Nausea in stomach, rarely in throat.
Urine seldom and scanty	Urine often, but scanty; copious after strong doses.
Sediment of urine red	Sediment of urine oftener white than red.
Catamenia of too long duration	Catamenia generally of short duration.
Voice hoarse or raised; stronger than usual, *or* low.	Voice hoarse or deep; low.
Expectoration infrequent; morning	Expectoration not constant; morning and during day; rarely at night.
Complaints predom. in lower part of chest	Complaints predom. in upper part of chest.
Remission of complaints during day	Remission *afternoon* and before midnight.
Worse during new moon	Worse during full moon.
Worse from growing cold, better from growing warm.	Better (resp. worse) from growing cold *or* warm.
Better in bed	Worse *or* better in bed.
Worse when turning in bed	*Worse or* better when turning in bed.
Worse when lying on back, better when lying on side.	*Generally* better when lying on back, worse when lying on side.
Worse when looking upwards	Worse when looking down, partic. at running water.
Worse when stooping, and when rising	Worse *or* better when stooping and rising.
Worse from touch	*Worse or* better from touch.
Worse when swallowing drink	Worse when swallowing *food* and saliva.
Worse after stool	Better *or* worse after stool.
Ailments from Aurum or Mercur.	Ailments from abuse of metals generally, and from abuse of Cinchona.
Worse from being awake at night	Worse from sleeping too long.
Worse after mental exertion	Worse after bodily exertion. C.Hg.

Predomin. worse —— **Predomin. better**

During continued motion, when sitting erect, from uncovering, from warm diet, and from pressure.

Predomin. better —— **Predomin. worse**

During rest, when standing,† after lying down, while lying, from warmth of bed, from wrapping up, when sitting bent forward, from cold diet, from drinking cold water, on inspiration, and when sweating.

---

* Cuprum has over-sensitiveness to pain much oftener than Sulph., which latter has sensation of numbness and insensibility in suffering parts, much oftener than Cuprum.

† On the other hand, Sulphur has improvement of complaints *when standing still after motion.*

Cuprum.	Veratrum.
Left side predominant, particularly *lower left, upper right side.*	*Right* side, particularly *lower right, upper left side.*
Crawling sensation in internal parts . . .	Crawling sensation in external parts.
Warts	Corns. C Hg.
Dry heat predominaut	Sweat, with heat predominant.
Thirst, particularly during heat and sweat .	Thirst not constant, rarely during sweat.
Chill lessened by drinking and after meals .	Chill increased by drinking and after meals.

Cheerfulness predominant — Irritability or haughtiness more rare than with Veratr.	Cheerfulness *or* dejection Distrust—Amorousness.
Fear of loss of reason	Fear of being poisoned, or of apoplexy.
Ailments from hearing bad news	Ailments from anger or grief.
Difficult comprehension	Easy *or* difficult comprehension.
Pupils dilated Cataracta	Pupils generally contracted—Amaurosis.
Sensitive smell	Loss of smell.
Saliva generally increased	Saliva generally diminished.
Nausea in throat, stomach, or abdomen . .	Nausea in stomach.
Intussusception of bowels with singultus, violent colic, stercorous vomiting, and great agony.	Intussusception of bowels with anxiety, forcing to pace the room, pressing abdomen with hands. C.Hg.
Catamenia too late	Catamenia too soon *or* too late.
Voice stronger than usual *or* low	Voice low.
Expectoration infrequent; in morning . .	Expectoration not constant; particularly during day.
Complaints predominant in lower part of chest and on fore-arm.	Complaints predominant in upper part of chest and on upper arm.

REMISSION of complaints during day . .	REMISSION during day and evening.
Worse from laughing and from mental exertion.	Worse from weeping and from bodily exertion.
Worse from touch and pressure	*Worse* from touch, *better* from pressure.
Better after meals	Worse *or* better after meals.
Worse from being over-hurried	Worse when idle.
Ailments from Aurum or Mercurius . . .	Ailments from Arsenic, Iron, or abuse of Cinchona.
Worse from being awake at night . . .	Worse from sleeping too long.

Predomin. worse ⏤ **Predomin. better**

When lying on back, from warm diet, from uncovering, from ascending, when moving and walking, and from pressure.

Predomin. better ⏤ **Predomin. worse**

When lying on side, from drinking cold water, from cold diet generally, from wrapping up, descending, during rest, when standing and lying, particularly in bed.

N.B. Cuprum has over-sensitiveness to pain much oftener than Veratr.; Veratr., on the other hand, has sensation to numbness in suffering parts much oftener than Cuprum.

Cyclamen.	Pulsatilla.
Complaints predominant in external parts, and on *left* side.†	Complaints predominant in internal parts, and on *right* side.
Want of irritability	Increased bodily irritability.
Light hair—Pain pressing inwards	Light *or* dark hair—Pain pressing outwards.
Itching, lessened *or* changed to another place by scratching.	Itching, unchang'd *or* aggravated by scratching.
Painless eruptions	Painful cutaneous eruptions.
Scars from varicelli, which have nearly disappeared, become dark-red, and the forehead is covered with similar spots.	A place formerly burned, now healed, becomes sore to the touch.*
Cold swelling of glands	Hot, painful swelling of glands.
Pulse generally unchanged; sometimes double.	Pulse generally frequent, small, and weak; sometimes intermitting or imperceptible.
Sweat sometimes only on lower part of body.	Sweat sometimes only on head; chill on lower part of body.
Want of thirst during all stages	Thirst only during heat.
Thirst only between heat and sweat‡	Want of thirst predom., but constant only dur'g chill; thirst appears *before* & *after* the chill, more rarely after the hot stage.

Cyclamen.	Pulsatilla.
Phlegmatic temperament	Cheerful disposition, inclining to phlegma and melancholy.
Obstinate, irritable, fault-find'g disposition.	Mild, yielding, lachrymose disposition.*
Dread of the past or future (neglected duties, sins committed, a misfortune threatening.	Anxious care about the present (his health, domestic affairs; religious doubt of his salvation).*
Serene humour changes suddenly into seriousness or peevishness.	Calm sadness; boldness; distrust – Greediness—Amorousness.
Aversion to work; will do nothing	Extreme irresolution, does not know what he wants.*
Ailments from grief	Ailments from fright, grief, mortification, or from excessive joy.
Memory active *or* weak	Weak mem'y—Unconsciousness—Delirium.
Mental labor impossible on account of dullness or stupefaction.	Mental labor very fatiguing.*
Vertigo, better when sitting in-doors, worse when moving in the open air.	Vertigo, worse when sitting in-doors, better when moving in the open air.
Apoplexia nervosa: slumber or interrupted sleep, benumbed; heaviness of head, heat in head; rising up, with red face; dark before the eyes, roaring in the ears; vertigo, everything appears to reel as if his head were spinning; pulse hard, full, over 100 beats in the minute; squamishness; rumbling bellyache; watery stools; laming pressure from upper arm into the fingers; spasmodic bending of thumb to index; bad smelling sweat between the toes disappeared.*	Apoplexy: deep sleep, rattling breathing, chest and throat contracted; red, puffed face; violent palpitation; pulse nearly imperceptible; hiccoughing, squamish, greenish vomiting, diarrhœa, incontinence of urine, urine bloody; tearing pains in upper limbs, dying of fingers; trembling; numbness in sole of foot and toes, boring stitches in the heals. Pommerais.*

---

† According to the Vienna provings more on the right side in the head, and left side on the body.*
‡ Thirst also during heat and with headache; in the evening when growing warm; at night.*

(Continued.)

Cyclamen.	Pulsatilla.
Rush of blood to the head, with anxiety; general coldness; after dinner.	Rush of blood to the head, as after drunkenness or loss of sleep; yellowish face, chills over the whole body; worse evening, during heat, in warm room; better when walking in the open air, and when tying something around the head.*
Stupefying headache, mostly in the left temple, with darkness before the eyes; loss of vision; heaviness of head; loss of appetite.	Stupefying headache, with running chills; worse in the evening, in the warm room; better from walking out-doors and in cool air.*
Stitches in the head disappear by the touch; some complaints worse when lying on back or on painful side.	Headache improved by external pressure and when lying on back or on painful side.
Roaring in ears when walking out-doors for any length of time.	Roaring in the ears, better when walking out-doors.
Facial eruptions of children	Wings of the nose ulcerative, and scabs on external ear (Tragus).*
Complaints predom. on upper lip, on forearm, and on instep (ankle*).	Complaints predom. on under lip, on upper arm, and on sole of foot (knee-joint*).
Dislike to beer, which he usually is fond of.	Thirst for beer.
Hiccoughing eructation; generally after meals, partic. in pregnant women.	Eructation tasting of food eaten, or ineffectual.*
Generally constipation—Diarrhœa mucous; in the evening.	Diarrhœa green, at night and partic. in the morning.*
Urine often and copious, only exceptionally scanty; sour (with iridescent cuticle on surface*)—Painless urging to urine.	Urine unfrequent and scanty, alkaline—Painful urging to urine.
Sexual desire lessened	Tormenting sexual desire with young girls.*
Catamenia too late *or* too soon	Catamenia predom. too late . . . .
Catamenia does not appear after being overheated or after exertion.	Catamenia does not appear after taking cold, from gett'g wet, or after sitt'g steadily.*
Fluent coryza	*Fluent coryza or* dry coryza.
Cough, more in the open air	Cough, better in the open air, worse in-doors.
Cough without expectoration	Cough generally with expectoration.
Pain in small of back, ceases when rising from a seat.	Pain in small of back, worse after sitting.
AGGRAV. of symptoms *even'g* till midnight.	AGGRAVATION from noon till midnight.
Worse during full moon	Worse before a thunder-storm.
Increase of symptoms in the open air (better in-doors).	Decrease of symptoms in the open air (worse in-doors.) C.Hg.

N.B. Cyclamen lacks the over-sensitiveness of Pulsatilla to pain, generally also the sensation of numbness in suffering parts peculiar to Pulsatilla. H.Gr.—Cyclamen has it after itching stitches in the skin.*

N.B. The concurrence and coincidence of these two remedies, which neither supply nor neutralize one another, is very remarkable: In menstrual complaints, want of thirst, nausea in throat, disgust for fatty things, disagreeing of pork, sensation of fullness in internal parts, sore and bruised pain in external parts, chillblains, scurfy and pricking eruptions; at the same time, both have the same aggravation in the evening, aggravation during rest, partic. while sitting, lying and standing, and improvement when rising from a seat, when walking, and from motion generally.*

All marked * are additions by C.Hg.

Cyclamen.	Spigelia.
Pressure in external parts—Painless eruptions.	Pressure in internal parts—Painful eruptions.
Insensibility of skin	Sensitiveness of skin. C.Hg.
Itching, lessened *or* removed to another place by scratching.	Itching, often unchanged by scratching, often also better or worse.
Pulse unchanged, but sometimes double .	Pulse changed, slow, generally large and hard, sometimes trembling.
Sweat chiefly on lower part of body . . .	Sweat, chiefly on upper part of body.
Thirst only between heat and sweat . . .	Want of thirst predominant; only during hot stage there, sometimes, is thirst.

Cyclamen.	Spigelia.
Mood changing; indifferent and indolent—Inward grief and terrors of conscience.	Mood depressed more than with Cyclamen; quick-tempered.
Very active memory, which alternates with weak memory.	Weak memory.
Fine, sharp itching, stinging in the hairy scalp, which constantly re-appears in another place after scratching; worse in the evening and when at rest, better from motion.	Dull stitches from within outwards, on the top of head, in alternation with a soreness there; worse from the touch and after washing, but while washing relieved. C.Hg.
Short-sightedness	Far-sightedness.
Saliva predominantly diminished (after small doses).	Saliva predominantly increased.
Predominant loss of appetite	Predominant hunger (ravenous hunger).
Aversion to beer	Desire for *or* aversion to beer; desire for spirituous liquors.
Ineffectual urging to urinate	Ineffectual urging to stool.
Fluent coryza	Fluent *or* dry coryza.
No expectoration with the cough	Expectoration infrequent.
Complaints generally on back of hand and on leg.	Complaints generally in palm of hand and on thigh.

Cyclamen.	Spigelia.
Remission from midnight till afternoon .	Remission of complaints after midnight.
Worse in bed	Worse *or* better in bed.
Worse on inspiration, better on expiration .	*Generally* better on inspiration, worse on expiration.
Worse when leaning against anything . .	Better *or* worse when leaning against anything.
Generally improved by touch	Worse from touch.
Better from moistening diseased part . .	Worse *or* better from washing and moistening.

Predomin. worse —— **Predomin. better**

During rest, when sitting down, after lying down, while lying, after breakfast, after meals generally, and on inspiration.

Predomin. better —— **Predomin. worse**

From motion, when walking, when rising from a seat, after getting out of bed, before breakfast, on expiration, and from touch.

N.B. Cyclamen lacks the over-sensitiveness of Spigelia to pain.

Digitalis.	Arsenic.
Left side; particularly *lower left, upper right side.*	*Right* side; particularly *lower right, upper left side.*
Muscles lax—Gnawing sensation in external parts.	Muscles rigid—Gnawing sensation in internal parts.
Apoplexy oftener than paralysis	Paralysis oftener than apoplexy.
Pulse slow, but accelerated, full, and hard by every motion.	Pulse accelerated, small, and weak.
Pulse slower in morning, accelerated in evening.	Pulse sometimes accelerated in morn'g, slower in evening.*
Partial sweat on upper part of body . . .	Partial sweat on lower part of body.
Thirst during heat, none during sweat . . .	Thirst rare during chill, mostly during sweat; during heat desire for drink without thirst—Thirst often appears *before* chill, less frequently *after* it, as also after sweat.
Thirst, particularly for beer	Thirst for acid drinks.

Digitalis.	Arsenic.
Mood distrustful	Mood despondent; malicious—Avarice.
Mental excitement *or* incapacity for thought.	Mental dullness.
Rarely delirium	Delirium.
Dreams of water, falling, vexation, etc . .	Dreams of fire, thunder-storm, vexation, embarrassment, misfortunes, dead people, etc.
Complaints predominant on external ear . .	Predominant complaints of inner ear.
Saliva increased	Saliva predominantly diminished.
Nausea in stomach	Nausea in throat.
Urine infrequent and scanty	Urine scanty (with diarrhœa) *or* copious.
Catamenia too scanty and predominantly too late.	Catamenia too profuse and predominantly too soon.
Respiration slow	Respiration quick.
Expectoration not constant; in evening, less in morning.	Expectoration predominant, but not constant; during day, less in morning.
Complaints predominant on shin	Complaints predominant on calf of leg.

Digitalis.	Arsenic.
AGGRAV., particularly morning	AGGRAV., particularly after midnight.
REMISSION *forenoon* and night	REMISSION *during day* and before midnight.
Complaints from lying on the accustomed *left* side.	Complaints from lying on the accustomed *right* side.
Better in bed	In bed (rest) worse *or* (warmth) better.
Worse after sleep	Better after sufficient sleep, but worse on awaking when roused.
Worse from light, better in the dark . . .	Better *or* worse from light (resp. in the dark).
Worse after urinating	Better *or* worse after urinating.

Predomin. worse ——— **Predomin. better**

From motion, when moving diseased part, when walking, when bending diseased part, lying on side, after sleep, and when setting the teeth.

Predomin. better ——— **Predomin. worse**

During rest, after lying down, while lying, lying on back, when turning in bed, but also when exerting the body, when respiring deeply, from scratching, when swallowing.

N.B. With Digitalis we rarely find the sensation of numbness in suffering parts belonging to Arsenic.

---

* According to provings, thus far, Arsen. metallicum always has this. C.Hg.

Digitalis.	Bellad.
Left side; partic. *lower left, upper right side.*	*Right* side; partic. *lower right, upper left side.*
Light hair—Skin and muscles lax . . .	Dark hair—Skin and muscles rigid.
Desire for open air — Apoplexia nervosa; apoplexia serosa.	Aversion to open air—Apoplex. sanguinea.
Blood uncoagulable	Blood coagulates easily.
Pulse slow, but accelerated, full, and hard, by every motion; irregular.	Pulse generally quick, full, hard, and tense.
Ascending heat	Descending heat.
Thirst during heat, not during sweat . .	Thirst not constant; most rare during chill; often *before* chill, and *after* sweat.
Dreams of water, falling, vexation, &c. . .	Dreams of fire, animals, falling, misfortunes, or business of the day

---

Fear of loss of reason	Fear of being poisoned, or of apoplexy.
Sensitive disposition	Mood changing; malicious — Insensibility of disposition predom.
Rarely delirium	Absent-mindedness -- Fancies — Unconsciousness.
Weak memory	Memory active *or* weak.
Dropsy of brain with wabbling in head, better when lying and stooping, worse when bending back, or shaking the head.	Dropsy of brain with wabbling in head, aggrav. partic. in the evening, and when lying, better when bending head back, and from pressure upon it.
Every thing looks red or green	Every thing looks red. C.Hg.
Pupils generally contracted . . .	Pupils generally dilated.
Complaints predom. on soft palate . . .	Complaints predom. on roof of mouth.
Appetite for sour things . . .	Aversion to sour things.
Nausea in stomach	Nausea in throat or in abdomen, more rarely in stomach.
Catamenia scanty and predom. too late . .	Catamenia too soon and profuse.
Voice raised or shrieking, less frequently failing.	Voice raised or low; aphony.
Expector. evening, less frequently morning.	Expector. morning, during day, evening.
Complaints predom. in lower part of chest, and on inner side of thigh	Complaints predom. in upper part of chest, and on outer side of thigh.

Remission night and *forenoon*	Remission after midnight and *forenoon.*
Worse when lying on side, better when lying on back.	Better (resp. worse) when lying on side or on back.
Worse when lying on painful side; better when lying on unpainful side.	Better (resp. worse) when lying on painful or on unpainful side.
Better *or* worse when getting out of bed .	Worse when getting out of bed.
Worse when bending diseased part . . .	Better *or* worse when bending diseased part.
Worse from spirituous liquors	Better *or* worse from spirituous liquors.
Worse when looking into distance . . .	Worse when looking at something near by.

Predomin. **worse** — Predomin. **better**

When bending diseased part backwards, when bending head back, and when sitting bent forward.

Predomin. **better** — Predomin. **worse**

From weeping, when swallowing, from bodily exertion, walking fast, running, and when sitting erect.

Digitalis.	China.
Upper right, lower left side	Upper left, lower right side.
Aversion to motion — Inclination for open air.	Inclination for motion — Aversion to open air.
Light hair—Inflammation of external parts.	Dark hair—Inflammation of internal parts.
Very rarely paralysis	Paralysis of limbs.
Pulse slow, but accelerated, full, and hard, by every motion.	Pulse quick, small, and hard; more quiet after meals.
Internal chill with external heat predom. .	External chill with internal heat predom.
Thirst during heat, not during sweat .	Thirst most prominent during sweat, and *before*, *between*, and *after* the different stages.
With drunkards congestion of blood to head and heart.	With drunkards, weak sight, liver complaint, dropsy, or consumption.

Sensitive disposition	Insensibility of disposition predom.
Mood cheerful *or* dejected	Mood sad and despondent.
Ecstacies *or* incapacity for thought — Insanity.	Mental excitability—Absent-mindedness—Fancies.
Optical illusions in bright or prismat. colors.	Optical illusions in black or in dark colors.
Nausea in stomach	Nausea in the throat or stomach.
Catamenia predom. too late and scanty . .	Catamenia too soon and profuse.
Voice hoarse, or raised and shrieking . .	Voice hoarse, or deep and low.
Expectoration evening, less in morning . .	Expectoration during day and evening.

Remission night and *forenoon*	Remission *afternoon* and evening.
Worse when lying on side, better when lying on back.	*Generally* better when lying on side; worse when lying on back.
Worse when lying on left side; better when lying on right side.	*Generally* better when lying on left side; worse when lying on right side.
Worse when sweating	Generally aggravated *after* sweat.
Worse after sleep	Better after sufficient sleep; but worse on awaking when roused.
Worse *or* better after getting out of bed .	Better after getting out of bed.
Worse when moving or bending diseased part.	Better or worse when moving and bending diseased part.
Worse when shaking the head	Worse *or* better from shaking the head.
Generally better when swallowing . . .	*Generally* worse when swallowing.
Worse after meals	Worse *or* better after meals.
Better on inspiration; worse on expiration.	Better *or* worse on in- and expiration.

Predomin. **worse** ——— Predomin. **better**

When lying on side, partic. on left side; when bending diseased parts backwards, and after sleep.

Predomin. **better** ——— Predomin. **worse**

When lying on back, lying on right side, after lying down, in bed, when turning in bed, when swallowing, from eructation, from weeping, walking fast, running, and bodily exertion generally.

Digitalis.	Nux vom.
Left side—Skin and muscles lax	*Right* side—Skin and muscles rigid.
Light hair—Desire for open air	Dark hair—Aversion to open air.
Pulse predom. slow, partic. slower in morning, more frequent at night; or intermitting the 3rd, 5th or 7th beat; accelerated, full, and hard, by every motion.	Pulse predom. frequent, partic. in the morning, and slow in the evening, or intermitting the 4th, 5th beat; full and hard, partic. during hot stage.
Thirst during heat, not during sweat . .	Thirst mostly during chill; also frequent *before* chill, before heat and sweat, and *after* sweat.
Coldness, left side	Coldness—right side.

Mood cheerful *or* dejected—Solicitude concerning the future.	Mood sad — Solicitude concerning the present. C. Hg.
Distrust—Rage	Amorousness—Malice.
Rarely delirium	Absent-mindedness — Fancies — Unconsciousness.
Dim-sightedness	Clearsightedness predom.
Complaints predom. on external ear, and on soft palate.	Complaints predom. in inner ear, and on roof of mouth.
Appetite for sour things and for beer . .	Predom. aversion to sour things — Desire for *or* aversion to beer.
Diarrhœa predom.	Constipation predom.
Catamenia too scanty and predom. too late.	Catamenia too soon and profuse.
Respiration retarded	Respir. accelerated oftener than retarded.
Expectoration evening, less morning. . .	Expector. morning, during day, evening.
Complaints predom. on shin	Complaints predom. on calf of leg.

REMISSION night and *forenoon*	REMISSION evening till midnight.
Worse when lying on side; better when lying on back.	*Generally* better when lying on side; worse when lying on back.
Worse after sleep	Better after sufficient & not too long sleep; but worse on awaking when roused.
Better *or* worse when getting out of bed .	Worse when getting out of bed.
Better before breakfast, worse afterwards .	Worse (resp. better) before *or* after breakfast.
Improv. oftener than aggrav. when swallowing.	Aggrav. oftener than improv. when swallowing.
Worse after drinking	*Worse or* better after drinking.
Better from eructation	Better *or* worse from eructation.
Better *or* worse when assuming an erect position.	Almost always aggrav. when assuming an erect position.
Worse when bending diseased part backwards.	*Generally* better when bending diseased part backwards.
Better *or* worse in the open air, (resp. indoors.)	Worse in the open air, better in doors.

Predomin. **worse** — Predomin. **better**

When closing the eyes, lying on left side, after sleep, and when bending diseased part backwards.

Predomin. **better** — Predomin **worse**

When opening the eyes, lying on right side, when respiring deeply, from bodily exertion, when turning in bed, and when swallowing.

Digitalis.	Pulsatilla.
Left side; partic. *lower left, upper right side.*	*Right* side; partic. *lower right, upper left side.*
Discharged blood coagulates slowly or not at all.	Discharged blood coagulates easily.
Pulse slow, but accelerated, full and hard, by every motion.	Pulse generally accelerated, small, and weak; sometimes imperceptible.
Cold, heat, &c., often confined to left side .	Cold, heat, &c., often confined to right side.
Thirst during heat, not during sweat . .	Want of thirst predom., but constant only during chill.
Mood cheerful *or* despondent—Rage . .	Calm sadness of mild dispositions — Mood changing; boldness; greediness—Amorousness.
Ment. excitability *or* incapacity for thought.	Absent-mindedness; sometimes mental dulness—Fancies.
Rarely unconsciousness	Insensibility.
Complaints predom. on external ear, and on soft palate.	Complaints generally in inner ear, and on roof of mouth.
Loss of appetite predom.	Generally hunger.
Nausea in stomach	Nausea in throat, stomach, or abdomen.
Coryza dry oftener than fluent	Coryza fluent oftener than dry.
Voice hoarse or screeching, rarely failing .	Voice hoarse or low.
Respiration slow	Respiration quick.
Expectoration not constant; evenings, less mornings.	Expectoration predom., but not constant; morning and during day.
Aggravation chiefly in the morning, also afternoon and evening.	Aggravation from noon till midnight.
Worse when moving or bending diseased part.	Better *or* worse when moving and bending diseased part.
Generally improved when standing . . .	Worse when standing.
Better when sitting down	Worse *or* better when sitting down.
Better after rising from a seat	*Better or* worse after rising from a seat.
Worse when lying on side, better when lying on back.	*Generally* worse when lying on side, better when lying on back.
Worse after sleep	Aggrav. oftener than improv. after sleep.*
Worse after breakfast	Generally better after breakfast.
Improved oftener than aggrav. when swallowing.	Aggravated oftener than improv. when swallowing.
Worse from cold diet	Generally better from cold diet.
Better from eructation	*Worse or* better from eructation.
Worse after meals	*Worse or* better after meals.
Worse after stool	*Better or* worse after stool.

Predomin. worse — **Predomin. better**

From cold, from growing cold, and in cold weather; from cold diet, when walking out-doors, from motion generally; lying on side, partic. on painful side.

Predomin. better — **Predomin. worse**

From warmth, from growing warm, and in warm air; in bed, during rest, after lying down; while lying, partic. on back, or on unpainful side; when turning in bed, when standing; from scratching, and from eructation.

N.B. We very rarely find the sensation of numbness in suffering parts belonging to Pulsat. with Digit.

* The aggrav. after sleep is only a supposition of Bœnninghausen, because Pulsat. has many troublesome symptoms interrupting sleep; the lessening of sweat after awaking from sleep, is characteristic of Pulsat. C.Hg.

Digitalis.	Sulphur.
Upper right, lower left side	Upper left, lower right side.
Sensation of numbness* in internal parts .	Sensitiveness in internal parts.
Desire for open air	Aversion to open air.
Apoplexy more frequent than paralysis . .	Paralysis more frequent than apoplexy.
External parts grow black	Red parts grow white.
Pulse slow, but accelerated, full and hard, by every motion; partic. slow in morning, and quicker at night.	Pulse accelerated, full, and hard; partic. quick night and morning, slower during day and evening.
Thirst during heat, not during sweat . .	Th. not constant, except perhaps dur'g sweat.
Dreams of water, falling, vexation, etc. . .	Dreams of fire, vexat., misfortunes, also merry dreams or about business of the day.
Mood distrustful—Rage	Mood changing; serious; gentle.
Solicitude concerning the future	Solicitude concerning the present. C.Hg.
Rarely delirium	Absent-mindedness — Fancies — Unconsciousness.
Desire for beer	Desire for *or* aversion to beer and spirituous liquors.
Urine infrequent and scanty	Urine often, but scanty; sometimes (after strong doses) copious.
Voice hoarse or raised and screeching, less frequently failing.	Voice hoarse or deep and low.
Respiration slow	Respiration quick.
Expectoration in the evening, less in the morning.	Expectoration morning and during day, less frequently at night.
Complaints predominant in lower part of chest. on front part of thigh and on shin.	Compl. predom. in upper part of chest, on back part of thigh, and on calf of leg.
REMISSION night and *forenoon*	REMISSION *afternoon* and before midnight.
Worse from grow'g cold & in cold weather, better from grow'g warm and in warm air.	Bett. (resp. worse) fr. grow'g cold & in cold weather, *or* fr. grow'g warm in warm air.
Worse when lying on side, better when lying on back.	Generally worse when lying on side, better when lying on back
Better on an empty stomach; worse after breakfast.	Worse (resp. better) on an empty stomach, *or* after breakfast.
Improv. oftener than aggrav. when swallow.	Aggrav. oftener than improv. when swallow.
Worse after stool	Better *or* worse after stool.
Better chang'g position while ly'g or stand'g.	*Worse or* better from change of position.
Improv. oftener than aggrav. when assuming an erect position.	Aggrav. oftener than improv. when assuming an erect position.
Better (resp. worse) when stretching out or drawing up diseased limb.	Almost always aggrav. by stretching out the limb, improved when drawing it up.
Predominant better in bed	*Worse or* better in bed.
Worse from touch.	*Worse or* better from touch.

Predomin. **worse** —— Predomin. **better**

From cold, from motion, and on expiration.

Predomin. **better** —— Predomin. **worse**

From warmth, during rest, when standing,† after lying down, while lying, in bed, also from bodily exertion, when walking fast, and running, on inspiration, from change of positioo, when assuming an erect position, when swallowing.

---

* Digitalis has over-sensitiveness to pain, oftener than Sulphur — Sulphur has sensation of numbness in suffering parts oftener than Digitalis.

† When standing still after (fatiguing) motion, Sulphur also has improvement.

Drosera.	Ipecacuanha.
Complaints (cutting pain, etc.) predominant in external parts.	Complaints (cutting pain, etc.) predominant in internal parts.
Itching, lessened by scratching	Itching, unchanged by scratching.
Pulse unchanged	Pulse changed, generally small and accelerated, sometimes imperceptible.
Heat of upper part of body	Coldness of upper part of body.
Thirst is generally wanting during chill, but appears *after* chill and during heat, also during sweat.	Thirst not constant.
Apoplexy not yet observed.	Apoplexy.

Mood more depressed than with Ipecac — Distrust.	Mood dejected
Pupils generally contracted	Pupils dilated.
Catamenia too late and scanty.	Catamenia too soon and profuse.
Fluent coryza predominant	Dry coryza.
Expectoration not constant; particularly in the morning.	Expectoration infrequent; morning and during day.
Complaints predominant on thigh and on shin.	Complaints predominant on leg and on calf of leg.

REMISSION *during day* and before midnight.	REMISSION of complaints during day.
Worse after sleep	Better *or* worse after sleep.
Worse after drinking	Improved oftener than aggravated after drinking.

Predomin. worse ⸺ **Predomin. better**

During rest, when standing, sitting and lying, in bed, on expiration, and after drinking.

Predomin. better ⸺ **Predomin. worse**

From motion, when walking, after getting out of bed, on inspiration,* when sitting down, and from touch.

N.B. Drosera lacks the over-sensitiveness of Ipecacuanha to pain, which is only apparently in contradiction to its character of want of irritability. Explained in preface.

---

* When respiring deeply, both remedies have predominant aggravation.

Drosera.	Nux vomica.
Complaints (pressure, throbbing, cutting pain, etc.) predominant in external parts.	Complaints (pressure, throbbing, cutting pain, etc.) predominant in internal parts.
Crawling sensation in internal parts—Hæmorrhages, blood light-red.	Crawling sensation in external parts—Hæmorrhages, blood dark.
Pulse unchanged	Pulse changed; generally hard, full, quick, sometimes intermitting.
One-sided chill or coldness, predom. left side.	One-sided chill or coldn., predom. right side.
Sweat sometimes only on front part of body.	Sweat often only on back part of body.
Thirst does not appear until *after* the cold stage.	Most thirst during chill, besides this *before* the chill, *before* and *after* the sweating stage.
No apoplexy—Very rarely paralysis . . .	Apoplexy—Paralysis.

Mood distrustful	Dejection — Mood irritable; malicious — Amorousness.
Anxious feeling in hypochondria	Anxious feeling in præcordia.
Pupils generally contracted.	Pupils generally dilated.
Diarrhœa predominant	Constipation predominant.
Catamenia too late and scanty.	Catamenia too soon and profuse.
Coryza predominantly fluent	Coryza generally dry, partic. in the open air; in-doors, on the other hand, it is fluent.
Respiration prevalently slow	Respiration quick oftener than slow.
Expectoration in the morning	Expectoration in the morning and during day.
Complaints predominant in hollow of elbow and on shin.	Complaints predominant in hollow of knee and on calf of leg.

REMISSION during day and before midnight.	REMISSION evening till midnight.
Worse when perspiring	*Worse or* better when perspiring.
Worse when lying on painful side, better when lying on unpainful side.	Generally as with Drosera, but often also the opposite.
Worse after sleep	Better after sufficient and not too long sleep, but worse on awaking when roused from sleep.
Better after getting out of bed	Worse *or* better after getting out of bed.
Worse when stooping	Better *or* worse when stooping.
Worse after drinking.	*Worse or* better after drinking.
Worse when sneezing	*Worse or* better from sneezing.
Aggravated oftener than improved by pressure.	Improved oftener than aggravated by pressure.

Predomin. worse — **Predomin. better**

From warmth, growing warm and in warm air, in bed, during rest, after lying down, while lying, sitting and standing, when lifting diseased limb, from pressure, and after sleep.

Predomin. better — **Predomin. worse**

From cold, growing cold and in cold weather, from motion, when walking, from touch, when letting diseased limb hang down, and from cold diet.

N.B. Drosera lacks the over-sensitiveness of Nux vomica to pain.

Drosera.	Pulsatilla.
Hæmorrhages, blood light-red	Hæmorrhages, blood dark—Apoplexy.
Complaints predominant in external parts .	Complaints predominant in internal parts.
Itching, generally lessened by scratching .	Itch'g, unchang'd *or* aggravat'd by scratching.
Sleeplessness after midnight	Sleeplessness before midnight.
Pulse unchanged	Pulse changed, sometimes intermitting; generally frequent, small, and weak.
One-sided coldness, predom. left side* . .	One-sided coldness, predom. right side.
Partial sweat on front part of body . . .	Partial sweat on back part of body.
Thirst does not appear till after chill . .	Want of thirst predominant, but constant only during chill—Thirst frequently appears *before* and *after* chill, less frequently between heat and sweat.

Drosera.	Pulsatilla.
Mood irritable; irascible	Mood indifferent—Calm sadness of gentle dispositions.
Anxious feeling in the hypochondria. . . .	Anxious feeling in præcordia—Unconsciousness—Delirium.
Far-sightedness	Short-sightedness.
Respirat. slow; predom. with moist sound.	Respirat'n quick; predom. with dry sound.
Expectoration not constant; morning . . .	Expectoration predominant, but not constant; morning and during day.
Complaints predominant on thigh . . .	Complaints generally on leg.

Drosera.	Pulsatilla.
REMISSION *during day* and before midnight.	REMISSION from midnight till noon.
Worse after sleep	*Worse or* better after sleep.
Better after getting out of bed	*Better or* worse after getting out of bed.
Worse when rising from a seat	*Worse or* better when rising from a seat.
Better *after* rising from a seat	*Better or* worse after rising from a seat.
Worse when stooping and when rising . .	Better *or* worse when stooping.
Worse when bending diseased part . . .	Better *or* worse when bending diseased part, partic. when holding it bent or bending it sideways; worse when bending it backwards.
Worse after meals	*Worse or* better after meals.
Worse after stool	*Better or* worse after stool.

Predomin. worse —— **Predomin. better**

Out-doors, when lying on painful side, when lifting diseased limb, when walking fast and running, from bodily exertion generally, from vinegar and sour things, from pressure, and after stool.

Predomin. better —— **Predomin. worse**

In-doors, when lying on unpainful side, when letting diseased limb hang down, from touch, and from scratching.

N.B. Drosera lacks both the over-sensitiveness of Pulsatilla to pain and the sensation of numbness in suffering parts.

---

* All other symptoms predom. on right side, like Pulsatilla.

Drosera.	Sulphur.
Right side—Cutting or ulcerative pain in external parts.	*Left* side—Cutting and ulcerative pain in internal parts.
Epilepsy, with rigidity — Hæmorrhages, blood, light-red.	Epilepsy, generally with convulsions—Hæmorrhages, blood dark.
Pulse unchanged — No apoplexy — Very rarely paralysis.	Pulse changed, generally full, hard, and accelerated, sometimes intermitting or imperceptible.
Heat often confined to upper part of body.	Heat on lower part of body or general, with exception of head.
Sweat on front part of body	Sweat on back part of body.
Thirst does not appear until *after* the chill.	Thirst greater during heat, but most constant during sweat.

Drosera.	Sulphur.
Mood not so depressed as with Sulphur—Distrust—Anxious feeling in hypochondria.	Mood depressed; indifferent; serious; gentle *or* irritable—Anxious feeling in præcordia.
Far-sightedness	Short-sightedness predominant.
Saliva increased	Saliva *generally* diminished.
Bitter vomit	Vomit sour oftener than bitter.
Respiration predominantly slow	Respiration quick.
Voice deep, hollow, without resonance . .	Voice deep.
Expectoration in the morning	Expectoration in the morning and during day, less frequently at night.
Complaints predominant on shin . . .	Complaints predominant on calf of leg.

Drosera.	Sulphur.
Remission *during day* and before midnight.	Remission *afternoon* and before midnight.
Worse when alone, better in company . .	*Generally* better when alone, worse in comp.
Worse in the open air, better in-doors . .	Better (resp. worse) in the open air *or* in-doors; partic. worse in crowded rooms, but better from warmth of stove.
Better from growing cold and in cold weather, worse from growing warm and in warm air.	Worse (resp. better) from growing cold and in cold weather, or from growing warm and in warm air.
Worse in bed and when turning in bed . .	*Worse or* better in bed, the same when turning in bed.
Better after getting out of bed	Worse *or* better after getting out of bed.
Worse when stooping and when rising . .	Worse *or* better when stooping and when rising.
Worse *or* better when stretching out diseased limb and when drawing it up.	Generally aggrav. when stretching out diseased limb, improv. when drawing it up.
Worse when sitting	Worse *or* better when sitting.
Worse after drinking	*Worse or* better after drinking.
Worse after stool	Better *or* worse after stool.
Worse from sneezing	*Worse or* better from sneezing.
Improv. oftener than aggravated by touch.	Aggrav. oftener than improved by touch.
Aggrav. oftener than improv. by pressure .	Improv. oftener than aggrav. by pressure.

Predomin. worse ——— **Predomin. better**

From pressure, on expiration, when holding the breath, when alone.

Predomin. better ——— **Predomin. worse**

From the touch, on inspiration, from cold diet, and when in company.

N.B. Drosera lacks the sensation of numbness in suffering parts peculiar to Sulph.

Dulcamara.	Belladonna.
Left side; partic. *lower left, upper right side.*	*Right* side; partic. *lower right, upper left side.*
Ematiation—No apoplexy	Obesity—Apoplexy.
Generally dry eruptions—Skin callous	Humid erupt. predom.—Skin chafed. C.Hg.
Painless swelling of glands	Painful swelling of glands.
Sleeplessness after midnight	Sleeplessness before midnight.
Pulse tense, hard, but small, partic. at night.	P. generally tense, hard and accel., but full.
Partial sweat on back part of body	Partial sweat on front part of body.
Thirst pred. during chill, rare during heat.	Thirst not constant; most rare during chill; often *before* chill and *after* sweat.
Hunger with dislike for food	Thirst, with disgust for drink.
Vomiting of drink	Vomiting of food.
Complaints of spleen predom.	Liver complaints predominant.
Inflammation of intestines predom.	Inflammation of throat predominant. C.Hg.
Fetid flatus	Scentless flatus.
Diarrhœa preval. painful	Diarrhœa generally painless.
Catamenia too late and scanty	Catamenia too soon and profuse.
Milk diminished	Milk increased.
Catarrh on the chest	Nasal catarrh. C.Hg.
Cough generally with expectoration	Cough generally without expectoration.

Dulcamara.	Belladonna.
Remission *forenoon* and before midnight	Remission forenoon and after midnight.
Worse during waning moon	Worse during full moon.
Worse *or* better when growing cold (resp. growing warm).	Predominantly worse when growing cold, better when growing warm.
Worse *or* better from warmth of bed	Better from warmth of bed.
Better or worse when getting out of bed	Worse when getting out of bed.
Better *or* worse *after* getting out of bed	Almost always improved *after* getting out of bed.
Worse *or* better when stretching out diseased limb and when drawing it up.	Predom. better when stretching out diseased limb, worse when drawing it up.
Worse or better while speaking	Worse when speaking.
Generally better after stool	Worse after stool.
Ailments from abuse of Cuprum	Ailments from Mercur., Iodine, Plumb., Cinchona, and from sting of insects or contagious Anthrax.
Similarity of symptoms more with Stannum.	Similarity of symptoms more with Mercurius. CHg.

Predomin. worse — **Predomin. better**

In wet weather, during rest, after lying down, in bed, when lying, sitting and standing, when stooping and sitting bent forward, and when bending diseased part backwards.

Predomin. better — **Predomin. worse**

In dry weather, from motion, when moving suffering part, when walking, when walking out-doors, when sitting erect, when rising from a seat, when getting out of bed, and after stool.

N.B. Dulcamara, whose constitutional character is want of irritability, lacks the over-sensitiveness of Belladonna to pain.

N.B. Both remedies have a great many symptoms worse when sitting, and both pain in the joints worse during rest. C.Hg.

Dulcamara.	Lycopodium.
Left side—Dark hair—Muscles rigid	*Right* side - Light hair—Muscles lax.
Sensitiveness in internal parts	Sensitiveness in external parts; sensation of numbness in internal parts.
Pain pressing inwards—Rending pain upwards.	Pain pressing outwards — Rending pain downwards.
Hæmorrh., blood light-red—No apoplexy.	Hæmorrhages, blood dark—Apoplexy.
Pulse small, hard, and tense, particularly at night; frequent at night, slow during day.	Pulse somewhat accelerated only in the evening and after meals; frequent in the evening, slow in the morning.
Thirst predominant during chill; rare during heat.	Thirst predominant; is wanting only dur'g chill; often appears *after* the sweat.
Skin callous, hardening	Skin predom. chafed and sore. C.Hg.
Eruptions generally dry	Eruptions generally humid.
Sleeplessness after midnight	Sleeplessness preval. before midnight.

Dulcamara.	Lycopodium.
Imbecility more frequent than insanity	Insanity more frequent than imbecility.
Vomiting of drink	Vomiting of food.
Bitter vomit	Vomit sour oftener than bitter.
Complaints of spleen predominant—Fetid flatus.	Liver complaints predominant—Flatus predominantly scentless.
Diarrhœa preval. painful	Painless diarrhœa.
Urine scanty; sediment red	Urine often, but scanty; sediment red (sandy) *or* whitish.
Incontinence more frequent than retention of urine.	Retention of urine more frequent than incontinence.
Catamenia generally of too short duration.	Catamenia generally of too long duration.
Complaints predom. on front side of thigh.	Complaints predom. on back part of thigh.

Dulcamara.	Lycopodium.
Remission *forenoon* and before midnight.	Remission *forenoon* and after midnight.
Worse during waning moon	Worse during new moon.
Worse in cold weather; better in warm air.	Better (resp. worse) in cold weather *or* in warm air.
Worse during sweat	Worse *or* better when perspiring.
Worse *or* better after getting out of bed	Almost always better after gett'g out of bed.
Better when rising from a seat	*Worse or* better when rising from a seat.
Worse *or* better when stretching out diseased limb, or when drawing it up.	Predom. worse when stretching out diseased limb, better when drawing it up.
Worse when stooping	Generally improved when stooping.
Worse when sitting bent forward, better when sitting erect.	*Generally* better when sitting bent forward, worse when sitting erect.
Worse from bend'g diseased part backwards.	Worse when bend'g diseased part sideways.
Worse *or* better from talking	Worse from talking.
Generally improved after stool	Generally aggravated after stool.
Ailments from abuse of Cuprum	Ailments from abuse of Mercurius.

Predomin. worse — **Predomin. better**

From cold, lying on back, when stooping and sitting bent forward, and on expiration.

Predomin. better — **Predomin. worse**

From warmth, lying on side, when sitting erect, from pressure, after stool, and when rising from a seat.

N.B. Dulcamora lacks the over-sensitiveness of Lycopodium to pain, and generally also the sensation of numbness in suffering parts.

Dulcamara.	Mercurius.
Upper right, lower left side—Dark hair—Muscles rigid.	Upper left, lower right side—Light hair—Muscles lax.
Want of bodily irritability	Increased bodily irritability.
Pain pressing inwards—Rending pain upwards.	Pain pressing outwards — Rending pain downwards.
No apoplexy	Rarely paralysis.
Skin callous, hardening	Skin chafed and sore. C.Hg.
Painless swelling of glands	Hot swelling of glands.
Pulse small, hard, and tense, particularly at night.	Pulse irregular; generally full and accelerated; sometimes trembl'g or intermitt'g.
Partial sweat on back of body	Partial sweat on front of body.
Thirst predominant during chill; quite rare during heat.	Thirst predominant in all stages, but not constant.
Sleeplessness after midnight	Sleeplessness prevalent before midnight.
Delirium	Rarely delirium.
Vomiting of drink	Vomiting of food.
Complaints of spleen predominant . . .	Liver complaint predominant.
Urine predominantly pale; scanty . . .	Urine dark; often and copious.
Dry coryza	Coryza fluent oftener than dry.
Cough generally with expectoration . . .	Expectoration not constant.
Complaints predominant on front part of thigh.	Complaints predominant on back part of thigh.
REMISSION *forenoon* and before midnight .	REMISSION of complaints during day.
Aggravation in the Spring	Aggravation in the Fall.
Better *or* worse from warmth of bed . .	Worse from warmth of bed.
Worse when lying on back, better when lying on side.	Generally better when lying on back, worse when lying on side.
Worse *or* better after getting out of bed .	Better after getting out of bed.
Better when rising from a seat	Worse *or* better when rising from a seat.
Worse when swallowing	Worse *or* better when swallowing (saliva or fluids).
Worse during and after meals	Worse *or* better during and after meals.
Generally improved after stool	Worse after stool.
Worse or better from talking	Worse from talking.

Predomin. worse — **Predomin. better**

During rest, when standing, sitting and lying, when sitting bent forward, when lying on back, and on expiration.

Predomin. better — **Predomin. worse**

From motion, when moving diseased part, when walking, when walking out-doors, from pressure, after stool, when sitting erect, and when lying on side.

Dulcamara.	Rhus.
Left side predominant, particularly *lower left, upper right side.*	*Right* side, particularly *lower right, upper left side.*
Dark hair—Aversion to motion	Light hair—Inclination for motion.
Complaints (sensitiveness, tension, etc.) predominant in internal parts.	Complaints (sensitiveness, tension, etc.) predominantly in external parts.*
Pain pressing inward	Pain pressing outwards.
Apoplexy not yet observed	Apoplexy.
Eruptions generally dry	Eruptions generally humid.
Painful ulcers, with scanty discharge . .	Painless ulcers, with much suppuration, particularly on the œdematic legs, with steady spontaneous discharge of the water.
Painless swelling of glands	Hot, painful swelling of glands.
Pulse sometimes slower than beating of heart; generally small, hard, and tense.	Pulse sometimes oftener than beating of heart; generally frequent, soft, and full.
Partial sweat on back of body	Partial sweat on front of body.
Thirst predominant during chill, tolerably rare during heat.	Thirst not constant.
Sleeplessness after midnight; awaking too early.	Sleeplessness prevalent before midnight; awaking too late.

Dulcamara.	Rhus.
Mood irritable	Mood anxious, depressed—Ailments from vexation with fear.
Urine scanty—Sediment red.	Urine too often and copious—Sedim. white.
Catamenia too late and scanty, generally also of too short duration.	Catamenia too soon, profuse, and of long duration.
Milk diminished	Milk generally increased.
Dry coryza	Fluent coryza.
Cough with expectoration	Cough generally dry.
Complaints predominant in upper part of chest, in palm of hand, and on front part of thigh.	Complaints predominant in lower part of chest, on back of hand, and on back part of thigh.

Dulcamara.	Rhus.
Remission *forenoon* and before midnight.	Remission of complaints during day.
Worse during waning moon	Worse during increase of moon.
Worse (resp. better) when growing cold *or* warm.	Worse when growing cold; better when growing warm.
Aggravated oftener than improved in bed .	Improved oftener than aggravated in bed.
Worse *or* better when stretching out diseased limb and when drawing it up.	Predom. better when stretching out diseased limb, worse when drawing it up.
Better when moving diseased part . . .	*Better or* worse when moving diseased part.
Worse when bending diseased part . . .	Worse *or* better when bend'g diseased part.
Better while and after rising from a seat .	Worse *or* better while and after rising from a seat.
Worse after meals	Worse *or* better after meals.
Worse or better from talking	Worse from talking.

Predomin. worse ⁀ **Predomin. better**

On expiration.

---

* Sensation of numbness, chiefly in the suffering parts, is often found with Rhus., rarely with Dulcamara.

† This difference of Rhus. can be traced back to another, according to which complaints are aggravated in the beginning of motion, but improved by continued motion.

Dulcamara.	Sepia.
Sensitiveness and other compl. predom. in internal parts.*	Sensitiveness and other compl. predom. in external parts.
Skin callous	Skin callous or chafed. C.Hg.
Pain pressing inward — Pain rending upwards.	Pain pressing outward — Pain rending downwards.
Hæmorrhages, blood light-red — No apoplexy.	Hæmorrhages, blood dark — Apoplexy.
Pulse small, hard, and tense, partic. at night.	Pulse quick and full, and then often intermitting at night, slow during day — Pulse accelerated, partic. by vexation & motion.
Thirst predom. during chill; tolerably rare during heat.	Want of thirst predom.; thirst is constant only during chill.
Sleeplessness after midnight	Sleeplessness preval. before midnight.

Dulcamara.	Sepia.
Delirium	Fancies.
Pupils dilated	Pupils contracted.
Mucous vomit — Vomiting of drink	Predom. vomiting of food.†
Affections of spleen predom.	Liver compl. predom.
Discharge of urine often, but scanty	Discharge of urine too seldom.
Urine preval. pale	Urine dark.
Catamenia too scanty, generally also of too short duration.	Catamenia of too long duration, generally also too profuse.
Expector. tolerably constant	Expector. predom., but not constant.
Compl. predom. on front part of thigh	Compl. predom. on back part of thigh.

Dulcamara.	Sepia.
REMISSION *forenoon* and before midnight.	REMISSION of complaints in the afternoon.
Worse during waning moon	Worse during new moon.
Worse in cold weather, better in warm air.	Better (resp. worse) in cold weather *or* in warm air.
Better (resp. worse) when growing cold or warm.	Predom. worse when growing cold, better when growing warm.
Worse when perspiring	*Worse or* better when perspiring.
Almost always improv. when walking in the open air.	Worse *or* better when walking in the open air.
Worse on awaking	Better after sufficient sleep; but worse on awaking, when roused from sleep.
Better when rising from a seat	Worse *or* better when rising from a seat.
Worse *or* better when stretching out diseased limb and when drawing it up.	Worse when stretching out diseased limb;—better when drawing it up.
Worse or better while talking	Worse while talking.
Worse after meals	Worse *or* better after meals.

Predomin. worse — **Predomin. better**

During wet weather, from dancing, and after sleep.

Predomin. better — **Predomin. worse**

In dry weather, from pressure, and after stool.

---

* In accordance with its constitutional wants of irritability, Dulcamara lacks the over-sensitiveness of the Sepia-patient to pain.

† We find *vomiting of bile* with both remedies.

Dulcamara.	Sulphur.
Upper right, lower left side — Hæmorrhages, blood light-red.	Upper left, lower right side — Hæmorrhages, blood dark.
Pain pressing inward — Pain rending upwards.	Pain pressing outward — Pain rending downwards.
Skin callous, hard	Skin predom. chafed and sore. C.Hg.
Painful ulcers	Painless ulcers.
Sleeplessness after midnight—Awaking too early.	Sleeplessness before midnight — Awaking too late.
Pulse small, hard, and tense, partic. at night; frequent at night, slow during day.	Pulse full, hard and accelerated, sometimes intermitting; frequent night and morning, slower during day and evening.
Chill increased in warm room	Chill abating in warm room.
Thirst predom. during chill; more rare during heat.	Thirst greatest during hot stage, but most constant during sweating stage.

Dulcamara.	Sulphur.
Solicitude concerning the future	Solicitude concerning the present. C.Hg.
Imbecility more frequent than insanity . .	Insanity more frequent than imbecility — Fancies.
Delirium	
Pupils dilated	Pupils contracted.
Saliva generally increased	Saliva generally diminished.
Vomiting of bile	Vomit sour oftener than bitter.
Vomiting drink.	Vomiting food.
Bellyache better after stool	Bellyache worse after stool.
Urine scanty	Urine often, but scanty; sometimes (after massive doses) copious.
Oppression worse when stooping . . .	Oppression predom. better when stooping.
Expectoration almost constant	Expectoration not constant.
Compl. predom. on front part of thigh . .	Compl. predom. on back part of thigh.

Dulcamara.	Sulphur.
REMISSION *forenoon* and before midnight.	REMISSION *afternoon* and before midnight.
Worse during waning moon	Worse during full moon.
Worse during cold weather, better in warm air.	Better (resp. worse) in cold weather *or* in warm air.
Worse when lying on back, better when lying on side.	Generally worse when lying on side.
Worse when sitting	Better *or* worse when sitting.
Worse when stooping	Better *or* worse when stooping.
Worse from the touch	*Worse or* better from the touch.
Better when moving diseased part . . .	*Worse or* better when moving the part.
Worse *or* better when stretching out diseased limb, and from drawing it up.	Predom. worse when stretching out diseased limb; better when drawing it up.
Worse or better while talking	Worse from talking.
Generally improved after stool	Worse *or* better after stool.
Ailments from Cuprum	Ailments from abuse of metals generally, and from abuse of Cinchona, &c.

Predomin. worse — **Predomin. better**

From cold, and when lying on back.

Predomin. better — **Predomin. worse**

From warmth, when lying on side, when rising from a seat, and when walking in the open air.

N.B. With Dulc. we very rarely find the sensation of numbness in suffering parts belonging to Sulph.

Euphrasia.	N. vomica.
Left side — Neither apoplexy nor paralysis.	*Right* side — Apoplexy — Paralysis.
Complaints (cramping, pinching, &c.) predominant in external parts.	Complaints (cramping, pinching pain, etc.) predominant in external parts.
Warts	Corns. C.Hg.
Pulse unchanged	Pulse changed in frequency and strength; generally hard, full, and quick.
Sweat often confined to front part of body.	Sweat often confined to back part of body.
Thirst has very rarely been observed	Thirst greatest during chill, also often between hot and sweating stage, *before* the cold, and *after* sweating stage.
Sweat increased during sleep	Sweat lessened during sleep.
Pupils contracted — Short-sightedness — Dimsightedness.	Pupils dilated — Far-sightedness — Predom. clearsightedness.
Optical illusions black, or in dark colors.	Optical illusions predominant in light colors.
Urine too often and copious	Urine infrequent and scanty.
Catamenia too scanty, of short duration and late.	Catamenia too profuse, of long duration and too soon.
Fluent coryza	Coryza generally dry, partic. in the open air; in-doors, on the other hand, it is fluent.
Cough predominant with expectoration	Cough generally dry.
Expectoration in the morning	Expector. morning, during day, evening.
Cough only during day, not at night	Cough evening and morning. C.Hg.
REMISSION of complaints during day	REMISSION evening till midnight.
Predominant worse after sleep	Better after sufficient and not too long sleep, but worse on awaking when roused.
Better after getting out of bed	Worse *or* better after getting out of bed.
Worse when stooping	*Better or* worse when stooping.
Better *or* worse from touch	Worse from touch.
Generally worse on inspiration, better on expiration.	Generally better on inspiration, worse on expiration.

Predomin. worse ⁓⁓⁓ **Predomin. better**

During rest, in bed, after lying down, while lying, sitting, and standing, on inspiration in-doors,* and after sleep.

Predomin. better ⁓⁓⁓ **Predomin. worse**

From motion, when walking, on expiration, in the open air, from drinking cold water, and from coffee.

N.B. Euphrasia lacks the over-sensitiveness of the N. vomica-patient to pain.

---

* In single cases we also find the symptoms of Euphrasia *improved in-doors.*

Euphrasia.	Phosphor.
Left side—Neither apoplexy nor paralysis.	*Right* side—*Paralysis*—Apoplexy.
Complaints (cramping, pinching pain, etc.) predominant in external parts.	Complaints (cramping, pinching pain, etc.) in internal parts.
Pulse unchanged	Pulse differs, irregular, generally accelerated, full and hard; sometimes intermitting.
Heat descending	Heat ascending.
Sleeplessness prevalent after midnight . .	Sleeplessness before midnight.
Weakness of memory	Memory predominant active.
Urine too often and copious	Urine often but scanty.
Catamenia too late, weak, and of short duration.	Catamenia too soon, profuse, and long duration, *or* too late, scanty and of short duration.
Expectoration rather constant; morning.	Expectoration not constant; morning and during day.
Complaints predominant on front part of thigh, and on calf of leg.	Complaints predominant on back part of thigh and on shin.

Euphrasia.	Phosphor.
Remission of complaints during day . .	Remission after midnight.
Worse in bed	*Worse or* better in bed.
Predominant worse after sleep	Better after sufficient sleep, but worse on awaking when roused and after the siesta.
Better after getting out of bed	Worse *or* better after getting out of bed.
Worse when stooping	Better *or* worse when stooping.
Better while riding	*Generally* worse while riding.
Worse *or* better from touch	Almost always improved by touch
Worse after meals	Worse *or* better after meals, particularly better after a satisfying meal.
Better from eructation	Worse *or* better from eructation.

Predomin. worse — **Predomin. better**

During rest, when standing, sitting and lying, and after sleep.

Predomin. better — **Predomin. worse**

From motion*, when walking, when riding, and from washing and moistening diseased part.

N.B. Euphrasia lacks the over-sensitiveness of the Phosphor-patient to pain, and generally also the sensation of numbness in suffering parts.

---

* The "*improvement by motion*," which sometimes occurs with Phosphor, seems to be exclusively confined to pain in joints, therefore it is an improvement, when moving suffering part.

Euphrasia.	Pulsatilla.
Left side, particularly *lower left, upper right side.*	*Right* side, particularly *lower right, upper left side.*
Complaints (cramping, pinching pain, etc.) predominant in external parts.	Complaints (cramping, pinching pain, etc.) predominant in internal parts.
Warts	Corns. C.Hg.
Pulse unchanged	Pulse changed, sometimes intermitting; generally frequent, small, faint.
Sweat often confined to front part of body.	Sweat often confined to back part of body.
Thirst very rarely observed.	Want of thirst predominant, but constant only during chill; thirst often *before* and *after* chill, less frequently between heat and sweat.
Sleeplessness prevalent after midnight . .	Sleeplessness before midnight.
Apoplexy or paralysis not yet observed .	*Apoplexy*—Paralysis.

Euphrasia.	Pulsatilla.
Optical illusions predominantly black, or in dark colors.	Optical illusions in bright colors.
Nasal complaints predominantly internal .	Nasal complaints external oftener than internal.
Constipation predominant	Generally diarrhœa.
Urine too often and copious	Urine not often enough and scanty.
Expectoration almost constant; morning .	Expectoration predominant, but not constant; morning and during day.
Complaints predominant in upper part of chest.	Complaints predominant in lower part of chest.

Euphrasia.	Pulsatilla.
AGGRAVATION from evening till morning .	AGGRAVATION from noon till midnight.
Better *or* worse from touch	Worse from touch.
Worse after meals	*Worse or* better after meals.
Better from eructation	*Worse or* better from eructation.
Better after getting out of bed	*Better or* worse after getting out of bed.
Worse when rising from a seat	Better *or* worse when rising from a seat.
Better *after* rising from a seat	*Better or* worse after rising from a seat.
Worse when looking into distance . . .	Worse when looking upwards.

Predomin. worse ——— **Predomin. better**

When opening the eyes, on inspiration, from bodily exertion, running, etc., and when bending diseased part sideways.

Predomin. better ——— **Predomin. worse**

When closing the eyes, from drinking coffee, and from eructation.

N.B. Euphrasia lacks the over-sensitiveness of the Pulsatilla-patient to pain, and generally also the sensation of numbness in suffering parts.

Euphrasia.	Sulphur.
Upper right, lower left side	Upper left, lower right side.
Paralysis not yet observed	Paralysis.
Pulse unchanged	Pulse generally hard, full, and accelerated; sometimes intermitting or imperceptible.
Heat descending	Heat ascending.
Sweat often confined to front part of body.	Sweat often confined to back part of body.
Thirst rarely observed	Thirst greatest during heat, but most constant during sweat.

Euphrasia.	Sulphur.
Sleeplessness predominant after midnight	Sleeplessness prevalent before midnight.
Complaints predominant on inner angle of eye.	Complaints predominant on external angle of eye.
Urine too often and copious	Urine often, but scanty; sometimes (after strong doses) copious.
Expectoration nearly constant, morning	Expectoration not constant; morning and during day, less frequently at night.
Complaints predominant on front part of thigh.	Complaints predominant on back part of thigh.

Euphrasia.	Sulphur.
Remission of complaints during day	Remission of complaints *afternoon* and before midnight.
Worse while sitting	Better *or* worse while sitting.
Worse in bed	*Worse or* better in bed.
Better after getting out of bed	Worse *or* better after getting out of bed.
Worse when stooping	Better *or* worse when stooping.
Better from eructation	*Almost always* improved by eructation.

Predomin. better — **Predomin. worse**

From coffee, from drinking cold water, from washing and moistening diseased part, and when riding.

N.B. With Euphrasia we very rarely find the numb sensation in suffering parts peculiar to Sulph.

Ferrum.	Calcarea.
Left side predominant—Increased irritability.	*Right* side predominant—Want of bodily irritability.
Dark hair—Pain rending downwards . .	Light hair—Pain rending upwards.
Apoplexy more frequent than paralysis . .	Paralysis more frequent than apoplexy.
Pulse full and hard; sometimes intermitting.	Pulse full and accelerated; often trembling.
Thirst, particularly during chill	Thirst is wanting only sometimes during chill.
Chill, lessened after getting out of bed . .	Chill, increased after getting out of bed.
Sweat, lessened while talking and after meals.	Sweat, increased when talking and after meals.

Changing mood; particularly merry one evening, sad the next—Haughtiness—Vehemence—Quarrelsomeness—Fear of apoplexy.	Silly merriment *or* dejection—Peevishness—Fear—Hopelessness—Amorousness—Fear of loss of reason—Unconsciousness—Fancies—Imbecility.
Ailments from anger	Consequences of vexation with fright or fear, or of hearing bad news.
Generally loss of appetite	Generally hunger.
Aversion for sour things	Appetite for sour things.
Urine alkaline	Urine sour.
Catamenia predominantly too late . . .	Catamenia in most cases too soon.
Expectoration predominant; is loosened only in the morning, particularly when moving.	Expectoration predominant, but not constant; is loosened in the morning and during day.
Complaints predominant on upper arm . .	Complaints predominant on fore-arm.

REMISSION before midnight and *during day.*	REMISSION of complaints before midnight.
Better when ascending, *worse* when descending.	*Worse* when ascending.
Better from wine, when it is not acid* . .	*Worse* from spirituous liquors.
Consequences of bodily exertion, of long marches, while moderate mental exertion improves.	Mental exertion aggravates much more than bodily exertion. C.Hg.
Ailments from Iodine or Arsenic	Ailments from Phosph., Digitalis, or Nitric acid.

Predomin. worse —— **Predomin. better**

When lifting diseased limb, after lying down, while sitting and standing, when assuming an erect position, from the touch, and when descending.

Predomin. better —— **Predomin. worse**

When letting the diseased limb hang down, after getting out of bed, after rising from a seat, when straining the eyes, when writing, (mental exertion), and when ascending.

N.B. We very rarely find the over-sensitiveness of Ferrum to pain with Calcarea; this is quite in accordance with the constitutional character of both remedies.

---

* Yet Ferrum as well as Calcarea will cure delirium tremens in conformable cases, which, however, is caused by alcoholic drinks oftener than by wine.

Ferrum.	Iod.
Left side — Dark hair — Increased irritability.	*Right* side*—Light hair†—Want of irritability.
Apoplexy—Aversion to open air	Very rarely paralysis—Inclination for open air.
Tension in internal, rending pain in external parts.	Tension in external, rending pain predom. in internal parts.
Warts	Corns. C.Hg.
Pulse full and hard; sometimes intermitting.	Pulse different; generally quick, full, and hard, particularly accelerated by every motion.
Thirst, particularly during chill	Thirst, particularly during sweat.
Sweat, lessened when speaking	Sweat, increased while speaking.

Alternating cheerful one evening, dejected the next — Haughtiness - *Quarrelsomeness*—Consequences of anger.	Cheerfulness *or* depression of spirits - Fear —*Gentleness* — Consequences of amorousness.
Temperament sanguine choleric	Temperament phlegmatic.
Generally loss of appetite	Hunger predominant.
Aversion to meat	Inclination for meat.
Predominant sterility	Predominant impotence.
Catamenia prevalently too late	Catamenia prevalently too soon.
Respiration predom. with dry sound. . . .	Respiration predom. with moist sound.
Expectoration in the morning	Expectoration in the evening.
Complaints predom. on ankle	Complaints predominant on wrist.

REMISSION *during day* and before midnight.	REMISSION *forenoon* and before midnight.
Worse while perspiring	*Worse after* perspiring.

Predomin. worse — **Predomin. better**

In the open air, from cold and in cold weather, during rest, while standing and sitting, particularly when sitting bent forward, after lying down,‡ and when lying on side.

Predomin. better — **Predomin. worse**

In-doors, from warmth and in warm air, from motion, running and bodily exertion, when sitting erect, and when lying on back.

N.B. With Iodine we very rarely find the over-sensitiveness of Ferrum to pain, and rarely also the numb sensation in suffering parts.

---

* Ferrum as well as Iodium seem to have the direction of symptoms from left to right side. C.Hg.

† According to Boeninghausen. But Iodium corresponds much more to the complaints of persons with black eyes and dark hair, while Bromium much oftener is indicated with blue eyes and light hair. C.Hg.

‡ Both remedies have aggravation *in bed*, but with Ferrum this is more a consequence of rest, with Iodine of warmth of bed.

Ferrum.	Lycopodium.
Left side—Dark hair—Inclinat. for motion.	*Right* side—Light hair—Aversion to motion
Hæmorrhages, blood light-red—Pain in the parts lain on.	Hæmorrhages, blood dark—Pain arises on the side not lain on.
Merriness predominant; also alternating merry one evening, sad the next.	Mood cheerful *or* sad; anxious; serious; peevish; distrustful; malicious; avaricious; amorous.
Vehemence—Quarrelsomeness	Unconsciousness — Absent-mindedness — Fancies—Insanity—Imbecility.
Pulse full & hard; sometimes intermitting.	Pulse accelerated somewhat only in the evening and after meals.
Thirst, particularly during chill	Thirst is wanting only during chill, often appears after sweat.
Capability of hysteric patients to see at night in the dark.	Nocturnal blindness.
Diarrhœa predominant	Costiveness predominant.
Involuntary discharge of urine predom. . .	Retent. of urine more freq. than incontinence.
Respiration preval. with dry sound . . .	Respiration preval. with moist sound.
Expectoration in the morning	Expectoration morning and evening.
Complaints predominant on upper arm . .	Complaints predominant on fore-arm.
Remission *during day* and before midnight	Remission *forenoon* and after midnight.
Worse when looking at running water . .	Worse when look'g at anyth'g turn'g round.
Almost always aggrav. in bed	Worse *or* better in bed.
Alm. always improv. when gett'g out of bed.	Worse *or* better when getting out of bed.
Better when sitting down	Better *or* worse when sitting down.
Worse when rising from a seat	*Worse or* better when rising from a seat.
Worse when sitting bent forward; better when sitting erect.	*Generally* better when sitting bent forward, worse when sitting erect.
Worse when stooping	*Generally* better when stooping.
Almost always aggrav. when assuming an erect position.	Better *or* worse when assuming an erect position.
Worse when descend'g; bett. when ascend'g.	*Generally* as with Ferr.; somet's the oppos.
Worse when bend'g diseas'd part backwards.	Pred. worse when bend diseas'd part sidew's.
Better *or* worse when stretching out diseased limb, and when drawing it up.	Worse when stretching out diseased limb; better when drawing it up.
Worse when lifting diseased limb, better when letting it hang down.	*Generally* better when lifting diseased limb, worse when letting it hang down.
Better or worse after meals	Predominant worse after meals.
Worse or better after drinking	Worse after drinking.
Better from wine, when it is not acid . .	Worse from drinking wine.
Better or worse from smoking	Worse from smoking.
Worse *or* better from talking	Worse from talking.
Worse growing cold, better growing warm.	Bett. (resp. worse) fr. grow'g cold *or* warm.
Worse in cold weather; better in warm air.	Better (resp. worse) in cold weather *or* in warm air.

Predomin. worse — **Predomin. better**

From cold, on an empty stomach, from warm diet,* out-doors, and when walking out-doors, when stooping, and setting bent forward, when lifting diseased limb, and when closing the eyes.

Predomin. better — **Predomin. worse**

From warmth, after breakfast, from cold diet, after meals, in-doors, when sitting erect, when letting diseased limb hang down; when opening the eyes, from drinking wine, from mental exertion, reading and writing, from straining the eyes, and from bodily exertion, walking fast, running, etc.

---

* With Lycopodium the formula "internal chill with external heat" corresponds to the improvement from cold, and from warm diet, while the formula "external chill with internal heat" is more applicable to Ferrum.

Ferrum.	Pulsatilla.
Left side; part. *lower left, upper right side.*	*Right* side; partic. *lower right, upper left side.*
Inclination for motion — Aversion to open air.	Aversion to motion — Inclination for open air.
Warts	Corns. C.Hg.
Hæmorrhages, blood light-red—Apoplexia sanguinea.	Hæmorrhages, blood dark—Apoplexia nervosa.
Pulse full and hard	Pulse generally frequent, small, and weak.
Thirst, partic. during chill	Want of thirst predom., but constant only during chill; thirst, partic. *before* and *after* chill; less frequently between heat and sweat.

Ferrum.	Pulsatilla.
Alternating, cheerful one evening, sad the next—Haughtiness—Irritability—Vehemence.	Fear — Calm, lachrymose sadness of mild dispositions — Indifference — Distrust — Peevishness — Boldness — Avarice — Amorousness.
Ailments from anger	Consequences of excessive joy, fright, grief, mortification, or of vexation with fright, dread or fear — Unconsciousness — Absent-mindedness—Fancies.
Faculty of hysterical patients to see at night in the dark.	Nocturnal blindness.
Styes on upper lids	Styes on upper and lower lids. C.Hg.
Generally loss of appetite	Generally hunger.
Aversion to sour things	Appetite for sour things.
Vomit sour	Vomit, bitter oftener than sour.
Diarrhœa painless	Diarrhœa generally painful.
Catamenia generally too profuse and of long* duration.	Catamenia too scanty and of short duration.
Expectoration predom.; morning. . . .	Expectoration predom.; morning and during day.
Worse after midnight, morning and evening.	*Worse* afternoon, evening, and before midnight.
Worse after coughing	*Worse while coughing.*
Worse after bodily exertion	Often aggrav. by mental exertion. C.Hg.
Better from wine when it is not acid, but worse from beer.	Worse from spirituous liquors, mostly from brandy.
Worse after sleep	*Worse or* better after sleep.

Predomin. worse ——— **Predomin. better**

Out-doors, in cold weather, from growing cold, from washing and moistening diseased part, and from sour things.

Predomin. better ——— **Predomin. worse**

In-doors, on warm days, from growing warm, and from drinking wine.

---

* Both remedies, given in X^0 after Catamenia, brought it on again. C.Hg.

Ferrum.	Sulphur.
Upper right, lower left side—Increased irritability.	Upper left, lower right side—Want of bodily irritability.
Painful ulcers—Hæmorrhages, blood light-red.	Painless ulcers—Hæmorrhages, blood dark.
Ferrum aggravates syphilis, like the Sulphates.	Sulphur acts curatively on syphilis complicated with psora.
Chill, lessened after getting out of bed . . .	More chill after getting out of bed.
Sweat often confined to lower part of body .	Sweat often confined to upper part of body.
Sweat lessened after meals and when talking .	Sweat increased after meals and when talking.
Thirst, particularly during chill	Thirst greatest during heat, but most constant during sweat.
Mood predominantly cheerful; also alternating merry one evening, sad the next; haughty; vehement; quarrelsome.	Mood anxious; indifferent; despondent; sad; gentle; serious and solemn; peevish.
Ailments from anger	Ailments from hearing bad news, from shame, mortification, or from vexation with fright, dread, or fear—Unconsciousness—Absentmindedness—Fancies—Insanity—Imbecility.
Apoplexy more frequent than paralysis . .	Paralysis more frequent than apoplexy.
Appetite for bread	Aversion to bread, particularly to rye-bread.
Urine alkaline—Spasmodic labor-pains . . .	Urine sour—Labor-pains weak or ceasing.
Catamenia too profuse and of long duration; watery.	Catamenia generally too scanty and of short duration; blood dark.
Expectoration predominant; morning . . .	Expectoration not constant; morning and during day, less frequently at night.
Complaints predominant on upper arm . . .	Complaints predominant on fore-arm.
Remission *during day* and before midnight .	Remission afternoon and before midnight.
Worse from growing cold and in cold weather, better when growing warm and in warm air.	Better (resp. worse) fr. grow'g cold & in cold weather, *or* fr. grow'g warm & in warm air.
Worse out-doors, better in-doors	Better (resp. worse) out-doors *or* in-doors.
Almost always aggravated in bed	*Worse or* better in bed.
Worse when lying on side, better when lying on back.	Generally as with Ferrum, but often the opposite.
Worse when turning in bed, and from change of position when lying or standing.	*Worse or* better from change of position.
Better after getting out of bed	Worse *or* better after getting out of bed.
Worse on an empty stomach, better after breakfast.	Better (resp. worse) on an empty stomach *or* after breakfast.
Better from wine when it is not acid . . .	Predominantly worse from wine.
Better *or* worse after meals	Worse after meals.
Better *or* worse from smoking	Worse from smoking.
Worse when looking up	Worse when looking down.
Worse when stooping	Worse *or* better when stooping.
Better when sitting down	*Better or* worse when sitting down.
Predominantly worse when sitting	Better *or* worse when sitting.
Worse *or* better when stretching out diseased limb or when drawing it up.	Predominantly worse when stretching out diseased limb, better when drawing it up.
Better when moving diseased part	Worse *or* better when moving diseased part.
Worse from the touch	*Worse or* better from the touch.
Worse *or* better when speaking	Worse from speaking.
Ailments from Iodine and Arsenic	Ailments from abuse of metals.

Predomin. worse —— **Predomin. better**

From cold, from warm diet, and when descending.

Predomin. better —— **Predomin. worse**

From warmth, from cold diet, when ascending, from drinking wine, straining the eyes, reading and writing, from mental or bodily exertion, when walking fast and running.

N.B. We very rarely find the over-sensitiveness of Ferrum to pain with Sulphur.

Fluor. acid.	Nitr. acid.
Right side—Irritability increased	*Left* side—Want of irritability.
Pain pressing outward	Pain pressing inward.
Dry cutaneous eruptions	Humid eruptions.
Scars redden and itch	Scars hurt with changes of weather; break open. C.Hg.
Pulse somewhat accelerated only by motion.	Pulse unequal; double; intermitting.
Sweat, lessened after meals	Sweat, increased after meals.
Neither vertigo, chill, nor spasms	Chill—Very rarely paralysis.

Moodiness in the evening	Moodiness in the morning—Distrust—Maliciousness.
No delirium	Unconsciousness.
In the morning, on awaking from short sleep, he feels as though he had slept all night.	In the morning, on awaking, feels as though he had not slept enough.
Sensation of warmth in the teeth	Sensation of coldness in the teeth.
Thirst	Thirst is wanting during chill and is not constant during heat; (often in the morning on awaking.) C.Hg
Hunger predominant	Loss of appetite predominant.
Diarrhœa painful	Diarrhœa preval. painless.
Urine too often	Urine scanty.
Erections predominant, with strong sexual desire.	Erections with weak sexual desire.
No expectoration with cough	Expectoration with cough not constant.
Complaints predominant on upper arm and on tip of elbow.	Complaints predominant on fore-arm and on patella.

Remission morning and before midnight .	Remission of complaints in forenoon.
Oppression of chest, better when bending back.	Oppression of chest, worse when bending back.
Worse while riding	*Better* while riding, *worse afterwards.*
Better *or* worse after urinating	Worse after urinating.
Ailments from Silicea	Ailments from Calcarea or Digitalis.

Predomin. worse ——— **Predomin. better**

When riding, from crossing the limbs, during rest, and when lying on unpainful side.

Predomin. better ——— **Predomin. worse**

When lying on painful side, when moving, when perspiring, and from washing with cold water.

Fluor. acid.	Pulsat.
Often indicated with old people	Often indicated with children and women.
Paralysis more frequent than with Pulsatilla.	Apoplexy.
Itching, lessened by scratching	Itching unchanged *or* aggrav. by scratching.
Pulse somewhat accelerated only by motion.	Pulse generally frequent, small, and weak; sometimes intermitting or imperceptible.
Sweat on suffering part	Heat on diseased part.
One-sided sweat, left side	One-sided sweat, right side.
Thirst	Want of thirst predom., but constant only during chill; often thirst *before* and *after* chill, less frequently between heat & sweat.
Heat increased by motion	Heat abating when moving.
Fixed pain in limbs	Pain in limbs, leaping from place to place.
Sensation of going to sleep of side not lain on.	Sensation of going to sleep of side lain on
Inclination for washing with cold water* .	Aversion to washing with cold water.

Fluor. acid.	Pulsat.
Cheerfulness—Irritability	Calm sadness of mild dispositions.
Neither vertigo, chill, nor spasms	Consequences of suppressed vexation—Unconsciousness.
	Delirium
Urine too often	Urine infrequent and scanty.
Cough without expectoration	Cough generally with expectoration.
	Expectoration mornings and during day.
Complaints predominant on inside of nose, on tip of elbow, on the inside of hands & fingers, and on instep, also in upper part of chest.	Nasal complaints external, oftener than internal; complaints predominant in hollow of elbow, on back of hand, and generally on sole of foot; also in lower part of chest.
Dryness in larynx and trachea	Accumulation of mucus in larynx & trachea.
Difficult respiration, better when lying bent backwards.	Difficult respiration, worse when lying with head low.

Fluor. acid.	Pulsat.
REMISSION mornings and before midnight.	REMISSION from midnight till noon.

Predomin. worse — **Predomin. better**

From walking in the open air,† from bodily exertion, from stretching out diseased limb, from acids, and from pressure.

Predomin. better — **Predomin. worse**

In-doors, during sweat, from rubbing and scratching, and when drawing up diseased limb.

N.B. Fluor. acid seems to lack the over-sensitiveness of Pulsat. to pain.

---

* With both remedies complaints are prevalently improved by washing.

† Only the exertion of walking aggrav., enduring the coldest weather as well as tropical heat extraordinarily well, is characteristic for Fluor. acid. C. Hg.

Fluor. acid.	Silicea.
Upper left, lower right side—Muscles rigid.	Upper right, lower left side—Muscles lax.
Insensibility — Often indicated with old people.	Over-sensitiveness — often indicated with children.
Scars redden and itch	Scars painful, break open. C. Hg.
Ulcers, worse from warmth, better from cold.	Ulcers, better from warmth, worse from cold.
Discharge from ulcers very copious. . . .	Discharge scanty or copious. C.Hg.
Atrophy of brain	In children, large head and open sutures.
Pricking itching, lessened by rubbing, brushing, etc., more on warm days.	Pricking itching, worse from scratching, sometimes unchanged, more in cold weather.
Apoplexy not yet observed	Vertigo—Chill—Spasms.
Pulse somewhat accelerated only by motion.	Pulse quick, small, and hard; often irregular.
Sweat increased in-doors, abating after meals.	Sweat abating in-doors, increased after meals.
Heat with inclination to uncover	Heat with aversion to uncover.
Sweat on diseased part	Coldness on suffering part.

Fluor. acid.	Silicea.
Irritable mood	Dejection—Gentleness—Amorousness.
Meutal excitability	Unable to think—Fancies.
Forgetfulness every evening, on the other hand, good memory in the morning.	Forgetfulness every morning.
Toothache, worse from cold drink; *or* improved, until the water becomes warm in the mouth.	Toothache worse from *warm* diet.
Hunger predominant	Want of appetite predominant.
Diarrhœa—Bellyache after stool	Constipation more frequent than diarrhœa—Remission of bellyache after stool.
Expectoration not yet observed	Expectoration predominant; during day.
Compl. predom in upper part of chest, on upper arm, on surface of hands and on top of foot.	Compl. predom. in lower part of chest, on fore-arm, back of hand and on sole of foot.
Lameness of upper limbs	Lameness of lower limbs. C.Hg.

Fluor. acid.	Silicea.
Remission mornings and before midnight.	Remission before midnight.
Pain, *better during* sweat	Pain, *worse after* sweat.
Worse in wet-cold weather	Worse in dry-cold weather.
Worse from bodily exertion	Better *or* worse from bodily exertion.
Some symptoms worse in-doors, others out-doors.	Worse out-doors; better in-doors.

Predomin. **better** 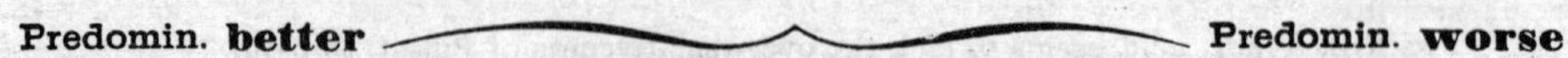 Predomin. **worse**

In dry weather, from uncovering, from cold, washing with cold water, when lying on painful side, and from rubbing and scratching.

Predomin. **worse** 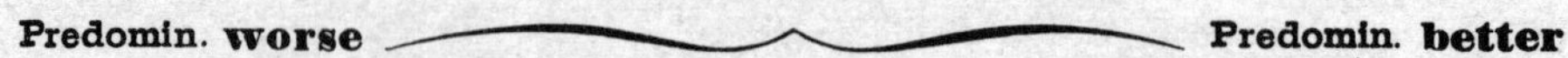 Predomin. **better**

In wet weather, from wrapping up, from warmth, and when lying on unpainful side.

Fluor. acid.	Sulphur.
Right side predom.—Increased irritability.	*Left* side—Want of irritability.
Ulcers painful	Ulcers, painless, itching.
Sensation of going to sleep of side not lain on.	Sensation of going to sleep of side lain on.
Pulse somewhat accelerated only by motion.	Pulse quick, full, and hard; sometimes intermitting.
Sweat on suffering part	Coldness on suffering part.
Heat lessened by washing	Heat increased by washing.
Sweat lessened after meals	Sweat increased after meals.
Heat on upper part of body	Heat on lower part of body, or general, with exception of head.
Thirst	Thirst greatest during hot stage, but most constant during sweating stage.
In the evening in bed loss of sleepiness by crowding of thoughts.	In the evening, in bed, when closing eyes, stupefaction and torpor.
In the morning on awaking from short sleep, it seems to him as though he had slept all night.	In the morning on awaking, feeling of not having had sufficient sleep.

Fluor. acid.	Sulphur.
Cheerfulness	Sadness — Hopelessness — Fear—Solemn, serious mood—Gentleness.
Alternation of active and weak memory .	Weakness of memory—Unconsciousness — Delirium—Fancies—Insanity.
Atrophy of brain	In children large head and open sutures.
Sensation of heaviness in the teeth . . .	Sensation of looseness of teeth. C.Hg.
Complaints predominant on inner angle of eye, on upper arm, on tip of elbow, and on top of foot.	Compl. predom. on external angle of eye, on fore-arm, in hollow of elbow, patella and sole of foot.
Hunger predominant	Generally want of appetite.
Desire for wine	Inclination *or* aversion for beer and spirituous liquors.
Urine alkaline	Urine sour.
Dryness in larynx and trachea	Larynx and trachea filled with mucus.
Cough dry	Cough either loose *or* dry.

Fluor. acid.	Sulphur.
Remission mornings and before midnight.	Remission *afternoon* and before midnight.
Worse after stool	Better *or* worse after stool.
Worse in the open air	Better *or* worse in the open air.
Better during sweat	*Worse during and after* sweat.
Worse from being awake at night . . .	Worse from sleeping too long.

Predomin. worse — **Predomin. better**

From external pressure, and when lying on unpainful side.

Predomin. better — **Predomin. worse**

During sweat, from washing with cold water, bending diseased part backwards, and when lying on painful side.

N.B. Fluor. acid seems to lack the numb sensation in suffering parts peculiar to Sulphur.

Gelseminum.	Aconitum.
Hæmorrhages, crimson blood, in drops . . .	Hæmorrh., light-red blood; brief; in streams.
Muscles relaxed, inaction of motory nerves .	Muscles rigid, inaction of sensitive nerves.*
Slow pulse predom.; is accelerated by moving the body, lessened after lying down.	Quick pulse pred.; acceler. mostly by emotions or coughing, or wh. lying, part. on left side.*
Pulse omitting every 10th beat; during the interval double beat of heart. B. Fincke.†	During three beats of pulse the point of heart touches wall of chest only once. Pereira.‡
Chills moderate; heat severe—Tendency to remit or intermit—Skin hot and dry in gastric and nervous fevers—Profuse sweat relieves in gastric fevers—Tendency to sleep in fever.	Rigors; inflammatory heat—Tendency to continuation—Skin hot & dry, with agony, tossing about; in inflammatory fevers*—Profuse sweat relieves in rheumatic fevers.*
Wakening from sleep by headache or colic .	Wakening from sleep by nightmare.*
Supersensitive; languid	Anxious; restless.
Cannot follow an idea for any length of time.	Ideas haunt him, cannot get rid of them.*
Gr't irritability, does not wish to be spoken to.	Gr't anguish or sadness, likes to be spoken to.*
Short, sharp cries in teething	Anxious lamentations.
Solicitude about the present*—Fear of falling.	Solicitude about the future*—Fear of death.
Complaints after hearing bad news, part. diarrhœa, chilliness, threatening abortion, &c.	Complaints following fright or vexation with fear, vehemence, rage, or anger.*
Ailm. fr. fright & fear following *immediately*.	Ailments from fright or fear following *later*.*
Vertigo *during chill* or while walking . . .	V. during fever or when getting up from seat.*
Head too light (Tilde) or too heavy; the latter disappears after urinating (Hale).	Head too heavy, worse after moving.*
Headache, every step aggravates	Headache, sunlight or least noise aggravates.*
Head feels too big	Forehead feels too full.
Fulln'ss, princip. in sinciput, heavin. in occiput.	Heaviness in sinciput, fulln. in the whole head.
Aversion to light, partic. candle-light . . .	Aversion or desire to light, partic. sunlight.*
Sight of distant objects confused	Sight dazzled by light.
Lateral oscillation of eye-balls	Distorted appearance of the eyes.
Eyes heavy and suffused	Eyes reddened; lachrymation.
Face crimson, w. fev.; leaden palen'ss w. pains.	Cheeks uneqally red, or red, hot, and bloated.
Face pale, with sickness and faintness from seeing wounded persons.	Face red while lying, turns pale, with faintness, from assuming an erect position.*
Expression of suffering—Lips crimson . . .	Expression of terror or of apathy—Lips livid.
Toothache in decayed teeth—Foul taste . .	Toothache in sound teeth—Bitter taste.
Pharynx feels as if filled up—Paral. dysphagia.	Pharynx feels dry. — Urging to swallow.*
Moderate thirst—Vomiting of ingesta . . .	Viol. th. pred.—Vomit. of mucus, blood or bile.
Windy wandering colic	Great tenderness of abdomen; stitching pains.
Curdled, or tea-green, or yellow stools . . .	Stools like chopped herbs, or black, or watery.
Congestions in chest; labored, painf. breath'g.	Cong. in chest, stitches, rattling, short breath.
Aching in the back and extremities	Pain in back and extremities as if bruised.
Aggrav. pred. afternoon, or all night, or all day.	**Aggravation** pred. forenoon and after midnight.
Aggr. ab't noon, fr. 11—3 o'cl. P.M. W.P.Wesselh.	Remission all day.*
Worse from warmth of bed	Better when growing warm; from warmth in general.*
Better from warm drink	Better from cold drink.*
Worse in the open air (pains)	Better in the open air (nervous symptoms).*
Worse in damp weather, before a thunder-storm, S.E. wind.*	Worse in dry weather, during clear weather and dry winds, N.W. wind.*
Better when sitting (headache)	Better when sitting still (rheumatism).*
Worse when looking sideways	Worse when looking downwards.*
Worse after breakfast	Worse before breakfast.*
Wine aggravates, partic. headache; also smoking (headache).	Desire for wine, and it betters; worse fr. smoking (palpitation).*

Predomin. **worse** ———— Predomin. **better**

From warm coverings, after sleeping, in the afternoon, J. C. M.; after *breakfast*, walking in open air, and drinking wine.*

Predomin. **better** ———— Predomin. **worse**

By gentle motion, *when erect*, from pressure, J. C. M.; after *urinating* and after sleep.*

N.B. Aconit. lacks the dullness and giddinesss accompanying the pains of Gelseminum, while Gelseminum has not the thirst and red face as a concomitant of pains like Aconit.*

† Omission of the pulse after ten to twenty beats has been observed thus far only from Agaric., Laches., Oxal. ac.; a double beat of the heart during this omission only with Gelsem.*

‡ Aconit. may be indicated by pulsus dicrotus, but not the Gelseminum.*

N B. Communicated by Dr. J. C. Morgan as a contribution to this work, * added by C. Hg.

Gelseminum.	Belladonna.
Upper right, lower left side predom.—From above downwards.	*Upper left, lower right side*—Rush of blood upwards.
Pulse accelerated with the pains	Pulse accelerated *or* retarded with the pains.
Fever all night; all day; more in afternoon. M.	Fever predom. afternoon, but especially in the evening. C.Hg.
With the sweat great relief of all symptoms.	With the sweat many mental and bodily symptoms appear. C.Hg.
Itching of skin preventing early sleep; otherwise more sleepless after midnight .	Sleeplessness, preval. especially before midnight.
Delirious while falling asleep	Dreams immediately as soon as he falls asleep. C.Hg.
Sensitive disposition; irritability; does not like to be spoken to or to speak; dejected; out of humor; indolent—Mental dullness.	Predom. insensibility of disposition; cheerfullness *or* dejection; loquacity *or* taciturnity—Predom. hastiness in all movements *—Ecstacies *or* mental dullness.
Cataleptic immobility with dilated pupils, closed eyes; but conscious of all that transpires. M.	Unconsciousness, also with stupefaction and loss of sight, dilated pupils and delirium.
Ailments from hearing bad and exciting news; chilliness (upper r. s.) headache, threatening of diarrhœa.	Ailments from fright, anger, mortification, or from vexation with fright, fear or vehemence.
Muscular pains, (especially in back, thighs, and calves, M.) better by gentle motions, worse fr. warmth of bed & after midnight.	Pain, partic. before midnight and when moving; generally *better by the warmth* of the bed.
Sensation in the head of lightness—of vertigo—(of bigness, M.)	Heaviness of head.
Headache increases with the sun; abates during first hours of afternoon and first *after* midnight;—better after sleep. M.	Remission of complaints after midnight and in the *forenoon*—Aggravation (during and) after sleep. M.
Nocturnal sore pain in eyes	Pain in eyes predom. in day time.
Dim and confused or double outlines apparent in distant objects. M.	Aggrav. when looking at near objects.
Crimson hue of the cheeks	Scarlet redness of the face. M.
Soon gets enough while eating	Want of feeling satisfied when eating.
Cramp in stomach better by riding . . .	Complaints aggrav. by concussion.
Gastr. oppres., worse by pressure of clothes.	Complaints predom. improved by pressure.
Bland fluent coryza	Predom. dry coryza.
Pains (in occiput, M.) and nape of neck worse when lying, H.Gr.—with the head low, better when on high pillows, with the eyes closed. M.	Pains in nape of neck better by lying on back—Predom. improvement by lying down; worse (illusions) on closing the eyes. M.
Complaints predom. in fore-arm and calf .	Complaints predom. in upper arm and shin.
Complains caused by thunder-storm . . .	Aggrav. during full moon.
Worse *or* (nausea, trembl'g) bett. in op. air.	Predom. worse in open air, better in doors

Predomin. worse —— **Predomin. better**

During rest † and from warmth of bed, also when looking at distant objects.

Predomin. better —— **Predomin. worse**

From (gentle) motion, from turning (shaking) the head and after sleep, from concussion and when looking at near objects.

N.B. All that is marked M. has been added by Dr. J. C. Morgan.

---

* Yet we also find aversion to motion and work with Bellad.

† Gelseminum has amelioration of the muscular pains and headache during *perfect rest* in certain positions, relaxing muscles. M

Glonoin.	Belladonna.
Left side predominant—Paraplegia . . .	*Right* side—Hemiplegia.
The more frequent the pulse, the more violent the headache.	The pulse is retarded quite as often as accelerated or unchanged with the pain.
Pulse sometimes double (compare Digit.) or intermitting.	Pulse sometimes intermitting.
Walking up and down at night on account of headache.	Running about at night because of insane fear.
Anxious feeling in pit of stomach with pain there.	Anxious feeling around the heart.
Yawning and inclination to bend head and spine backwards.	Yawning and stretching.
Weak memory	Memory active *or* weak.
Vertigo when stepping out-doors	Vertigo, better when stepping out-doors.
Vertigo or cramping in the back of the neck when bending head back.	Complaints better when bending head back.
Coldness, sometimes general with exception of head.	Sweat, sometimes general with exception of head.
Throbbing in head from back to front part.	Beating in head from front to back and to sides.
Headache *worse* after lying down and when stooping, and in *damp weather*, better after sufficient sleep, out-doors, and after vomiting.	Headache generally *better* after lying down, and when stooping; generally *aggrav.* in *dry weather; worse* after sleep, out-doors and by vomiting.
In megrim one sees everything half light and half dark.	Double sight.
Faceache, worse from warmth of bed . .	Faceache, better from warmth of bed.
Under-lip feels swollen	Swelling and sensation as of swelling of the lips, particularly upper lip.
Nausea, better during sweat	Complaints worse during sweat, better after it.
Respiration (partic. expiration) accelerated.	Respiration either accelerated *or* retarded; particularly often quick inspiration and slow expiration.
Palpitation of heart, ceases after getting up from lying, and when walking about.	Palpitation of heart worse when moving.
Coldness of the hands	Heat *or* coldness of hands.
Complaints *better* after drinking water . .	*Worse* when and after drinking.
Walking* eases pain in limbs and palpitation of heart.	Walking, motion in general, aggrav. all symptoms.

Predomin. better — **Predomin. worse**

In dry weather, in cold open air, from uncovering,† particularly uncovering the head, from drinking coffee, after sleep, after vomiting, during motion and sweat.

Predomin. worse — **Predomin. better**

In wet weather, in-doors, from wrapping up, partic. wrapping up head, when bending the head back, when stooping, after lying down, when holding the breath, from warmth of bed, and during rest.

* Other symptoms of Glon. like those of Bell. grow worse from motion, better during rest.

† Only the *sensation of coldness* of Glon. is increased by uncovering.

Graphit.	Calcarea.
Complaints predom. in external parts	Complaints predom. in internal parts.
Pain pressing outward—Pain rending downwards.	Pain pressing inward—Pain rending upwards.
Eruptions generally humid	Eruptions generally dry.
Pulse full and hard, but not perceptibly accelerated.	Pulse full and accelerated, often trembling.
Heat or sweat with aversion to uncover	Heat or sweat with inclination to uncover.
First chill, then heat	First heat, then chill.
Want of thirst, partic. during heat	Thirst is wanting only sometimes during chill.
Dreams of water, embarrassment, misfortunes, &c.; also dreams that exert the mind.	Dreams of fire, sickness, vexation, and quarrel, also phantastic ones.

Graphit.	Calcarea.
Mood changing; sad and despondent	Dejection *or* silly merriness.
Ailments from grief	Ailm. from hearing bad news, or from vexation with fright, dread or fear.
Neither fancies, unconsciousness, nor delirium.	Insanity—*Imbecility*.
Vertigo, inclining to fall forward	Vertigo, inclining to fall backwards or sideways.
Complaints predom. on inner angle of eye	Complaints predom. on external angle of eye.
Optical illusions in bright colors	Optical illusions black or in dark colors.
Acute smell predom.	Loss of smell.
Eruption on upper lip	Eruption predom. on under lip.
Complaints predom. on lower jaw and lower teeth, on inside of gums and in hollow of knee.	Complaints predom. on upper jaw and upper teeth, on outside of gums, and on patella.
Urine scanty	Urine too often.
Catamenia too scanty, of short duration, and late.	Catamenia too profuse, of long duration, and generally too soon.
Nasal secretion watery	Nasal secretion thick.
Expectoration almost constant; during day and evening.	Expector. predom., but not constant, mornings and during day.

Graphit.	Calcarea.
Remission of complaints during day	Remission before midnight.
Worse *or* better from warmth of bed	Worse from warmth of bed.
Worse when hungry	Worse after a satisfying meal.
Generally better when swallowing	Worse when swallowing.
Generally better after drinking	Worse after drinking.
Worse from washing or moistening	*Worse or* better* from moistening.
Worse from cold diet; better from warm diet.	Worse (resp. better) from cold *or* warm diet.
Worse while perspiring	*Worse or* better when perspiring.
Worse when looking up	Worse when looking up *or* down.
Worse from light; better in the dark	Better (resp. worse) from light *or* in the dark.
Worse from sneezing	*Worse or* better from sneezing.

Predomin. worse —— **Predomin. better**

In-doors, when lying on painful side, from uncovering, from the touch, when sitting, when lifting or resting diseased limb on anything, and after breakfast.

Predomin. better —— **Predomin. worse**

Out-doors,† when lying on unpainful side, from wrapping up, from pressure, after sweat, when‡ riding, when letting diseased limb hang down, *before* breakfast, when swallowing, from spirituous liquors, and *after* drinking.

N.B. With Calcarea, which bears the character of want of irritability, we very rarely find the over-sensitiveness to pain peculiar to Graphit.

---

* "*Improvement by moistening*" we only find with the abdominal inflammation of Calcarea.

† "*When walking out-doors*" both remedies have predom. aggrav.; therefore, the influence of the open air is not decisive for Graph., but that of motion.

‡ "*After* riding" the complaints of Graph. are aggrav.

Graphit.	Natr. carb.
Trembling sensation in internal parts . .	Trembling of external parts.
Discharge from ulcers copious or scanty .	Discharge from ulcers copious. C.Hg.
Pulse full and hard, but accelerated only somewhat in the morning.	Pulse frequent at night, slow during day.
Want of thirst, particularly during heat .	Thirst predominant, but generally not until *after* chill.
Chill increased after meals	Chill lessened after meals.

Graphit.	Natr. carb.
Mood changing; sad.	Mood glad *or* dull; serious; irritable; malicious—Avarice.
Ailments from grief	Ailments from vexation with fright—*Imbecility*—Insanity.
Optical illusions in bright colors	Optical illusions in dark colors.
Nasal complaints predom. internal . . .	Nasal complaints predom. external.
Sour vomit	Predom. bitter vomit.
Constipation predominant—When diarrhœa occurs, it is preval. painless.	Painful diarrhœa predominant.
Urine scanty.	Urine too often and copious.
Catamenia too late and scanty	Catamenia too soon and profuse.
Leucorrhœa watery	Leucorrhœa thick.
Nasal secretion watery	Nasal secretion thick.
Expectoration during day and evening . .	Expectoration morning and evening.

Graphit.	Natr. carb.
REMISSION of complaints during day . .	REMISSION before midnight.
Worse when hungry	Worse after a satisfying meal.
Worse after stool	Worse *or* better after stool.
Worse *or* better from growing cold (resp. growing warm).	Predom. worse from growing cold, better from growing warm.
Worse after sleep	*Worse or* better after sleep.
Worse *or* better after getting out of bed .	Predom. better after getting out of bed.
Worse when rising from a seat	Better *or* worse when rising from a seat.
Worse from straining the eyes	Better *or* worse from straining the eyes.
Worse during sweat	Better *or* worse when sweating.
Ailments from Arsenic	Ailments from abuse of Cinchona.

Predomin. worse ——— **Predomin. better**

From motion, when walking, when getting out of bed, from the touch, and in-doors.

Predomin. better ——— **Predomin. worse**

During rest, after lying down, when lying and standing, out-doors, from spirituous liquors, after drinking, and after sweat.

N.B. Natr. carb. lacks the sensation of numbness in suffering parts peculiar to Graphit.

Graphit.	Petroleum.
Sensitiveness or tension in internal parts .	Sensitiveness or tension in external parts.
Eruptions generally humid—Itch humid .	Eruptions dry *or* humid—Dry itch.
Pulse full and hard, but not perceptibly accelerated, except in the morning.	Pulse slow during rest, but stronger, full and accelerated by every motion, partic. in the evening.
Want of thirst, particularly during heat .	Thirst during heat, but not during chill.
Chill increased after meals, lessened in the open air.	Chill lessened after meals, increased in the open air.
Sweat often confined to the front part of body.	Sweat often confined to the back part of body.

Graphit.	Petroleum.
Mood changing—Amorousness	Mood malicious—Mental dullness.
Ailments from grief	Ailments from fright, or from vexation with fright.
Nasal complaints internal, and complaints on inside of gums predom.	Nasal complaints external, and complaints on exterior of gums predom.
Burning sensation in the teeth.	Sensation of coldness in the teeth. C.Hg.
Sour vomit	Predom. bitter vomit.
Diarrhœa quite rare, and, when it occurs, painless.	Diarrhœa generally painful.
Urine scanty	Urine too often, but scanty.
Catamenia too late and scanty.	Catamenia too late and scanty, *or* too soon and profuse.
Respiration with dry sound	Respiration predom. with moist sound.
Expectoration almost constant; during day and evening.	Expectoration infrequent; during day.

Graphit.	Petroleum.
AGGRAVATION from evening till morning .	AGGRAVATION morning and evening till midnight.
Worse during full moon	Worse before thunder-storm.
Worse (resp. better) from growing cold *or* warm.	Predom. worse from growing cold, better from growing warm.
Worse *or* better after getting out of bed .	Better after getting out of bed.
Worse when stretching out diseased limb, better when drawing it up.	Worse *or* better when stretching out the limb and when drawing it up.
Worse from touch.	Worse *or* better from touch.
Worse from straining the eyes	*Worse or* better from straining the eyes.
Generally better when swallowing and after drinking, but particularly worse when swallowing saliva.	Worse when swallowing and after drinking, partic. worse when swallowing food.

Predomin. worse — **Predomin. better**

When sitting, in-doors, and after breakfast.

Predomin. better — **Predomin. worse**

When standing and riding, out-doors, before breakfast, when swallowing, after drinking, particularly spirituous liquors, and after sweat.

Graphit.	Silicea.
Sensitiveness of internal parts; crawling sensation in external parts.	Sensitiveness of external parts; crawling sensation in internal parts.
Eruptions generally humid—Humid itch	Eruptions generally dry—Dry itch.
Scars burn, break open	Scars sore to the touch, break open. C.Hg
Distention of veins of feet	Distention of veins of hands.
Pulse full and hard, but not perceptibly accelerated, except mornings.	Pulse small, hard, and quick, often irregular; quick at night, slow during day.
Want of thirst, partic. during heat	Thirst predom., partic. during heat.
Sweat often confined to front part of body.	Sweat often confined to back part of body.
Chill lessened in the open air	Chill increased in the open air.
Rarely paralysis - No apoplexy	*Paralysis*—Apoplexy.
Mood changing	Gentleness—Fancies.
Optical illusions in bright colors	Optical illusions in black or in dark colors.
Complaints of inner ear predom.	Complaints of external ear most frequent.
Predom. acute smell	Loss of smell.
Hunger predom.	Generally loss of appetite.
Sour vomit	Bitter vomit.
Belly-ache after stool	Remission of belly-ache after stool.
Urine scanty—Sediment whitish	Urine too often—Sedim. reddish or yellow
Catamenia too late and scanty	Catamenia generally too late and scanty, but often also too soon and profuse.
Hard scars, remaining after mammary abscesses, are absorbed. Guernsey.	Hard-edged fistulous ulcers, remaining after mammary abscesses. W. Gross.
Expectoration during day and evening	Expectoration during day.
Complaints predom. on shoulder joint	Complaints predom. on hip joint.
Remission of complaints during day	Remission before midnight.
Worse (resp. better) from growing cold *or* warm.	Predom. worse from growing cold; better from growing warm.
Worse from washing and moistening diseased part.	*Worse or* better from washing.
Worse in bed	*Better or* worse in bed.
Worse or better from warmth of bed	Better from warmth of bed.
Worse when hungry	Worse after a satisfying meal.
Better *or* worse after meals	Almost always aggrav. after meals.
Improv. oftener than aggrav. after drinking.	Aggrav. oftener than improv. after drinking.
Worse *or* better from weeping	Worse from weeping.
Worse from bodily exertion	Worse *or* better from exertion.
Ailments from Arsenic	Ailments from Sulph., Mercur., or from sting of insects.

Predomin. worse —— **Predomin. better**

In-doors, in bed and from warmth of bed; also during continued motion.

Predomin. better —— **Predomin. worse**

Out-doors,* when lying, when riding, after perspiring, from pressure, when swallowing, after drinking, partic. spirituous liquors, and during rest.

---

* "*When walking out-doors*" both remedies have predom. aggrav.; therefore the influence of motion, and not that of the open air, must decide for Graphit.

Helleb. nig.	Arsenic.
Muscles lax—Gnawing pain in external parts.	Muscles rigid—Gnawing pain in intern. parts.
Itching, unchanged by scratching	Itching, aggrav. by scratching.
Humid eruptions	Eruptions generally dry.
Loosing hair from the eye-brows and pudenda.	Loosing hair from the head, partic. the anterior part. C. Hg.
Very rarely paralysis of limbs	Paralysis.
Pulse slow, small, and weak	Pulse very mucn accelerated, small, and weak; sometimes intermitting.
Pulse often slower than beating of heart	Pulse suppressed, with strong beating of heart.
Want of thirst predom.	Least thirst during chill, most during sweat; patient drinks often, but little at a time during heat.
First heat, then chill	First chill, then heat.
Chill increased after getting out of bed	Chill lessened after getting out of bed.

Helleb. nig.	Arsenic.
Insensibility of disposition	Sensitive disposition.
Distrust	Mood anxious, peevish, irritable, malicious—Avariciousness.
Absent-mindedness—Fancies	Delirium—Insanity.*
Complaints of external ear predom.	Complaints of inner ear predom.
Thirst with disgust for drink	Desire for drink without thirst.
Generally hunger	Generally loss of appetite.
Nausea, partic. in the stomach	Nausea, partic. in the throat.
Urine often, but scanty	Urine scanty (with diarrhœa) *or* copious.
Retention of urine	Incontinence oftener than retention of **urine**.
Respiration slow	Respiration quick.
Cough, without expectoration	Cough generally *with* expectoration.
Complaints predom. on thigh	Complaints predom. on leg.
Vesicles around the joints	Erysipelas around the joints.

Helleb. nig.	Arsenic.
Remission of complaints during day	Remission *during day* and before midnight.
Generally better during sleep	Worse during sleep.
Better after sleep	Better after sufficient sleep; but worse on awaking when roused.
Worse in bed	In bed (warmth) better *or* (rest) worse.
Worse *or* better when getting out of bed	Almost alw. improv. when getting out of bed.
Better after perspiring	*Worse or* better after perspiring.
Worse (resp. better) on an empty stomach, *or* after breakfast.	Predom. better on an empty stomach; worse after breakfast.
Worse after stool	*Worse or* better after stool.
Worse *or* better from pressure	Predom. improv. by pressure.
Worse from light, better in the dark	Worse (resp. better) from light *or* in the dark.

Predomin. worse — **Predomin. better**

In a warm room, in company, from warm diet, from warmth of bed, from motion, when walking, when sitting down, when bending diseased limb, and when biting.

Predomin. better — **Predomin. worse**

Out-doors,† when alone, from cold diet, during rest, when sitting and lying, during sleep, and after sweat.

N.B. Helleb. very rarely has the over-sensitiveness to pain which Ars. often has.

---

* "*Imbecility*" is found with both remedies.
† "*When walking out-doors,*" Helleb. has—chiefly in consequence of motion—predominately aggravation.

Helleb. nigr.	Belladonna.
Anæmie	Plethora predominant.
Skin and muscles lax—Inclination for open air.	Skin and muscles rigid Aversion to open air.
Painless cutaneous eruptions	Painful eruptions.
Pulse slow, small, and weak	Pulse generally quick, full, hard, and tense
Chill, lessened out-doors	Chill, increased out-doors.
Sweat, lessened after sleep	Sweat, increased after sleep.
Want of thirst	Thirst not constant; quite rare during chill; often *before* chill, and *after* sweat.

Calm sadness	Mood cheerful *or* sad; changing; anxious; peevish; irritable; malicious.
Ailments from grief, or from vexation with reserved displeasure.	Ailments from fright, anger, mortification, or from vexation with fright, fear, or vehemence.
Weakness of memory	Memory active *or* weak.
Mental dullness – No delirium	Ecstasies *or* mental dullness—Delirium—Insanity.
No apoplexy—Very rarely paralysis . . .	Apoplexy—Paralysis of limbs.
Nausea in stomach, less frequently in abdomen.	Nausea in throat or abdomen, less frequently in stomach.
Red parts become white	External parts become black.

Remission of complaints during day . .	Remission *forenoon* and afternoon.
Worse from light, particularly daylight . .	Worse from light, particularly candle-light
Generally better during sleep	Worse during sleep.
Better *or* worse when getting out of bed .	Worse when getting out of bed.
Better *or* worse after getting out of bed .	Almost always improved after getting out of bed.
Worse when bending diseased part . . .	Worse *or* better when bending diseased part, particularly worse when bending it sideways; better when bending it inwards or backwards, and when holding it bent.
Worse *or* better from pressure.	Predom. better from pressure.
Better after sweat	Worse *or* better after sweat.

Predomin. worse ——— **Predomin. better**

In-doors, in bed and from warmth of bed, when sitting down, when stooping, and when bending diseased part backwards.

Predomin. better ——— **Predomin. worse**

Out-doors,* during sleep, and on awaking.

N.B. With Helleb. we very rarely find the over-sensitiveness of Belladonna to pain; mere sensitiveness (to touch, etc.), on the other hand, is found with "both" remedies.

---

* "When walking out-doors," both remedies have predominant aggravation; therefore, it is chiefly the influence of motion which must decide for Helleb.

Helleb. nigr.	Pulsatilla.
Constitutional want of irritability . . .	Increased irritability.
Pain pressing inwards—No apoplexy . . .	Pain pressing outwards—Apoplexy.
Itching, unchanged by scratching . . .	Itching, aggrav. *or* unchanged by scratching.
Painless cutaneous eruptions	Painful eruptions.
Pulse often slower than beating of heart; generally slow	Pulse sometimes suppressed with strong beating of heart; generally quick.
Chill increased by motion, lessened in warm room.	Chill lessened by motion, increased in warm room.
Heat lessened during sleep	Heat increased during sleep.
Want of thirst constant.	Want of thirst predom., but constant only during chill.

Helleb. nigr.	Pulsatilla.
Insensibility of disposition	Sensitive disposit.—Mood changing; anxious; peevish — Boldness — Avarice — Amorousness.
Ailments from vexation with reserved displeasure.	Ailments from excessive joy, fright, mortification, or from vexation with fright, dread, or fear—Delirium.
Pupils predom. dilated	Pupils generally contracted.
Complaints predom. on external ear, and on upper lip.	Complaints on inner ear and under lip predom.
Appetite for bread	Aversion to bread.
Nausea in stomach, less frequently in abdomen.	Nausea in throat, stomach, or abdomen.
Diarrhœa predom. painless	Diarrhœa generally painful.
Urine often, but scanty	Urine seldom and scanty.
Retention of urine	Incontinence more frequent than retention of urine.
Respiration slow—Cough dry	Respiration quick—Cough generally with expectoration.
Complaints predom. on thigh	Complaints predom. on leg.

Helleb. nigr.	Pulsatilla.
Aggravation from evening till morning . .	Aggravation from noon till midnight.
Worse when respiring deeply	Better *or* worse when respiring deeply.
Worse when swallowing	Better *or* worse when swallowing, partic. worse when swallowing saliva.
Worse after stool.	*Better or* worse after stool.
Better after sweat	*Worse or* better after sweat.
Better after sleep	*Worse or* better after sleep.
Worse from uncovering; better from wrapping up.	*Generally* better from uncovering, worse from wrapping up.
Worse when bending diseased part	Better *or* worse when bending diseased part, partic. better when bending it sideways, or when holding it bent.
Worse when sitting down	Worse *or* better when sitting down.
Better after rising from a seat	*Better or* worse after rising from a seat.

Predomin. worse — **Predomin. better**

From cold, from growing cold and in cold weather, from uncovering, motion, walking, when walking out-doors,* from bodily exertion, after stool, and on inspiration.

Predomin. better — **Predomin. worse**

From warmth, growing warm and in warm air, from wrapping up, during rest, when standing, sitting and lying,† during and after sleep, after sweat, and on expiration.

N.B. The over-sensitiveness of Pulsat. to pain is very rarely found with Helleb.—Mere sensitiveness (to touch, &c.), on the other hand, is found with both remedies.

---

* Both remedies have predom. improv. of complaints "*out-doors*, aggrav. in-doors.

† The symptoms of both remedies are predom. aggrav. "*in bed*" and "*from warmth of bed.*"

Helleb. nig	Veratr. alb.
Want of bodily irritability predominant . .	Increased bodily irritability.
No apoplexy—Very rarely paralysis . . .	Apoplexy—Paralysis.
Epilepsy, with consciousness	Epilepsy, generally with loss of consciousness.
Humid, painless eruptions—Painless ulcers.	Dry, painful eruptions – Painful ulcers.
Pulse regular	Pulse irregular, sometimes intermitting.
Heat or sweat, with aversion to uncover .	Heat or sweat, with inclination to uncover.
Chill increased after getting out of bed .	Chill lessened after getting out of bed.
First heat, then chill	First chill, then heat.
Want of thirst constant	Thirst not constant; least thirst during sweat.

Insensibility of disposition	Sensitive disposition.
Calm sadness—Indifference	Cheerfulness *or* dejection — Fear — Maliciousness—Irritability—Amorousness.
Ailments from vexation with reserved displeasure.	Ailments from fright, anger, grief, or from vexation with dread or fear.
No delirium — Difficult comprehension—Mental dullness—Imbecility.	Delirium—Easy *or* difficult comprehens'n—Rarely mental dullness – Ecstasies—Insanity.
Melancholy, with apathy and stupor . . .	Melancholy with lamentation and disconsolateness.
Pupils predominantly dilated	Pupils generally contracted.
Saliva generally increased	Saliva generally diminished.
Urine often, but scanty	Urine seldom and scanty; only exceptionally copious.
Respiration slow—Cough dry	Respiration quick—Expectoration not constant.
Complaints predom. on thigh	Complaints predom. on leg.

Remission of complaints during day . .	Remission *during day* and evening.
Predom. worse from growing cold, better from growing warm.	Better (resp. worse) from growing cold or from growing warm.
Better *or* worse when assuming an erect position.	Worse when assuming an erect position.
Better after rising from a seat	*Better or* worse after rising from a seat.
Worse *or* better from pressure	*Generally* improved by pressure.
Worse after stool	Worse *or* better after stool.

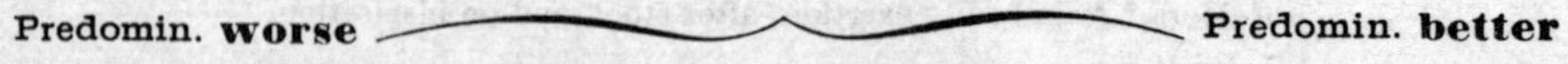

From uncovering, from warm diet, from motion, when walking, when ascending, and when bending diseased part backwards.

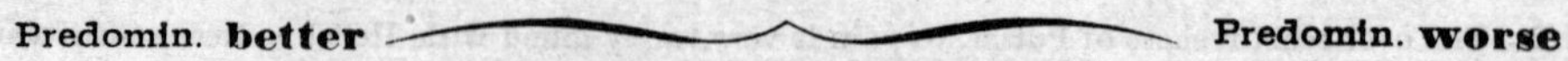

From wrapping up, from cold diet, during rest, when standing, sitting and lying, when descending, during sleep, and on awaking.

Hepar s. c.	Belladonna.
Light hair—Emaciation	Dark hair—Obesity.
Rarely apoplexy or paralysis	Apoplexy—Paralysis.
Sweat increased when and after getting out of bed.	Sweat lessened when and after getting out of bed.

Hepar s. c.	Belladonna.
Sensitive disposition	Insensibility of disposition predominant.
Dejection	Cheerfulness *or* dejection—Indifference.
Ailments of vexation with vehemence . . .	Consequences of anger, mortification, or from vexation with fear or vehemence.
Weak memory.	Memory active *or* weak.
Rarely fancies	Insensibility—Ecstasies or mental dullness.
Complaints predominant in external angle of eye.	Complaints predominant in inner angle of eye.
Short-sightedness—Objects appear too light in dark parts of the room.	Far-sightedness—Objects appear too light in the candle-light.
Mucus or fetid pus discharges from the ears .	Discharge chiefly of blood from the ears.
Appetite for sour things	Aversion to sour things.
Fetid flatus	Scentless flatus.
Discharge of succus prostaticus, particularly with stool and after urinating.	Pollutions predominant.
Expectoration not constant; in morning and during day.	Expectoration infrequent; morning, during day, evening.
Complaints predominant on fore-arm, on tip of elbow, on inner side of thigh, and on top of foot.	Complaints predominant on upper arm, in hollow of elbow, on patella, on outside of thigh, and on sole of foot.

Hepar s. c.	Belladonna.
REMISSION of complaints afternoon	REMISSION *forenoon* and after midnight.
Worse when lying on painful side, better when lying on unpainful side.	Better (resp. worse) when lying on painful *or* on unpainful side.
Generally better when lifting diseased limb and when resting it on anything, worse when letting it hang down.	Worse when lifting diseased limb and when resting it on anything, better when letting it hang down.
Worse when leaning against anything . . .	When leaning against anything worse *or* (against anything hard) better.
Better after sweat	Worse *or* better after perspiring.
Worse *or* better from speaking	Worse from speaking.
Worse when eating or swallowing	*Worse or* better when eat'g or when swallow'g.
Worse when swallowing food and saliva . .	Worse when swallowing, partic. drink.
Worse from spirituous liquors.	Worse *or* better from spirituous liquors.
Worse from eructation	Generally better from eructation.
Worse or better after stool	Worse after stool.
Almost always improved by smoking	Worse from smoking.
Ailments from sleeping on damp ground . .	Ailments from sleeping in the sun *or* moonlight.

Predomin. worse ⟶ **Predomin. better**

On an empty stomach, from cold diet, when stretching out diseased limb or letting it hang down, after getting out of bed, when stooping, from eructation, from pressure, and when turning in bed.

Predomin. better ⟶ **Predomin. worse**

After breakfast, from warm diet,* when drawing up diseased limb, lifting or resting it on anything, and from smoking.

N.B. Both remedies have the symptoms of drinking eagerly, hastily; Bellad. with trembling haste. CHg.

---

* Yet we also find "aggravation by drinking cold water" with Belladonna; this is on account of the difficulty of "swallowing drink."

Hepar s. c.	Lachesis.
Heat, with thirst	Heat, generally without thirst.
Thirst predominant, but not constant; least thirst during chill.	Thirst *before* chill, but not during chill; not very frequent during heat.
Rarely apoplexy	Apoplexy.
Pulse hard, full, and accelerated	Pulse small, weak, and accelerated; often alternating with full and strong beats, generally very unequal.
Anxious dreams	Pleasant dreams.

Hepar s. c.	Lachesis.
Reserve—Mood changing; depressed	Loquacity — Cheerfulness — Haughtiness — Amorousness—Distrust.
Ailments from vexation with vehemence . .	Ailments from jealousy.
Difficult comprehension	Easy comprehension—Ecstasies.
Complaints predominant on upper eyelids . .	Complaints predominant on lower eyelids.
Mucous vomit	Vomiting of food.
Urine seldom and scanty	Urine too often.
Sexual desire too weak	Sexual desire too strong.
Catamenia too soon and profuse	Catamenia too scanty, at the same time too late *or* too soon.
Dry coryza predominant	Fluent coryza predominant.
Expectoration not constant with the cough .	Expectoration infrequent.

Hepar s. c.	Lachesis.
Remission of complaints afternoon	Remission from midnight till noon.
Worse in cold weather; better in warm air .	Generally better in cold weather, worse in warm air.
Worse when lying on painful side, better when lying on unpainful side.	Better (resp. worse) when lying on painful *or* unpainful side.
Worse during sleep and on awaking	*Worse or* better during sleep and on awaking.
Worse when stooping	*Better or* worse when stooping.
Better *or* worse when assuming an erect position.	Worse when assuming an erect position.
Better after rising from a seat	*Better or* worse after rising from a seat.
Worse when swallowing, particularly when swallowing saliva and food.	*Better or* worse when swallowing, particularly worse when swallowing saliva and drink.
Worse during and after meals	Better *or* worse during and after meals.
Worse after drinking	Worse *or* better after drinking.
Worse from spirituous liquors	Better *or* worse from spirituous liquors.
Worse from eructation	Worse *or* better from eructation.
Worse *or* better from speaking	Worse from speaking.
Worse from sneezing	Worse *or* better when sneezing.
Ailments from Silicea or Metals, (Iod or Iodate of Potassium. C.Hg.)	Ailments from abuse of Cinchona, or from sting of insects. (Mercurius. C.Hg.)

Predomin. worse — **Predomin. better**

In cold dry weather, from cold diet, from motion, when walking, shaking the head, respiring deeply, when letting diseased limb hang down, from drinking coffee, when swallowing food, and when stooping.

Predomin. better — **Predomin. worse**

In warm and damp air, from warm diet, during rest, when standing and lying, when lifting diseased limb, and when smoking.

N.B. **Lachesis has the predominant characteristic of increased constitutional irritability; Hepar s. c., on the other hand, at least in chronic complaints, prevalent want of irritability.**

Hepar s. c.	Mercur.
Humid cutaneous eruptions	Eruptions generally dry.
Rarely apoplexy	Apoplexy.
Thirst predom., but not constant; most rare during chill.	Thirst almost constant during all stages of the fever.
Chill lessened in warm room	Chill increased in warm room.
Sweat increased when and after getting out of bed, abating when speaking.	Sweat lessened when and after getting out of bed; increased when speaking.
Congestion of blood to eyes	Congestion of blood to ears.
Dreams of fire, sickness, quarrel, or business of the day.	Dreams of water, thieves, animals, shooting, and misfortunes.
Ailments from fright, or from vexation with vehemence.	Seriousness—Amorousness—Ailments from mortification.
Scrofulous inflammation of eyes, of a torpid character.	Scrofulous inflammation of eyes of an erethic character.
Optical illusions in red colors	Optical illusions in green colors. C.Hg.
Desire for wine or brandy	Aversion to wine or brandy; but appetite for beer.
Urine too seldom and scanty	Urine too often and copious.
Sexual desire too weak	Sexual desire too strong.
Discharge of succus prostaticus	Pollutions.
Catamenia predom. too soon and profuse	Catamenia too late; at the same time scanty *or* profuse.
Dry coryza predom.	Coryza fluent oftener than dry.
Expectoration morning and during day	Expectoration during day.
REMISSION of complaints in the afternoon	REMISSION during day.
Worse when getting out of bed	Better *or* worse when getting out of bed.
Worse or better *after* getting out of bed	Better *after* getting out of bed.
Worse *or* better when sitting	Almost always improv. when sitting.
Generally better when bending diseased part.	Worse when bending diseased part.
Better from scratching	Worse *or* better from scratching.
Worse when blowing nose	Worse when blowing nose; but better afterwards.
Worse *or* better from speaking	Worse from speaking.
Worse from growing cold; better from growing warm.	Better (resp. worse) from growing cold *or* warm.
Worse from cold, better from warm diet	Worse *or* better from cold diet, and in the latter case, worse from warm diet
Worse when swallowing	Better *or* worse when swallowing, partic. worse when swallowing saliva and drink.
Worse during and after meals	Worse *or* better during and after meals.
Worse or better after stool	Worse after stool.

Predomin. worse — **Predomin. better**

In dry weather, after getting out of bed, when leaning against anything, when letting diseased limb hang down, and when swallowing food.

Predomin. better — **Predomin. worse**

In wet weather, in bed and from warmth of bed, after perspiration, when lifting diseased limb, and when bending suffering part.

Hepar s. c.	Silicea.
Predominantly *upper left, lower right side.*	Predom. *upper right, lower left side.*
In chronic complaints predom. want of irritability; in recent cases, on the other hand, often great irritability.	Increased bodily irritability.
Constriction in inward parts	Constriction in external parts.
Crawling sensation in external parts . . .	Crawling sensation in inward parts.
Humid cutaneous eruptions	Dry eruptions.
Ulcers, also lardaceous, with thick pus . .	Ulcers with watery herpetic discharge, sometimes with proud flesh, or local sensation of coldness.
Pulse accelerated, hard and full; sometimes intermitting.	Pulse quick, hard, but small; often irregular.
Congestion of blood to eyes	Congestion of blood to ears.
Thirst predom., but not constant; most rare during chill.	Thirst predom., partic. during hot stage.
Chill lessened in warm room	Chill increased in warm room.
Dreams anxious, partic. of falling, fire, quarrel, &c.	Dreams sometimes anxious (of water, animals, thieves, ghosts), sometimes pleasant, erotic, imaginative.

Mood irritable, malicious	Mood indifferent, gentle; amorous.
Consequences of fright, or of vexation with vehemence.	Consequences of vexation — Apoplexy and paralysis much more freq. than with Hep.
Delirium—Fancies rarely	Fancies.
Compl. predom. on external angle of eye .	Complaints predom. on inner angle of eye.
Short-sightedness—Pupils dilated . . .	Far-sightedness—Pupils contracted.
Vomiting of mucus	Vomiting predom. of food or drink.
Urine seldom and scanty; sediment whitish.	Urine too often—Sedim. reddish or yellow.
Sexual desire lessened or weak	Sexual desire increased or strong.
Catamenia too soon and too profuse . .	Catamenia generally too late and scanty.
(In fevers) finger seem like dead	(In fevers) heat in fingers.

REMISSION of complaints afternoon . . .	REMISSION before midnight.
Some symptoms *aggrav.* by weeping . .	*Aggrav.* by weeping *or* laughing.
Worse when moving; better during rest, when lying,* and standing.	*Worse* when idle, and in the beginning of motion; *better* during continued moderate motion.
Worse when opening the mouth	*Worse* when opening *or* closing the mouth.
Worse *or* better when assuming an erect position.	Better when assuming an erect position.
Worse after drinking	Better *or* worse after drinking.
Better *or* worse when speaking	Worse when speaking.
Ailments from Silicea or Metals, from Nitric acid, Iodine, Arsenic, or Belladonna.	Ailments from Sulphur or the sting of insects, H.Gr.; the most important in all complaints following vaccination. C.Hg.

Predomin. worse ——— **Predomin. better**

From motion, eructation, and on an empty stomach.

Predomin better ——— **Predomin. worse**

During rest, after sweat, from scratching and rubbing, from smoking, and after breakfast.

---

* With both remedies the warmth of the bed improves.

Hepar s. c.	Spongia.
Predominant want of irritation (torpor) in chronic diseases; in recent cases, on the contrary, often increased irritability.	Predominantly increased bodily irritability.
Aversion to open air	Inclination for open air.
Chill lessened in warm room	Chill increased in warm room.

Hepar s. c.	Spongia.
Anxious dreams	Pleasant dreams.
Mood depressed; irritable; malicious . .	Cheerfulness—No insanity.
Congestion of blood to eyes	Congestion of blood to ears.
Saliva increased	Saliva diminished.
Croup, with deep, rough, barking cough; with hoarseness or aphony with slight suffocating spasms; respiration not without rattling of mucus.	Croup, with piping, crowing, very dry sounding cough, rough, crowing cry, and sensitiveness of the larynx to the touch.
Cough, excited by cold diet and when lying.	Cough, *improved* by eating and drinking; worse when sitting erect, from motion and exertion.
Expectoration in morning and during day .	When there is expectoration, it is only in morning.

Hepar s. c.	Spongia.
Remission of complaints in afternoon.	**Aggravation** afternoon and night, partic. before midnight.
Worse after singing	*Worse while* singing.
Worse when swallowing.	Better when swallowing, *worse* when not swallowing.
Worse when lying with head low, *better* with head high.	*Better* in horizontal position.

Predomin. worse — **Predomin. better**

With head lying low, out-doors, and when eating and swallowing.

Predomin. better — **Predomin. worse**

With head lying high, in-doors, when growing warm in bed, from smoking, from bending suffering part, from bending head backwards, and from rubbing and scratching.

Hepar s. c.	**Sulphur.**
Eruptions humid	Eruptions generally dry.
Painful eruptions and d° ulcers	Painful eruptions and d° ulcers.
Heat or sweat with aversion to uncover .	Heat or sweat with inclination to uncover.
Sweat lessened when speaking	Sweat increased when speaking.

Mood malicious	Mood changing; serious, indifferent, gentle.
Fancies much more seldom than with Sulph.	Unconsciousness.
Ailments from fright, or from vexation with vehemence.	Ailments from mortification, hearing bad news, or from vexation with dread or fear; more rarely from anger.
Very rarely paralysis	Paralysis.
Complaints predom. on external ear, on tip of elbow, and on top of foot	Complaints predom. in inner ear, in hollow of elbow, on patella, and on sole of foot.
Eyes protruding—Pupils dilated	Eyes generally sunken—Pupils contracted.
Saliva predom. increased	Saliva *generally* diminished.
Appetite for spirituous liquors	Inclination for or aversion to beer and spirituous liquors.
Vomit predom. on bile	Vomit sour oftener than bitter.
Urine infrequent and scanty	Ur. often & scanty, but sometimes copious.
Sediment of urine white	Sediment whitish *or reddish*.
Catamenia too soon and profuse	Catamenia *generally* too late and scanty.

Remission of complaints afternoon . . .	Remission afternoon and before midnight.
Worse when moving; better during rest .	*Worse* in the beginning of motion, from walking fast and running, *better* during continued moderate motion.
Wórse when turning in bed	*Worse or* better when turning in bed.
Worse on an empty stomach	Better *or* worse on an empty stomach.
Worse *after* singing	Worse *while* singing.
Worse out-doors,* *better* in-doors . . .	*Better or* worse out-doors; worse in-doors, if the room is crowded, but *better* from warmth of stove.
Better *or* worse when talking	Worse when speaking.

Predomin. worse —— **Predomin. better**

In dry weather, from cold,‡ uncovering, eructation, from external pressure, and when moving.

Predomin. better —— **Predomin. worse**

In damp weather, from warmth, wrapping up, after lying down, while lying, from warmth of bed, after sweat, from smoking, when standing, when bending suffering part, and during rest.

N.B. With Sulph. we rarely find the over-sensitiveness of Hepar s. c. to pain,—rarely with Hepar s. c. the sensation of numbness of suffering parts peculiar to Sulph.

---

* Both remedies have aggrav. "*when walking out-doors.*"

† We find aggrav. "from cold weather" with both remedies,—with Sulph. also "from hot weather."

Hepar s. c.	Zincum.
Light hair—Constriction in internal parts .	Dark hair—Constriction in external parts.
Rarely paralysis	Paralysis of limbs.
Hydrocephalus	Hydrocephaloid. C.Hg.
Pulse accelerated, full, and hard; frequent at night, slow during day.	Pulse small and frequent in evening, slower in the morning and during day.

Hepar s. c.	Zincum.
Mood dejected; malicious	Mood cheerful; indifferent; changing—Amorousness.
Optical illusions dark or in red colors—Cataract.	Optical illusions bright; principally green, or blue, or yellow—Amaurosis.
Mucous vomit	Vomiting predom. of food.
Urine almost always dark—Sediment whitish.	Urine predom. pale—Sediment yellow.
Sexual desire too weak	Sexual desire too strong.
Discharge of succus prostaticus predom. .	Pollutions predominant.
Scrotum relaxed	Scrotum contracted. C.Hg.
Catamenia too soon and profuse	Catam. predom. too late and scanty.
Cough generally without expectoration . .	Cough generally with expectoration.
Expectoration morning and during day .	Expectoration partic. mornings.
Complaints predominant on tip of elbow, on hip-joint, on thigh, partic. on the inner side of thigh.	Complaints predominant in hollow of elbow, on patella, on shoulder-joint, on leg, and on outer side of thigh.

Hepar s. c.	Zincum.
Remission of complaints in the afternoon .	**Aggravation** afternoon and evening, rarely at night.
Worse or better after getting out of bed .	Better after getting out of bed.
Worse *or* better when assuming an erect position.	Worse when assuming an erect position.
Better *or* worse when sitting	Predom. worse when sitting.
Almost always aggravated when stretching out diseased limb, better when drawing it up.	Better when stretching out diseased limb, worse when drawing it up.
Almost always aggravated by touch . . .	Better *or* worse from touch.
Worse when swallowing	*Generally* better when swallowing.
Worse from eructation	*Worse or* better from eructation.
Worse or better after stool.	Worse after stool.
Ailments from Silicea or Metals, from Nitr. acid, Arsenic, Iodine, or Belladonna.	Ailments from Baryt.

Predomin. worse ——— **Predomin. better**

In dry weather, out-doors, when closing the eyes, when and after getting out of bed, when stretching out diseased limb, from pressure, on an empty stomach; but also when eating, when swallowing, from cold diet, when blowing the nose, and when tying the clothes tight around the hips.

Predomin. better ——— **Predomin. worse**

In wet weather, in-doors, when opening the eyes, after lying down, in bed, when standing, when drawing up diseased limb, when bending diseased part, after breakfast, from warm diet, and from loosening the clothes.

Hyoscyamus.	Nux vomica.
Light hair—Skin and muscles lax . . .	Dark hair—Skin and muscles rigid.
Complaints (pinching, &c.) predom. in external parts.	Complaints (pinching pain, &c.) predom. in internal parts.
Crawling sensation in internal parts—Obesity.	Crawling sensation in external parts—Emaciation.
Want of bodily irritability	Increased bodily irritability.
Painless eruptions and ulcers	Painful eruptions and ulcers.
Painless paralysis, partic. of one side only .	Paral. generally of both sides (paraplegia).
Hæmorrhages, blood light-red	Hæmorrhages, blood dark.
Epilepsy with unconsciousness	Epilepsy with full consciousness.
Partial sweat on lower part of body . . .	Partial sweat on upper part of body.
Sweat increased during sleep	Sweat lessened during sleep.
Thirst is wanting only during cold stage .	Thirst greatest during chill.
Insensibility of disposition	Sensitiveness.
Cheerfulness – Changing mood—Distrust .	Sadness—Peevishness—Irascibility.
Consequences of jealousy oftener than with Nux vom.	Ailments from mortification or contradiction.
Mental dullness	Mental dullness much more rare.
Hunger predom.	Generally loss of appetite.
Diarrhœa, painless	Costiveness—When there is diarrhœa, it is painful.
Catamenia too late and profuse	Catamenia too soon and profuse.
Expectoration infrequent; during day . .	Expectoration not constant; morning, during day, evening.
Complaints predom. on wrist	Complaints predom. on ankle.
Remission of complaints during day . .	**Remission** evening till midnight.
Worse after sleep	Better after sufficient and not too long sleep; but worse on awaking when the sleep is interrupted.
Predom. worse after getting out of bed . .	Worse *or* better after getting out of bed.
Better on an empty stomach (before breakfast).	Worse *or* better on an empty stomach.
Worse when swallowing drink	*Worse or* better when swallowing; partic. worse when swallowing food or swallowing saliva.
Worse after drinking	*Worse or* better after drinking.
Worse when perspiring	*Worse or* better when perspiring.
Worse when bending diseased part	*Worse or* better wh. bending diseased part.
Generally improv. when assuming an erect position.	Almost always aggrav. when assuming an erect position.
Ailments from Belladonna	Ailments from Arsenic or Copper vapors, from Sulph., Calc., Phosph., Iodine, Petroleum, Graphit, from Coffea, Cocculus, Colchicum, Digitalis, Pulsatilla, Stramonium, or Lachesis.
Complaints following inhalation of ether .	Complaints following the use of aromatics, ginger, onions, &c. C. Hg.

Predomin. worse —— **Predomin. better**

After lying down, when lying generally, partic. in a bent posture, after sleep, and when swallowing drink.

Predomin. better —— **Predomin. worse**

When assuming an erect position, in extended posture, when getting out of bed, from drinking coffee, and from smoking.

Hyoscyamus.	Pulsatilla.
Complaints (pinching pain, etc.) predominant in external parts.	Complaints (pinching pain, etc.) predominant in internal parts.
Want of bodily irritability—Painless erupt's.	Increased irritability—Painful eruptions.
Hæmorrhages, blood light-red	Hæmorrhages, blood dark.
Pulse generally quick, full, hard, strong . .	Pulse generally frequent, but small and weak.
Heat abating in bed	Heat increased in bed.
Thirst generally wanting only during cold stage.	Want of thirst predominant, but constant only during chill.

Hyoscyamus.	Pulsatilla.
Insensibility of disposition	Sensitive disposition.
Mood irritable; malicious; haughty	Calm sadness of mild dispositions — Indifference—Peevishness—Boldness—Avarice.
Ailments from (fright, grief, vexation) anger, disappointed love or jealousy.	Ailments from (fright, grief, vexation) excessive joy or from mortification.
Memory active *or* weak—Mental dullness . .	Weak memory—Mental dullness more rarely.
Eyes protruding — Pupils predom. dilated—Clear-sightedness more frequent than dim-sightedness.	Eyes sunken—Pupils generally contracted—Dim-sightedness.
Nasal complaints predom. internal	Nasal compl. external oftener than internal.
Painless diarrhœa	Diarrhœa generally painful.
Catamenia predom. profuse	Catamenia predom. scanty.
Expectoration infrequent; during day . . .	Expectoration predominant, but not constant; morning and during day.
Complaints predom. on fore-arm and thigh .	Complaints predom. on upper arm and on leg

---

Hyoscyamus.	Pulsatilla.
AGGRAVAT. from evening till morning . . .	AGGRAVAT. from noon till midnight.
Worse when looking upwards or sideways . .	Worse when looking upwards.
Better after perspiring	*Generally* worse after perspiring.
Worse from uncovering, better from wrapping up.	*Generally* better from uncovering, worse from wrapping up.
Worse after sleep	*Worse or* better after sleep.
Generally worse after getting out of bed . .	Generally improved after getting out of bed.
Generally improved when stooping	Generally aggravated when stooping.
Worse when bending diseased part	Better *or* worse when bending diseased part, partic. better when bending it sideways; worse when bending it back.
Worse when swallowing drink	*Worse or* better when swallowing, particularly worse when swallowing saliva.
Worse after meals	*Worse or* better after meals.
Worse after stool	*Better or* worse after stool.
Ailments from Plumbum	Ailments from Copper vapors, and from Sulph., Mercur., or Cinchona, etc.

Predomin. worse ⁀ **Predomin. better**

Out-doors, from cold, growing cold and in cold weather, from drinking cold water, uncovering, lying in bent posture, when lying on painful side, "after" getting out of bed, from walking fast and from bodily exertion generally, from pressure, and after stool.

Predomin. better ⁀ **Predomin. worse**

In-doors, from warmth, from growing warm and in warm air, from drinking coffee and smoking, from wrapping up, after sweat, in extended position, when lying on unpainful side, in bed generally, when sitting, and when stooping.

N.B. Pulsatilla has numb sensation in suffering parts oftener than Hyoscyamus.

Hyoscyamus.	Stramonium.
Crawling sensation in internal parts — Parched skin – Obesity.	Crawling sensation in external parts — Perspires easily—Emaciation.
Painless paralysis, generally of one side .	Painless paralysis, generally of both sides.
Hæmorrhages, blood light-red	Hæmorrhages, blood dark.
Pulse generally regular	Pulse very irregular, sometimes trembling.
Thirst is wanting only during chill . . .	Thirst, as with Hyosc.; but often also between heat and sweat.

Aversion to light and company	Inclination for light and company.
Fear of being poisoned	Fear of loss of reason.
Ailments from anger, grief, or disappointed love.	Ailments from hearing bad news.
Memory very active *or* weak	Weak memory.
Delirium tremens or convulsions with unconsciousness and with aversion to light and company.	Delirium tremens or convulsions with full consciousness and desire for light and company.
Clear-sightedness oftener than dim-sightedness.	Dim-sightedness.
Optical illusions in bright colors	Optic. illusions in dark or prismatic colors.
Objects predominant appear too large . .	Objects appear too small.
Puerperal convulsions with grinding of teeth.	Puerperal convulsions with copious sweat'g. Lippe.
Secretion of milk diminished	Secretion of milk increased.
Expectoration infrequent	Expectoration not yet observed.
Horse refuses to be mounted	Horse getting restless from every noise, inclining to run off, biting & attacking with great agility.

Remission of complaints during day . .	Remission during day and evening.
Ailments from heat of sun	Improvement of complaints in sun-light.
Worse from light; better in the dark . .	Better *or* worse fr. light (resp. in the dark.)
Worse in company; better when alone . .	*Generally* bett. in comp., worse when alone.
Worse *or* better from pressure	Worse from pressure.
Worse when lying on painful side, better when lying on unpainful side.	*Generally* better when liyng on painful side, worse when lying on unpainful side.
Generally better when getting out of bed.	Worse when getting out of bed.
Predominant worse *after* getting out of bed.	Worse *or* better after getting out of bed.
Better or worse when stooping, and when assuming an erect position.	Worse when stooping, and when assuming an erect position.
Ailments from Belladonna or Plumbum . .	Ailments from Mercurius or Plumbum.

Predomin. worse ——— **Predomin. better**

In the sun, in company, after lying down, while lying, partic. when lying on painful side, & after stool.

Predomin. better ——— **Predomin. worse**

When alone, when getting out of bed, when lying on unpainful side, when stooping, & when assuming an erect position.

N.B. Stramonium lacks the over-sensitiveness to pain of Hyoscyamus.

Ignatia.	Nux vomica.
Predom. *left* side*—Sanguine temperament .	*Right* side—Sanguine choleric temperament.
Painless ulcers and swelling of glands . . .	Painful ulcers and swelling of glands.
Pulse very changeable†	Pulse sometimes intermitting or imperceptible
Coldness, easily overcome by external warmth.	Coldness, which cannot be overcome by external warmth. C.Hg.
Chill, lessened after getting out of bed and after meals.	Chill, increased after getting out of bed and after meals.
Thirst only during chill	Thirst *greatest* during chill.
Heat, with inclination to uncover	Heat, with aversion to uncover.
Heat, lessened while eating	Heat, increased while eating.
Sweat, lessened by exertion	Sweat, partic. when exerting the body.
Sleeplessness before midnight	*Sleeplessness predom. after midnight.*
Sleepless after depressing emotions	Sleepless after exertions of mind. C.Hg.
Mood changing; anxious; capricious . . .	Mood peevish; irascible.
Taciturnity	Loquacity—Unconsciousness.
Ailments from mortification, grief, and disappointed love.	Ailments from outbursts of passion, partic. in the morning.
Epilepsy with unconsciousness	Epilepsy with full consciousness.
Appetite for sour things—Aversion to wine and brandy.	Aversion to sour things—Desire for brandy
Diarrhœa predominant	Constipation predominant.
Urine often and copious	Urine seldom and scanty.
Sexual desire weak	Sexual desire strong.
Catamenia too soon and scanty (or profuse. C.Hg.)	Cat. too soon and profuse (or scanty. C.Hg.)
Expectoration in the evening	Expectoration morning and during day.
Remission of complaints before midnight . .	Remission evening till midnight.
Worse from inflating the belly	*Worse* from drawing in the belly.
Worse when not swallowing and when swallowing liquids; *better* when swallowing food.	*Worse* when swallowing, partic. when swallowing food and saliva; often better when swallowing (drink).
Often worse when lying, particularly aggrav. by lying on side oftener than on back, which latter position often improves.	Better when lying, partic. on side; aggrav. by lying on back. C.Hg.
Antidote to Zink	Aggravates the symptoms of Zink. C.Hg.

Predomin. worse —— **Predomin. better**

From wrapping up, after lying down, in bed, partic. when lying on unpainful side, "between" respiration, when lying on left side, and when swallowing drink.

Predomin. better —— **Predomin. worse**

From uncovering, after rising from seat, (when lying on painful side), from deep respiration, from drawing in the belly, from bodily exertion,‡ and generally after eating, particularly sour things, when lying on right side and from change of posture, when swallowing food.

---

* According to Bönninghausen; but it is quite undecided. According to the value and number of the symptoms the sides are alike with both remedies; N. vom. perhaps upper left, lower right side; Ignat perhaps upper right, lower left side. In the head, Ignat. has symptoms going from right to left; in the chest, from left to right. C.Hg.

† The predom. condition of the pulse is the same with both remedies.

‡ The improvement with Ignat. is predom. caused by bodily exertion; yet we sometimes find aggrav. from exertion with this remedy. H.Gr.—Both remedies have consequences of too great mental exertion. C.Hg.

Ignatia.	Phosph. acid.
Over-sensitiveness to pain	Painlessness predom.
Upper right, lower left side—Aversion to motion.	*Upper left, lower right side*—Inclination for motion.
Tension in internal parts; inflammation in external parts.	Tension in external parts; inflammation in internal parts.
Pain piercing inwards—Apoplexy	Pain piercing outwards—No apoplexy.
Pulse very changeable; generally quick, full, and hard.	Pulse irregular, intermitting; generally frequent, but small and weak.
Internal chill with external heat* predom. .	External chill with internal heat predom.
Cold feet and hot hands.	Cold hands and warm feet.
Heat or sweat pred. with inclinat. to uncover.	Heat or sweat with aversion to uncover.
Thirst only during cold stage, and after sweat.	Want of thirst predom.; no thirst during chill, rare during heat, & preval. only dur'g sweat.
Sensitive disposition and acute feeling—Mood changing; bold—Amorousness.	Insensibility of disposition (and of body).
Ailments from hearing bad news, fright, or from vexation with fear. H. Gr.	Ailments from grief and sorrow, or homesickness, or disappointed love, partic. with drowsiness, night-sweats towards morning, emaciation. C. Hg.
Incapacity for thought in the evening—Insanity.	Incapacity for thought in the morning—Unconsciousness.
Complaints predom. on external angle of eye, in inner ear, on inside of nose, and on roof of mouth.	Complaints frequent on inner angle of eye, on external ear, on outside of nose, and on soft palate.
Secretion of saliva increased	Saliva predom. diminished.
Aversion to warm food	Inclination for warm food.
Aversion to spirituous liquors or milk . . .	Appetite for wine, beer, or milk.
Appetite for bread, partic. rye bread . . .	Aversion to bread.
Generally bitter vomit, less frequently sour vomit.	Sour vomit.
Predom. emission of succus prostaticus . .	Pollutions more frequent than prostatorrhœa.
Catamenia too soon, but scanty	Catamenia too soon and profuse.
Voice trembling	Voice nasal.
Expectoration seldom; evenings	Expector. almost constant; partic. mornings.
Frequent complaints on upper arm and on calf of leg.	Complaints predom. on fore-arm and on shin.
Remission of complaints before midnight . .	Remission afternoon and before midnight.
Better from scratching	Worse *or* better from scratching.
Generally worse from wrapping up; better from uncovering.	Better from wrapping up, worse from uncovering.
Generally better when lying on painful side; worse when lying on unpainful side.	Worse when lying on painful side, better when lying on unpainful side.
Better *or* worse when getting out of bed . .	Worse when getting out of bed.
Better *or* worse when stooping, & when rising.	Predom. worse when stooping and when rising.
Better or worse from exertion	Worse from bodily exertion.
Worse from straining the eyes	Better *or* worse from straining the eyes.
Worse when swallowing drink	Worse when swallowing food.
Ailments from Coffea, Chamom., Pulsatilla, Nux vomica, or Zinc.	Ailments from Lachesis.

Predomin. worse — **Predomin. better**

Out-doors, when lying on unpainful side, from wrapping up, when opening the eyes, before breakfast, from cold diet,† and when moving diseased part.

Predomin. better — **Predomin. worse**

In-doors, when lying on painful side, from uncovering, when closing eyes, after breakfast, from warm diet, vinegar and acids; after meals, and when rising from a seat.

* Therefore worse from wrapping up and from *cold* diet, &c. Comp. Zincum—Sulphur.

† Yet we find "aggrav. from drinking cold water" with both remedies.

Ignatia.	Pulsatilla.
Predom. *left* side; partic. *lower left and upper right.*	*Right* side; partic. *lower right, upper left side.*
Aversion to open air	Inclination for open air.
Itching, lessened *or* locality changed by rubbing and scratching	Itching, aggrav. *or* unchanged by scratching.
Painless swelling of glands	Painful, hot, swelling of glands.
Pulse very changeable; generally quick, full, and hard; sometimes frequent in morning, slower during day or evening.	Pulse predom. accelerated, but small and weak, partic. frequent in evening, slower in the morning; sometimes intermitting or imperceptible.
Chill increased out-doors, lessened in warm room and after meals.	Chill, lessened out-doors, increased in warm room and after meals.
Heat often general, with exception of feet.	Coldness often general, with except. of feet.
Partial chill on back of body	Partial chill on front part of body.
Thirst only during chill	Want of thirst predom., but *constant* only during chill.
Sleepless after depressing emotions . . .	Sleepless after eating too much. C.Hg.

Ignatia.	Pulsatilla.
Mood depressed *or* cheerful	Sadness—Distrust – Avarice.
Fear of loneliness	Love's to be alone.
Ailments from (fright, vexation, grief) shame, hearing bad news, disappointed love or jealousy.	Ailments from (fright, vexation, grief) excessive joy—Unconsciousness.
Compl. predom. on external angle of eye, in inside of nose, in spleen, and in palms of hands.	Compl. predom. in inner angle of eye, on outside of nose, in liver, and on back of hand.
Generally want of appetite	Generally hunger.
Desire for rye-bread	Disgust for rye-bread.
In drunkards, aversion to spirituous liquors.	Inclination for spirituous liquors.
Urine often and copious	Urine infrequent and scanty.
Catamenia too soon and of long duration .	Catam. pred. too late and of short duration
Milk diminished	Milk generally increased.
Expector. infrequent; only in the evening when cough is worse.	Expectoration predom., but not constant; morning and during day.

Ignatia.	Pulsatilla.
REMISSION of complaints before midnight.	*Aggrav.* afternoon, even'g & bef. midnight.
Worse dur'g *passive* mot. (rid'g) & after it.	Better during *active* motion, *worse after* it.
Worse when hold'g diseased parts together.	*Better* when lying in bent posture.
Worse when swallowing drink	Worse when swallowing saliva.
Better when respiring deeply	Worse *or* better when respiring deeply.
Ailments from Pulsatilla, Coffea, Nux vomica or Zink.	Ailments from Ignatia, Bellad., Cinchona, Colchicum, Cantharides, Sabad., Argent., Mercur., Platina, Ferrrum, Stannum, Sulph., Sulph. acid. and Tartar. emetic.

Predomin. worse — **Predomin. better**

Out-doors, from cold, in cold weather, from cold diet, when opening the eyes, and from tying the clothes tight.

Predomin. better — **Predomin. worse**

In-doors, from warmth, in warm air, from warm diet, when closing the eyes, when lying, when sitting bent forward, from change of posture, eructation, loosening the clothes, and from rubbing and scratching.

N.B. Ignatia has the numb sensation in suffering parts less frequently than Pulsatilla.

Ignatia.	Rhus.
Left side, partic. *lower left, upper right side.*	*Right* side, part. *lower right, upper left side.*
Complaints (tension, etc.) predom. in internal parts.	Complaints (tension, etc.) predom. in external parts.
Aversion to motion — Hæmorrhages, blood dark.	Inclination for motion—Hæmorrhages, blood light-red.
Apoplexy oftener than paralysis	Paralysis oftener than apoplexy.
Itching, lessen'd *or* locality chang'd by scratching.	Itching, lessened (or unchanged) by scratching.
Painless swelling of glands	Painful, hot swelling of glands.
Pulse very changeable; generally quick, full, hard.	Pulse irregular; generally accelerated, but faint and soft; sometimes intermitting.
Chill lessened after meals—Sweat lessened by exertion.	Chill increased after meals—Sweat by exertion.
Heat or sweat, with inclination to uncover	Heat or sweat, with aversion to uncover.
Thirst only during cold stage	Thirst not constant.
Aversion to being alone	Inclination for being alone.
Fear of loss of reason	Fear of being poisoned.
Mood changing; cheerful *or* depressed; gentle; indifferent; bold.	Mood hopeless—Rarely amorousness—Rarely absent-mindedness—Insensibility.
Nasal complaints internal	Nasal complaints external oftener than intern.
Eruption on under lip	Eruption on upper lip.
Catamenia too scanty—Milk diminished	Catamenia profuse—Milk generally increased.
Expectoration infrequent; evening	Expectoration not constant; morning.
Complaints predom. on upper arm and palm of hand.	Complaints predom. on fore-arm and back of hand.
Remission of complaints before midnight	Remission during day.
Predom. worse in bed and from warmth of bed.	*Better or* worse in bed and from warmth of bed.
Generally worse when lying on side, better when lying on back.	Better when lying on side; worse when lying on back.
Better or worse from exertion	Worse from bodily exertion.
Worse from moving or bending diseased part.	Better *or* worse from moving and bending diseased part.
Generally better when lifting diseased limb or resting it on anything; worse when letting it hang down.	Worse when lifting diseased limb or when resting it on anything; better when letting it hang down.
Better *or* worse when assuming an erect position.	Almost always aggravated when assuming an erect position.
Better when and after rising from a seat	Worse *or* better when and after rising from a seat.
Almost always improved after meals	*Worse or* better after meals.
Worse after drinking	*Worse or* better after drinking.
Predom. worse after stool	*Generally* better after stool.
Often worse after mental exertion	Worse *after* bodily exertion. C.Hg.

Predomin. **worse** ——— Predomin. **better**

On expiration, from wrapping up, after sweat, when lying on side, when sitting erect, when moving suffering part, when letting diseased limb hang down, and after stool.

Predomin. **better** ——— Predomin. **worse**

On inspiration and when respiring deeply, from uncovering, when lying on back, when sitting bent forward, from washing with cold water and moistening the suffering part, when lifting or resting diseased limb on anything, from change of posture when lying or standing, when swallowing,* and from eructation.

N.B. Rhus lacks the over-sensitiveness of Ignatia to pain; on the other hand, Ignatia rarely has the numb sensation in suffering parts peculiar to Rhus.

---

* But worse when swallowing drink. Rhus worse when swallowing food and saliva.

Ignatia.	Sulphur.
Upper right, lower left side — Pain piercing inwards.	Upper left, lower right side — Pain piercing outwards.
Ulcerative pain in external parts; pinching pain in internal parts.	Ulcerative pain in internal parts; pinching pain in external parts.
External parts become black	Red parts become white — Rarely over-sensitiveness.
Itching, lessened *or* locality changed by scratching.	Itching, lessened by scratching—Want of irritability predom.
Apoplexy more frequent than paralysis . .	Paralysis more frequent than apoplexy.
In the morning on awaking concussion of the body, (on falling asleep, starting up.)	Concussions or starting up, on falling asleep.
Chill lessened after getting out of bed . . .	Chill increased after getting out of bed.
Heat general, with exception of feet . . .	Heat general, with exception of the head.
Sweat lessened by bodily exertion	Sweat increased by exertion.
Thirst only during cold stage — Pulse very changeable.	Th. mostly during heat; during chill generally want of thirst—Pulse sometimes intermitt'g.
Mood *depressed* or cheerful—Boldness . . .	Depression — Embarrassment — Rarely amorousness.
Ailments from hearing bad news, from shame, grief, disappointed love or jealousy, and from vexation with reserved displeasure.	Ailments from anger or vexation with vehemence.
Eruption on lower lip	Eruption predom. on upper lip.
Saliva predom. increased	Saliva *generally* diminished.
Appetite for bread, partic. rye bread . . .	Dislike for bread, partic. rye bread.
Dislike for wine and brandy	Appetite or dislike for wine and spirituous liquors.
Vomit bitter oftener than sour	Vomit sour oftener than bitter.
Urine too often and copious	Urine often, but scanty.
Catamenia too soon and of long duration . .	Catam. *generally* too late & of short duration.
Expectoration seldom; evening	Expectoration not constant; morning and during day, less at night.
Complaints predom. on upper arm	Complaints predom. on fore-arm.
Remission of complaints before midnight . .	Aggravation *afternoon* and before midnight.
Predom. worse in the open air, better in doors.	Bett. *or* worse in the open air (resp. in-doors), partic. better from warmth of stove, but worse in crowded rooms.
Predom. worse from cold and in cold weather, better from growing warm and in warm air.	Better (resp. worse) fr. growing cold & in cold weather, *or* fr. growing warm & in warm air.
Worse after perspiring	*Worse or* better after perspiring.
Predom. worse in bed	Worse *or* better in bed.
Better from change of position when lying or standing.	*Worse or* better from change of position.
Worse *or* better when getting out of bed . .	Better when getting out of bed.
Predom. worse when opening the eyes; better when closing them.	Better *or* worse when opening the eyes and when closing them.
Worse on an empty stomach; better after breakfast.	Better or worse on an empty stomach (resp. after breakfast).
Better from eructation	*Better or* worse from eructation.
Almost alw. improv. by taking a deep breath.	Worse *or* better when taking a deep breath.
Better from weeping	*Worse or* better from weeping.
Worse from touch	*Worse or* better from touch.
Worse from moving the diseased part . . .	Worse *or* better from moving the part.
Better or worse from exertion	Almost always aggrav. by bodily exertion.
Worse after drinking	*Worse or* better after drinking.

Predomin. worse — **Predomin. better**

From cold, on expiration, when sitting erect, wh. letting diseased limb hang down, or wh. drawing it up.

Predomin. better — **Predomin. worse**

From warmth, on inspiration, when sitting bent forward, when lifting diseased limb, and when stretching it out, from washing the suffering part with cold water, or moistening it, when rising from a seat, from vinegar and sour things, when swallowing,* and after meals.

* Yet Ignat. has aggrav. when swallowing drink; Sulph., on the other hand, has aggr. when swallowing *food* & saliva.

Ignatia.	Zincum.
Complaints (constriction, &c.) predom. in internal parts.	Complaints (constriction, &c.) predom. in external parts.
Hæmorrhages, blood dark—Apoplexy .	Hæmorrh., blood light-red—No apoplexy.
External parts become black	Red parts become white.
Pain in glands, pressing outward	Pain in glands, inward pressing.
Itching, lessened *or* locality changed by scratching.	Itching lessened *or* locality changed by scratching, *or* unchanged.
Pulse very changeable; frequent in morning, slower during day and evening.	Pulse sometimes intermitting; small and frequent in morning, & slower during day.
Congestion of blood to head	Congestion of blood to feet.
Thirst only during chill	Often want of thirst during chill.
Chill lessened after meals	Chill increased after meals.
Internal chill with external heat predom. .	External chill with internal heat predom.
Sweat often confined to upper part of body.	Sweat often confined to lower part of body.

Ignatia.	Zincum.
Mood anxious; *depressed* or cheerful—Boldness.	Mood cheerful.
Ailments from shame, reserved grief or disappointed love.	Ailments from vexation.
Absent-mindedness—Fancies	No fancies.
Eruption on under lip	Eruption on upper lip.
Diarrhœa predom.	Constipation.
Emission of succus prostaticus predom.	Pollutions predom.
Catamenia too soon	Catamenia generally too late, less frequently too soon.
Fluent coryza predom.	Dry coryza predom.
Expectoration infrequent; partic. in the evening.	Expectoration almost constant; partic. in the morning.
Complaints predom. on upper arm . . .	Complaints predom. on fore-arm.

Ignatia.	Zincum.
REMISSION of complaints before midnight .	AGGRAVATION afternoon and *evening.*
Worse from touch	Worse *or* better from touch.
Better *or* worse when sitting	Predom. worse when sitting.
Predom. worse when lying	Better *or* worse when lying.
Worse *or* better when and after getting out of bed.	Better when and after getting out of bed.
Better *or* worse when assuming an erect position.	Worse from assuming an erect posture.
Better or worse from exertion	Worse from bodily exertion.
Ailments from Zinc., Coffea, Chamom., Nux vomica or Pulsatilla	Ailments from Baryt.
Worse when swallowing drink	Worse when swallowing food.*

Predomin. worse ——— **Predomin. better**

Out-doors, *before* breakfast, from drinking cold water and from cold diet, when swallowing drink and tying clothes tight.

Predomin. better ——— **Predomin. worse**

In-doors, *after* breakfast, after meals, from warm diet, from eructation, from drawing in the belly, from washing and moistening the suffering part with cold water,—when swallowing food and loosening the clothes.

---

* Generally both remedies have *improvement* of complaints when swallowing.

Iodium.	Hepar s. c.
Upper right, lower left side	Upper left, lower right side.
Inclination for open air	Aversion to open air.
Diseases of the periosteum oftener than of the bones.	Diseases of the bones.
Heat or sweat, with inclination to uncover.	Heat or sweat, with aversion to uncover.
Chill increased in warm room	Chill abating in warm room.
Sweat increased when speaking, abating when and after getting out of bed.	Sweat abating when speaking, increased when and after getting out of bed.
Thirst, particularly during sweat	Thirst predominant, but not constant; most rare during chill.
Cheerfulness more frequent than dejection—Mood rarely irritable or peevish; chang'g.	Mood dejected.
Phlegma	Restlessness and haste—Insanity.
Eyes sunken	Eyes protruding.
Optical illusions in bright colors	Optical illusions in dark colors.
Coryza fluent oftener than dry.	Coryza oftener dry than fluent.
Expectoration almost constant; evening; tasting saltish, sweetish, or putrid.	Cough generally dry—Expectoration morning and during day; tasting sweetish or sour.
Vomiting predom. of food	Mucous vomit.
Urine pale—Sexual desire strong.	Urine dark—Sexual desire weak.
Complaints predom. on wrist	Complaints predom. on ankle.
REMISSION *forenoon* and before midnight.	REMISSION of complaints afternoon.
Worse when swallowing food and drink	Worse when swallowing food and saliva.
Worse when drinking	*Worse after* drinking.
Better on inspiration, *worse* on expiration.	Worse when respiring, particularly when respiring deeply.
Worse when speaking	Better *or* worse when speaking.
Ailments from Mercurius, Arsenic, Nitrate of Silver, Calcarea.	Ailments from Calcarea or abuse of Metals, Arsenic, Nitric acid, Iodine, or Belladonna.

Predomin. worse ——— **Predomin. better**

In-doors, from wrapping it up, from warmth, warmth of bed, after sweat, and from smoking.

Predomin. better ——— **Predomin. worse**

Out-doors, from uncovering, from cold, growing cold, in (dry) cold weather, after getting out of bed. from eructation, on inspiration and deep respiration.

N.B. Over-sensitiveness to pain is often found with Hepar s. c., hardly ever with Iodine.

Iodine.	Mercur.
Upper right, lower left side—Want of irritability.	Upper left, lower right side — Increased bodily irritability.
Inclination for open air—No apoplexy . .	Aversion to open air—Apoplexy.
Humid eruptions	Eruptions generally dry.
Itching, unchanged by scratching . . .	Itching, lessened *or* aggrav. by scratching.
Gnawing pain in internal parts	Gnawing pain in external parts.
Sleeplessness after midnight	Sleeplessness prevalent before midnight.
Pulse accelerated, mostly by every motion; at the same time oftener large and hard, than weak and threadlike.	Pulse irregular, sometimes intermitting; it is oftener accelerated and full, than slow and faint.
Chill lessened after getting out of bed . .	Chill increased after getting out of bed.
Thirst, particularly during sweat	Thirst predom. during all stages, but not constant.
Mood cheerful *or* depressed; rarely irritable.	Mood dejected; peevish; malicious.
Rarely fancies	Absent-mindedness—Unconsciousness.
Atrophy of brain	In children large head and unclosed sutures, with precocious mental development.
Eyes sunken*	Eyes protruding.
Optical illusions in bright colors	Optical illusions in dark colors.
Hunger predominant	Generally want of appetite.
Appetite for meat	Aversion to meat.
Desire for wine or brandy	Aversion to wine or brandy, but appetite for beer.
Urine predominant pale; scanty; smelling like ammoniac.	Urine dark; frequent and copious, having sour smell.
Catamenia too soon and profuse	Catamenia too late; at the same time scanty *or* profuse.
Expectoration almost constant; evenings .	Expectoration not constant; during day.
Complaints predom. in lower part of chest.	Complaints predom. in upper part of chest
REMISSION *forenoon* and before midnight.	REMISSION of complaints during day.
Ailments from Mercurius, Argent. nitricum, Arsenic or Calcarea.	Ailments from Arsenic or Copper vapors, Aurum, Sulph., Antimon., Coffea, Lachesis, Bell., Opium, Valeriana, Cinchona, Dulcamara or Mezereum.
Worse when lying on back, better when lying on side.	*Generally* better when lying on back, worse when lying on side.
Worse from wrapping up, better from uncovering.	*Generally* better from wrapping up, worse from uncovering.
Better when growing cold	Better *or* worse when growing cold.
Worse when swallowing drink and food .	Worse when swallowing drink and saliva.

Predomin. worse — **Predomin. better**

In warm air, in-doors, from wrapping up, when lying on back, on expiration from smoking, and when swallowing food.

Predomin. better — **Predomin. worse**

In cold weather, out-doors, from uncovering, when lying on side, on inspiration, and from sweets.

* From emaciation, the loss of fat around the eye-balls; but in some cases the eye-balls protrude as if enlarged after abuse of Iodine, particularly where mercurial preparations had also been given. Hepar is the principal antidote in such cases. C.Hg.

Iodium.	Sulphur.
Right side, partic. *upper right, lower left side.*	*Left* side, partic. *upper left, lower right side.*
Inclination for open air—Very rarely paralys.	Aversion to open air—Paralysis.
Dry gangræna—Humid eruptions	Gangræna humida—Eruptions generally dry.
Itching, unchanged by scratching	Itching, lessened by scratching.
Diseases of the periosteum predominant . .	Diseases of the bones.
Painful swelling of glands	Painless, but generally hot swelling of glands.
Pulse accelerated, partic. by every motion; at the same time large and hard oftener than weak and thread-like.	Pulse quick, full, and hard; sometimes intermitting.
Sweat on lower part of body	Heat on lower part of body; sweat above.
Chill worse in warm room, lessened after getting out of bed and after meals.	Chill lessened in warm room, increased after getting out of bed and after meals.
Sleeplessness after midnight	Sleeplessness before midnight.

Iodium.	Sulphur.
Mood oftener happy than depressed; rarely peevish or irritable.	Mood anxious; serious; solemn; sad; indifferent; peevish; irritable.
Very rarely fancies	Absent-mindedness—Insanity.
Atrophy of brain	In children, large head and open sutures.
Optical illusions in bright colors	Optical illusions in dark colors.
Saliva predom. increased	Saliva *generally* diminished.
Hunger predominant.	Generally loss of appetite.
Appetite for meat or spirituous liquors . .	Aversion to meat; inclination for *or* aversion to spirituous liquors.*
Urine smelling like Ammoniac	Urine having sour smell.
Catamenia too soon and profuse	Catamenia generally too late and scanty.
Expectoration almost constant; evening . .	Expectoration not constant; morning and during day; more rare at night.
Complaints predominant in lower part of chest.	Complaints predom. in upper part of chest.

Iodium.	Sulphur.
Remission *forenoon* and before midnight . .	Remission *afternoon* and before midnight.
Worse in-doors; better out-doors†	Better (resp. worse) in-doors *or* out of doors.
Worse in warm air; better in cold weather .	Better (resp. worse) in warm *or* cold air.
Better when growing cold; worse when growing warm.	Better (resp. worse) when growing cold *or* warm.
Worse after sweat	*Worse or* better after sweat.
Almost always aggravated in bed	*Worse or* better in bed.
Worse from warmth of bed	*Worse or* better from warmth of bed.
Worse when lying on back, better when lying on side.	Generally better when lying on back, worse when lying on side.
Better after getting out of bed	Worse *or* better after getting out of bed.
Worse when moving diseased part	Worse *or* better when moving diseased part.
Worse from being touched	*Worse or* better from being touched.
Worse when fasting; better after breakfast .	Better (resp. worse) on an empty stomach; predom. worse after breakfast.
Worse when hungry; better after a satisfying meal.	Worse after a satisfying meal.
Improved oftener than aggrav. after meals .	Worse after meals.
Worse after stool	Worse *or* better after stool.
Worse from weeping	Worse *or* better from weeping.
Worse when swallowing food and drink . .	Worse when swallowing food and saliva.

Predomin. worse —— **Predomin. better**

On expiration, from motion, when sitting erect, when lying on back, and from pressure.

Predomin. better —— **Predomin. worse**

On inspiration, during rest, when standing, after lying down, while lying, partic. on side, when sitting bent forward, after meals, partic. after a satisfying meal, and from sweets.

---

* With immoderate wine-drinkers a disgust for wine sometimes follows the administration of Sulphur (Hahnemann); in some cases it creates an irresistable desire for alcoholic drinks even with boys. C.Hg.

† Both remedies have predominant aggravation " when walking out-doors."

Ipecacuanha.	Antimon. tartar.
Right side—Want of bodily irritability	*Left* side—Increased irritability.
Pain pressing outwards—Skin parched	Pain pressing inwards — Disposition to sweat.
Apoplexy - Plethora	Very rarely apoplexy—Anæmie
Sleeplessness	Somnolence predominant.
Pulse very much accelerated, but often imperceptible.	Pulse quick, full, and strong, sometimes trembling; very much accelerated by every motion; when the fever abates, it is often slow and imperceptible.
Thirst not constant	Thirst only sometimes during heat and between heat and sweat.
Thirst predom. during chill	Want of thirst during chill.
Chill moderated by drinking	Chill increased by drinking.

Ipecacuanha.	Antimon. tartar.
Mood peevish; irritable	Mood despondent—Boldness—Mental dullness.
Nausea predominant in stomach, less frequently in abdomen.	Nausea in stomach or abdomen, rarely in throat.
Vomit bitter oftener than sour	Vomit predom. sour.
Difficult expiration	Short, gasping inspiration, and long, sighing expiration.
Expectoration infrequent	Expectoration not constant.

Ipecacuanha.	Antimon. tartar.
Worse *or* better on awaking	Worse on awaking.
Worse after getting out of bed	Almost always improved after getting out of bed.
Worse when stooping	Almost always improved when stooping.
Generally better after drinking	Worse after drinking.
Ailments from Tartar emetic, Ferrum, Cuprum, Arsenic, Alumina, Arnica, Cinchona, Dulcamara, or Opium.	Ailments from Baryt. or Sepia.

Predomin. worse 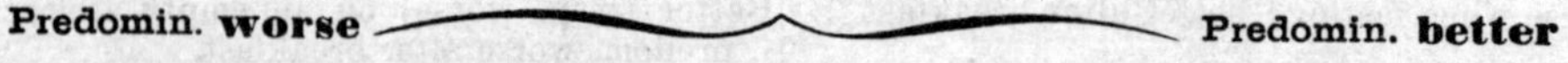 **Predomin. better**

In dry weather, after getting out of bed, when stooping, and on inspiration.

Predomin. better — **Predomin worse**

In wet weather, when lying and sitting, after drinking, and on inspiration.

N.B. Apparently in contradiction to the constitutional character of both remedies, we find oversensitiveness to pain less frequently with Antimon. tart. than with Ipecacuanha. Compare preface.

Ipecacuanha.	Nux vomica.
Want of bodily irritability—Light hair. .	Increased irritability—Dark hair.
Skin and muscles lax—Hæmorrhages, blood light-red.	Skin and muscles rigid — Hæmorrhages, blood dark.
Epilepsy, with loss of consciousness . . .	Epilepsy, with full consciousness.
Pulse very much accelerated, but often imperceptible.	Pulse generally quick, full, and hard; sometimes intermitting or imperceptible.
Chill lessened out-doors	Chill increased out-doors.
Chill lessened after drinking	Chill predom. worse after drinking. C.Hg.
Heat increased in-doors	Heat lessened in-doors.
Coldness on upper part of body	Coldness on lower part of body.
Taciturnity	Loquacity — Fear — Malice — Amorousness — Absent-mindedness — Fancies—Delirium.
Very rarely paralysis	Paralysis of limbs.
Aversion to bacon	Appetite for fatty things.
Inguinal hernia, easily reduced	Inguinal hernia, difficult to reduce.
Diarrhœa predominant; generally painless.	Constipation predominant; when diarrhœa occurs, it is painful
Urine dark	Urine generally pale.
Respiration with moist sound	Respiration with dry sound.
Expectoration very infrequent; *morning* and during day.	Expectoration not constant; from morning till evening.
AGGRAVATION from evening till morning .	AGGRAVATION after midnight, morning and dnring day.
REMISSION during day	REMISSION evening till midnight.*
Although better in-doors, worse when the room is too warm.	Better in warm room.
Better after drinking	Worse *or* better after drinking.
Worse from light, partic. candle-light .	Worse from light, partic. daylight.
Ailments from Alum., Antimon. tart., Ferrum, Arnica, or Opium.	Ailments from Calcarea, Sulphur, Phosphor, Iodine, Plumbum, Graphites, Petroleum, Lachesis, Coffea, Chamomilla, Pulsatilla, Cocculus, Colchicum, Digitalis, Stramonium.

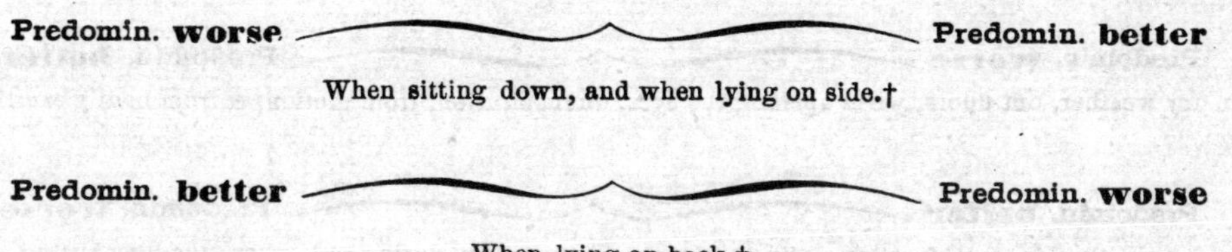

* Nux vomica "fevers" also occur in the "evening," but, as a rule, "not" in the forenoon, when other Nux vomica complaints are predominant.

† With Nux vomica there is also an aggrav. when lying on side and improv. when lying on back, but much more seldom than the reverse

Ipecacuanha.	Pulsatilla.
Want of bodily irritability — Aversion to open air.	Increased irritability—Inclination for open air.
Hæmorrhages, blood light-red — *Upper right, lower left side.*	Hæmorrhages, blood predom. dark—*Upper left, lower right side.*
Dropsy predominant in internal parts . .	Dropsy predominant in external parts.
Itching, unchanged by scratching . . .	Itching, aggrav. *or* unchanged by scratch'g.
No affection of glands, & very rarely of bones.	Very rarely muscular spasms.
Coldness, partic. of upper part of body . .	Coldness, part. of feet or right side.
Sweat smells sour	Sweat often smells musty or like musk.
Thirst not constant, but predominant during chill.	Want of thirst predominant, but constant only during chill.
Chill moderated by drinking	Chill increased by drinking. C.Hg.

Ipecacuanha.	Pulsatilla.
Dejection less prominent than with Pulsatilla.	Fear — Indifference — Gentleness — Amorousness—Rarely irritability—Boldness—Avarice—Distrust.
Rarely unconsciousness or delirium . . .	Absent-mindedness – Fancies.
Pupils predominant dilated	Pupils generally contracted.
Want of appetite predominant	Generally hunger.
Nausea predominant in stomach, less frequently in abdomen.	Nausea in throat, stomach or abdomen.
Qualmishness after eating what disagrees with the stomach, and of use when the stomach is empty again.	Qualmishness after eating what disagrees with the stomach, and of use while the stomach still contains the food.
Vomiting, first water, then food.	Vomiting, first food then water.
Diarrhœa predominant painless	Diarrhœa generally painful.
Catamenia too soon and profuse	Catamenia too late and predom. scanty.
Dry coryza	Coryza fluent, partic. right side, oftener than dry.
Voice hollow	Voice hoarse or aphony.
Respiration quick, *or* slow, and sighing .	Respiration quick or unequal.
Rattling of mucus	Respiration with dry sound.
Expectoration infrequent; morning	Expector. predom.; morning & during day.
Complaints predominant in palm of hand .	Complaints predominant on back of hand.

Ipecacuanha.	Pulsatilla.
Aggravation from evening till morning .	Aggravation from noon till midnight.
Worse in dry-cold weather	*Worse* in wet-cold or warm air.
Worse from bodily exertion	Worse from mental exertion; oftener improv. than aggrav. by bodily exertion.
Worse *during* sweat, better *after* it . .	Worse during and after sweat
Worse when lying on side, better when lying on back.	Sometimes better when lying on side and sometimes when lying on back.

Predomin. worse — **Predomin. better**

In dry weather, out-doors, when opening the eyes, on inspiration, from motion, & from bodily exertion.

Predomin. better — **Predomin. worse**

In wet weather, in-doors*, when closing the eyes, on expiration, during rest, when standing, sitting, and lying, after drinking, and after sweat.

N.B. Ipecac. seems to lack the sensation of numbness in suffering parts peculiar to Pulsatilla.

---

* However, in too hot a room Ipecacuanha also has aggravation.

Ipecacuanha.	Veratrum.
Upper right, lower left side—Want of irritability.	Upper left, lower right side—Bodily irritability increased.
Rending pain or dropsy in internal parts .	Rending pain or dropsy in external parts.
Pulse very much accelerated	Pulse irregular; generally slow, small, and weak; sometimes slower than beating of heart.
Thirst not constant, but very predom. during chill.	Thirst predom., but not constant, most rare during sweat.
Chill moderated by drinking	*Chill increased by drinking.*
Very rarely paralysis	Paralysis.

Wrapt in thought	Being besides one's self.
Very rarely haughtiness	Cheerfulness *or* dejection—Distrust—Fear — Malice — Amorousness; very rarely peevishness — Absent-mindedness — Fancies—Delirium—Insanity.
Pupils predom. dilated	Pupils generally contracted.
Saliva generally increased	Saliva generally diminished.
Urine scanty	Urine seldom & scanty; sometimes copious.
Catamenia too soon	Catamenia too soon *or* too late.
Expectoration; morning and during day .	Expector. not constant; partic. during day.

Remission of complaints during day . .	Remission during day and evening.
Better (resp. worse) in cold *or* warm air .	Worse in cold weather; better in warm air.
Worse when growing warm; better when growing cold.	Better (resp. worse) when growing cold *or* warm.
Worse *or* better on awaking	Worse on awaking.
Worse after getting out of bed	Worse *or* better after getting out of bed.
Predom. worse on inspiration, better on expiration.	Predom. worse on in- and expiration.
Worse after meals	Worse *or* better after meals.
Generally better after drinking	Worse after drinking.
Worse from being awake at night . . .	Worse from sleeping too long.

Predomin. worse — **Predomin. better**

In dry weather, out-doors, but also from warmth of stove, from motion, and when walking.

Predomin. better — **Predomin. worse**

In wet weather, in-doors, during rest, when standing, sitting, and lying, after drinking, particularly drinking cold water.

N.B. Apparently in contradiction to the constitutional character of both remedies, we find over-sensitiveness to pain oftener with Ipecac. than with Veratr.—Comp. preface.

Kali bichrom.	Arsenic.
Complaints predom. in external parts . . .	Complaints predom. in internal parts.
First right, then left side	First left, then right side.
Deep ulcers—Periostitis	Shallow ulcers—Inflammation of periosteum.
Thirst predom.	Thirst occurs mostly during sweat, and least during chill.

Kali bichrom.	Arsenic.
Taciturnity	Loquacity oftener than taciturnity.
Misanthropy	Fear of being alone oftener than misanthropy.
Saliva increased	Saliva diminished.
Complaints predom. on soft palate	Complaints predom. on roof of mouth.
Diphtheria, fauces with ulcers, deep eating in, tongue coated thick yellow, edges red and full of small, painful ulcers; nose discharging tough, stringy phlegm; swelling of parotid glands with pain in ears; croup-like cough; eruption like measles—Sensation of a hair on the root of the tongue.	Diphtheria, ulcers extending to the roof of mouth; tongue white; nose watering; the characteristic restlessness, thirst & aggrav. after midnight; hoarse cough with restlessness after midnight, with putrid diarrhœa disposed to nettle-rash—Sensation of a hai in the throat. Lipp(
Urine scanty	Urine scanty (with diarrhœa) *or* copious.
Voice nasal	Voice trembling.

Kali bichrom.	Arsenic.
Aggravation morning and noon	Aggravation from evening till morning, particularly after midnight.
Generally aggrav. by motion	Generally improv. by motion.
Better after lying down	*Worse* after lying down.
Worse when getting out of bed	*Better* when getting out of bed; worse *or* better *after* getting out of bed.
Worse on inspiration	Often worse on expiration.
Consequences of immoderate drinking of malt-liquors. Lippe.	Consequences of immoderate drinking of spirituous liquors. Wahle.
Ailments from Arsenic vapors or Mercurius.	Ailments from contagious Anthrax, Plumb., Iod., Cinchona, Digit., Strychnine, Phosph.

Kali bichrom.	Mercurius.
Muscles rigid	Muscles lax.
Deep ulcers	Ulcers shallow oftener than deep.
Nasal complaints predom. internal	Nasal compl. *external* oftener than internal.
Complaints predom. in lower part of chest .	Complaints predom. in upper part of chest.
Urine scanty	Urine often and copious.
Emission of succus prostaticus (with the stool).	Pollutions.
Catamenia too soon	Catamenia too late.
Expectoration viscid	Expectoration sharp and acrid.

Kali bichrom.	Mercurius.
Aggravation morning and noon	Aggravation from evening till morning.
Improved by running of nose, nose-bleed, and soft stool.	Aggravated by loss of animal fluids.

Worse — **Better**

From smoking.

Better — **Worse**

From Vomiting.

Kali bichrom.	Natr. mur.
Light hair	Dark hair.
Pain in the limbs shifting from place to place.	Fixed pain in limbs.
Internal nasal complaints predom. — Compl. on *lower* teeth.	External nasal complaints ,predom. — Complaints on *upper* teeth.
Neither unconsciousness nor delirium . . .	Unconsciousness—Delirium.
Diphtheria—Pain in the ear extending to the swelled parotid glands and to the head; tongue coated yellow, especially at the root; pricking in the tonsils and scraping with stitches in the throat; burning in the throat; after abuse of Iod. of Mercury. Lippe.	Diphtheria—Swelling of submaxillory glands; tongue like a map, marked with red lines; burning in throat; dryness in the throat with thirst after abuse of nitrate of silver. Raue.
Vomiting of viscous mucus	Vomiting of food oftener than mucus.
Urine scanty—Sediment whitish	Urine too often—Sediment reddish.
Catamenia too soon	Catamenia predom. too late.
Eluent coryza—Nasal secretion watery or viscous, or in hard lumps.	Dry coryza—Nasal secretion thick.
Expectoration not constant	Expectoration infrequent.
Aggravation morning and noon	Remission of complaints afternoon.
Ailments from Arsenic vapors or Mercurius.	Ailments from abuse of Cinchona.

Predomin. worse ——— **Predomin. better**

From cold, from cold* diet, and when sitting down.

Predomin. better ——— **Predomin. worse**

From warmth, and after getting out of bed.

Kali bichrom.	Nitr. acid.
Light hair — Itching aggrav. by scratching .	Dark hair—Itching, relieved by scratching.
Complaints predom. on *lower* teeth, on soft palate and in lower part of chest.	Complaints predom. on *upper* teeth, on roof of mouth, and in upper part of chest.
Thirst predom..	Thirst predom., except during chill.
Diphtheria—Ulcers, deep eating in the fauces and on the palate, phagedenous; tough, stringy discharge from the nose; swelling of parotid glands. Lippe.	Diphtheria—Ulcers in the mouth with stinging as from splinters; corroding discharge from the nose; swelling of parotid glands. Raue.
Bleeding fr. the nose, blood thick & dark-red; pulse irregular, small, contracted. Lippe.	Bleeding from the nose, blood acid like vinegar; intermitting pulse. Lippe.
Vomiting of viscous mucus	Vomiting of food.
Urinal sediment whitish	Urinal sediment *reddish* or whitish.
Expectoration not constant	Expect. not constant; morning & during day.
Pain in chest predom. right side	Pain in chest predom. left side.
Aggravation morning and noon	Remission forenoon.
Ailments from Mercurius or Arsenic vapors.	Ailments from Mercur., Calcar., or Digitalis.
Worse when swallowing saliva	Worse when swallowing food.

Predomin. worse ——— **Predomin. better**

In cold weather, when stooping, when sitting down, in the side not lain on, and from scratching.

Predomin. better ——— **Predomin. worse**

In warm air, after getting out of bed, and in the side lain on.

* Natr. mur. has also sometimes improv. from warm diet.

Kali bichrom.	Pulsatilla.
Complaints predom. in external parts . . .	Complaints predom. in internal part
Complaints from Arsenic vapors	Complaints from Copper vapors.
Pains appear and disappear suddenly, or increase and decrease gradually.	Pains appear suddenly and disapp. gradually.
Pains attack first one part, then re-appear in another.	Pains (rheumatic) shift from one place to another without an intermission.*
Aversion to bodily and mental exertion . .	Desire to walk slowly, and relief from it.*
Ulcers: overlapping edges, a red areola around, a hard bottom with a blackish spot in the middle.	*Ulcers*: swollen red surroundings, bleed easily, and suppurate profusely.*
Moderately cold air is felt very unpleasantly .	Desire for the open air, and amelioration in the cold, open air.*
Thirst predom.	Want of thirst predom.
Headache, better when lying down	Headache, worse when lying down.
Photophobia by daylight, not by candle-light.	Photoph. by candle-light, not by dim daylight.
Flow of water from the eyes with burning when opening them.	Lachrymation in the cold, open air and in the wind.*
Pustules on the cornea	Obscuration of the cornea.*
Stitches in the (left) ear, extending into the neck, head.	Stitches and tearing with inflamm., swelling, heat & redness of the intern. & extern. ear.*
The nose feels too heavy	The nose feels sore internally and externally.
Complaints of inner nose predom.	Nasal compl. external oftener than internal.
Watery discharge from the nose with great sensitiveness and ulceration of the nostrils.	Green fetid discharge.*
Hard, plug-like masses (klinkers) causing pain when removed.	Chronic coryza with yellow-green discharge from nose.
Bad smell from the nose	Subjective smell like old catarrh.*
Great dryness of mouth and lips, momentarily relieved by drinking.	The mouth feels dry, clammy, compelling him to moisten it at times.
Tongue dry, and heavily coated in the morning .	Tongue coated yellow (white) and is covered with tough mucus.
Tongue coated at the root and with a heavy yellow felt.	Tongue feels in the middle as if burned.*
Tongue red, smooth glossy (in dysentery) . . .	Tongue feels dry, clammy, without thirst.*
Throat and soft palate dark-red copper color . .	Inflammation of the throat with veins distended.*
Complaints predom. on soft palate	Complaints predom. on roof of mouth.
Burning in the throat	Sore feeling, stinging in the throat.*
Inflammation & ulceration of the palate & tonsils.	Tough mucus in the throat, esp. in the morning.*
Thirst with tongue and mouth dry	Thirstlessness with moist tongue.*
Vomiting of sour substances	Vomiting of bile.*
Vomiting of food after breakfast	Vomit. of food after each meal, esp. in the evening.
Watery diarrhœa followed by tenesmus (morning).	Watery diarrhœa preceded by rumbling in the abdomen (night).*
Urinal sediment whitish	Urinal sediment red.
Emission of succus prostat. (with the stool) .	Pollutions.
Catamenia too soon	Catamenia too late.
Hoarseness (evening)	Hoarseness when speaking aloud.*
Loud rattling cough with nausea and expectoration dragging to the feet in strings.	Cough with expectoration of much bitter, yellow, green, or blood-streaked mucus.*
Expectoration not constant, stringy	Expectoration predom., but not constant.
Like a heavy load laying on chest (when awaking from sleep).	Constriction of chest, (when awaking from sleep.)*
Stitches under the sternum through to the back.	Stitches in the chest.*
Sensation of coldness in the region of the heart.	Burning sensation in the region of the heart.
AGGRAVATION morning and noon	AGGRAVATION from noon till midnight.
Better from running of nose, nose-bleed, soft stools, (sometimes from vomiting).	*Worse* from loss of fluids.

Predomin. worse ——— **Predomin. better**

In cold weather, from cold, from cold diet, from motion, from bodily exertion, when lifting diseased limb, and on inspiration.

Predomin. better ——— **Predomin. worse**

In warm air, from warmth, during rest, when letting diseased limb hang down, and on expiration.

N.B. Kali bichrom. seems to lack both the over-sensitiveness of Pulsatilla to pain and the sensation of numbness in suffering parts.

N.B. * added by Dr. A. Lippe, wo first used Kali bichr. in *measles*.

Kali carb.	Arsenic.
Complaints (gnawing pain, etc.) predomin. in external parts.	Complaints (gnawing pain, etc.) predomin. in internal parts.
Pain rending downwards—Pred. plethora.	Pain rending upwards—Predom. anæmie.
Humid eruptions	Eruptions generally dry.
Ulcers, dicsharge rather copiously	Discharge pred. cop's., rarely scanty. C.Hg
In the scars tension, pressing, rending	In scars burning. C.Hg.
Dreams of water, thieves, ghosts, diseases (dead people, misfortunes), also erotic, imaginative, and phantastic dreams	Dreams of fire, thunder-storm (dead persons & misfortunes), vexation, embarrassment, etc.
Pulse very different; often slow and weak; often frequent and hard.	Pulse generally frequent, small, and weak.
Partial sweat on upper part of body	Sweat on lower part of body.
Sweat increased by motion	Sweat lessened by motion.
Thirst predominant, except perhaps during chill.	Least thirst during chill, most during sweat; drinks often, but little at a time during heat.

Kali carb.	Arsenic.
Absent-mindedness	Indifference—Irritability—Maliciousness—Avarice—Imbecility—Insanity.
Ailments from hearing bad news	Ailm. from vexat'n with fear or vehemence.
Complaints predominant on upper eyelids.	Complaints predominant on lower eyelids.
Aversion to bread, particularly rye-bread	Appetite for bread, particularly rye-bread.
Appetite for sweets	Aversion to sweats.
Nausea in stomach	Nausea, particularly in throat.
Constipation predominant	Diarrhœa predominant.
Urine often but scanty	Urine scanty (with diarrhœa) *or* copious.
Catam. too scanty, but of long duration	Catam. too profuse and of long duration.
Coryza dry oftener than fluent	Fluent coryza.
Expectoration is loosened in morning and during day, and is generally swallowed.	Expectoration during day.
Complaints predominant in hollow of elbow and on shin	Complaints predominant in hollow of knee and on calf of leg.

Kali carb.	Arsenic.
Worse after sweating	*Worse or* better after sweating.
Better *or* worse from warmth of bed	Better from warmth of bed.
Worse after sleep	Better after sufficient sleep; but worse on awaking when roused from sleep.
Worse when getting out of bed	Almost always improv. when getting out of bed
Worse from light, better in the dark	Better (resp. worse) from light or in the dark.
Worse when stooping; predom. better when assuming an erect position.	Better *or* worse when stooping and when assuming an erect position.
Better or worse from eructation	Better from eructation.
Worse after stool	*Worse or* better after stool.

Predomin. worse ——— **Predomin. better**

In wet weather, from washing and moistening diseased part, when bending it, from pressure, when lying on side, partic. on unpainful side, when getting out of bed, after sleep, when sitting down, when riding, and from warm diet.

Predomin. better ——— **Predomin. worse**

In dry weather, when lying on back, or on painful side, from scratching and rubbing, when riding on horseback, and from cold diet.

Kali carb.	Lycopodium.
Dark hair — Muscles rigid — Crackling in internal parts.	Light hair—Muscles lax—Crackling in the joints.
Spasms with full consciousness	Spasms with unconsciousness.
Pulse very different, often more frequent in the morning, slower in evening; rarely reversed; often unequal, irregular, intermitting; also slow and weak, or accelerated and hard; trembling.	Pulse somewhat accelerated only after meals and in the evening, partic. frequent in the evening, slow in the morning.
One-sided heat, right side	One-sided heat, left side.

Kali carb.	Lycopodium.
Mood sad	Mood changing; cheerful *or* depressed; serious; gentle *or* irritable; haughty; malicious; miserly; distrustful.
Solicitude concerning bodily welfare . .	Solicitude concern'g spiritual welfare. C.Hg.
Ailments from hearing bad news	Ailments from anger.
Very rarely fancies	Imbecility—Insanity.
Apoplexy not yet observed	Apoplexy.
Compl. predom. on external angle of eye, on outside of nose, on upper lip, in lower part of chest, and on upper arm.	Compl. predom. on inner angle of eye, on inside of nose, on under-lip, in upper part of chest, and on fore-arm.
Urinary sediment reddish	Urinary sediment red (sandy) *or* whitish.
Respiration predominant with dry sound .	Respiration predom. with moist sound.
Expectoration not constant; morning and during day.	Expectoration almost constant; morning and evening.

Kali carb.	Lycopodium.
Remission of complaints *during day* and before midnight.	Remission forenoon and after midnight.
Worse in cold weather, better in warm air.	Better (resp. worse) in cold *or* warm air.
Worse from growing cold, better from growing warm.	Better (resp. worse) from growing cold or warm.
Worse after perspiring	*Better or* worse after perspiring.
Better *or* worse after getting out of bed .	Almost always improved after getting out of bed.
Worse when hungry	Worse after a satisfying meal.
Better or worse from eructation	Better from eructation.
Worse from sneezing	Worse *or* better when sneezing.
Worse from needle-work and the like . .	Better when knitting.
Worse when alone, better when in company.	Better (resp. worse) when alone or in comp.
Worse after stool	Worse *or* better after stool.

Predomin. worse ⁀ **Predomin. better**

When lying on unpainful side, when lifting diseased limb, from cold, from warm diet, and from doing needle-work.

Predomin better ⁀ **Predomin. worse**

When lying on painful side, when letting diseased limb hang down, from warmth, in warm rooms, and from cold diet.

Kali carb.	Nitr. acid.
Ulcerative pain in external parts	Ulcerative pain in internal parts.
Crackling in internal parts	Crackling of joints.
In the scars tension, pressing, and rending.	Scars get sore, break open. C.Hg.
Rending pain downwards	Rending pain upwards.
One-sided heat, right side	One-sided heat, left side.
Peevishness not so frequent as with Nitr. acid.	Distrust—Maliciousness.
Absent-mindedness more frequent than with Nitr. acid.	Rarely paralysis.
Complaints predom. on *upper* eyelids, on outside of nose, on upper arm, in hollow of elbow, on shin, and in lower part of chest.	Complaints predom. on *lower* eyelids, on inside of nose, on fore-arm, in hollow of knee, on calf of leg, and in upper part of chest.
Urine hot, but often scanty; sediment reddish.	Urine cold *or* hot; scanty; sediment red *or* white.
Catamenia too scanty, at the same time too late *or* too soon.	Catamenia too profuse and too soon.
Sexual desire preval. strong	Sexual desire weak.
Respiration generally with dry sound . .	Respiration preval. with moist sound.
Expectoration not constant; is generally swallowed; morning and during day; less frequent in the evening.	Expectoration not constant; morning and during day.
Pleuro-Pneumonia, with dry, suppressed cough, when the stitching pain continues or returns.	Pleuro-Pneumonia, with copious greenish, blood-streaked expectoration, when the fever increases and the stitrhing pain disappears; in old, emaciated, choleric people.
REMISSION *during day* and before midnight.	REMISSION of complaints in the forenoon.
Worse when riding	*Better* when riding, *worse afterwards.*

Predomin. worse — **Predomin. better**

In cold weather, after perspiring, when stooping, when sitting down, when lying on unpainful side,* and when riding.

Predomin. better — **Predomin. worse**

In warm air, when assuming an erect position, when leaning against anything, and when lying on the painful side.

N.B. Nitr. acid. lacks the sensation of numbness in suffering parts peculiar to Kali carb.

*** In rare cases we also find aggravation with Kali carb. when lying on painful side, and improvement when lying on unpainful side.**

Kali carb.	Phosphor.
Complaints (sensitiveness, etc.) predominant in external parts.	Complaints (sensitiveness, etc.) predom. in internal parts.
Crackling in internal parts	Crackling of joints.
Humid eruptions	Dry (symptomatic) eruptions.
Ulcers discharge copiously	Ulcers, discharge copious or scanty. C.Hg.
Scars: tension, pressing, tearing	Scars: pinching contraction; break open; bleed. C.Hg.
Partial sweat on upper part of body . .	Partial sweat on lower part of body.
Thirst predominant, except during chill .	Want of thirst constant during all stages.
Chill increased out-doors, sweat also while eating.	Chill lessened out-doors — Sweat lessened while eating.
Complaints predom. on external angle of eye, on upper jaw and upper lip, and in lower part of chest.	Complaints predom. in inner angle of eye, on lower jaw, on under lip, and in upper part of chest.
Dreams of water, thieves, ghosts, misfortunes, diseases, dead people, erotic and sentimental dreams.	Dreams of fire, misfortunes, diseases, of dead people, embarrassment, quarrel and vexation, erotic, or concerning the business of the day, historical, or mentally exerting dreams.

Kali carb.	Phosphor.
Mood sad	Mood cheerful or depressed; changing; indifferent; irritable; haughty.
Ailments from vexation with reserved displeasure, and from hearing bad news.	Ailments from anger or vexation with vehemence.
Weak memory	Memory active—Rarely absent-mindedness.
Very rarely fancies	Ecstasies—Insanity.
Apoplexy not yet observed.	Apoplexy.
Appetite for sweets	Aversion to sweets.
Constipation predominant	Diarrhœa predominant; painless.
Catamenia too scanty	Catamenia too profuse *or* scanty.
Sputa generally swallowed	Sputa are expectorated.

Kali carb.	Phosphor.
REMISSION *during day* and before midnight.	REMISSION of complaints after midnight.
Worse when alone, better when in company.	Better (resp. worse) when alone *or* in comp.
Better *or* worse from warmth of bed.	Predom. worse from warmth of bed.
Worse (better) when lying on right *or* on left side.	Better when lying on right side, worse when lying on left side.
Worse during sleep	Worse *or* better during sleep.
Worse on awaking from sleep	Better after sufficient sleep; but worse on awaking when roused and after the siesta.
Worse when eating, partic. bread . . .	Worse *or* better when eating; partic. eating bread.

Predomin. worse — **Predomin. better**

When lying on side, particularly lying on unpainful side, when sitting down, when sitting erect and standing, when lifting diseased limb or when resting it on anything, and after sleep.

Predomin. better — **Predomin. worse**

When lying on back or on painful side, when sitting bent forward, when assuming an erect position, when letting diseased limb hang down, and in warm rooms.

Kali carb.	Pulsatilla.
Want of bodily irritability—Compl. predom. in external parts.	Increased irritability—Complaints predom. in internal parts.
Crackling in internal parts—Boring pain from without inwards.	Crackl'g of joints—Bor'g pain from within outwards.
Aversion to open air	Inclination for open air.
Pulse very different; often frequent in the morning, slower in the evening, rarely the reverse; often unequal, irregular or trembling; often slow and weak, often also accelerated and hard.	Pulse generally frequent, small, and weak; slow in the morning, frequent in the evening; sometimes imperceptible.
Heat on lower part of body	Heat on upper part of body.
Thirst predominant; but is often wanting during chill.	Want of thirst predominant, but constant only during chill.
Chill increased out-doors	Chill abated out-doors.
Itching, relieved by scratching	Itch'g, unchanged *or* aggrav. by scratch'g
Aversion to being alone	Desire to be alone.
Very rarely fancies	Mood changing; indifferent; gentle; bold; distrustful—Parsimony.
Ailments from hearing bad news	Ailments from excessive joy.
Paralysis—No apoplexy	Apoplexy—Very rarely paralysis.
Compl. predom. on external angle of eye, on upper lip, upper jaw, & upper teeth.	Compl. predom. in inner angle of eye, on under lip, lower jaw, and lower teeth.
Swelling of upper lip predominant	Swelling of under lip predominant.
Nausea in stomach	Nausea in throat, stomach, and abdomen.
Constipation predominant	Diarrhœa predominant.
Urine too often, but scanty	Urine infrequent and scanty.
Catamenía too scanty, but of long duration.	Catam. too scanty and of short duration.
Coryza dry oftener than fluent	Coryza fluent (partic. right side) oftener than dry.
Sputa are swallowed	Sputa are expectorated.
REMISSION *during day* and before midnight.	REMISSION from midnight till noon.
Worse from exertion, walking fast, etc.	Improv. oftener than aggrav. by exertion.
Worse when taking a deep breath	Better *or* worse when taking a deep breath.
Worse after stool	*Better or* worse after stool.
Better *or* worse from warmth of bed	Worse from warmth of bed.
Worse (better) when lying on right *or* left side.	Better when lying on right side, worse when lying on left side.
Worse after sleep	Worse *or* better after sleep.
Worse (better) when opening *or* closing the eyes.	Better when opening, worse when closing the eyes.
Almost always improved when rising (from a stooping posture).	Worse *or* better when rising.
Better *or* worse from being touched.	Worse from touch.

Predomin. worse — **Predomin. better**

From cold, growing cold and in cold weather, on inspiration, when sitting erect, when lifting diseased limb or resting it on anything, when washing, moistening, or bending suffering part sideways, from pressure, after stool, and from bodily exertion.

Predomin. better — **Predomin. worse**

From warmth, growing warm and in warm air, on expiration, when sitting bent forward, when letting diseased limb hang down, from sweets, in warm rooms, and from rubbing and scratching.

Kali carb.	Sepia.
Spasms with full consciousness	Spasms with unconsciousness.
Itching of skin, relieved by scratching . .	Itching, aggrav. by scratching.
Eruptions humid	Erupt'ons generally dry.
Ulcers, discharge copious	Ulcers, discharge very copious or scanty. C.Hg
Pulse very different; sometimes frequent in the morning, slower in the evening; rarely reversed.	Pulse accelerated, partic. by vexation and motion; frequent at night, slow during the day.
Heat with thirst	Heat without thirst.
Thirst predom.; but during chill want of thirst is predominant.	Want of thirst; only during chill thirst is constant.
Fear of being alone	Desire to be alone — Mood indifferent; apathetic; serious; irritable—Avarice.
Consequences of grief—Self-willed . . .	Consequences of anger.
Delirium	Insanity—Imbecility.
Very rarely fancies	Apoplexy.
Swelling, or eruption on *upper* lip predom.	Swelling or eruption on *under* lip predem.
Compl. predom. on upper arm & on shin .	Compl. predom. on fore-arm and on calf.
Discharge of urine too often, but scanty .	Discharge of urine not often enough.
Urinal sediment reddish	Urinal sediment *red or* whitish.
Catamenia scanty	Catamenia profuse oftener than scanty.
False labor-pains too weak or spasmodic; originating in the small of back, and extending to the uterus with bearing down.	Spasmodic labor too weak or *with oversensitiveness;* the os uteri is swollen and indurated, resists dilatation, and with pain along the spine. Lippe.
After-pains most in sacral region, drawing down and pressing on the genitals.	After-pains with backache. Lippe.
Cough, partic. at night (after midnight) and dry in evening and night, in the morning and during day with expectoration, which is generally swallowed.	Cough, partic. forenoon and evening till midnight; dry during day, in the morning (evening) and at night, with expectoration, which is generally swallowed.
Remission during day and before midnight.	Remission of complaints in the afternoon
Worse in cold weather, partic. when it is wet and cold.	Better *or* worse in cold weather, but preval. worse in *dry* cold weather.
Worse after sleep	Better *or* worse after sleep.
Worse when hungry	Worse after a satisfying meal.
Worse from bodily exertion	Improv. oftener than aggrav. by exertion.

Predomin. worse — **Predomin. better**

In wet weather, when alone, when moving, running, from bodily exertion generally, when sitting down, when sitting erect, when lying on side, and after breakfast.

Predomin. better — **Predomin. worse**

In dry weather, in company, during rest, when sitting bent forward, when lying on back, when leaning against anything, from riding on horseback, on an empty stomach, from rubbing and scratching.

Kali carb.	Sulphur.
Over-sensitiveness*—Crackling in internal parts.	Insensibility—Numb sensation—Crackling of joints.
Pinching pain in internal parts; ulcerative pain in external parts.	Pinching pain in external parts; ulcerative pain in internal parts.
Cutaneous eruptions humid	Eruptions generally dry.
Complaints predominant in lower part of chest, on upper arm, and on shin.	Complaints predominant in upper part of chest, on fore-arm, and on calf of leg.
Pulse different; sometimes frequent in the morning, slower at night; rarely reversed.	Pulse quick, full, hard; partic. frequent night and morning; slower during day and evening.
Dreams of water, thieves, ghosts, diseases, or very phantastical.	Dreams of fire, vexation, business of the day, or merry.

Rarely fancies	Mood chang'g; indifferent; gentle; serious; irritable—Insanity—Imbecility.
Solicitude concerning the future	Solicitude concerning the present. C.Hg.
Ailments from grief or fright	Ailments from mortification, shame; less frequently from anger.
Saliva generally iucreased	Saliva generally diminished.
Urinal sediment red	Urinal sediment white oftener than red.
Catamenia of long duration	Catamenia generally of too short duration.
Cough, loose in morning and during day—Sputa are swallowed.	Expectoration in the morning and during the day; sometimes also at night.

REMISSION of complaints during day and before midnight.	REMISSION afternoon and before midnight.
Worse in cold, better in warm air . . .	Better (worse) in cold weather *or* in warm air.
Worse from growing cold, better from growing warm.	Better (worse) when growing cold *or* warm.
Predom. better in warm room	Worse in crowded room, but better from warmth of stove.
Worse after perspiring	*Worse or* better after perspiring.
Better *or* worse from warmth of bed . .	Almost always aggrav. by warmth of bed.
Worse when turning in bed	*Worse or* better when turning in bed.
Better (resp. worse) when stretching out *or* when drawing up diseased limb.	Worse when stretching out diseased limb; better when drawing it up.
When rising (from stooping posture) almost always improved.	Aggravated oftener than improved when rising.
Worse when looking into the light . . .	Worse when looking at running water.
Worse when hungry	Worse after a satisfying meal.
Worse after stool	Worse *or* better after stool.

Predomin. worse — **Predomin. better**

From cold, from warm diet, when alone, when sitting down, when sitting erect, when lying on unpainful side, also from external pressure.

Predomin. better — **Predomin. worse**

From warmth, from cold diet, when in company, when sitting bent forward, when assuming an erect position, when lying on painful side, and from sweets.

---

* This is not in contradiction to the constitutional want of irritability. Compare preface.

Kreosot.	Arsenic.
Left side—Bodily irritability increased . .	*Right* side—Want of bodily irritability.
Tension or constriction in external parts .	Tension or constriction in internal parts.
Stitches downwards—Apoplexy	Stitches upwards—Paralysis—Rarely apoplexy.
Sleeplessness preval. before midnight . .	Sleeplessness preval. after midnight.
Eruptions generally humid	Eruption generally dry.
Thirst during heat, none during chill . .	Least thirst during chill, most during sweat; desire for drink without thirst, during heat—Frequently thirst *before* chill, less frequently after it, and after sweat.

According to observations up to the present time, the symptoms of mind and disposition are only such as Arsenic also has.	Mood anxious, indifferent, irritable, malicious—Avarice—Unconsciousness—Delirium—Insanity.
Complaints generally on external ear . .	Complaints of inner ear predom.
Constipation predom.	Diarrhœa predom.
Urine too often and copious	Urine scanty (with diarrhœa) *or* copious.
Sexual desire preval. weak	Sexual desire too strong.
Dry coryza predom.	Fluent coryza.
Expectoration morning and evening . . .	Expectoration partic. during day.
Complaints predom. on fore-arm, on elbow-joint, and on shin.	Complaints predom. on upper arm, on knee, and on calf of leg.

Remission forenoon and evening. . . .	Remiss. *during day* and before midnight.
Better *or* worse from scratching	Worse from scratching.
Better after stool	*Worse or* better after stool.
Worse after urination	Better *or* worse after urinating.
Generally improved on expiration . . .	Generally aggrav. on expiration.

Predomin. worse ——— **Predomin. better**

From motion, when walking, when sitting down, when sitting erect, when lying on side, and from washing or bathing with cold water.

Predomin. better ——— **Predomin. worse**

During rest, after lying down, while lying, when sitting bent forward, when lying on back, and on expiration.

N.B. Kreosot seems to lack the over-sensitiveness of Arsenic to pain, and generally also the sensation of numbness in suffering parts.—This relation is only apparently in contradiction with the constitutional character of each remedy; comp. preface.

Kreosot.	Nux vomica.
Left side—Inclination for motion . . .	*Right* side—Aversion to motion.
Pain pressing inward	Pain pressing outward.
Apoplexia sanguinea—No paralysis . . .	Apoplexia nervosa—Paralysis.
Pulse small and weak, with violent ebullition of blood.	Pulse generally quick, full, hard, partic. during hot stage of fever; sometimes intermitting.
Thirst during heat, worse during chill . .	Most thirst during chill, also between heat and sweat, and *before* and *after* the fever attack.
Chill increased while sitting, lessened by motion.	Chill lessened while sitting, increased by motion.
Sleeplessness preval. before midnight . .	Sleeplessness preval. after midnight.

Peevishness not so constant as with Nux vomica.	Fear; irritability; maliciousness; amorousness.
Very rarely absent-mindedness.	Unconsciousness—Delirium.
Ailments from emotion generally	Ailments from anger, fright, grief, disappointed love, and jealousy; from mortification, and from vexation with fright, dread, fear, indignation or vehemence.
Dim-sightedness	Clear-sightedness predominant.
Complaints generally on external ear, on upper jaw, and on shin.	Complaints generally on inner ear, on lower jaw, and on calf.
Diarrhœa infrequent and painless	Diarrhœa infrequent and painful.
Urine too often and copious	Urine infrequent and scanty.
Sexual desire too weak	Sexual desire too strong.
Nasal secretion thick	Nasal secretion watery.
Cough generally with expectoration; morning and evening.	Cough generally without expector.; morning, during day, evening.

REMISSION forenoon and evening	REMISSION evening till midnight.
Worse when lying on side, better when lying on back.	*Generally* better when lying on side, worse when lying on back.
Better (resp. worse) when lying on right *or* left side.	Worse when lying on right side, better when lying on left side.
Worse *or* better when getting out of bed	Worse when getting out of bed.
Better *after* getting out of bed	Worse *or* better after getting out of bed.
Worse from washing and bathing with cold water.	*Generally* better from washing and moistening with cold water.
Better from pressure	*Better* or worse from pressure.
Worse when swallowing	*Worse or* better when swallowing.
Worse when stooping	*Better or* worse when stooping.

Predomin. worse — **Predomin. better**

On inspiration,* when lying on side, when sitting down, when sitting erect, when lifting diseased limb, and from washing with cold water.

Predomin. better — **Predomin. worse**

On expiration, when lying on back, after stool, when sitting bent forward, and when letting diseased limb hang down.

N.B. Although both remedies have the characteristic of increased irritability, still Kerosot. seems to lack the over-sensitiveness of the Nux vomica-patients to pain.

---

* Booth remedies have aggrav. of complaints *when taking a deep breath.*

Kreosot.	Sulphur.
Increased irritability — Pain pressing inward.	Want of bodily irritability—Pain pressing outward.
Apoplexy	Paralysis more frequent than apoplexy.
Eruptions generally humid	Eruptions generally dry.
Painful ulcers	Painless ulcers.
Pulse mall and weak, with violent ebullition of blood.	Pulse quick, full, and hard, sometimes intermitting.
Thirst during heat, none during chill	Thirst appears already *before* the chill; is most prominent during hot stage.
Heat or sweat, with aversion to uncover	Heat or sweat, with inclination to uncover.
The pains are spreading to remote parts	The pains are excited by mov'g remote parts.

Kreosot.	Sulphur.
Peevishness and depression less frequent than with Sulph.—Rarely irritability.	Mood serious; indifferent; changing, gentle *or* irritable.
Neither unconsciousness nor delirium	Absent-mindedness—Insanity.
Ailments from emotion generally	Ailments from shame, mortification, or from vexation with fright, dread or fear.
Eyes protruding	Eyes generally sunken.
Complaints generally on external ear	Complaints of inner ear predominant.
Subjective putrid smell	Objective stench from nose predom.
Nasal secretion thick	Nasal secretion predom. watery.
Complaints predominant on upper gum	Complaints predominant on lower gum.
Urine too often and copious; smelling ammoniacal.	Urine often, but scanty; but sometimes copious; sour.
Sediment red oftener than white	Sediment white oftener than red.
Catamenia too soon, profuse, and of long duration.	Catamenia *generally* too late, scanty, and of short duration.
Expectoration predom., but not constant; morning and evening.	Expectoration not constant; morning and during day, less frequent at night.
Complaints predominant on shin	Complaints predominant on calf of leg.

Kreosot.	Sulphur.
Remission forenoon and evening	Remission *afternoon* and before midnight.
Worse from growing cold & in cold weather, better from growing warm and in warm air.	Better (resp. worse) from growing cold and in cold weather, *or* from growing warm and in warm air.
Worse when turning in bed	*Worse or* better when turning in bed.
Worse from touch	*Worse or* better from touch.
Better after stool	Worse *or* better after stool.

Predomin. worse — **Predomin. better**

From cold, from uncovering, from motion, when sitting down, and when sitting erect.

Predomin. better — **Predomin. worse**

From warmth, from wrapping up, during rest, after lying down, while lying, when standing, when sitting bent forward, and after sleep.

N.B. We rarely find the sensation of numbness in suffering parts peculiar to Sulph. with Kreosot.

Lachesis.	Helleborus.
Increased constitutional irritability predom.	Want of constitutional irritability predom.
Upper left, lower right side	Lower left, upper right side.
Aversion to open air—Apoplexy	Inclination for open air—No apoplexy.
Epilepsy with unconsciousness . . .	Epilepsy with full consciousness.
External parts become black	Red parts become white.
Painful eruptions — Painful ulcers, sometimes with proud flesh.	Painless eruptions and ulcers.
Pulse accelerated, small, and weak; often alternating with full and strong beats; unequal and intermitting.	Pulse generally slow, small, and weak.
First chill, then heat	First heat, then chill.
Want of thirst predom.; that is thirst *before*, but not during the chill; during heat it is not frequent.	Constant want of thirst.
Sweat increased when and after getting out of bed.	Sweat lessened when getting out of bed.
Sleeplessness	Somnolence predominant.

Sensitive disposition—Mood predominantly cheerful; irritable; malicious; haughty—Amorousness.	Insensibility of disposition — Indifference and dejection predominant.
Ailments from fright, disappointed love, or jealousy	Ailments from mortification, or from vexation with reserved displeasure.
Easy comprehension — Ecstasies — Rarely absentmindedness, fancies, or unconsciousness.	Difficult comprehension—Mental dullness—No delirium.
Insanity	Imbecility.
Want of appetite predominant	Generally hunger.
Urine too often	Urine often, but scanty.
Rarely expectoration with the cough . .	Cough always dry (without expectoration).

REMISSION from midnight till noon . . .	REMISSION during day.
Worse when getting out of bed	Better *or* worse when getting out of bed.
Worse from pressure	Better *or* worse from pressure.
Better when swallowing *or* worse (when *swallowing saliva* or drink).	Worse when swallowing.

Predomin. worse — **Predomin. better**

Out doors,* in warm air, after sleep, during rest, when standing, sitting and lying.

Predomin. better — **Predomin. worse**

In-doors and from warmth of stove, in cold weather, in bed, from motion and when walking, on inspiration and from deep respiration, when stooping, when shaking head, and when bending diseased part backwards.

---

* "When walking out-doors" both remedies have predominant aggravation; therefore the influence of motion, and not that of the open air, decides for Helleborus.

Lachesis.	Lycopodium.
Upper left, lower right side—Often indicated with young women.	Upper right, lower left side—Often indicated with old women.
Paralysis generally of one side and painful .	Paral. often of both sides; generally painless.
Sensitiveness of internal and external parts .	Insensibility or numb sensation in internal parts; sensitiveness in external parts.
Ulcers better from warmth, worse from cold .	Ulcers worse from warmth, better from cold.
Pulse frequent, small, and weak; often alternating with full and strong beats; often trembling, unequal, or intermitting.	Pulse somewhat accelerated only after meals; partic. frequent in the evening, slow in the morning.
Sweat lessened while eating	Sweat increased while eating.
Heat, without thirst and with aversion to uncover.	Heat, with thirst and inclination to uncover.
Want of thirst predom.; thirst partic. *before* chill.	Thirst predominant even *after* sweat.
Pleasant dreams	Anxious dreams.
Loquacity—Mood cheerful; rarely peevish .	Taciturnity — Mood changing; depressed *or* cheerful; serious; gentle—Avarice.
Ailments from disappointed love or jealousy.	Ailments from anger, vexation, mortification, or grief.
Easy comprehension — Mental excitability—Rarely absent-mindedness, fancies, or unconsciousness.	Difficult comprehension—Mental dullness.
Complaints predominant on lower eyelids . .	Complaints predominant on upper eyelids.
Urine too often	Urine often, but scanty.
Catamenia generally scanty; of short duration.	Catam. generally of too long duration; at the same time scanty *or* profuse.
With scanty catam., bleeding from the anus—Instead of suppressed catam., toothache.	At the time of the suppressed catam. the breasts fill with milk. C.Hg.
Respiration preval. slow	Quick respiration.
Expectoration infrequent; morning and during day.	Expectoration tolerably constant; morning and evening.
REMISSION from midnight till noon	REMISSION after midnight and in the *forenoon.*
Worse when getting out of bed or rising from a seat.	Worse *or* better when rising from bed or from a seat.
Worse *or* better *after* rising from a seat . .	Better after rising from a seat.
Worse from light, partic. from sunlight . .	Worse from light, partic. from candle-light.
Worse from heat of sun.	Worse in snowy air.
Worse before thunder-storm	Worse during new moon.
Better when swallowing, *or* worse (swallowing saliva and drink).	Worse when swallowing.
Generally improved when eating	Generally aggravated while eating.
Better *or* worse *after* meals	Almost always aggravated after meals.
Worse *or* better from spirituous liquors . .	Worse from spirituous liquors.
Worse or better from eruptation	Better from eructation.

Predomin. worse —— **Predomin. better**

Out-doors and when walking out-doors, from cold, from uncovering, after getting out of bed, before breakfast, from warm diet,* when ascending, and when lifting diseased limb.

Predomin. better —— **Predomin worse**

In-doors and from warmth of stove, from warmth in general, from wrapping up, during sleep, after breakfast, from cold diet, when descending, when letting diseased limb hang down, when bending suffering part backwards, on inspiration and deep respiration, and after pollutions.

N.B. Lachesis lacks the sensation of numbness in suffering parts peculiar to Lycopodium, often also the over-sensitiveness of the latter to pain. Mere sensitiveness, on the other hand, (to the touch, etc.) is found with both remedies.

* In "Diphtheria," where both are of the greatest importance, the choice often decides for Lachesis by swallowing saliva; not food; for Lycop., if worse when swallowing warm drinks (Raue); Lachesis has more exsudative patches on the tonsils, particularly on the left side; Lycop. a darkish hue on the fauces, partic. right side; with both the patients are worse after sleep, with Lachesis particularly in the morning, with Lycop. when awaking after every nap, (children are cross, naughty, kick about). Other characteristics of Lachesis are over-sensibility of throat to the touch, or croup-like symptoms; of Lycop. the breathing through the mouth, or dilatation of nostrils with every inspiration, or parotid swellings, etc. C.Hg.

Lachesis.	Mercur.
Hæmorrhages, blood dark	Hæmorrhages, blood pale.
Blood incoagulable	Blood coagulates easily.
Humid, cutaneous eruptions	Eruptions most frequently dry.
Scars redden, hurt, burn, break open, and bleed.	Scars redden. C. Hg.
Pulse accelerated, small, and weak, often alternating with full and strong beats.	Pulse generally accelerated and full.
Want of thirst constant during chill, pred. during heat; often thirst *before* the chill.	Thirst almost constant during all stages.
Chill abated in warm room	Chill increased in warm room.
Sweat increased when and after getting out of bed, lessened while eating.	Sweat abated when and after getting out of bed, increased while eating.
When asleep lying on back	When asleep lying on side.

Lachesis.	Mercur.
Loquacity—Mood cheerful, rarely peevish.	Taciturnity—Mood serious; dejected.
Ailments fr. disappointed love or jealousy.	Ailments from mortification.
Easy comprehension—Mental excitability.	Difficult comprehension—Mental dullness.
Rarely absent-mindedness, fancies, or unconsciousness.	Rarely delirium.
Insanity more frequent than imbecility	Imbecility more frequent than insanity.
Paralysis	Very rarely paralysis.
Nasal complaints predom. internal	Nasal compl. external oftener than internal.
Desire for spirituous liquors	Aversion to wine; but appetite for beer.
Urine smells like ammoniac	Urine smells sour.
Catamenia too soon *or* late; generally too scanty.	Catamenia too late; scanty and of short duration, *or* profuse and of long duration.
Instead of suppressed catamenia, toothache.	Instead of catam., milk in the breasts. C. Hg.
Respiration predom. slow	Respiration preval quick.
Expectoration infrequent; morning and during day.	Expectoration not constant; during day.

Lachesis.	Mercur.
AGGRAVATION from noon till midnight	AGGRAVATION from evening till morning.
Ailments from Mercurial vapors	Ailments from Copper or Arsenic vapors, and from Calc. or Sulph.
Worse in the Spring	Worse in the Fall.
Worse *or* better after sleep	Worse after sleep.

Predomin. worse — **Predomin. better**

In warm air, during rest, when standing, sitting, and lying; after getting out of bed, and from smoking.

Predomin. better — **Predomin. worse**

In cold weather, from motion, when walking, from shaking head, on inspiration and deep respiration, when stooping, in bed during sleep, after pollutions, and from drinking cold water.

Lachesis.	**Phosphor.**
Often indicated with women and children . .	Often indicated with old people.
Upper left, lower right side—Light hair . .	*Upper right, lower left side*—Dark hair.
Muscles lax — Hæmorrhages of dark blood .	Muscles rigid—Hæmorrh. of light-red blood.
Apoplexia sanguinea*—Ulcerative pain in internal parts.	Apoplexia nervosa—Ulcerative pain in external parts.
Apoplexy more frequent than paralysis . .	Paralysis more frequent than apoplexy.
Paralysis generally painful	Paralysis generally painless.
Epilepsy with unconsciousness	Epilepsy with full consciousness.
Black spots on the skin	White spots on the skin.
Eruptions generally humid	Eruptions generally dry.
Scars break open and bleed after reddening and burning.	Scars break open and bleed after a pinching contraction. C.Hg.
Pulse predom. small and weak	Pulse predom. full and hard.
Heat, with aversion to uncover	Heat, with inclination to uncover.
Want of thirst predom., mostly during chill; thirst *before* the chill.	Want of thirst constant during all stages.
Awaking too early	Awaking too late.
Desire to be alone—Loquacity	Fear of being alone—Reserve.
Disposition sensitive	Disposition *insensible or* sensitive.
Cheerfulness — Consequences of disappointed love or jealousy—Rarely peevishness.	Changing mood—Cheerfulness *or* melancholy — Consequences of anger or vexation with vehemence—Indifference.
Weakness of memory	Active memory.
Headache better from warmth; worse from touch or pressure.	Headache; worse from warmth, better from touch and pressure.
Complaints predom. on lower eyelids . . .	Complaints predom. on upper eyelids.
Desire for beer	Aversion to beer.
Flatus passing with difficulty	Flatus passing easily, generally scentless, often [hot.
Urine too often	Urine often, but scanty.
Catamenia generally scanty and of short duration.	Catamenia profuse *or* scanty, of too long *or* short duration.
Instead of catamenia, toothache	Catamenia suppressed and milk in the breasts C.Hg.
Nasal secretion watery	Nasal secretion thick and viscid.
Voice nasal—Respiration slow	Voice trembling or hissing — Respiration predomin. quick.
Cough almost always dry	Cough sometimes dry, sometimes with expectoration.
REMISSION from midnight till noon	REMISSION of complaints after midnight.
Oftener improv. than aggrav. by swallowing; but worse partic. when swallowing saliva and drink.	*Worse* when swallowing food and drink.
Generally worse in warm air; better in cold weather.	Predom. aggrav. in cold weather, predom. better in warm air.
Worse after sleep	*Better* after sleep, with exception of siesta; worse on awaking when roused.
Ailments from abuse of Cinchona or Mercur.	Ailments from abuse of table-salt or Iod.

Predomin. worse — **Predomin. better**

In warm air, out-doors, from uncovering, during rest, when standing and sitting, partic. sitting erect; on an empty stomach, from the touch,† and after sleep.

Predomin. better — **Predomin. worse**

In cold weather, in-doors, from wrapping up, from motion, shaking head, sitting bent forward, and after breakfast.

N.B. Lachesis lacks the sensation of numbness in suffering parts, peculiar to Phosphor.; the over-sensitiveness of the latter to pain is also found less frequently with Lachesis.

---

* Much oftener in formerly so-called Apoplexia nervosa, partic. after excessive mental excitement, and when it is precursory or preparatory to softening of the brain, when Phosphor. acid. or Ammon. carb. are of the greatest advantage after it. C.Hg.

† Yet we also find an *aggrav.* with Phosphor. "*from soft touch.*"

Lachesis.	Phosphor. acid.
Skin and muscles lax — Increased irritability.	Skin and muscles rigid—Want of bodily irritability.
Aversion to motion*	Inclination for motion.
Painful ulcers, with scanty discharge . . .	Painless ulcers, with copious discharge.
Paralysis generally of one side and painful.	Paralysis generally of one side and painless.
Apoplexy	Apoplexy not yet observed.
Pulse intermitting every tenth beat, or later up to the thirtieth beat.	Pulse intermitting one to two beats.
Internal chill, with external heat predom. .	External chill, with internal heat predom.
Thirst often only *before* chill	Thirst generally only during sweat.

Lachesis.	Phosphor. acid.
Sensitive disposition – Loquacity	Insensibility of disposition—Taciturnity.
Cheerfulness—Haughtiness—Distrust . .	Dejection *or* cheerfulness.
Rarely peevishness	Mood *indifferent;* rarely irritable.
Ailments from fright	Ailments from shame, disappointed love, grief, mortification, or from vexation with reserved displeasure.
Easy comprehension—Mental excitement .	Difficult comprehension—Mental dullness.
Rarely unconsciousness (except in fainting spells, epilepsy, etc.)	Unconsciousness.
Insanity	Imbecility.
Nasal complaints predom. internal . . .	Nasal complaints predom. internal.
Urine too often	Urine frequent and copious; sometimes scanty.
Sexual desire increased; too strong . . .	Sexual desire decreased; too weak.
Catamenia too soon *or* late; at the same time predom. scanty and of short duration.	Catamenia too soon and too profuse.
Expectoration tolerably infrequent; morning and during day.	Expectoration tolerably constant; morning.

Lachesis.	Phosphor. acid.
Aggravation from noon till midnight . .	Aggravation evening and from midnight till noon.
Worse from heat of sun	Worse in snowy air.
Almost always aggravated after getting out of bed.	Better *or* worse after getting out of bed.
Better or worse after rising from a seat .	Better after rising from a seat.
Better *or* worse after meals	Worse after meals.
Better *or* worse when swallowing, partic. worse when swallowing saliva or when drinking.	Predom. better when swallowing, partic. when swallowing saliva and when drinking; but worse when swallowing food.

Predomin. worse — **Predomin. better**

In warm air, in wet weather, out-doors and when walking out-doors, before breakfast, from pressure, when changing posture, when lying or standing, and when lifting diseased limb.

Predomin. better — **Predomin. worse**

In cold, dry weather, in-doors, after breakfast, when letting diseased limb hang down, when stooping, in bed, during sleep, after pollutions, and from drinking cold water.

---

* Yet there is generally an improvement with both remedies from motion.

Lachesis.	Pulsatilla.
Blood uncoagulable	Blood coagulates easily.
Apoplexia sanguinea* — Paralysis generally painful.	Apoplexia nervosa—Paralysis generally painless.
Ulcers with scanty discharge, sometimes proud flesh; better from warmth, worse from cold.	Ulcers with copious discharge; worse from warmth, better from cold.
Warts	Corns. C.Hg.
Pulse irregular	Pulse rather equal.
Thirst, often only *before* the chill	Thirst often only *before* and *after* the chill, and worse between heat and sweat.
Awaking too early	Awaking too late.

Satiety of life, with longing for death . . .	Satiety of life with fear of death.
Mood cheerful, haughty; irritable, malicious, jealous; rarely peevish.	Mood changing; gentle; bold; despondent and anxious; indifferent; good-natured — Calm sadness of mild dispositions—Parsimony.
Repugnance of women to marry	Aversion of men to women.
Ailments from disappointed love or jealousy.	Ailments from excessive joy, from grief, mortification, or vexation.
Mental excitability—Insanity	Mental dullness—Melancholy.
Rarely absent-mindedness, fancies or unconsciousness.	Unconsciousness, &c.
Nasal complaints predom. internal	Nasal compl. external oftener than internal.
Want of appetite predom.	Generally hunger.
Painless diarrhœa	Diarrhœa generally painful.
Urine too often	Urine seldom and scanty.
Catamenia too soon *or* too late	Catamenia too late.
Respiration preval. slow	Respiration quick.
Cough, generally without expectoration . .	Cough generally with expectoration.
Complaints generally on palm of hand . . .	Complaints predom. on back of hand.

Better or worse during sleep	Worse during sleep.
Worse when and after getting out of bed . .	*Better or* worse when & after gett'g out of bed.
Worse when rising from a seat	*Worse or* better when rising from a seat.
Worse when rising (from a stooping posture).	Worse *or* better when rising.
Better when taking a deep breath	Better *or* worse when taking a deep breath.
Worse *or* better from sneezing	Worse from sneezing.
Worse from bodily exertion	Improv. oftener than aggrav. by exertion.
Worse from pressure	*Better or* worse from pressure.
Generally improv. when eating	Almost always aggrav. when eating.
Worse *or* better from spirituous liquors . .	Worse from spirituous liquors.
Worse after stool	*Better or* worse after stool.

Predomin. worse —————— **Predomin. better**

From cold and growing cold, out-doors and when walking out-doors, from uncovering, lying on right side, when lying on painful side, when sitting erect, when holding suffering part bent, when stretching out or lifting diseased limb, from weeping, from tying clothes tight, from pressure, from vinegar and sour things, after stool, when and after getting out of bed, and from bodily exertion.

Predomin. better —————— **Predomin. worse**

From warmth and growing warm, in-doors and from warmth of stove, from wrapping up, in bed, lying on left side, when lying on unpainful side, when stooping and sitting bent forward, when bending diseased part backwards, when drawing up suffering limb or letting it hang down, from loosening the clothes, when eating, partic. fruit; after pollutions, and from shaking the head.

N.B. Lachesis lacks the sensation of numbness in suffering parts peculiar to Pulsat., often also the over-sensitiveness of Puls. to pain. Mere sensitiveness (to touch &c.), on the other hand, is found with both remedies.

---

* See note to Lachesis—Phosphor.

Lycopodium.	Graphites.
Sensitiveness in external parts	Sensitiveness in internal parts—No apoplexy.
Hæmorrhages, blood dark	Hæmorrhages, blood light-red.
Sweat around the joints.	Skin chopped around the joints.
Swelling of suffering parts	Emaciation of suffering parts.
Pulse somewhat accelerated only in the evening and after meals; frequent in the evening, slow in the morning.	Pulse full and hard, but somewhat accelerated only in the morn'g; frequent in the morning, slow during day or evening.
Thirst is wanting only during chill . . .	Want of thirst, partic. during heat.
Thirst, with disgust for drink	Desire for drink, without thirst.
Internal chill, with external heat predom. .	External chill, with internal heat.
Heat or sweat, with inclination to uncover.	Heat or sweat, with aversion to uncover.

Lycopodium.	Graphites.
Dejectedness *or* cheerfulness—Gentleness—Seriousness — Distrust — Haughtiness—Avarice—Maliciousness.	Sadness—Despondency.
Mental dullness—Imbecility—Insanity . .	Neither unconsciousness, delirium, nor fancies.
Consequences of grief, mortification, vexation, anger, (or fright).	Ailments from grief (or fright).
Optical illusions in black or in dark colors .	Optical illusions in bright colors.
Scentless flatus predominant	Fetid flatus.
Urine often, but scanty	Urine scanty.
Urinal sediment red (sandy) or whitish . .	Urinal sediment whitish.
Catamenia generally of too long duration; at the same time profuse *or* scanty.	Catamenia of too long duration and scanty.
With suppressed catamenia, milk in the breasts.	With suppressed catamenia, bleeding from anus. C.Hg.
Respiration with moist sound	Respiration with dry sound.
Difficult respiration better in bed	Difficult respiration worse in bed.
Expectoration morning and evening . . .	Expectoration during day and evening.

Lycopodium.	Graphites.
Remission after midnight and in the *forenoon.*	Remission of complaints during day.
Worse during new moon	*Worse* during full moon.
Worse when riding	*Better* while riding, *worse afterwards.*
Worse after a satisfying meal	Worse when hungry.

Predomin. worse ⏞ **Predomin. better**

From warmth, from wrapping up, when letting diseased limb hang down, during rest, when standing, sitting and lying, from pressure, from drinking wine, and when riding.

Predomin. better ⏞ **Predomin. worse**

From cold, from uncovering, when lifting up diseased limb, when moving, and when stooping.

Lycopodium.	Phosphor.
Light hair—Skin and muscles lax . . .	Dark hair—Skin and muscles rigid.
Hæmorrhages, blood dark — Apoplexia sanguinea.	Hæmorrhages, blood light-red—Apoplexia nervosa.
Sensitiveness of external parts	Sensitiveness of internal parts.
Sweat around the joints—Eruptions generally humid.	Vesicles around the joints — Eruptions generally dry.
Apoplexy more frequent than paralysis . .	Paralysis more frequent than apoplexy.
Spasms with unconsciousness	Spasms with full consciousness.
Distention of veins of feet	Distention of veins of hands.
Pulse somewhat accelerated only after meals and in the evening.	Pulse generally quick, full, and hard; regular; sometimes intermitting.
Sensation of coldness in the veins . . .	Burning in the veins.
Heat, then chill—Thirst wanting only during chill.	Chill, then heat—Want of thirst constant.
Chill or heat, predominant left side . . .	Chill or heat, predominant right side.
Chill lessened after getting out of bed . .	Chill increased after getting out of bed.
Sweat increased during meals	Sweat lessened during meals.

Sensitive disposition—Gentleness—Seriousness.	*Insensibility or* sensitiveness of disposition.
Sadness (predom.) *or* cheerfulness . . .	*Cheerfulness* or hypochondric mood.*
Depressed mood and timidity	Hypochondria with peevish irritability.
Consequences of mortification or of vexation with reserved displeasure.	Ailments from vexation with fright.
Weak memory—Mental dullness up to imbecility.	Active memory—Mental excitement—Ecstasies.
Pupils dilated	Pupils contracted.
Complaints generally in inner ear, and predominant on under lip.	Complaints generally on external ear, and predominant on upper lip.
Appetite for sweets	Aversion to sweets.
Constipation predominant	Diarrhœa predominant.
Retention of urine more frequent than incontinence.	Involuntary discharge of urine.
Catamenia predominant too late	Catamenia generally too soon.
Expectoration almost constant; particularly morning and evening.	Expectoration not constant; morning and during the day.
Milk diminished, but often running from the breast.	Running out of the milk; the quantity generally increased.

REMISSION after midnight and in forenoon.	REMISSION of compl. after midnight.
Better after eructation	Worse *or* better after eructation.
Worse *or* better after stool	*Better* after stool.
Worse during new moon	Worse before a thunder-storm.

Predomin. worse ——— **Predomin. better**

During rest, when standing and sitting, partic. sitting erect, from warmth, from cold diet, from beer, coffee or wine, after drinking in general, from eating a satisfying meal, after sleep,† from touch,‡ and when lying on side.

Predomin. better ——— **Predomin. worse**

During continued moderate motion,§ partic. of the diseased limb, when sitting bent forward, from cold,** from warm diet, after sweating, when lying on back, and from needle-work.

---

* A sudden change of mood is found with both remedies.

† Yet Phosph. has aggravation as well as improvement "*on awaking.*"

‡ We also find aggrav. "*from soft touch*" with Phosphor.

§ In the beginning of motion and when walking fast both remedies have aggrav.

** Growing cold and cold weather (as well as warmth) exert a very varied influence on the symptoms of Lyc.; Phosphor-symptoms, on the other hand, are preval. aggrav. by growing cold and in cold weather, and improv. by growing warm and in warm air.

Lycopodium.	Phosph. acid.
Upper right, lower left side—Muscles lax .	Upper left, lower right side – Muscles rigid.
Aversion to motion	Desire for motion.
Pulse somewhat accelerated only in the evening and after meals.	Pulse generally frequent, small, and weak; irregular, intermitting.
Heat, with thirst and inclination to uncover.	Heat, without thirst and with aversion to uncover.
Thirst is wanting only during chill . . .	Want of thirst predominant; thirst almost only during sweat.
Anxious dreams	Pleasant dreams predom.

Lycopodium.	Phosph. acid.
Sensitive disposition	Insensibility of disposition.
Distrust — Malice — Haughtiness — Amorousness—Insanity.	Mood rarely irritable.
Consequences of (grief, mortification), fright, anger, or from vexation with fear or vehemence.	Ailments from (grief, mortification), shame, disappointed love, or jealousy.
Apoplexy	Very rarely paralysis.
Paralysis often of both sides	Paralysis generally of one side.
Vertigo, inclining to fall forwards . . .	Vertigo, inclining to fall forwards or backwards.
Complaints generally in inner ear, on upper lip; also predom. on upper eyelids, in upper part of chest, in hollow of elbow, on inner side of thigh, and on calf of leg.	Complaints generally on external ear and on under lip; also predom. on lower eyelids, in lower part of chest, on tip of elbow, on external side of thigh, and on shin.
Nausea in stomach—Costiveness	Nausea partic. in throat—Diarrhœa.
Urine often, but scanty	Urine often and copious; only exceptionally scanty.
Retention of urine oftener than incontinence.	Involuntary discharge of urine predom.
Catamenia too late; at the same time scanty *or* profuse.	Catamenia too soon and profuse.
Expectoration morning and evening; with hooping-cough, however, there is expectoration in the morning and during day.	Expectoration in the morning.

Lycopodium.	Phosph. acid.
Remission *forenoon* and after midnight .	Remission afternoon and before midnight.
Worse while and after passing urine . .	*Worse before and while* passing urine.
Worse from change of posture	Improved oftener than aggravat'd by change of posture.

Predomin. worse — **Predomin. better**

In wet weather, from cold diet, on inspiration, from wrapping up, from pressure, and when swallowing.

Predomin. better — **Predomin. worse**

In dry weather, from warm diet, on expiration, from uncovering, when stooping, and "after" sweat.

N.B. Over-sensitiveness to pain is frequent with Lycopodium, rare with Phosph. acid.

Lycopodium.	Pulsatilla.
Upper right, lower left side—Chill or heat on left side.	*Upper right, lower left side*—Chill or heat on right side of body.
Cold shudders on upper part of body	Chill on lower part of body; heat on upper part of body.
Thirst often after sweat	Thirst often *before* the chill.
Apoplexia sanguinea—Paralysis	Apoplexia nervosa—Rarely paralysis.
Sadness *or* cheerfulness—Haughtiness—Mood irritable; malicious.	Mood sad, quiet, gentle; rarely irritable; indifferent—Boldness.
Ailments from anger and from vexation with vehemence or reserved displeasure.	Ailments from excessive joy and from vexation with fright.
Vertigo, inclining to fall forwards	Vertigo, inclining to fall backwards.
Pupils dilated	Pupils generally contracted.
Optical illusions in dark colors	Optical illusions in bright colors.
Nausea in stomach	Nausea in throat, stomach, or abdomen.
Sour vomit predom.	Vomit is bitter oftener than sour.
Scentless flatus predom.	Hot, fetid flatus.
Constipat.; when diarrh. occurs, it is painless.	Diarrhœa predom., generally painful.
Urine often, but scanty	Urine seldom and scanty.
Urinal sediment red (sandy) *or* whitish	Urinal sediment reddish.
Retent. of urine more freq. than incontinence.	Incontinence more freq. than retent. of urine.
Catamenia generally of too long duration	Catamenia of too short duration.
Emission of scantily secreted milk	Emission of milk, the secretion of which is generally increased.
Coryza dry oftener than fluent	Coryza fluent (right side) oftener than dry.
Respiration preval. with moist sound	Respiration predom. with dry sound.
Expector. nearly constant; morning & even'g.	Expector. not constant; morn. & during day.
Complaints predom. in upper part of chest, on fore-arm, in palm of hand, on inside of nose, and on upper lip.	Complaints predom. in lower part of chest, on upper arm, on back of hand, on outside of nose and on under lip.
With Horses: Swelling of the hind-legs	With Horses: swelling of the front-legs.
Remission after midnight and in the *forenoon*.	Remiss. aft. midnight, in the morn. & forenoon.
Worse during new moon	Worse before a thunder-storm.
Better (worse) in cold *or* warm air	Better in cold weather, worse in warm air.
Better (worse) when growing cold *or* warm	Bett. wh. grow'g cold, worse wh. grow'g warm.
Worse from bodily exertion	Generally improv. by exertion.
Better *or* worse while and after perspiring	Worse while and after perspiring.
Better *or* worse in bed and fr. warmth of bed.	Alm. alw. aggrav. in bed & fr. warmth of bed.
Worse after sleep	*Worse or* better after sleep.
Worse from pressure	*Better or* worse from pressure.
Better when moving diseased part	*Better or* worse when moving the part.
Better after rising from a seat	*Better or* worse after rising from a seat.
Worse when swallowing	Better when swallowing, *or* worse (when swallowing saliva); in the first case often worse *after* swallowing.
Better from eructation	*Worse or* better from eructation.
Worse or better from sneezing	Worse from sneezing.
Worse when taking a deep breath	Better *or* worse when taking a deep breath.
Better or worse from weeping	Better from weeping.
Worse when looking at anything which turns.	Worse when looking up.

Predomin. worse — **Predomin. better**

When lying in a contracted posture, lying on painful side, when sitting erect, when stretching out diseased limb, on bending it sideways, washing or moistening suffering part, tying clothes tight, on inspiration, when opening the eyes, from drinking cold water and from cold diet in general, from bodily exertion and pressure.

Predomin. better — **Predomin. worse**

In extended posture, lying on unpainful side, when sitting bent forward, drawing up diseased limb, loosening the clothes, on expiration, when closing the eyes, from warm diet, from eructation, and when stooping.

Lycopodium.	Sepia.
Light hair—Skin and muscles lax	Dark hair—Skin and muscles rigid.
Eruptions generally humid	Eruptions generally dry.
Pulse somewhat accelerated only in the evening and after meals, slow in the morning.	Pulse frequent and full at night, slow during day; is accelerated, partic. by vexation and motion.
Thirst is wanting only during chill, frequently appears after sweat.	Want of thirst predom.; thirst is constant only during chill, and frequently appears also *before* and *after* chill.
Heat with thirst	Heat without thirst.

Lycopodium.	Sepia.
Taciturnity	Loquacity.
Mood dull *or* cheerful, gentle; amorous; haughty; distrustful, malicious.	Dejection of spirits.
Delirium	No delirium.
Ailments from grief, mortification, or from vexation with reserved displeasure.	Ailments from disappointed love, or vexation with fright.
Pupils dilated	Pupils contracted
Complaints predom. on upper lip	Complaints predom. on under lip.
Vomit sour oftener than bitter	Bitter vomit predom.
Scentless flatus—Urine too often, but scanty.	Fetid flatus—Discharge of urine too infrequent.
Retention of urine oftener than incontinence.	Incontinentiæ urinæ predom.
Catamenia scanty oftener than profuse . . .	Catamenia profuse oftener than scanty.
Respiratien preval. with moist sound . . .	Respiration preval. with dry sound.
Expectoration nearly constant; morning and evening.	Expectoration predom., but not constant; is loosened night and morning, and generally swallowed.
Toothache with the cough	Cough with the toothache. C.Hg.

Lycopodium.	Sepia.
Remission after midnight and *forenoon* . .	Remission of complaints afternoon.
Worse (better) when alone *or* in company . .	Better when alone, worse when in company.
Worse during new moon	Worse before a thunder-storm.
Better (worse) from growing cold *or* warm .	Predom. worse from growing cold; better when growing warm.
Better or worse after sweat	Worse after sweat.
Worse (better) when lying on right *or* left side.	Better when lying on right side, worse when lying on left side.
Worse after sleep	Better after sufficient sleep, but worse on awaking when roused from sleep.
Worse or better when sneezing	Worse when sneezing.
Worse on inspiration and deep respiration .	Better *or* worse on inspiration and deep respiration.
Worse *or* better when rising (after stooping).	Almost always improv. when rising.
Worse *or* better when sitting down . . .	Better when sitting down.
Worse from bodily exertion	Generally improv. by exertion.
Worse when looking at anything which turns.	Worse when looking up, or over a large surface.

Predomin. worse — **Predomin. better**

From warmth, wrapping up, in wet weather, from drinking cold water and from cold diet in general, when lying on side, partic. on painful side; when turning in bed, after sleep, when sitting erect, when descending, from bodily exertion, and after breakfast.

Predomin. better — **Predomin. worse**

From cold, from uncovering, in dry weather, from warm diet, when lying on back or on unpainful side, when sitting bent forward, when kneeling, when ascending, when stooping, on expiration, on an empty stomach, and from eructation.

N.B. With Sepia we very rarely find the sensation of numbness in suffering parts peculiar to Lycop.

Lycopodium.	Silicea.
Apoplexia sanguinea	Apoplexia nervosa.
Apoplexy more frequent than paralysis . .	Paralysis more frequent than apoplexy.
Aversion to motion—Eruptions predominantly humid.	Inclination for motion—Eruptions predom. dry.
Ulcers worse from warmth, better from cold .	Ulcers better from warmth, worse from cold.
Pulse somewhat accelerated only after meals and in the evening; slow in the morning.	Pulse generally small, hard, and quick, partic. frequent at night, slower during the day.
Distention of veins of feet	Distention of veins of hands.
Heat, with inclination to uncover	Heat, with aversion to uncover.

Lycopodium.	Silicea.
Mood *sad or* cheerful; serious; haughty; malicious; parsimonious; distrustful.	Dejection—No delirium—No insanity.
Pupils dilated	Pupils contracted.
Complaints generally in inner ear, in palm of hand, and in upper part of chest.	Complaints generally on external ear, on back of hand, and in lower part of chest.
Vomit sour oftener than bitter; mucous . .	Bitter vomit — Vomiting food oftener than mucus.
Bellyache after stool	Remission of bellyache after stool.
Urine often, but scanty	Urine too often.
Urinal sediment red (sandy) *or* whitish . .	Urinal sediment reddish *or* yellowish.
Retention of urine more frequent than incontinence.	Incontinentia urinæ predom.
Respiration preval. with moist sound . . .	Respiration with dry sound.
Expectoration morning and evening	Expectoration during day.
In fevers: hands and fingers become like dead.	Heat in the fingers (in fevers).

Lycopodium.	Silicea.
Remission after midnight and *forenoon* . .	Remission before midnight.
Aggravation during new moon	Aggravation more frequent during full moon than new moon.
Worse (better) in warm *or* cold air	Better in warm air, worse in cold weather.
Worse (better) when growing warm *or* cold	Predom. better when growing warm; worse when growing cold.
Better or worse after perspiring	Worse after perspiring.
Worse *or* better from warmth of bed . . .	Better from warmth of bed.
Worse (better) when lying on right or left side.	Better when lying on right side, worse when lying on left side.
Worse *or* better when getting out of bed . .	Worse when getting out of bed.
Almost always improved after getting out of bed.	Worse *or* better after getting out of bed.
Better *or* worse when sitting down	Better when sitting down.
Worse or better when rising from a seat . .	Worse when rising from a seat.
Worse *or* better when rising (after stooping).	Better when rising.
Worse from bodily exertion	Worse *or* better from exertion.
Worse or better when riding on horseback .	Worse when riding on horseback.
Worse after drinking	*Worse or* better after drinking.
Better or worse from weeping	Worse from weeping.
Worse when looking at anything which turns.	Worse when looking up.
Worse (better) when alone *or* in company . .	Worse when alone; better in company.

Predomin. **worse** ⏜ Predomin. **better**

In wet weather, from warmth, from wrapping up, in-doors and from warmth of stove, when lying on side, when letting diseased limb hang down, and when descending.

Predomin. **better** ⏜ Predomin. **worse**

In dry weather, from cold, from uncovering, out-doors and when walking out-doors, when lying on back, when lifting diseased limb, when ascending, when stooping, from needle-work, and from weeping.

Lycopodium.	Sulphur.
Right side; partic. *upper right, lower left side.*	*Left* side, part. *upper left, lower right side.*
Sensation of numbness predominant; sensitiveness only external.	Sensitiveness predom; sensation of numbness only external.
Pinching pain in internal parts—Eruptions predominantly humid.	Pinching pain in external parts—Eruptions generally dry.
Apoplexy more frequent than paralysis.	Paralysis more frequent than apoplexy.
Pulse somewhat accelerated only after meals and in the evening; slow in the morning.	Pulse quick, full, & hard, partic. accelerated night & morn'g, slower dur'g day & even'g.
Thirst is wanting only during chill; often appears after sweat	Thirst predomin., but not constant; often appears already *before* chill.
Chill lessened after getting out of bed	Chill increased after getting out of bed.
Dejection or cheerfulness—Haughtiness—Maliciousness—Miserliness—Distrust.	Mood despondent—Rarely amorousness.
Ailments from grief or vexation with reserved displeasure.	Ailments from shame or vexation with fright, rarely from anger.
Pupils dilated	Pupils contracted.
Complaints predom. in inner angle of eye	Compl. predom. on external angle of eye.
Swelling of under lip predominant	Swelling of upper lip predom.
Scentless flatus	Fetid flatus.
Catamenia of too long duration	Catam. *generally* of short duration.
With suppressed Catamenia, milk in breasts.	With suppr. hæmorrhoidal tumors. C.Hg.
Expectoration almost constant; morning and evening	Expector. not constant; morning and during day, less frequent at night.
Sweat around the joints	Itch'g, erysipelas or vesicles around the joints.
Remission *forenoon* and after midnight	Remission *afternoon* & before midnight.
Worse during new moon	Worse during full moon.
Worse *or* better when perspiring	Worse when perspiring.
Better or worse from warmth of bed	Generally aggrav. by warmth of bed.
Almost always improv. after getting out of bed.	Worse *or* better after getting out of bed.
Worse *or* better when sitting down	Almost always improv. when sitting down.
Worse or better when rising from a seat	Worse when rising from a seat.
Worse from change of posture	*Worse or* better from change of posture.
Better when moving diseased part	Worse *or* better when mov'g diseased part.
Worse when looking at anything which turns.	Worse from looking at running water and from looking down in general.
Generally improv. by weeping	Predominant aggrav. by weeping.

Predomin. **worse** ⸻ Predomin. **better**

When sitting erect, when descending, when letting diseased limb hang down, and from pressure.

Predomin. **better** ⸻ Predomin. **worse**

When sitting bent forward, when ascending, when lifting diseased limb, from warmth of bed, from weeping, and needle-work.

N.B With Sulph., whose predom. characteristic is want of irritability, we very rarely find the over-sensitiveness of Lycopodium to pain. On the other hand, mere sensitiveness (to touch, etc.) is found with both remedies.

Magnesia carb.	Calcarea.
Left side predom. – Inclination for open air.	*Right* side—Aversion to open air.
Hæmorrhages, blood dark—Neither apoplexy nor paralysis.	Hæmorrh., blood light-red – Apoplexy—Paralysis.
Epilepsy with full consciousness	Epilepsy with unconsciousness.
Pulse generally unchanged; only at night somewhat accelerated.	Pulse different, sometimes trembling; generally full and quick.
Heat or sweat, with aversion to uncover	Heat or sweat, with inclination to uncover.
One-sided heat, right side—First chill, then heat.	One-sided heat, left side—First heat, then chill.
Want of thirst predominant, partic. during heat.	Thirst predominant; only during chill it is sometimes wanting.
Ulcers, with scanty discharge	Ulcers, with much pus—Caries.
Warts become atrophic	Warts removed by suppuration and forming of crusts.

Compl. predom. in inner angle of eye, on upper lip, on lower jaw and lower teeth, in lower part of chest, on front part of thigh, and in hollow of knee.	Compl. predom. in external angle of eye, on under lip, upper jaw and upper teeth, in upper part of chest, on back part of thigh, and on patella.
Generally desire for meats	Disgust for meat.
Sexual desire weak	Sexual desire strong.
Catamenia too late, scanty, of short duration.	Catamenia predominantly too soon, profuse, and of long duration.
Nasal secretion watery	Nasal secretion thick, often of a bad odor.
Expectoration predominant	Expectoration predom., but not constant.
Heat in the fingers (in fever)	(In fever) fingers become as though dead.

Aggravation evening and night, partic. after midnight.	Remission before midnight.

Predomin. worse —— **Predomin. better**

During rest, after lying down,* when lying on painful† side, when sitting down, when sitting and standing, in-doors, and from uncovering.

Predomin. better —— **Predomin. worse**

From motion, when lying on unpainful side, out-doors, from wrapping up, from anything wet, washing and moistening diseased part,‡ and from drinking cold water.

N.B. Magnesia seems to lack the sensation of numbness in suffering parts peculiar to Calcarea; on the other hand, the over-sensitiveness of Magnesia to pain is only rarely found with Calcarea.

---

* Both remedies have aggrav. from warmth of bed.

† With Calcarea we sometimes find, though less frequently, aggrav. by lying on painful side, and improv. by lying on unpainful side.

‡ Calcarea has an exception to this in case of Enteritis, which are improved by cold applications.

Magn. c.	Phosphor.
Left side—Light hair—Skin and muscles lax.	*Right* side—Dark hair—Skin and muscles rigid.
Often indicated with children	Often indicated with old people.
Inclination for motion — Hæmorrhages, blood dark.	Aversion to motion—Hæmorrhages, blood light-red.
Apoplexy or paralysis not yet observed . .	Apoplexy, and more frequently paralysis.
Pulse generally unchanged, only at night somewhat accelerated.	Pulse very different; irregular, intermitting; generally accelerated, and at the same time oftener full and hard than small and weak.
Heat or sweat, with aversion to uncover .	Heat or sweat, with inclination to uncover.
Causes atrophy of warts	Cures warts, etc., by suppuration.

Complaints predominant on lower eyelids, on upper lip, in lower part of chest, and on front part of thigh.	Complaints predominant on upper eyelids, on lower lip, in upper part of chest, and on back part of thigh.
Appetite for bread, particularly bread and butter, predominant.	Aversion to bread predominant.
Sexual desire too weak	Sexual desire preval. strong.
Catamenia predominantly too late, scanty, and of short duration.	Catamenia predominantly too soon; at the same time too profuse and of long duration, *or* too scanty and of short duration.
Nasal secretion watery	Nasal secretion thick or viscid.
Expectoration predom. with the cough . .	Expectoration not constant.

Aggravation evening and night, partic. after midnight.	Remission of complaints after midnight.
Worse during sleep	Worse *or* better during sleep.
Worse on awaking from sleep.	Better after sufficient sleep, but worse on awaking when roused and after the siesta.
Better *or* worse when getting out of bed .	Worse when getting out of bed
Worse when riding	*Worse or* better when riding.
Worse in company, better when alone . .	Better (worse) in company *or* when alone.

Predomin. worse — **Predomin. better**

From uncovering (partic. the head), during rest, when sitting down, when standing, sitting and lying, when lifting or drawing up diseased limb, from touch, and after sleep.

Predomin. better — **Predomin. worse**

From wrapping up (partic. the head), from motion, when walking, when rising from seat, when rising (after stooping), when letting diseased limb hang down or when stretching it out, from washing and moistening, and from warmth of stove.*

* Both remedies have predom. aggravation "in-doors" in general, and improvement of symptoms in the open air.

Magn. c.	Pulsatilla.
Left side, particularly *lower left, upper right side.*	*Right* side, particularly *lower right, upper left side.*
Want of bodily irritability—Inclination for motion.	Increased irritability—Aversion to motion (which, however, improves).
Itching, lessened by scratching.	Itching, unchang'd *or* aggrav. by scratch'g.
Cutaneous eruptions predominantly dry.	Eruptions rather humid.
Ulcers, with scanty discharge	Ulcers, with copious discharge.
Awaking too early	Awaking too late.
Pulse often unchanged; only at night somewhat accelerated; frequent at night, slow during day.	Pulse accelerated, small, and weak; frequent in the evening, slow in the morning; sometimes intermitting or imperceptible.

Optical illusions in black or dark colors.	Optical illusions in bright colors.
Complaints predominant on upper lip	Complaints predominant on under lip.
Appetite for bread, partic. bread and butter, predominant.	Aversion to bread, partic. rye-bread, predominant.
Diarrhœa predominantly painless	Diarrhœa generally painful.
Dry coryza	Coryza fluent (partic. right side) oftener than dry.
Cough, generally with expectoration	Cough, with expectoration oftener than without it.
Complaints predominant in palm of hand.	Complaints predominant on back of hand.
(In fevers) heat in the fingers	(In fevers) fingers become as though dead.

AGGRAVATION evening and after midnight.	AGGRAVATION from noon till midnight.
Worse on awaking from sleep	*Worse or* better after sleep.
Predominantly worse from pressure	*Generally* improved by pressure.
Generally worse from moving the part	Generally improved by moving diseased part.
Worse when bending diseased part	Better *or* worse when bend'g diseased part.
Worse when sitting down	Better *or* worse when sitting down.
Better when rising from a seat	*Better or* worse when rising from a seat.
Better *after* rising from a seat	*Better or* worse after rising from a seat.
Worse (better) from cold *or* warm diet.	Better from cold diet; worse from warm diet.
Better from eructation	*Worse or* better from eructation.
Worse after stool	*Better or* worse after stool.

Predomin. worse ——— **Predomin. better**

From cold, growing cold and in cold weather, from uncovering, from pressure, from moving diseased part, when lifting diseased limb, when lying on painful side, and after stool.

Predomin. better ——— **Predomin. worse**

From warmth, warmth of stove,* growing warm and in warm air, from wrapping up, letting diseased limb hang down, lying on unpainful side, and from rubbing and scratching.

---

* Both remedies have predominant aggravation "in-doors" in general, and improvem. of symptoms in the open air

Magn. c.	Sepia.
Light hair—Skin and muscles lax . . .	Dark hair—Skin and muscles rigid.
Pinching pain in internal parts—Rending pain upwards.	Pinching pain in external parts—Rending pain downwards.
Inclination for open air	Aversion to open air.
Epilepsy, with full consciousness	Epilepsy, with unconsciousness.
Itching, generally lessened by scratching .	Itching, aggravated by scratching.
Complaints predominant on upper lip, in hollow of knee, and on front part of thigh.	Complaints predom. on under lip, in hollow of elbow, and on back part of thigh.

Magn. c.	Sepia.
Apoplexy or paralysis not yet observed. .	Apoplexy—Paralysis.
Pulse generally unchanged	Pulse accelerated, partic. by vexation and motion; sometimes intermitting.
First chill, then heat	First heat, then chill.
Want of thirst predominant	Thirst only during chill.
Chill lessened in the open air	Chill increased in the open air.
Appetite for bread, partic. bread and butter, predom.; also for meat.	Aversion to bread and meat.
Burning sensation in the teeth	Cold sensation in teeth. C.Hg.
Sexual desire lessened	Sexual desire generally lessened, but even when increased, less ability.
Catamenia too scanty and of short duration.	Catamenia lasting too long; at the same time profuse *or* scanty.
Expectoration predominant; morning and during day.	Expectoration predominant, but not constant; is loosened night and morning, and generally swallowed.
(In fevers) heat in the fingers	(In fevers) fingers become as though dead.

Magn. c.	Sepia.
AGGRAVATION evening and night, partic. after midnight.	REMISSION of complaints afternoon.
Worse in cold weather; better in warm air.	Better (worse) in cold weather *or* in warm air.
Worse from warmth of bed	*Better or* worse from warmth of bed.
Worse on awaking from sleep	Better after sufficient sleep; but worse on awaking when roused from sleep.
Better when rising from a seat	Worse *or* better when rising from a seat.

Predomin. worse —————— **Predomin. better**

In wet weather, from warmth of bed, when turning in bed, when lying on painful side, after sleep, when drawing up diseased limb, when moving suffering part, when sitting down, and from smoking.

Predomin. better —————— **Predomin. worse**

In dry weather, from warmth of stove, when lying on unpainful side, when stretching out diseased limb, from washing and moistening suffering part, from scratching, and from eructation.

Magn. c.	Silicea.
Left side—Rending pain upwards . . .	*Right* side—Rending pain downwards.
Pinching pain in internal parts, constriction the same.	Pinching pain in external parts, constriction the same.
Want of bodily irritability—Inclination for open air.	Increased irritability — Aversion to open air.
Epilepsy, with full consciousness	Epilepsy, with unconsciousness.
Itching, lessened by scratching	Itching, unchanged *or* aggrav. by scratching.
Causes atrophy of warts	Cures warts, etc., by suppuration.
Apoplexy or paralysis not yet observed .	Apoplexy, and oftener paralysis.
Pulse unchanged	Pulse changed, generally accelerated, hard, small, or imperceptible.
Chill lessened out-doors	Chill increased out-doors.
Want of thirst predominant	Thirst predominant.

Magn. c.	Silicea.
Complaints predominant on lower eyelids, in palm of hand, and on front part of thigh.	Complaints predominant on upper eyelids, on back of hand, and on back part of thigh.
Appetite for meat predominant	Aversion to meat.
Mucous vomit predominant	Vomiting of food predominant.
Sexual desire too weak	Sexual desire too strong.
Catamenia of short duration and scanty .	Catamenia lasting too long; at the same time profuse *or* scanty.
Expectoration morning and during day .	Expectoration during day.
(In fevers) heat in the fingers	(In fevers) blue finger-nails.

Magn. c.	Silicea.
AGGRAVATION evening and night, partic. after midnight.	REMISSION of complaints before midnight.
Worse when getting out of bed	Better *or* worse when getting out of bed.

Predomin. worse — **Predomin. better**

In wet weather, in-doors, in company, from warmth of bed, and when sitting down.

Predomin. better — **Predomin. worse**

In dry weather, out-doors and when walking out-doors, when alone, when rising from a. seat, from scratching, and from washing and moistening diseased part.

Magn. mur.	Calcarea.
Upper left, lower right side—Inclination for open air.	Upper right, lower left side—Aversion to open air.
Itching, generally unchanged by scratching.	Itching, improved oftener than aggravated by scratching.
Pulse generally unchanged	Pulse changed, sometimes trembling; generally quick and full.
Heat or sweat, with aversion to uncover .	Heat or sweat, with inclination to uncover.
Chill lessened in bed	Chill increased in bed.
Thirst constant	Only sometimes during chill want of thirst.

Complaints predominant on upper lip and on top of foot.	Complaints generally on under lip and sole of foot.
Loss of appetite predominant	Generally hunger.
Erections	Impotence, with increased sexual desire.
Catamenia predominantly too scanty and of short duration.	Catamenia predominantly too profuse and of long duration.
Nasal secretion watery	Nasal secretion thick.
Expectoration not constant; during day .	Expectoration predominant, but not constant; morning and during day.

REMISSION of complaints during day . .	REMISSION before midnight.
Worse from light; better in the dark . .	Better (worse) from light *or* in the dark.
Almost always aggravated when closing the eyes, better when opening them.	Better (worse) when opening *or* when closing eyes.
Worse when lying on right side; better when lying on left side.	*Generally* better when lying on right side; worse when lying on left side.
Worse from being awake at night . . .	Worse from sleeping too long.
Better from moving diseased part . . .	Worse *or* better from moving the part.

Predomin. worse — **Predomin. better**

In-doors, during rest, after lying down, when lying, sitting and standing, partic. when lying on painful or on right side, but also when lifting diseased limb, when rising (from stooping), from touch, and from uncovering.

Predomin. better — **Predomin. worse**

Out-doors and when walking out-doors, when walking and from motion in general, when lying on unpainful or on left side, when letting diseased limb hang down, from pressure, wrapping up, after sweat, and in bed.

N.B. With Magn. mur. we rarely find the sensation of numbness in suffering parts peculiar to Calc.

Magn. mur.	Lycopodium.
Upper left, lower right side	*Upper right, lower left side.*
Inclination for motion	Aversion to motion, (which, however, improves).
Pulse generally unchanged	Pulse somewhat accelerated only in the evening and after meals.

Magn. mur.	Lycopodium.
Heat or sweat, with aversion to uncover .	Heat or sweat, with inclination to uncover.
Chill lessened in bed	Chill increased in bed.
Thirst during all stages of the fever . . .	Thirst is wanting only during chill.
Catamenia predominantly of too short duration and scanty; at the same time too soon *or* too late.	Catamenia of too long duration; at the same time scanty *or* profuse; generally too late.
Fluent coryza more frequent than stoppage of nose.	Stoppage of nose more frequent than fluent coryza.
Expectoration not constant; during day .	Expectoration almost constant; morning and evening.

Magn. mur.	Lycopodium.
Aggravation from evening till morning .	Aggravation morning and *from noon till midnight.*
Worse in cold weather, better in warm air .	Better (worse) in cold weather *or* in warm air.
Worse when growing cold, better when growing warm.	Better (worse) when growing cold *or* warm.
Better after sweating	*Better or* worse after sweating.
Predominantly better in bed	Worse *or* better in bed.
Worse (better) when lying on back *or* on side.	Predominantly better when lying on back, worse when lying on side.
Worse *or* better after sleep	Worse after sleep.
Worse from being awake at night . . .	Worse from sleeping too long.
Worse when getting out of bed	Better *or* worse when getting out of bed.
Worse when rising from stooping . . .	Better *or* worse when rising.
Worse when riding on horseback	*Worse or* better when riding on horseback.
Worse (better) from warm *or* cold diet . .	Better from warm, worse from cold diet.
Worse after stool	*Worse or* better after stool.

Predomin. worse ⸻ **Predomin. better**

From cold, uncovering, in extended posture, after getting out of bed, before breakfast, when closing the eyes, when ascending, when lifting diseased limb, when stooping, and from needle-work.

Predomin. better ⸻ **Predomin. worse**

From warmth, wrapping up, in contracted posture, after breakfast, when opening the eyes, when descending, letting diseased limb hang down, and from external pressure.

N.B. With Magn. mur. we rarely find the over-sensitiveness of Lycopod. to pain, and rarely also the sensation of numbness of suffering parts. Mere sensitiveness (to touch, etc.), on the other hand, occurs with both remedies.

Magn. mur.	Phosphor.
Upper left, lower right side—Inclination for motion.	Upper right, lower left side—Aversion to motion.
Itching unchanged, rarely lessened by scratching.	Itching, lessened oftener than aggrav. by scratching.
Apoplexy or paralysis not yet observed .	Apoplexy, and still oftener paralysis.
Pulse generally unchanged, only a little accelerated.	Pulse accelerated, often irregular, intermitting; oftener full & hard than small & faint.
Heat or sweat, with aversion to uncover .	Heat, etc., with predom. inclinat'n to uncov.
Chill lessened in bed	Chill increased in bed.
Sweat increased when eating	Sweat lessened when eating.
Thirst during all stages of the fever . . .	Want of thirst during all stages of the fever.

Magn. mur.	Phosphor.
Compl. predom. on upper lip, upper jaw, upper teeth, and on top of foot.	Compl. predom. on lower lip, jaw, & teeth, also on sole of foot.
Appetite for sweets	Aversion to sweets.
Catamenia too scanty	Catamenia too profuse *or* too scanty.
Labor-pains weak or ceasing	Labor-pains spasmodic, too painful.
Nasal secretion watery	Nasal secretion thick.
Expectoration during day	Expectoration morning and during day.

Magn. mur.	Phosphor.
REMISSION of complaints during day . .	REMISSION after midnight.
Worse in cold weather; better in warm air.	Worse (better) in cold weather *or* in warm air.
Worse when growing cold; better when growing warm.	Worse (better) when growing cold *or* warm.
Worse (better) from cold *or* warm diet .	Better from cold diet,* worse from warm diet.
Better from eructation	Worse *or* better from eructation.
Worse during and after meals, partic. worse after a satisfying meal.	Worse *or* better during and after meals, partic. better after a satisfying meal.
Worse during sleep	Worse *or* better during sleep.
Predominantly worse when closing eyes, better when opening them.	Better (worse) when closing *or* opening the eyes.
Better *or* worse when sneezing	Worse when sneezing.
Worse from mental exertion	Better *or* worse from mental exertion.
Improv. by moving diseased part	Worse *or* better from moving diseased part.

Predomin. **worse** — Predomin. **better**

During rest, when standing, sitting and lying, partic. lying on right side, when lifting diseased limb or resting it on anything, when uncovering, from touch, and after a satisfying meal.

Predomin. **better** — Predomin. **worse**

From motion, when walking, lying on left side, letting diseased limb hang down, from wrapping up, from pressure, and after sweat.

N.B. The over-sensitiveness of Phosphor to pain, as well as sensation of numbness in suffering parts, are both rarely found with Magn. mur.

---

* Drinking cold water alleviates Phosphor-gastrosis only until the water has become warm in the stomach.

Magn. mur.	Pulsatilla.
Inclination for motion	Aversion to mot'n (which, however, improv.)
Itch'g, *unchanged or* lessened by scratch'g.	Itch'g, unchanged or aggrav. by scratch'g.
Pulse unchanged	Pulse changed, sometimes intermitting, generally frequent, small, weak.
Chill lessened in bed	Chill increased in bed.
Thirst during all stages of fever . . .	Want of thirst predom., but constant only during chill.

Magn. mur.	Pulsatilla.
Compl. predom. on upper lip, upper jaw, and upper teeth, on outside of gum, and on top of foot.	Compl. predom. on lower lip, lower jaw, and lower teeth, on inner side of gum, & on sole of foot.
Paralysis or apoplexy not yet observed .	Paralysis, and still oftener apoplexy.
Predominant loss of appetite	Generally hunger.
Nausea in stomach	Nausea in throat, stomach or abdomen.
Catamenia too soon *or* too late	Catamenia too late.
Expectoration not constant; morning . .	Expectoration predom., but not constant; morning and during day.

Magn. mur.	Pulsatilla.
REMISSION of complaints during day . .	REMISSION from midnight till noon.
Better from pressure	*Better or* worse from pressure.
Worse when stooping and when rising .	*Worse or* better when stooping and when rising.
Better from moving diseased part . . .	*Better or* worse from moving the part.
Worse when getting out of bed	*Better or* worse when getting out of bed.
Predominantly worse *after* gett'g out of bed.	*Better or* worse after getting out of bed.
Better after rising from a seat	*Better or* worse after rising from a seat.
Better *or* worse when sneezing	Worse when sneezing.
Worse when swallowing	*Worse or* better when swallowing.
Worse (better) from cold *or* warm diet . .	Better from cold, worse from warm diet.
Worse after meals	*Worse or* better after meals.
Better from eructation	*Worse or* better from eructation.
Worse after stool	*Better or* worse after stool.

Predomin. worse — **Predomin. better**

From cold, growing cold and in cold weather, from uncovering, lying on right side or on painful side, when lifting diseased limb or resting it on anything, from tying the clothes tight, when and after getting out of bed, and on inspiration.

Predomin. better — **Predomin. worse**

From warmth, growing warm and in warm air, from wrapping up, lying on left side or on unpainful side, when letting diseased limb hang down, from loosening the clothes, in bed, after perspiring, and from eructation.

N.B. We rarely find the over-sensitiveness of Pulsatilla to pain with Magn. mur., rarely also the sensation of numbness in suffering parts peculiar to Pulsatilla. Mere sensitiveness (to touch, etc.), on the other hand, occurs with both remedies.

Magn. mur.	Sepia.
Inclination for open air	Aversion to open air.
Itching unchanged, less frequently relieved by scratching.	Itching aggrav. by scratching.
Pulse generally unchanged, only a little accelerated.	Pulse accelerated, partic. by vexation and motion; unequal, trembling; quick and full, also intermitting, at night; slow during day.
Chill lessened in the open air	Chill increased in the open air.
Heat with thirst	Heat without thirst
Thirst during all stages of the fever	Want of thirst; only during chill thirst is constant.
Apoplexy or paralysis not yet observed	Apoplexy, and still oftener paralysis.

Magn. mur.	Sepia.
Taciturnity	Loquacity—Unconsciousness.
Complaints predom. on upper lip	Complaints predom. on under lip.
Erections	Impotence, with changing sexual desire.
Catamenia too scanty and of too short duration.	Catamenia lasting too long; at the same time too profuse *or* too scanty.
Expectoration not constant; during day	Expectoration predom., but not constant; is loosened, partic. at night and in morning, and is generally swallowed.

Magn. mur.	Sepia.
Remission of complaints during day	Remission afternoon.
Worse in cold weather; better in warm air.	Better (worse) in cold weather *or* in warm air.
Worse after lying down	*Worse or* better after lying down.
Predom. better in bed	*Worse or* better in bed.
Worse (better) when lying on side or on back.	Predom. better when lying on side; worse when lying on back.
Predom. worse when and after getting out of bed.	*Better or* worse when and after getting out of bed.
Worse (better) from cold *or* warm diet	Predom. better from cold, worse from warm diet.
Worse after meals	*Worse or* better after meals.
Better *or* worse from sneezing	Worse from sneezing.

Predomin. worse —— **Predomin. better**

When lying on right or on painful side, when closing the eyes, when rising (after stooping), when and after getting out of bed.

Predomin. better —— **Predomin worse**

When lying on left or on unpainful side, when opening the eyes, after sweat, from pressure, from clenching the teeth, and from eructation.

N.B. The over-sensitiveness of Sepia to pain is very rarely found with Magn. mur. — Mere sensitiveness (to touch &c.), on the other hand, is found with both remedies.

Mercurius.	Nitr. acid.
Light hair—Skin and muscles lax . . .	Dark hair—Skin and muscles rigid.
Increased irritability — Pain pressing outwards.	Want of bodily irritability — Pain pressing inwards.
Rending pain, downwards—Eruptions generally dry.	Rending pain upwards—Eruptions humid.
Scars redden	Scars hurt with change of weather; break open. C.Hg.
Sore pain in external parts	Sore pain in internal parts.
Hot swelling of glands	Painless (cold) swelling of glands.
Pulse generally full and accelerated; sometimes imperceptible or trembling.	Pulse more irregular than with **Mercurius**.
Sweat smelling sour and mouldy	Sweat smelling sour or like urine.
Thirst predom. during all stages of fever .	Thirst is wanting during chill.
Often indicated with children and women .	Often indicated with old people.
Loosing of hair, partic. on fore-head and temples.	Loosing of hair, part. on top of head.

Mood serious—Amorousness	Distrust.
Ailments after mortification	Ailments after mental excitement in general.
Absent-mindedn.—Imbecility—Apoplexy .	Very rarely apoplexy.
Nasal complaints external oftener than internal; complaints predom. on lower jaw, soft palate, tip of elbow, and on shin.	Internal nasal complaints predom. — Complaints frequent also on upper jaw, roof of mouth, patella, and on calf of leg.
Aversion to greasy food	Appetite for fatty things.
Nausea in œsophagus or stomach	Nausea, principally in stomach.
Diarrhœa predom. painful	Diarrhœa predom. painless.
Urine often and copious; hot; smelling sour (comp. sweat).	Urine scanty; cold *or* hot; generally smelling like ammoniac (comp. sweat).
Sexual desire too strong	Sexual desire too weak.
Catamenia too late; blood light-red . . .	Catamenia too soon; blood dark.
Expectoration during day	Expectoration morning and during day.
Sweating of feet scentless	Sweating of feet fetid.

Remission of complaints during day . .	Remission forenoon.
Worse during and after sweat	*Worse* during sweat, *better after* it.
Worse when swallowing saliva and drink; frequently improv. when swallowing food.	Worse when swallowing food.
Ailments from Sulph., Antimon., Cuprum, Aurum, Lachesis, Coffea, Cinchona, Bellad., Op., Valer., Dulc., Mezer.	Ailments from Mercur., Calcarea, or Digitalis.

Predomin. worse ——— **Predomin. better**

In cold weather,* in warm bed, when stooping, and after perspiring.

Predomin. better ——— **Predomin. worse**

In warm air, after getting out of bed, when leaning against anything, and when swallowing food

---

* Cold and warmth *in general* sometimes cause improvement and sometimes aggravation.

Mercurius.	Opium.
Increased bodily irritability	Want of bodily irritability.
Sensitiveness predominant in internal parts; insensibility (numbness) in external parts.	Insensibility (numbness) in internal and external parts.
Sleeplessness predominant	Somnolence predominant.
Heat, with aversion to uncover	Heat, with inclination to uncover.
Thirst predominant, but not constant . . .	Want of thirst; thirst almost only between heat and sweat.
Very rarely paralysis	Paralysis.
Taciturnity—Mood despondent, embarrassed, fretful; irritable; malicious.	Loquacity—Mood cheerful; gentle; indifferent—Boldness—Rage.
Ailments from mortification	Ailments from joy, fright, fear, vexation, or anger.
Difficult comprehension — Weak memory — Mental dullness.	Easy *or* difficult comprehension — Memory oftener active than weakened — Ecstasies *or* mental dullness.
Complaints predominant on upper lip . . .	Complaints predominant on under lip.
Secretion of saliva increased*	Saliva diminished.
Aversion to wine, but appetite for beer. . .	Desire for spirituous liquors.
Nausea, partic. in stomach and œsophagus .	Very rarely nausea.
Diarrhœa predominantly painful	Constipation; when diarrhœa occurs, it is painless.
Urine often and copious	Urine infrequent and scanty; sometimes copious.
Incontinentia urinæ predominant.	Retention of urine oftener than incontinence.
With Horses, from overexertion, profuse urination.	With Horses, from overexertion, retention of urine.
Catamenia too scanty *or* too profuse . . .	Catamenia too profuse.
Coryza fluent oftener than dry	Dry coryza.
Respiration predominantly quick.	Respiration generally slow.
Remission of complaints during day	Remission during day and evening.
Worse (better) from cold and growing cold, *or* warmth and growing warm.	Better from cold and growing cold, worse from warmth and growing warm.
Worse during and after sweat.	Worse during sweat, better *after* it.
Better when swallowing, *or* worse (when swallowing saliva and drink).	Worse when swallowing.
Worse from spirituous liquors	Worse *or* better from spirituous liquors.
Worse after stool.	Worse *or* better after stool.
Better *or* worse when assuming an erect position.	Worse when rising from stooping.
Ailments from Copper or Arsenic vapors, from abuse of Cinchona, Calcarea, or Sulphur.†	Ailments from Mercurius, Plumb., Strychnine, or Digitalis.

Predomin. worse ⁓ **Predomin. better**

In cold weather, from uncovering, out-doors, from motion, when walking, from pressure, in contracted posture, from drinking coffee, after urinating, and after sweat.

Predomin. better ⁓ **Predomin. worse**

In warm air, from wrapping up, in-doors, during rest, when standing, sitting and lying, partic. in extended posture, and from smoking.

* This is to be understood cum grano salis; for in molecular doses, Mercurius causes dryness of the mouth.

† Compare the preceding diagnosis Mercur. and Nitr. acid.

Mercurius.	Pulsatilla.
Aversion to open air—Sweat on front part of body.	Inclination for open air — Sweat on back part of body.
Heat left side—Coldness or sweat on suffering part.	Heat right side—Heat on suffering part.
Thirst during all stages of the fever.	Want of thirst predom., but constant only during chill.
Sweat general, with exception of feet	Sweat only on head.
Pulse irregular, generally full and accelerated; quick at night, slow during day.	Pulse accelerated, small, and weak; quick in the evening, slow in the morning.
Itching relieved *or* aggravated by scratching.	Itching unchanged *or* aggrav. by scratching.
Lying on side during sleep	When asleep, lying on back, the arms over the head (or lying on belly).

Mercurius.	Pulsatilla.
Dreads being alone — Mood irritable; malicious—Embarrassment.	Desire to be alone—Mood good-natured, indifferent; distrustful—Avarice—Boldness.
Ailments from mortification—Rarely delirium.	Ailments from excessive joy, fright, grief, mortification, or vexation.
Pupils dilated—Optic. illusions in dark colors.	Pupils generally contracted—Optical illusions in bright colors.
Styes on upper eyelid	Styes on upper and lower eyelids. C.Hg.
Eyes protruding	Eyes sunken.
Swelling of upper lip predom.	Swelling of lower lip predom.
Complaints predom. on soft palate, in upper part of chest, on tip of elbow, fore-arm, and palm of hand.	Complaints predom. on roof of mouth, in lower part of chest, in hollow of elbow, on upper arm, and on back of hands.
Generally loss of appetite	Generally hunger.
Aversion to wine and brandy, but appetite for beer and for milk	Appetite for wine, brandy, or beer; but aversion to milk.
Nausea in œsophag. or stom., rarely in throat.	Nausea in throat, stomach, or abdomen.
Urine smelling sour; often and copious	Ur. smelling like ammoniac; infreq. & scanty.
Catamenia too scanty and of short duration, *or* profuse and of long duration; blood light-red, serous—Milk diminished.	Catamenia too scanty and of short duration; blood dark—Milk generally increased.
Expectoration not constant; during day	Expectoration predom., but not constant; morning and during day.

Mercurius.	Pulsatilla.
Aggravation from evening till morning	Aggravation from noon till midnight.
Worse (better) when growing cold *or* warm	Better when growing cold; worse when growing warm.
Worse after sweat	*Worse or* better after sweat.
Worse on awaking from sleep	*Worse or* better after sleep.
Better after rising from bed or a seat	*Better or* worse after rising from bed or a seat.
Worse from moving diseased part	*Better or* worse from moving diseased part.
Generally worse from pressure	*Generally* improv. by pressure.
Worse *or* better when eating	Almost always aggrav. when eating.
Worse from cold *or* from warm diet; when the latter aggravates, better from cold diet.	Better from cold, worse from warm diet.
Worse after stool	*Better or* worse after stool.
Worse while blowing nose, but bett. *afterw.*	Worse when blowing nose.
Worse when taking a deep breath	Better *or* worse when taking a deep breath.

Predomin. worse — **Predomin. better**

In cold weather, out-doors and when walking out-doors, on inspiration, from uncovering, from washing and moistening suffering part, from drinking cold water,* from sour things, pressure, tying the clothes tight, when lying on right or on painful side, when sitting erect, from motion, when walking, when lifting or stretching out diseased limb, from bodily exertion, and after stool.

Predomin. better — **Predomin. worse**

In warm air, in-doors, on expiration, from wrapping up, loosening the clothes, when lying on left or on unpainful side, when sitting bent forward, during rest, when standing, sitting and lying, when letting diseased limb hang down, or when drawing it up.

N.B. With Mercurius we find the over-sensitiveness of Pulsatilla to pain quite as rarely as sensation of numbness in suffering parts.—Mere sensitiveness (to touch, &c.), on the other hand, is found with both remedies.

---

* On the other hand, Pulsatilla cures complaints which appear some time after, but are caused by taking a cold drink when overheated.

Mercurius.	Staphisagria.
Light hair—Skin and muscles lax	Dark hair—Skin and muscles rigid.
Pain pressing outward—Trembling of the limbs—Apoplexy.	Pain pressing inward - Internal trembling, trembling sensation.
Itching, lessened *or* aggrav. by scratching.	Itching, aggrav. by scratching, or appears in another place.
Painful eruptions—Dry itch	Painless eruptions—Humid itch.
Erysipelas around the joints	Crusts around the joints.
A pressure outward in the glands	Painful pressing inward in the glands.
Pulse irregular, generally full & accelerated.	Pulse small and accelerated
Heat or sweat, with aversion to uncover	Heat or sweat, with inclination to uncover.*
Sweat smelling sour or mouldy	Sweat smelling like rotten eggs.
Thirst predominant, but not constant	Want of thirst predom., except during heat.
Mood irritable; malicious—Absent-mindedness.	Indifference.
Ailments from mortification	Ailments from mortification, misbehavior of others, shame, grief, disappointed love, or vexation with indignation or reserved displeasure.
Styes on upper eyelid	Styes on upper and lower lids. C.Hg.
Eyes protruding	Eyes sunken.
Generally loss of appetite	Hunger predominant.
Aversion to wine—Appetite for beer	Desire for wine or brandy.
Nausea in œsophagus or stomach, rarely in throat.	Nausea in throat, less frequently in œsophagus or abdomen.
Diarrhœa	Constipation predominant.
Urine often and copious	Urine often, but scanty.
Catamenia profuse *or* scanty	Catamenia scanty.
Nasal secretion watery	Nasal secretion thick.
Expectoration not constant; during day	Expector. predom.; is loosened at night, and is generally swallowed.
Compl. predom. on tip of elbow and on shin.	Compl. predom. on patella & in calf of leg.
Remission during day.†	Remission undecided.‡
Worse from light; better in the dark	Better (worse) from light *or* in the dark.
Worse from bodily exertion	*Worse* from bodily exertion, and still ***more*** from mental exertion.
Ailments from Sulph., Antimon., Cuprum, Aurum, Lachesis, Cinchona, Coffea, Belladonna, Opium, Valer., Dulcam., Mezer.	Ailments from Mercurius or Thuya.

Mercurius		Staphisagria
Predomin. worse	**On inspiration, and in contracted posture.**	**Predomin. better**
Predomin. better	**On expiration, and in extended posture.**	**Predomin. worse**

* However, the symptoms of Staphisagria are aggrav. as often as improv. by uncovering, resp. wrapping up.

† Mercury also has a peculiar toothache, which torments all day but ceases at night. C.Hg.

‡ Staphisagria has its gastric symptoms, nausea, pressure in stomach, pain in abdomen, and diarrhœa only in the morning; its colic, morning and evening, not in the night. Other pains the same; only the headache, evening, *night* or morning, and the toothache, night and morning. The cough commences in the morning, increases during forenoon and noon, and continues during the evening. The itching somewhat in the morning, mostly in the evening; the ulcers are most painful in the evening. The chill only appears at all parts of the day, the heat night & morning, the sweat only at night. To one symptom in the forenoon there are three in the afternoon, seven in the evening, five at night, and ten in the morning. C.Hg.

Mercurius.	Sulphur.
Increased irritability—Pinching pain in internal parts.	Want of bodily irritability—Pinching pain in external parts.
Itching relieved *or* aggrav. by scratching	Itching relieved by scratching.
Painful eruptions	Painless eruptions.
Apoplexy more frequent than paralysis	Paralysis more frequent than apoplexy.
Heat or sweat with aversion to uncover	Heat or sweat with inclination to uncover.
Sweat on front part of body—Pulse irregular, trembling, imperceptible.	Sweat on back of body—Pulse quick, full, and hard.
Chill increased in warm room	Chill abating in warm room.
Dreams of water, thieves, animals, shooting, &c.	Dreams of fire, vexation, also imaginative, merry or mentally exciting dreams.
Mood malicious	Mood changing; gentle; indifferent.
Ailments from mortification	Ailments from shame, mortification, or vexation with fright or fear; less frequently after anger.
Imbecility oftener than insanity	Insanity oftener than imbecility.
Pupils dilated—Eyes protruding	Pupils contracted—Eyes generally sunken.
Secretion of saliva increased	Saliva *generally* diminished.
Aversion to wine or brandy, but appetite for beer and for milk.	Predom. appetite for (wine or) *brandy*, but avers. to milk; desire for *or* avers. to beer.
Vomiting bile	Vomit is sour oftener than bitter.
Nausea in œsophagus or stomach	Nausea in stomach.
Urine too often and copious	Urine often, but scanty; sometimes copious.
Expectoration during day	Expectoration morning and during day; less frequent at night.
Complaints predom. on tip of elbow and on shin.	Complaints predom. in hollow of elbow, on patella, and on calf of leg.
Remission of complaints during day	Remission *afternoon* and before midnight.
Worse in the Fall	Worse in the Spring.
Almost always worse in cold weather, better in warm air.	Better (worse) in cold weather *or* in warm air.
Predom. worse out-doors, better in-doors; but worse from warmth of stove.	Predom. better out-dors, worse in-doors, particularly worse in room filled with people, but better from warmth of stove.
Worse when turning in bed	*Worse or* better when turning in bed.
Better after getting out of bed.	Worse *or* better after getting out of bed.
Worse *or* better when rising from a seat	Worse when rising from a seat.
Worse when moving diseased part	Worse *or* better when moving the part.
Worse from touch	*Worse or* better from touch.
Worse after sweat	*Worse or* better after sweat.
Worse when swallowing drink*	Worse when swallowing food (dry).
Worse from cold *or* warm diet; in the latter case better from cold diet.	Better from cold diet; worse from warm diet.
Worse from spirituous liquors	*Worse or* better from spirituous liquors.
Better *or* worse after meals	Worse after meals.
Worse after drinking	*Worse or* better after drinking.
Worse after stool	Worse *or* better after stool.
Worse when sneezing	*Worse or* better when sneezing.
Worse when taking a deep breath	Better *or* worse when taking a deep breath.
Worse when looking into light	Worse when looking at running water.

Predomin. worse — **Predomin. better**

Out-doors, but also from warmth of stove, from uncovering, lying on right side, when sitting erect, from motion, when walking, from holding the breath, and from pressure.

Predomin. better — **Predomin. worse**

In-doors, from wrapping up, lying on left side, when sitting bent forward, during rest, when standing and lying, from smoking and when swallowing food.

* Both remedies have predom. aggrav. when swallowing saliva; Mercurius often has improv. when swallowing food.

Mercurius.	Thuya.
Sensitiveness in internal parts	Insensibility or sensation of numbness in internal parts
Itching, relieved *or* worse from scratching.	Itching, relieved by scratching.
Scars redden	In the scars stinging. C.Hg.
Hot swelling of glands	Cold swelling of glands.
Erysipelas around the joints	Œdema around the joints.
Involuntary motions, which can be momentarily suppressed by volition.	Involuntary motions, aggrav. by trying to suppress them.
Pulse irregular, generally full and accelerated; slow during day, quick at night.	Pulse slow and weak in morning, accelerated and full in evening.
Congestion of blood to ears	Congestion of blood to eyes.
Chill, with thirst—Heat, with aversion to uncover.	Chill, without thirst—Heat, with inclination to uncover.
Chill during day, heat at night	Heat dur'g forenoon, chilliness in afternoon.
Thirst predominant, but not constant	Thirst wanting during chill; is predom. during heat, not constant during sweat.
Clonic spasms during chill	Clonic spasms during heat or sweat
Sweat increased when walking out-doors	Sweat lessened when walking out-doors.

Dreads being alone	Desire to be alone—Haughtiness.
Ailments from mortification	Ailments from vexation or anger—Very rarely unconsciousness.
Imbecility	Ecstasies *or* imbecility.
Apoplexy more frequent than paralysis	Paralysis more frequent than apoplexy
Complaints predominant on lower jaw and on tip of elbow.	Compl. most frequent on upper jaw, and predom. in hollow of elbow & on patella.
Pupils dilated	Pupils generally contracted.
Saliva increased*	Saliva generally diminished.
Aversion to wine	Desire for wine.
Diarrhœa	Constipation.
Catam. too late; at the same time scanty *or* profuse.	Catamenia predominantly too soon and too scanty.
Expectoration not constant; during day	Expectoration almost constant; evening.

Aggravations from evening till morning.	Aggravations, partic. *afternoon* & *after midnight*, also in mornings & evenings.
Remission of complaints during day	Remission *forenoon* and before midnight.
Worse during and after sweat	*Worse* during sweat, *better after* it.
Ailments from Arsenic or Copper vapors, Calcarea, Cinchona, or the sting of insects.	Ailments from abuse of Mercurius or Iodine.

Predomin. worse — **Predomin. better**

When moving, when walking, from touch, from scratching & from pressure, from drinking cold water, after stool, and after sweat.

Predomin. better — **Predomin. worse**

During rest, when lying and sitting, generally also when standing, and from smoking.

---

* Compare note to diagnosis of Mercurius and Opium.

Mezereum.	Mercurius.
Upper right, lower left side — Inclination for open air.	Upper left, lower right side—Aversion to open air.
Crawling sensation or jerking pain in internal parts.	Crawling sensation or jerking pain in external parts.
Emaciation of suffering parts	Swelling of suffering parts.
Tearing stitching in the muscles	Tearing stitching in the joints.
Eruptions generally humid	Eruptions generally dry.
Itching, aggrav. by scratching, *or* changed to another place.	Itching, aggrav. *or* lessened by scratching.
Vesicular erysipelas—Softnesss of skin . .	Erysipelas, with smooth skin—Hardness of skin.
In the scars, a stinging	Scars redden. C.Hg.
Sleeplessness preval. after midnight . . .	Sleeplessness preval. before midnight.
Pulse often unchanged; full and hard; *accelerated in the evening;* sometimes frequent in morning, slow in the evening.	Pulse changed, accelerated; sometimes irregular, trembling, or imperceptible; frequent at night, slow during day.
Chill lessened out-doors	Chill increased out-doors.
Thirst, partic. during cold stage	Thirst predominant during all stages, but not constant.

Mezereum.	Mercurius.
Joyousness *or* dejection—Boldness . . .	Dejection of spirits — Seriousness — Maliciousness—Amorousness—Embarrassm't.
No fancies	Apoplexy.
Complaints predominant on upper jaw, upper teeth, roof of mouth, in lower part of chest, on upper arm, and on the outer side of thigh.	Complaints predominant on lower jaw, lower teeth, on soft palate, in upper part of chest, on fore-arm, and on inner side of thigh.
Nasal complaints internal oftener than external	Nasal complaints external oftener than internal.
Swelling or breaking out of under lip predominant.	Swelling or breaking out of upper lip predominant.
Appetite for coffee, wine, bacon	Aversion to coffee, greasy (fat) dishes, and wine; but appetite for beer.
Urine often, but scanty	Urine often and copious.
Catamenia too soon	Catamenia too late.
Lack of voice, failing, interrupted . . .	Lack of voice, not clear or trembling.
Expectoration infrequent; morning . . .	Expectoration not constant; during day.

Mezereum.	Mercurius.
Remission *during day* and after midnight.	Remission during day.
Ailments from Phosphorus, Mercurius, or Nitric. acid.	Ailments from Sulphur., Antimon., Cupr., Aurum, Lachesis, Bell., Cinchona, Opium, Coffea, Valeriana, Mezereum, or Dulcam.

Predomin. worse — **Predomin. better**

In-doors, when closing mouth and when keeping it closed.

Predomin. better — **Predomin. worse**

Out-doors, when opening mouth and keeping it open, and when stooping.

Mezereum.	Nitric acid.
Upper right, lower left side—Light hair .	Upper left, lower right side—Dark hair.
Inclination for open air—Emaciation, particularly of the face.	Aversion to open air—Emaciation, partic. of feet.
Cutting pains in external parts	Cutting pains in internal parts.
Pain pressing outwards	Pain pressing inwards.
Vesicular erysipelas—Itching, aggrav. *or* changed to another place by scratching.	Erysipelas with smooth skin—Itching lessened by scratching.
Stinging in scars	Scars, sensitive to changes of weather, break open. C.Hg.
Pulse often unchanged; generally full and hard; frequent in evening, slow in the morning; less often the opposite.	Pulse unequal, dicrotus, &c.
Chill lessened out-doors	Chill increased out-doors.
Thirst, particularly during chill	Thirst is wanting during chill.
Anxious dreams predom.	Pleasant dreams predom.
Complaints predom. in lower part of chest, on upper arm, on elbow-joint, on outer side of thigh, and on shin.	Complaints predom. in upper part of chest, on fore-arm, on knee-joint, on inner side of thigh, and on calf of leg.

Mezereum.	Nitric acid.
Joyousness *or* dejection—Boldness . . .	Dejection of spirits—Malice—Delirium.
Swelling of under lip predom.	Swelling of upper lip predom.
Vomiting, principally slime	Vomiting, principally food.
Urine often, but scanty; hot	Urine scanty; cold *or* hot.
Urinal sediment reddish	Urinal sediment red *or* white.
Sexual desire increased, strong	Sexual desire diminished, weak.
Expectoration infrequent; morning . . .	Expectoration not constant; morning and during day.

Mezereum.	Nitric acid.
Remission *during day* and after midnight.	Remission of complaints forenoon.
Ailments from Nitric acid. or Phosphor. .	Ailments from Calcar. or Digitalis.
Worse from drinking beer	Worse *or* better from spirituous liquors.
Better or worse when swallowing, partic. worse when swallowing saliva.	*Worse or* better when swallowing, partic. worse when swallowing food.

Predomin. worse — **Predomin. better**

On an empty stomach, when not swallowing, in cold weather,* in-doors, from warmth of bed, and from rubbing and scratching.

Predomin. better — **Predomin. worse**

After breakfast, during and after meals, when swallowing food, in warm air, out of doors, and when sucking with the tongue.

*** Cold and warm in general sometimes cause improvement, sometimes aggravation.**

Mezereum.	Phosphor.
Left side predominant – Light hair . . .	*Right* side predom. – Dark hair.
Emaciation, partic. of the face and suffering parts.	Emaciation, partic. of the hands – Swelling of suffering parts.
Cutting pain in external parts	Cutting pain in internal parts.
Twitching pain in internal parts	Twitching pain in external parts.
Itching in external parts—Skin soft . . .	Itching in internal parts—Skin rough.
Scars sting	Scars break open or bleed. C. Hg.
Itching, aggrav. *or* changed to another place by scratching.	Itching, *lessened or* aggrav. by scratching.
Humid eruptions predominant	Dry eruptions predom.
Compl. predom. in inner ear, on lower lip, upper jaw and upper teeth, and in lower part of chest.	Compl. generally on *external* ear, on upper lip, on lower jaw and lower teeth, and in upper part of chest.
Sleeplessness after midnight; awak'g early.	Sleeplessness before midnight & awak'g late.
Pulse often unchanged; generally full and hard.	Pulse accelerated, unequal, often intermitting.
Chill or heat descending	Chill or heat ascending.
One-sided heat, left side	One-sided heat, right side.
Thirst, particularly during chill	Want of thirst.

Boldness—Rarely indifference	Mood changing; haughty; amorous.
Mental dullness	Delirium—Fancies—Mental excitability—Ecstasies.
Imbecility—Weakness of memory	Insanity—Active memory.
Very rarely paralysis	Apoplexy.
Headache better from stooping	Headache worse from stooping. C. Hg.
Pupils predominantly dilated	Pupils predom. contracted.
Vomit predominantly bitter	Vomit predom. sour.
Toothache, better with mouth open & from drawing in the air.	Toothache, worse when opening mouth and drawing in air.
Nasal secretion watery	Nasal secretion thick.
Voice failing, interrupted	Voice trembling or hissing.
Expectoration infrequent; morning . . .	Expector. not constant; morn'g & dur'g day.

Remission *during day* and after midnight.	Remission of compl. after midnight.
Ailments from Mercurius, Nitric. acid., or Phosphor.	Ailments from Iodine or abuse of table-salt.
Worse when alone; better in company . .	Better (worse) when alone *or* in company.

Predomin. worse — **Predomin. better**

When sitting erect, when lifting or drawing up diseased limb, from rubbing, on an empty stomach, after drinking, partic. drinking wine, from sweets, and when growing warm.

Predomin. better — **Predomin. worse**

When sitting bent forward, when letting diseased limb hang down, when swallowing,* when growing cold, and after breakfast.

N.B. Over-sensitiveness to pain as well as sensation of numbness in suffering parts is found much oftener with Phosphor. than with Mezereum.

---

* Mezer., however, has aggrav. when swallowing saliva; Phosph. has aggrav. when swallowing food, and partic. drink.

Mezereum.	Pulsatilla.
Left side, part. *lower left*, *upper right side*	*Right* side, partic. *lower right*, *upper left side*.
Itching, aggrav. *or* changed to another place by scratching.	Itching, aggrav. *or* unchanged by scratching.
Vesicular erysipelas	Erysipelas with smooth skin.
Pulse often unchanged; generally full and hard.	Pulse generally frequent, small, and weak; sometimes imperceptible.
One-sided heat, left side	One-sided heat, right side.
Thirst, partic. during chill	Want of thirst, partic. during chill.
Sleeplessness after midnight — **Awaking too early.**	Sleeplessness after midnight — **Awaking too late.**
No apoplexy—**Phlegmatic temperament**	**Apoplexy—Sanguine phlegmat. temperament.**

Mezereum.	Pulsatilla.
Dreads being alone	Desires to be alone.
Mood cheerful *or* sad	Mood changing; good-natured—**Calm sadness of mild dispositions—Amorousn.—Avarice.**
Rarely unconsciousness	Fancies—Delirium.
Complaints of nose, **generally internal**; complaints on upper jaw, on upper teeth	Complaints of nose, **generally external**; complaints on lower jaw, on lower teeth.
Appetite for bacon	Aversion to fatty (greasy) food.
Urine often, but scanty	Urine infrequent and scanty.
Catamenia too soon and of long duration	**Catamenia too late and of short duration.**
Larynx and trachea dry	**Larynx and trachea filled with mucus.**
Expectoration infrequent; **morning**	Expectoration **predom., but not constant; morning and during day.**

Mezereum.	Pulsatilla.
Aggrav. morning and *evening* till midnight	Aggrav. afternoon and evening till midnight.
Better (worse) in wet *or* dry weather	**Worse in wet weather; better in dry weather.**
Worse from bodily exertion	Improv. oftener than aggrav. by exertion.
Worse when taking a deep breath	Better *or* worse when taking a deep breath.
Worse from tying the clothes tight	*Generally* improv. by tying clothes tight.
Generally worse from pressure	*Generally* better from pressure.
Worse when bending diseased part	Better *or* worse when bending the part.
Worse on awaking from sleep	*Worse or* better after sleep.
Worse when getting out of bed	*Better or* worse when getting out of bed.
Better after rising from a seat	*Better or* worse after rising from a seat.
Predom. better when swallowing	*Worse or* better when swallowing.
Better from eructation	*Worse or* better from eructation.
Almost always aggrav. after stool	*Better or* worse after stool.

Predomin. worse — **Predomin. better**

From cold and in cold weather,* from motion and when walking, from washing and moistening diseased part, when lifting or stretching out diseased part, when sitting erect, on inspiration, from pressure, from tying the clothes tight, when lying on painful side, after stool, when closing the mouth, when getting out of bed, and from bodily exertion.

Predomin. better — **Predomin. worse**

From warmth and in warm air, during rest, when standing, sitting and lying. when letting diseased limb hang down or drawing it up, when stooping and sitting bent forward, from loosening the clothes, lying on unpainful side, when opening the mouth, when swallowing, during and after meals, and from eructation.

N.B. We rarely find either the sensitiveness of Pulsatilla to pain, or the sensation of numbness of suffering parts, with Mezereum.

* Both remedies have predom. improv. "*when growing cold*," aggrav. "*when growing warm*."

Mezereum.	Rhus.
Left side, partic. *lower left, upper right side.*	*Right* side, partic. *lower right, upper left side.*
Inclination for open air—Aversion to motion.	Aversion to open air—Inclination for motion.
Emaciation of diseased parts	Swelling of diseased parts.
The whole left side goes to sleep	The right side goes to sleep.
Very rarely paralysis—No apoplexy . . .	Paralysis of limbs—Apoplexy.
Softness of skin	Hardness of skin with thickening of the same.
Painful ulcers	Painless ulcers.
Itching, aggrav. *or* changed to another place by scratching.	Itching relieved by scratching.
Sleeplessness after midnight — Awaking too early.	Sleeplessness preval. before midnight—Awaking too late.
Pulse often unchanged; generally full and hard.	Pulse generally quick, small and weak, often irregular, sometimes imperceptible or trembling.
Chill lessened out-doors	Chill increased out-doors.
Thirst, partic. during cold stage of fever . .	Thirst not constant.

Dreads being alone — Mood sad *or* cheerful; irritable—Boldness.	Desires to be alone — Dejection of spirits predomin.—Fancies—Delirium.
Nasal complaints internal oftener than external.	Nasal complaints external oftener than internal.
Swelling of lower lip or an eruption predom.	Swelling of upper lip predom., or herpes labialis.
Complaints predom. on upper jaw and upper teeth.	Complaints predom. on lower jaw and lower teeth.
Sensation in the teeth as if lifted up	Sensation in the teeth as if drawn in. C.Hg.
The tartar on teeth becomes rough	Crusty caries of the teeth.
Desire for wine	Aversion to wine.
Urine often, but scanty; sediment red . . .	Urine often and copious; sediment white.
Nasal secretion watery	Nasal secretion thick.
Expectoration infrequent	Expectoration not constant.
Complaints predom. on upper arm, shin, and sole of foot.	Complaints predom. on fore-arm, calf of leg, and top of foot.

Remission after midnight and during day . .	Remission of complaints during day.
Better (worse) in wet *or* in dry weather .	Worse in wet, better in dry weather.
Worse or better from washing and moistening.	Worse from washing and moistening.
Predom. worse in bed	*Better or* worse in bed.
Worse when getting out of bed	Worse *or* better when getting out of bed.
Better after rising from a seat	Worse *or* better after rising from a seat.
Better *or* worse when assuming an erect position.	Almost always aggrav. when rising (from stooping).
Worse when bending diseased part	*Worse or* better when bending the part.
Better while eating	Worse *or* better when eating.
Better from warm *or* cold diet, and in the latter case worse from warm diet.	Predom. worse from cold, better from warm diet.
Worse after drinking	*Worse or* better after drinking.
Almost always aggrav. after stool . .	*Better or* worse after stool.
Ailments from Phosphor. or Nitric. acid. . .	Ailments from Bryonia, Ranunculus, Rhododendron, or Tartarus emeticus.

Predomin. **worse** — Predomin. **better**

In-doors and from warmth of stove, when growing warm, from pressure, when lying on painful side, when sitting erect, from motion, when walking, when stretching out diseased limb, when closing the mouth, after stool, and from rubbing and scratching.

Predomin. **better** — Predomin. **worse**

Out-doors, when growing cold, lying on unpainful side, when sitting bent forward, during rest, when standing and sitting, when drawing up diseased limb, when opening the mouth, stooping, swallowing, drinking cold water, and from eructation.

Mezereum.	Thuya.
Upper right, lower left side—Inclination for open air.	Upper left, lower right side—Aversion to open air.
No apoplexy	Apoplexy.
Internal inflammations—Twitch'g pains predominant in internal parts.	External inflammations — Twitch'g pains predom. in external parts.
Diseases in the middle part of cylindrical bones.	Pains, partic. in the middle (thickest part) of muscles.
Softness of skin	Hardness and thickening of skin.
Stinging in the scars	Stinging and digging in scars. C.Hg.
Itching, aggrav. *or* changed to another place by scratching.	Itching, relieved by scratching.
Pulse often unchanged	Pulse changed, unequal.
Chill lessened out-doors	Chill increased out-doors.
Thirst, particularly during chill . . .	Thirst is wanting during chill, is predom. during heat, not constant during sweat.

Mezereum.	Thuya.
Weakness of reasoning powers	Mental excitability (ecstasies) *or* weakness of reasoning powers.
Pupils predominantly dilated	Pupils predom. contracted.
Teeth decay on the side, above the gums .	Painful affection of the roots of teeth inside of the gums, with healthy crown of tooth; loosening, decaying from the side, and falling out.
Secretion of saliva almost always increased.	Saliva generally diminished.
Vomit bitter-sour	Vomit fatty, like oil.
Urine scanty	Urine copious and often.
Erections with sexual inclination	Erections with aversion.
Catamenia too soon and profuse	Catam. too scanty and of short duration.

Mezereum.	Thuya.
AGGRAVATIONS morning and *evening* till midnight.	AGGRAVATIONS morning, *afternoon*, evening, and *after midnight*.
Better when swallowing, *worse* when not swallowing.	Worse when swallowing.
Better when sitting, partic. when sitting bent forward.	Worse when sitting.
Ailments from Nitric. acid. or Phosphor. .	Ailments from Iodine or Sulph.
Worse from spirituous liquors	Worse *or* better from spirituous liquors.

Predomin. worse —— **Predomin. better**

From motion,* when lifting diseased limb, when closing the mouth, in-doors,† from cold, on an empty stomach, after stool, from touch and pressure, and from rubbing and scratching

Predomin. better —— **Predomin. worse**

During rest, when sitting and standing, letting diseased limb hang down, when opening the mouth, out-doors, from warmth, when stooping, and after breakfast.

---

* When moving diseased limb or when bending it, Thuya sometimes has improv. and sometimes aggrav.
† We also find aggrav. with Thuya in the room, that is when it is to warm.

Moschus.	Phosphor.
Cramping pain in external parts—Pain pressing inwards.	Cramping pain in internal parts — Pain pressing outwards.
Complaints predominant in lower part of chest and in thigh.	Complaints most frequent in upper part of chest and on leg.
Itching, relieved by scratching.	Itching, lessened oftener than aggrav. by scratching.
Anæmie	Plethora more frequent than anæmie.
Apoplexy more frequent than paralysis . .	Paralysis more frequent than apoplexy.
Pulse very full and accelerated; but sometimes imperceptible.	Pulse various, different, unequal, irregular, intermitting; generally frequent, at the same time full & hard oftener than small and faint.
Chill or heat descending	Chill or heat ascending.
Respiration preval. slow	Respiration generally accelerated.
Expectoration not yet observed	Expector. not constant with the cough.

REMISSION morning and forenoon . . .	REMISSION of complaints after midnight.
Worse from touch	Almost always improv. by touch.
Better from moving diseased part . . .	Better *or* worse from moving the part.
Better when rising (from stooping) . . .	Almost always aggrav. when assuming an erect position.
Worse in bed	Worse *or* better in bed.
Worse during sweat	*Worse or* better during sweat.
Worse during sleep	*Worse or* better during sleep.
Worse on awaking from sleep	Better after sufficient sleep, but worse on awaking when roused from sleep & after the siesta.
Better after getting out of bed	Worse *or* better after getting out of bed.
Better from eructation	Worse *or* better from eructation.

Predomin. worse — **Predomin. better**

Out-doors, during rest, when standing, sitting and lying, partic. when sitting erect, lying on side, from touch, and after sleep.

Predomin. better — **Predomin. worse**

In-doors and from warmth of stove, but also when walking,* out-doors, from motion, when walking, sitting bent forward, lying on back, from *warmth* of bed, and when rising (after stooping).

---

* It is evident from the foregoing, that, in this case, it is not the influence of the open air which improv. or aggrav., but that of motion.

Muriat. acid.	Arsenic.
Left side, particularly *lower left, upper right side.*	*Right* side, particularly *lower right, upper left side.*
Complaints (throbbing, etc.) predominant in external parts.	Complaints (throbbing, etc.) predominant in internal parts.
Bruised pain in internal parts	Bruised pain in external parts.
Paralysis generally of one side	Paralysis generally of both sides.
Itching, generally relieved by scratching .	Itching, aggravated by scratching.
Deep ulcers	Superficial ulcers, often with proud flesh.
Somnolence predominant; when sleeplessness occurs, it is preval. before midnight.	Sleeplessness predominant, particularly after midnight.
Pulse slow and weak; partic. slow during day, more frequent at night.	Pulse very much accelerated, small, and weak; partic. frequent in the morning, slower in evening.
Heat or sweat, with inclination to uncover.	Heat or sweat, with aversion to uncover.
Want of thirst; only sometimes thirst during chill.	Least thirst during chill, most during sweat; during heat drinks often, but little at a time.
Taciturnity during the sweat	Loquacity during the sweat. C.Hg.
Mental excitability *or* dullness—Unconsciousness—Taciturnity.	Mood despondent; irritable; malicious—Avarice—Mental dullness—Insanity—Rarely unconsciousness—Talkativeness predom.
Perpendicular half-sight	Horizontal half-sight.
Hunger predominant	Generally loss of appetite.
Urine too often and copious	Urine scanty (with diarrhœa) *or* copious.
Sexual desire too weak	Sexual desire too strong.
Coryza predominantly dry	Fluent coryza.
Expectoration infrequent; morning and evening.	Expectoration predominant, but not constant; during day.
Complaints predominant on thigh . . .	Complaints predominant on leg.
Aggravation aftern'n & before midnight.	**Remission** *during day* and before midnight.
Worse from light, better in the dark . .	Better (worse) from light *or* in the dark.
Better (worse) when growing cold *or* warm.	Worse on grow'g cold, bett. on grow'g warm.
Predominantly worse in bed	Worse in bed (rest) *or* (warmth) better.
Worse on awaking from sleep	Better after sufficient sleep, but worse on awaking when roused from sleep.
Worse *or* better from washing, etc. . . .	Predom. better from washing and moistening diseased part.
Better (worse) when stretching out diseased limb *or* when drawing it up.	Worse when stretching out the limb, better when drawing it up.
Worse when rising (from stooping) . . .	Better *or* worse when assum'g an erect posit.

Predomin. **worse**	Predomin. **better**

In wet weather, from warmth of bed, wrapping up the head, and after sleep.

Predomin. **better**	Predomin. **worse**

In dry weather, from uncovering the head, when sneezing, from touch, and from rubbing and scratching.

N.B. Mur. acid. lacks the sensitiveness of Arsenic to touch, and generally also to pain, as well as the sensation of numbness in suffering parts peculiar to Arsenic.

Muriat. acid.	Bryonia.
Left side—Want of bodily irritability . .	*Right* side—Increased bodily irritability.
Complaints predominant in external parts .	Complaints predominant in internal parts—Apoplexy.
Paralysis generally one-sided	Paralysis generally of both sides.
Itching, relieved by scratching.	Itching, relieved *or* unchanged by scratch'g.
Painful ulcers	Painless ulcers.
Pulse slow and weak	Pulse quick, full, hard, and tense.
Want of thirst; only sometimes thirst during chill.	Thirst predominant, but not constant.

Muriat. acid.	Bryonia.
Mood indifferent	Mood *irritable;* despondent.
Rarely fancies—Ecstasies or mental dullness.	Fancies—Mental excitability.
Diarrhœa predominant	Constipation predominant.
Urine pale; too often and copious . . .	Urine dark; often, but scanty; sometimes copious.
Catamenia too soon	Catamenia too soon *or* too late.
Respiration with dry sound	Respiration preval. with moist sound.
Expectoration infrequent; morning and evening.	Expectoration not constant; morning and evening; sometimes also during day.

Muriat. acid.	Bryonia.
Aggravation afternoon and before midnight.	Aggravation *evening*, night, and morn'g.
Worse in cold weather; better in warm air.	Worse (better) in cold weather *or* in warm air.
Worse on awaking from sleep.	Aggravated oftener than improved after sleep.
Better or worse from stooping	Worse from stooping.
Worse from assuming an erect position . .	*Worse or* better from assuming an erect position.
Better *or* worse when bending the part . .	Worse when bending diseased part.
Worse (better) when stretching out diseased limb *or* when drawing it up.	Worse when stretching out diseased limb, better when drawing it up.
Almost always improved by touch . . .	*Worse or* better from touch.
Better after drinking	Worse *or* better after drinking.

Predomin. worse — **Predomin. better**

In wet weather, from drinking cold water, from cold diet in general, after stool, during rest, after lying down, when lying and sitting, in bed and from warmth of bed, when lying on painful side.

Predomin. better — **Predomin. worse**

In dry weather, from warm diet, from motion, when walking and from moving diseased part, after getting out of bed or rising from a seat, when lying on unpainful side, from touch, from stooping, and from sneezing.

N.B. Mur. acid. lacks the sensitiveness of Bryonia to touch, and generally also to pain.

Muriat. acid.	Lycopodium.
Left side — No apoplexy — Paralysis generally one-sided.	*Right* side — Apoplexy — Paralysis often of both sides.
Compl. predom. in lower part of chest, in thigh, partic. on front part of it.	Compl. predom. in upper part of chest, on leg, and on back part of thigh.
Pulse slow and weak; sometimes intermitting; slow during day, more frequent at night.	Pulse somewhat accelerated only in the evening and after meals; frequent in the evening, slow in morning
Thirst only sometimes during chill . . .	Thirst is wanting only during chill
Mood indifferent	Mood *sad or* cheerful; serious; irritable; malicious; haughty — Amorousness — Avarice — Distrust.
Rarely fancies — Ecstasies *or* mental dullness.	Absent-mindedness — Fancies — Mental dullness.
Imbecility	Insanity more frequent than imbecility.
Pupils contracted — Compl. predom. on external angle of eye.	Pupils dilated – Compl. predom. in inner angle of eye.
Diarrhœa	Constipation.
Urine too often and copious	Urine often, but scanty.
Incontinence predominant	Retention of urine more frequent than incontinence.
Catamenia too soon and profuse	Catamenia too late; at the same time too scanty *or* profuse.
Respiration with dry sound	Respiration preval. with moist sound.
Expectoration infrequent	Expectoration almost constant.
AGGRAVATION afternoon & before midnight.	AGGRAVATION morning and from *noon till midnight.*
Worse in cold weather, better in warm air.	Bett. (worse) in cold weather *or* in warm air.
Better *or* worse from washing, etc. . . .	Worse from washing and moistening diseased part.
Better *or* worse from bending the part . .	Worse from bending diseased part.
Better (worse) when stretching out diseased limb *or* when drawing it up.	Worse when stretching out diseased limb, better when drawing it up.
Better when sitting down	Worse *or* better when sitting down.
Worse when rising from a seat	*Worse or* better when rising from a seat.
Worse when rising (from stooping) . . .	Worse *or* better when rising.
Worse after stool	Worse *or* better after stool.
Worse when perspiring	Better *or* worse when perspiring.
Better when sneezing	*Worse or* better when sneezing.

Predomin. **worse** — Predomin. **better**

From cold, out-doors, and when ascending.

Predomin. **better** — Predomin. **worse**

From warmth, in-doors, when descending, when standing, from touch and pressure, when sneezing.

N.B. Mur. acid. almost always lacks the sensitiveness of Lycopod. to touch or to pain, and also the sensation of numbness in suffering parts.

Muriat. acid.	Pulsatilla.
Left side, partic. *lower left, upper right side.*	*Right* side; partic. *lower right, upper left side.*
Complaints predominant in external parts.	Compl predom. in internal parts.
Want of bodily irritability — Aversion to open air.	Increase of irritability — Inclination for open air.
Apoplexy not yet observed	Apoplexy.
Itching, generally lessened by scratching .	Itching, unchanged *or* aggrav. by scratching.
Pulse slow and weak, only at night somewhat accelerated.	Pulse frequent, small, and weak; frequent in the evening, slower during the day.
Want of thirst; only sometimes during cold stage there is thirst.	Want of thirst predom., but constant only during chill.
Awaking too early	Awaking too late.
Very rarely imaginations — Ecstasies or mental dullness.	Imaginations — Absent-mindedness — Mental dullness.
Imbecility	Melancholy.
Compl. predom. on outer angle of eye . .	Compl. predom. on inner angle of eye.
Secretion of saliva predom. diminished . .	Saliva generally increased.
Urine too often and copious	Urine not often enough and scanty.
Sexual desire too weak	Sexual desire too strong.
Dry coryza	Coryza fluent (partic. right side) oftener than dry.
Expector. infrequent; morning & evening.	Expector. predom., but not constant; morning and during day
Complaints predominant on thigh . . .	Compl. predom. on leg.
AGGRAVATION afternoon & before midnight.	AGGRAVATION afternoon and evening till midnight.
Worse (better) when growing cold or warm.	Better when growing cold; worse when growing warm.
Worse on awaking from sleep	*Worse or* better after sleep.
Worse from bodily exertion	*Generally* improv. by exertion.
Worse when rising (from stooping) . . .	*Worse or* better when rising.
Better when sitting down	Worse *or* better when sitting down.
Worse when rising from a seat	Worse or better when rising from a seat.
Better after rising from a seat	*Better or* worse after rising from a seat.
Better from moving diseased part . . .	*Better or* worse from moving the part.
Worse (better) when stretching out diseased limb or when drawing it up.	Predom. better when stretching out diseased limb, worse when drawing it up.
Worse *or* better from washing, etc. . . .	Predom. better from washing & moistening diseased limb.
Worse after meals	*Worse or* better after meals.
Worse after stool	*Better or* worse after stool.

Predomin. worse — **Predomin. better**

From cold and in cold weather, out-doors, from drinking cold water and from cold diet generally, when lying on painful side, after stool, and from bodily exertion.

Predomin. better — **Predomin. worse**

From warmth and in warm air, in-doors, from warm diet, when lying on unpainful side, when standing, when stooping, when sneezing, from touch, and from rubbing and scratching.

N.B. Mur. acid. almost always lacks the over-sensitiveness of Pulsatilla to pain or touch, and the sensation of numbness in suffering parts peculiar to Pulsatilla.

Natr. carb.	Calcarea.
Complaints of external parts predom.	Complaints of internal parts predom.
No apoplexy—Very rarely paralysis	Apoplexy—Paralysis.
Complaints predom. on outside of nose, on lower jaw, on lower teeth, on lower gum, in lower part of chest, and in hollow of knee.	Frequent complaints on inside of nose, on upper jaw, upper teeth, and on upper gum, in upper part of chest, and on patella.
Itching relieved by scratching	Itching *relieved or* aggrav. by scratching
Pulse generally unchanged; only at night somewhat irritated.	Pulse changed, sometimes trembling, generally quick and full.
One-sided heat, right side	One-sided heat, left side.
First chill, then heat	First heat, then chill.
Heat or sweat, with aversion to uncover	Heat or sweat, with inclination to uncover
Heat or chill lessened after meals	Heat or chill increased after meals.
During sleep lying on side	During sleep, lying on back, generally the hands over the head; *or* lying on belly.

Natr. carb.	Calcarea.
Dread of apoplexy	Dread of loss of reason.
Joyousness or dejection — Seriousness — Avarice—Maliciousness.	*Sadness or* silly merriment.
Rarely unconsciousness	Illusions—Delirium.
Eruption on upper lip	Eruptions predom. on lower lip.
Vomit predom. bitter	Vomit predom. sour.
Diarrhœa painful	Diarrhœa generally painless.
Expectoration almost constant; morning and evening.	Expectoration predom., but not constant; morning and during day.

Natr. carb.	Calcarea.
Worse during full moon *or* before a thunderstorm.	Worse during *full or* during new moon.
Worse from light; better in the dark	Better (worse) from light *or* in the dark.
Better *or* worse when straining the sight	Worse when straining the sight.
Worse from bodily exertion	*Worse or* better from exertion.
Predom. better after getting out of bed	*Worse or* better after getting out of bed.
Worse from sneezing	*Worse or* better from sneezing.
Worse on in- and expiration	Worse on inspiration; better on expiration.
Better from smoking	*Worse or* better from smoking.
Better *or* worse when swallowing	Worse when swallowing.
Better *or* worse after stool	Worse after stool.
Worse *or* better when perspiring	Almost always aggrav. when perspiring.

Predomin. worse — **Predomin. better**

From uncovering, during rest, after lying down, when lying, sitting and standing; also when lifting diseased limb, and after breakfast.*

Predomin. better — **Predomin. worse**

From wrapping up, from motion, when walking, when letting diseased limb hang down, when and after getting out of bed, *before* breakfast, from smoking, from pressure, from boring in ears and nose with the finger, and from mental exertion.

N.B. Natr. carb. lacks the sensation of numbness in suffering parts peculiar to Calcar.; on the other hand, the over-sensitiveness of Natr. carb. to pain is very rarely found with Calcarea.

* **Both remedies have aggrav. after a satisfying meal.**

Natr. carb.	Lycopodium.
Sensitiveness predominant in internal parts	Insensibility or sensation of numbness in internal parts.
No apoplexy—Rarely paralysis	*Apoplexy*—Paralysis.
Pulse irritated and accelerated at night, slow during day.	Pulse somewhat accelerated only in the evening and after meals, slow in the morning.
Thirst often between chill and heat	Thirst frequently *after* the sweat.
Heat or chill right side	Heat or chill left side.
Heat or chill less after meals	Heat or chill increased after meals.
Chill lessened in bed	Chill increased in bed.
Heat or sweat, with aversion to uncover	Heat or sweat, with inclination to uncover.
Mood rarely irritable; rarely distrustful	Mood gentle *or* irritable—Distrust.
Solicitude concerning bodily welfare	Solicitude concerning spiritual welfare. C.Hg.
Ailments from vexation with fright	Ailments from vexation with vehemence.
Rarely absent-mindedness — Rarely unconsciousness.	Illusions—Delirium.
Imbecility more frequent than insanity	Insanity more frequent than imbecility.
During sleep lying on side	During sleep lying on back.
Nasal complaints predom. external	Nasal complaints predom. internal.
Vomit predom. bitter	Vomit sour, oftener than bitter.
Fetid flatus	Scentless flatus predom.
Painful diarrhœa	Painless diarrhœa.
Urine too often and copious	Urine often, but scanty.
Catamenia too soon and profuse	Catamenia too late; at the same time scanty *or* profuse.
Coryza fluent oftener than dry	Stoppage of nose more frequent than fluent coryza.
Complaints predominant in lower part of chest.	Complaints predominant in upper part of chest.
Remission of complaints before midnight	Remission after midnight and *forenoon.*
Worse during full moon, and before a thunder-storm.	Worse during new moon.
Worse from light, partic. sunlight	Worse from light, partic. candle-light.
Worse in cold weather, better in warm air	Better (worse) in cold weather *or* in warm air.
Predom. worse when growing cold, better when growing warm.	*Generally* better when growing cold, worse when growing warm.
Worse after perspiring	*Better or* worse after perspiring.
Predom. worse in bed and from warmth of bed.	Better *or* worse in bed and from warmth of bed.
Worse or better after sleep	Worse after sleep.
Better when getting out of bed	Worse *or* better when getting out of bed.
Better when rising (from stooping)	Worse *or* better when rising.
Better when sitting down	Worse *or* better when sitting down.
Better *or* worse when swallowing	Worse when swallowing.
Better from eating bread	Worse from bread, partic. rye-bread.
Better or worse after meals	Almost almost aggravated after meals.
Worse when sneezing	*Worse or* better when sneezing.
Worse on inspiration and expiration	Worse on inspiration, better on expiration.
Worse when riding on horseback	*Worse or* better when riding on horseback.
Better when alone, worse when in company	Worse (better) when alone *or* in company.
Better *or* worse from straining the sight	Worse from straining the sight.

Predomin. worse —— **Predomin. better**

From cold and when growing cold, in the open air, from uncovering, lying on left side, when ascending, when lifting diseased limb, and when stooping.

Predomin. better —— **Predomin. worse**

From warmth and when growing warm, in-doors, from wrapping up, lying on right side, when descending, when letting diseased limb hang down, from touch and pressure, from eating bread, smoking, and from mental exertion.

Natr. carb.	Natr. mur.
Upper right, lower left side – Inflammation of external parts.	Upper left, lower right side—Inflammation of internal parts.
Aversion to open air—Skin & muscles lax.	Inclinat'n for open air—Skin & muscles rigid.
Dryness of skin—Often indic. with children.	Perspir'g easily—Oft. indic. with old people.
No apoplexy—Very rarely paralysis . .	Apoplexy—Paralysis.
Compl predom on upper eyelids, on lower jaw, lower teeth, lower gums, and on back of hands.	Compl. predom. on lower eyelids, on upper jaw, upper teeth, on upper gums, and in palm of hands.
Pulse generally unchanged	Pulse unequal, irregular, intermitting, sometimes trembling.
Thirst predom., but generally not until after the chill.	Thirst during the attack of fever, and also when there is no fever.
Chill lessened in bed and after meals . .	Chill increased in bed and after meals.

Natr. carb.	Natr. mur.
Fear of apoplexy	Fear of loss of reason.
Mood joyous *or* serious; anxious; despondent; peevish—Avarice.	Mood changing; indifferent; sad; irritable.
Ailments from excessive joy, grief, or vexation with fright.	Ailm. from fright, anger, mortific., or vexat'n with reserved displeasure—Delirium.
Hunger predominant	Loss of appetite predominant.
Catamenia predom. too soon and profuse .	Catam. too late; at the same time scanty *or* profuse.
Fluent coryza more freq. than stopp. of nose.	Stoppage of nose predom.
Expector. almost constant; morn'g & even'g.	Expector. infrequent; morning.
Palpitation of heart equal	Palpitation of heart, with intermitting beats of heart and pulse.

Natr. carb.	Natr. mur.
REMISSION of compl. before midnight . .	REMISSION afternoon.
Worse when in company; better when alone.	Better (worse) when in company *or* alone.
Worse or better after sleep	Worse on awaking from sleep.
Worse from wash'g and moisten'g the part.	Worse *or* better from washing, etc.
Worse after perspiring	*Better or* worse after perspiring.
Predom. worse from growing cold, better from growing warm.	Better (worse) from growing cold or warm.
Worse from cold, better from warm diet .	Better (worse) from cold *or* warm diet.
Better *or* worse when swallowing . . .	Worse when swallowing.
Better or worse after meals	Worse after meals.
Worse after drinking	*Worse or* better after drinking.
Better *or* worse after stool	Predom. worse after stool.
Better *or* worse when straining the sight .	Worse when straining the sight.
Worse from speaking	*Worse or* better from speaking.
Worse or better when writing	Worse when writing.
Worse when stooping; better when rising.	*Worse or* better when stoop'g & when rising.
Worse *or* better when rising from a seat .	Worse when rising from a seat.
Better after rising from a seat	Worse *or* better after rising from a seat.

Predomin. worse —— **Predomin. bette[r]**

From cold, out of doors, during rest, after lying down, when lying, sitting and standing, & after sweat.

Predomin. better —— **Predomin. worse**

From warmth, in-doors, from motion, when walking, when and after getting out of bed, from mental exertion, from touch and pressure, from eating bread, and smoking.

N.B. Natr. mur. lacks the over-sensitiveness of Natr. carb. to pain. — Natr. carb. has not the sensation of numbness in suffering parts peculiar to Natr. mur.

Natr. carb.	Phosphor.
Complaints predom. in external parts	Complaints predom. in internal parts.
Skin and muscles lax — Often indicated with children.	Skin and muscles rigid—Often indicated with old people.
No apoplexy—Very rarely paralysis	Apoplexy—*Paralysis.*
Itching, relieved by scratching	Itching, *lessened or* aggrav. by scratching.
Pulse generally unchanged; only at night somewhat accelerated.	Pulse accelerated, irregular; intermitting.
Heat descending	Heat ascending.
Chill or heat lessened after meals	Chill or heat increased after meals.
Sweat increased during meals	Sweat lessened during meals.
Heat or sweat, with aversion to uncover	Heat or sweat, with inclination to uncover.
Thirst, but generally not until *after* the chill.	Want of thirst during all stages of the fever.
Fear of apoplexy	Fear of loss of reason *or* apoplexy.
Mood serious—Avarice	Mood indifferent—Haughtiness.
Ailments from excessive joy	Ailments from fright or anger.
Difficult comprehension—Mental dullness	Easy *or* difficult comprehension—Mental excitability predom.
Rarely unconsciousness—Imbecility	Unconsciousness — Delirium — Fancies — Insanity.
Pupils dilated	Pupils contracted.
Bad objective smell from nose	Putrid subjective smell predom.
Complaints predom. on upper lip	Complaints predom. on under lip.
Appetite for sweets and for beer	Aversion to sweets and to beer.
Vomit predom. bitter	Vomit predom. sour.
Fetid flatus	Scentless, often hot flatus.
Painful diarrhœa	Generally painless diarrhœa.
Urine smells sour; too often and copious	Urine smells like ammoniac; often, but scanty.
Catamenia too profuse	Catamenia profuse *or* scanty.
Labor-pains weak or ceasing	Labor-pains spasmodic, too painful.
Expectoration almost constant; morning and evening.	Expectoration not constant; morning and during day.
Complaints predom. in lower part of chest and on back of hand.	Complaints most frequent in upper part of chest, and in palms of hands.
Remission of complaints before midnight	Remission after midnight.
Ailments from abuse of Cinchona	Ailments from Iodine or Natr. mur.
Worse when in company; better when alone	Better (worse) when in company *or* when alone.
Worse when sleeping	Worse *or* better when sleeping.
Predom. better after getting out of bed	Worse *or* better after getting out of bed.
Better *or* worse when rising from a seat	Almost always aggr. when rising from a seat.
Worse from washing and moistening the part.	*Worse or* better from washing, &c.
Worse when stooping	Better *or* worse when stooping.
Worse or better when writing	Worse when writing.
Better *or* worse when straining the sight	Worse when straining the sight.
Better *or* worse when swallowing	Almost always aggrav. when swallowing.
Better from eructation	Worse *or* better from eructation.
Better *or* worse after stool	Worse after stool.

Predomin. worse — **Predomin. better**

Out of doors, from uncovering, during rest, when standing, sitting and lying, when lying on side, when lifting diseased limb, from cold diet, drinking cold water, from spirituous liquors, from sweets, after a satisfying meal, and after drinking.

Predomin. worse — **Predomin. better**

In-doors, from wrapping up, from motion,* when walking, lying on back, when letting diseased limb hang down, from warm diet, from eating bread, smoking, exerting the mind, when rising (from stooping , and from pressure.

* Both remedies generally have improv. when *moving diseased part.*

Natr. carb.	Pulsatilla.
Aversion to open air—*Upper right, lower left side.*	Inclination for open air—*Upper left, lower right side.*
Complaints predominant in external parts.	Compl. predom. in internal parts.
Compl. predom. on upper lip, on outside of gums, and on fore-arm.	Compl. predom. on under lip, on inside of gums, and on upper arm.
Apoplexy not yet observed	Apoplexy.
Itching lessened, rarely aggrav. by scratch'g.	Itching, unchanged *or* aggrav. by scratch'g.
During sleep lying on side	During sleep lying on back, generally the hands over the head.
Pulse often unchanged; irritated & accelerated at night, slow during the day.	Pulse generally accelerated, small, & weak; frequent in the evening, slow in the morning; sometimes intermitt. & imperceptible.
Chill lessened in bed and after meals	Chill increased in bed and after meals.
Thirst predom.; is wanting only during cold stage.	Want of thirst predom., particularly during chill.

Mood cheerful *or* despondent; serious; malicious.	Mood changing; indifferent; calm, achrymose sadness of mild dispositions.
Rarely unconsciousness	Fancies—Delirium.
Pupils dilated—Optical illusions in dark colors.	Pupils generally contracted; Optical illusions in bright colors.
Nausea in stomach	Nausea in throat, stomach, or abdomen.
Urine smells sour; too often and copious.	Urine smells like ammoniac; too seldom & scanty.
Catamenia too soon and profuse	Catam. too late and generally scanty.
Expectoration tolerably constant; morning and evening.	Expectoration predom., but not constant; morning and during day.

Remission of complaints before midnight.	Remission from midnight till noon.
Better *or* worse when straining the sight	Worse when straining the sight.
Worse when writing, or better (from mental exertion).	Worse when writing.
Better *or* worse during sweat	Worse during sweat.
Worse after sweat.	*Worse or* better after sweat.
Better when getting out of bed	*Better or* worse when getting out of bed.
Better when sitting down	Better when sitting down (motion) *or* (from change of posture) worse.
Better after rising from a seat	*Better or* worse after rising from a seat.
Worse when stooping; better when rising.	*Worse or* better when stoop'g & when ris'g.
Generally better after meals.	*Generally* worse after meals.
Worse when taking a deep breath	Better *or* worse from taking a deep breath.

Predomin. worse — **Predomin. better**

From cold, growing cold and in cold weather, out-doors, from uncovering, from washing and moistening diseased part, when lifting the suffering limb, from bodily exertion, drinking cold water, and from cold diet in general.

Predomin. better — **Predomin. worse**

From warmth, growing warm and in warm air, in-doors, from wrapping up, letting diseased limb hang down, from *mental exertion*, from warm diet, eating bread, after eating generally, from eructation, smoking, touch, and from rubbing and scratching.

Natr. carb.	Sepia.
Skin and muscles lax—No apoplexy	Skin and muscles rigid—Apoplexy
Very rarely paralysis—Itching, relieved by scratching.	Paralysis—Itching, aggrav. by scratching.
Pulse generally unchanged	Pulse accelerated, particularly by vexation and motion.
Heat descending	Heat ascending.
First chill, then heat	First heat, then chill.
Heat lessened by mental exertion and after meals.	Heat increased by mental exertion and after meals.
Heat with thirst	Heat without thirst—Want of thirst generally.
Thirst is wanting only during chill	Thirst is constant only during chill.
Mood cheerful *or* despondent—Amorousness.	Mood sad; indifferent.
Ailments from vexation with fright	Ailments from vexation with fear—Fancies.
Pupils dilated—Short-sightedness	Pupils contracted—Far-sightedness.
Bad objective smell from nose	Putrid objective smell predominant.
Eruption on upper lip	Eruption on under lip.
Toothache lessened by smoking	Toothache increased by smooking. C.Hg.
Hunger predominant—Urine too often and copious.	Generally loss of appetite—Discharge of urine too seldom.
Catamenia too soon—Leucorrhœa thick	Catamenia generally too late—Watery leucorrhœa.
Nasal secretion thick	Nasal secretion watery.
Expectoration almost constant, morning and evening.	Expectoration predominant, but not constant; is loosened night and morning, and is generally swallowed.
Complaints predominant in hollow of knee.	Complaints predominant in hollow of elbow
REMISSION before midnight	REMISSION afternoon.
Worse during full moon	Worse during new moon.
Worse in cold weather, better in warm air.	Better (worse) in cold weather *or* warm air.
Better when getting out of bed	*Better or* worse when getting out of bed.
Worse or better when writing	Worse when writing.
Worse from bodily exertion	Improved oftener than aggrav. by exertion.
Better *or* worse when swallowing	Worse when swallowing.
Generally better after meals	*Generally* worse after meals.*

Predomin. worse — **Predomin better**

In wet weather, from bodily exertion, lying on side, drinking cold water and from cold diet generally, after breakfast.

Predomin. better — **Predomin. worse**

In dry weather, from mental exertion, lying on back, before breakfast, but also after meals, partic. from warm diet and eating bread, from eructation, touch and pressure, and from rubbing and scratching.

* Both remedies have aggravation after a satisfying meal.

Natr. carb.	Sulphur.
Right side, partic. *upper right, lower left side.*	*Left* side, partic. *upper left, lower right side.*
Over-sensitiveness predom.	Loss of feeling or sensation of numbness predom.
Ulcerative pain in external parts—Pinching pain in internal parts.	Ulcerative pain in internal parts—Pinching pain in external parts.
Pulse generally unchanged	Pulse generally hard and accelerated; sometimes intermitting or imperceptible.
Heat descending	Heat ascending.
Heat or sweat, with aversion to uncover .	Heat or sweat, with inclination to uncover.
Chill lessened after meals	Chill increased after meals.
Boldness—Malice—Avarice	Embarrassment—Gentleness.
Mood cheerful *or* despondent	Mood serious, solemn; *sad;* indifferent—Fancies—Delirium.
Imbecility more frequent than insanity . .	Insanity more frequent than imbecility.
Pupils dilated	Pupils contracted.
Saliva generally increased	Saliva generally diminished.
Hunger predom.	Generally loss of appetite.
Appetite for beer	Desire *or* aversion for beer and spirituous liquors.
Vomiting of bile predom.	Vomit sour oftener than bitter.
Urine too often and copious	Urine often, but scanty; sometimes copious.
Catamenia too soon and profuse	Catamenia *generally* too late and scanty.
Nasal secretion thick	Nasal secretion watery.
Expectoration almost constant; morning and evening.	Expectoration not constant; morning and during day; rarely at night.
Complaints predom. in lower part of chest.	Complaints predom. in upper part of chest.
REMISSION of complaints before midnight .	REMISSION afternoon and before midnight.
Generally worse when growing cold and in cold weather; better when growing warm and in warm air.	*Generally* better when growing cold and in cold weather; worse when growing warm and in warm air.
Worse *or* better during sweat.	Almost always aggrav. during sweat.
Better after sweat	*Worse or* better after sweat.
Worse or better after sleep	Worse after sleep.
Predom. better after getting out of bed .	Worse *or* better after getting out of bed.
Better *or* worse when rising from a seat .	Worse when rising from a seat.
Better when rising (from stooping) . . .	*Worse or* better when rising.
Generally better from touch	*Generally* worse from touch.
Better *or* worse when straining the sight .	Worse when straining the sight.
Worse from sneezing	*Worse or* better from sneezing.
Better *or* worse after meals	Worse after meals.
Worse after drinking	*Worse or* better after drinking.

Predomin. worse — **Predomin. better**

From cold, growing cold and in cold weather, out-doors, and from uncovering.

Predomin. better — **Predomin. worse**

From warmth, growing warm and in warm air, in-doors,* from wrapping up, after sweat, from touch, from moving diseased limb, when rising (from stooping), after meals, partic. after eating bread, from smoking, and from mental exertion.

N.B. Natr. carb. lacks the sensation of numbness in suffering parts peculiar to Sulph. The latter generally has not the over-sensitiveness of Natr. carb. to pain.

* Both remedies have aggrav. in *hot, crowded rooms;* Sulphur has improv. from warmth of stove.

Natr. mur.	Phosphor.
Upper left, lower right side—Complaints predomin. in external parts.	Upper right, lower left side—Complaints predomin. in internal parts.
Complaints predom. on lower eyelids, on upper jaw and upper teeth, on inside of ear, lower part of chest, on front surface of thigh, and on calf of leg.	Complaints predom. on upper eyelids, on lower jaw and lower teeth, on outside of ear, upper part of chest, on back part of thigh, and on shin.
Paralysis with muscular atrophy — Humid eruptions.	Nervous paralysis—Dry (symptomatic) eruptions.
Scars redden and hurt	Scars break open and bleed. C.Hg.
Heat or sweat with aversion to uncover . .	Heat or sweat with inclination to uncover.
Sweat increased during meals	Sweat abated during meals.
Thirst during and without fever	Want of thirst during all stages.
Predisposition to sweat (sweating easily) . .	Dryness of skin predom.
Distentions of veins of feet.	Distention of veins of hands.
Desires to be alone	Dreads being alone.
Mood sad oftener than joyous*	Mood joyous oftener than sad.†
Weak memory — Weakness of will — Mental dullness—Imbecility.	Active memory—Mental excitability—Ecstasies—Fancies—Insanity.
Appetite for farinaceous food	Aversion to farinaceous food.
Urine too often (and copious) — Leucorrhœa greenish.	Urine often, but scanty—Leucorrhœa or nasal secretion yellow, like ochre.
Catamenia too late and of long duration . .	Catam. pred. too soon; too long *or* too short.
Labor-pains weak or ceasing	Labor-pains too painful.
Expectoration seldom; morning	Expector. not constant; morn. & during day.
Beating of heart and pulse intermitting . .	Palpit. of heart with equal, accelerated beats.
Remission of complaints afternoon	Remission after midnight.
Ailments from abuse of Cinchona	Ailments from Iodine or Natr. mur.
Aggrav. during the full moon, rarely with a thunder-storm.	Aggrav. before a thunder-storm or during a storm.
Generally better during and after sweat . .	*Generally* worse during and after sweat.
Worse during and on awaking from sleep . .	Worse *or* better during, bett. aft. sufic. sleep.‡
Worse or better when turning in bed . . .	Worse when turning in bed.
Generally worse after getting out of bed . .	Better *or* worse after getting out of bed.
Predom. worse when stooping	Better *or* worse when stooping.
Worse *or* better when assuming an erect posit.	Alm. alw. aggrav. when assum. an erect posit.
Worse (bett.) when sitting erect *or* bent forw.	Bett. wh. sitt. erect, worse wh. sitt. bent forw.
Worse from moving diseased part	*Better or* worse from moving the part.
Worse (better) when lifting diseased limb, *or* when letting it hang down	Predom. better when lifting diseased limb; worse when letting it hang down.
Worse or better from exertion	Worse from bodily exertion.
Worse when looking at anything white. . .	Worse when looking into light, or at shining [things.
Worse or better when speaking	Worse when speaking.
Worse when swallowing, during and after meals, partic. when eating bread.	*Worse or* better when swallowing, during and after meals, and from eating bread.
Worse (better) from cold or warm diet. . .	Better from cold, worse from warm diet.
Generally aggrav. after drinking	*Generally* better after drinking.
Worse or better after stool	Worse after stool.
Worse or better when turning in bed . . .	Worse from change (when lying or standing).

Predomin. worse — **Predomin. better**

From uncovering, but also from warmth, from spirituous liquors, after a satisfying meal, after drinking, when lying on the side, when lifting or drawing up diseased limb, loosening the clothes, when leaning back, from touch, during the evening twilight, and after sleep.

Predomin. better — **Predomin. worse**

From wrapping up, but also from cold, during and after sweat, when lying on back, stretching out diseased limb or letting it hang down, and from tying the clothes tight.

N.B. Natr. mur. lacks the over-sensitiveness of Phosph. to pain.

* Comp. "Mind and Ailments" in *Natr. mur.* — Sepia.
† The same with Phosphor. Comp. Amm. mur., or Asa fœt., or Baryt. — Phosphor., &c.
‡ Comp. "Sleep" in † to Phosph. — Sulph.

Natr. mur.	Sepia.
Inclination for open air—Spasms with consciousness.	Aversion to open air—Spasms with unconsciousness.
Thirst during the fever and when there is no fever.	Want of thirst; thirst is only constant during chill.
First chill, then heat	First heat, then chill.

Natr. mur.	Sepia.
Fear of loss of reason	Fear of apoplexy.
Mood changing; *sad or* joyous — Malice—Amorousness.	Mood serious; sad and despondent—Avarice.
Ailments from mortification or vexation with reserved displeasure—Delirium.	Ailments in consequence of disappointed love or vexation with fear—Fancies—Insanity.
Complaints predominant on upper lip, in hollow of knee, and on front surface of thigh.	Complaints predominant on lower lip, in hollow of elbow, and on back part of thigh.
Often indicated with old people	Often indicated with women.
Eruptions generally humid	Eruptions generally dry.
Urinal sediment red — Urine too often, but scanty.	Urinal sediment *red or* white—Discharge of urine too seldom.
Leucorrhœa thick—Nasal secretion the same.	Leucorrhœa watery—Nasal secret'n the same.
Expectoration infrequent; morning	Expectoration predominant, but not constant; is loosened night and morning, and generally swallowed.

Natr. mur.	Sepia.
Worse during full moon	Worse during new moon.
Worse (better) when alone *or* in company	Better when alone; worse when in company.
Worse when looking at anything white	Worse when looking over a large surface.
Worse when taking a deep breath	Worse *or* better when taking a deep breath.
Better *or* worse from washing, etc.	Almost always aggrav. by wash'g & moisten'g.
Better or worse from growing cold	Almost always aggrav. when growing cold.
Worse (better) from cold *or* warm diet	Predominantly better from cold diet, worse from warm diet.
Worse after meals	*Worse or* better after meals.
Worse or better after drinking	Worse after drinking.
Better from eructation	Almost always aggravated by eructation.
Worse or better when turning in bed	Better when turning in bed.
Worse when awaking from sleep	Better after sufficient sleep, but worse on awaking when roused from sleep.
Generally worse when and after getting out of bed.	*Generally* better when and after getting out of bed.
Worse (better) when sitting erect *or* bent forward.	Better when sitting erect; worse when sitting bent forward.
Worse when rising from a seat	Worse *or* better when rising from a seat.
Worse *or* better after rising from a seat	Better after rising from a seat.
Worse or better when assum'g an erect posit'n.	Almost always improv. on assum. an erect pos.
Predom. worse when bending diseased part sideways.	Predominantly worse when bending the part backwards.
Predominantly worse when swallowing drink.	Worse when swallowing food.

Predomin. worse — **Predomin. better**

From warmth and from growing warm,* lying on side, partic. lying on painful side, when turning in bed, when and after getting out of bed, after breakfast, from motion, from moving diseased part, when walking, from bodily exertion, when rising (from stooping), when drawing up diseasec limb, and from loosening the clothes.

Predomin. better — **Predomin. worse**

From cold and when growing cold, when lying on back or when lying on unpainful side, during and after sweat, "before" breakfast, from eructation, during rest, after lying down, when lying, sitting and standing, when stretching out diseased limb, and from tying the clothes tight.

N.B. Natr. mur. lacks the over-sensitiveness of Sepia to pain, whereas the latter generally lacks the sensation of numbness in suffering parts peculiar to Natr. mur. Mere sensitiveness to touch, etc., on the other hand, is found with both remedies.

* Both remedies have predominant improvement in the open air, aggravation in-doors.

Natr. mur.	**Sulphur.**
Right side—Inclination for open air	*Left* side—Aversion to open air.
Ulcerative pain in external parts; pinching pain in internal parts.	Ulcerative pain in internal parts; pinching pain in external parts.
Compl. predom. on lower eyelids, on upper gums, in lower part of chest, and on front surface of thigh.	Compl. predom. on upper eyelids, on lower gums, in upper part of chest, and on back part of thigh.
Eruption predominantly humid	Eruption generally dry.
Pulse very irregular, sometimes trembling.	P. quick, full, hard; but sometimes imperc.
Heat on upper part of body	Heat on lower part of body, or general, with exception of head.
Heat, with aversion to uncover	Heat, with inclination to uncover.
Thirst during the fever and when there is none.	Thirst mostly during heat; generally want of thirst during chill.
Mood *sad or* joyous; malicious	Mood serious, solemn or enthusiastic; sad; despondent; gentle.
Ailments from vexation with reserved displeasure.	Ailm. from shame, hear'g bad news, or vexation with fright, less frequently fr. anger.
Imbecility	Insanity more frequent than imbecility.
Secretion of saliva increased	Saliva *generally* diminished.
Urine alkaline; sediment red	Urine sour; sediment white oftener than red.
Urine too often and generally increased	Urine often, but scanty; sometimes copious.
Catamenia of too long duration	Catam. *generally* of short duration.
Nasal secretion thick	Nasal secretion watery.
Expectoration infrequent; morning	Expector. not constant; morning and during day, less frequently at night.
Remission of complaints afternoon	Remission *afternoon* and before midnight.
Predom. worse in cold weather, better in warm air.	*Generally* better in cold weather, worse in warm nir.
Generally better in bed*	*Generally* worse in bed.
Worse when looking at anything white	Worse when looking down.
Worse from sneezing	*Worse or* better from sneezing.
Worse when taking a deep breath	Worse *or* better when taking a deep breath.
Worse (better) when sitting erect or bent forward.	Predom. better when sitting erect, worse when sitting bent forward.
Better when bending the body towards the painful side.	Worse when bending the body towards the painful side.
Predom. worse when swallowing drink	*Worse or* better when swallowing, partic. worse when swallowing food and saliva.
Better on an empty stomach; worse after breakfast.	Worse (better) before *or* after breakfast.
Better *or* worse from coffee	Worse from drinking coffee.
Worse (better) from cold *or* warm diet	Predom. worse fr. cold, bett. fr. warm diet.
Predom. worse after stool	Worse *or* better after stool.
Worse from moving diseased part	*Worse or* better from moving the part.

Predomin. worse — **Predomin. better**

In cold weather, from uncovering, from motion, when walking, when getting out of bed, from pressure and when drawing up diseased limb, from loosening the clothes.

Predomin. better — **Predomin. worse**

In warm air, from wrapping up, during rest, after lying down, when lying, sitting and standing, when stretching out diseased limb, in bed,* during and after sweat, (drinking cold water), and from tying the clothes tight.

---

* The symptoms of both remedies are aggrav. by *warmth* of bed.

Natr. mur.	Thuya.
Right side—Dark hair—Muscles rigid . .	*Left* side—Light hair—Muscles lax.
Often indicated with old people—Internal inflammations.	Often indicated with children—External inflammations predom.
Inclination oftener than aversion to open air.	Aversion to open air.
Spasms with full consciousness.	Spasms with unconsciousness.
Complaints predom. on upper gums and in lower part of chest.	Complaints predom. on lower gum and in upper part of chest.
Pulsating in external parts	Pulsating in internal parts.
Scars redden and hurt	In scars stinging and digging. C. Hg.
Pulse very irregular; sometimes more frequent at night than during the day.	Pulse slow and weak in the morning, accelerated and full in the evening.
Congestion of blood to ears	Congestion of blood to eyes.
Chill with thirst—First chill, then heat . .	Chill without thirst—First heat, then chill.
Heat with aversion to uncover	Heat with inclination to uncover.
Thirst during fever and when there is none.	Thirt is wanting during chill, predom. during heat, not constant during sweat
Sweat increased when and after getting out of bed.	Sweat abated when and after getting out of bed.
Awaking too late	Awaking too soon.
Talkativeness—Changing mood—Amativeness.	Reserve—Haughtiness—Rarely amorousness.
Weak reasoning powers	Mental excitability *or* weakness of reasoning powers—Rarely unconsciousness—Fancies.
Headache: like a nail driven in, on left side.	Headache: like a nail driven in, on right side. C. Hg.
Things appear too large	Things appear too small.
Saliva increased	Saliva generally diminished.
Catamenia too late, of long duration, at the same time scanty *or* profuse.	Catamenia too soon, at the same time too scanty and of short duration.
Cough generally dry; expectoration in morning.	Cough predom. loose; expectoration particularly in the evening.
REMISSION of complaints afternoon—AGGRAVATION partic. morning.	REMISSION forenoon and before midnight—AGGRAVATION partic. afternoon and after midnight.
Worse when bending diseased part . . .	Improv. oftener than aggrav. by bending diseased part.
Generally better out-doors	Aggrav. oftener than improv. out-doors.
Generally better during and after sweat .	*Worse* during sweat; *better afterwards.*
Predom. better from tying the clothes tight.	Better from loosening the clothes.
Predom. worse when swallowing drink . .	Worse when swallowing saliva.
Ailments from abuse of Cinchona	Ailments from Sulph., Mercur., or Iodine.
Worse when looking at distant things . .	Worse when looking at anything which is near.

Predomin. worse — **Predomin. better**

From motion, when walking, when drawing up diseased limb, from uncovering, from touch, pressure, after stool, and from loosening the clothes.

Predomin. better — **Predomin. worse**

During rest, when standing, sitting, lying, in bed, when stretching out diseased limb, from wrapping up, when perspiring, and from tying the clothes tight.

Nitr. acid.	Petroleum.
Left side—Ulcerative pain in internal parts.	*Right* side—Ulcerative pain in external parts.
Stitching pain going outwards—Very rarely paralysis.	Stitching pain going inwards—Paralysis of limbs.
Dryness of skin—Ulcers, with copious discharge.	Perspiring easily—Ulcers, with scanty discharge.
Dark hair—Eruptions humid	Light hair—Eruptions dry *or* humid.
Complaints predominant on inside of nose, on upper gum, and in the kidneys.	Complaints predominant on outside of nose, on lower gum, and in the bladder.
Pulse very irregular; dicrotous; intermitting.	Pulse slow during rest, but stronger, full, and accelerated when moving.
Pleasant dreams predominant	Anxious dreams predominant.
Peevishness — Distrust — Maliciousness—Ailments from emotions generally—Unconsciousness—Delirium.	Ailments from vexation with fright—No delirium.
Loss of appetite predominant	Hunger predominant.
Appetite for fatty things	Aversion to fatty things.
Diarrhœa predominantly painless	Diarrhœa painful.
Urine scanty	Urine often, but scanty.
Catamenia profuse and too soon	Catamenia scanty and generally too late.
Expectoration not constant; morning and during day.	Expectoration infrequent; during day.
REMISSION of complaints forenoon. . . .	AGGRAVATION morning and evening, till midnight.
Better (worse) from cold *or* warmth .	Worse from cold, better from warmth.
Worse in hot rooms	Better from warmth of stove.
Worse *or* better from spirituous liquors .	Worse from spirituous liquors.
Worse or better after drinking . . .	Worse after drinking.
Worse from touch	Worse *or* better from touch.
Worse when straining the sight	*Worse or* better from straining the sight.

Predomin. worse —— **Predomin. better**

In warm air, in a warm room,* after getting out of bed, after breakfast, and when assuming an erect position.

Predomin better —— **Predomin. worse**

In cold weather,† in bed, after sweat, on an empty stomach, when stooping, and when riding.

N.B. With Nitr. acid., whose predominant characteristic is want of irritability, we very rarely find the over-sensitiveness of Petroleum to pain.

* Both remedies have predominant improvement "in-doors" generally, aggravation out-doors.
† Both remedies have predominant aggravation "when growing cold," improvement when growing warm

Nitr. acid.	Pulsatilla.
Left side — Aversion to open air — Want of bodily irritability.	*Right* side — Inclination for open air — Increased irritability.
Pain pressing inwards—Very rarely apoplexy.	Pain pressing outwards—Apoplexy.
Painless swelling of glands — Often indicated with old people.	Painful swelling of glands — Often indicated with women and children.
Awaking too early	Awaking too late.
Pulse very irregular—Heat left side . . .	Pulse generally quick, small and weak; sometimes imperceptible—Heat right side.

Nitr. acid.	Pulsatilla.
Mood irritable; malicious	Mood changing; good-natured; calm sadness of mild dispositions; indifference; boldness; amorousness; avarice.
Ailments from emotions in general	Ailments from excessive joy, fright, grief, mortification, or vexation with fear.
Complaints predom. on inside of nose, on upper lip, upper jaw and upper teeth, on outside of gums, in upper part of chest, in the kidneys, and on fore-arm.	Complaints predom. on outside of nose, on lower lip, lower jaw and lower teeth, on inner side of gums, in lower part of chest, in the bladder, and on upper arm.
Optical illusions in dark colors	Optical illusions in bright colors.
Loss of appetite predom.	Generally hunger.
Appetite for fatty things	Predom. aversion to fatty things.
Nausea, partic. in stomach, less frequently in the throat.	Nausea in throat, stomach, or abdomen.
Diarrhœa predom. painless	Diarrhœa generally painful.
Urinal sediment white *or* reddish	Urinal sediment red.
Sexual desire preval. weak	Sexual desire too strong.
Catamenia too soon and profuse	Catamenia predom. too late and scanty.
Milk diminished	Milk generally increased.
Stoppage of nose oftener than fluent coryza .	Fluent coryza (partic. right side) oftener than stoppage of nose.
Respiration predom. with moist sound . . .	Respiration preval. with dry sound.
Expectoration not constant	Expectoration predom., but not constant.

Nitr. acid.	Pulsatilla.
Remission of complaints forenoon	Remission from midnight till noon.
Worse (better) from cold *or* warmth . . .	Better from cold; worse from warmth.
Worse on awaking from sleep	*Worse or* better after sleep.
Predom. worse when and after getting out of bed.	*Generally* better when and after getting out of bed.
Worse when rising from a seat	*Worse or* better when getting up from a seat.
Better *after* rising from a seat	*Better* or worse after rising from a seat.
Better when stooping; worse when rising . .	*Worse or* better when stooping & when rising.
Worse when bending diseased part	Worse *or* better when bending the part.
Worse from pressure	*Generally* better from pressure.
Worse from drinking fast	Worse from eating fast.
Worse *or* better from spirituous liquors . .	Worse from spirituous liquors.
Worse or better after drinking	Worse after drinking.
Worse after stool	*Better or* worse after stool.
Predom. worse when swallowing, partic. when swallowing food.	*Worse or* better when swallowing, part. worse when swallowing saliva.

Predomin. worse ——— **Predomin. better**

When growing cold* and from cold diet, after stool, from washing and moistening suffering part, when lifting diseased limb, from motion, when walking, out-doors and when walking out-doors, on inspiration, from bodily exertion, when lying on painful side, when and after getting out of bed, from pressure, and from weeping.

Predomin. better ——— **Predomin. worse**

When growing warm and from warm diet, after sweat, when letting diseased limb hang down, during rest, when lying, in bed and from warmth of bed, in-doors,† when lying on unpainful side, when stooping, from eructation, and from rubbing and scratching.

N.B. Nitr. acid. lacks the sensation of numbness in suffering parts, generally also the over-sensitiveness of Puls. to pain. Mere sensitiveness (to touch, &c.), however, is found with both remedies.

---

* Both remedies have predom. improv "*in cold weather*," aggrav. in warm air.

† Both remedies have aggrav. "*in hot rooms.*"

Nitr. acid.	Sepia.
Itching, relieved by scratching	Itching, aggrav. by scratching
Ulcerative pain in internal parts	Ulcerative pain in external parts.
Pain pressing inwards	Pain pressing outwards.
Rending pain upwards	Rending pain downwards.
Sensation of softness in hard parts	Sensation of hardness in soft parts.
Eruptions humid	Eruptions generally dry.
Erysipelas with smooth skin—Ulcers with watery pus.	Erysipelas generally vesicular—Ulcers with viscid pus.
Epilepsy with full consciousness	Epilepsy with unconsciousness.
Compl. predom. in the kidneys, in hollow of knee, and on patella	Compl. predom. in the bladder, in hollow of elbow, and on tip of elbow.
Pulse very irregular	Pulse quick & full at night, slow dur'g day; accelerated by vexation and motion.
Thirst only during heat, none during chill.	Want of thirst, also during the hot stage—Only during chill thirst is constant.

Nitr. acid.	Sepia.
Distrust — Maliciousness — Obstinacy — Rarely absent-mindedness—Very rarely fancies.	Seriousness — Indifference — Avarice — Weakness of will — Insanity — Imbecility—No delirium.
Ailments from emotions in general	Ailments in consequence of anger, fright, or vexation with heat.
Very rarely apoplexy	Paralysis.
Short-sightedness	Far-sightedness.
Yellow around the eyes	Yellow around nose and mouth.
Upper lip swollen or an eruption on it	Under lip swollen or an eruption on it.
Appetite for fatty things	Aversion to fatty things.
Urine cold *or* hot	Urine hot.
Sexual desire weak	Sexual desire changing.
Respiration prevalently with moist sound.	Respiration predom. with dry sound.
Expectoration not constant; morning and during day.	Expector predom., but not constant; is loosened partic. night and morning, and generally swallowed.

Nitr. acid.	Sepia.
REMISSION of complaints forenoon	REMISSION afternoon.
Ailments from Calcarea or Digitalis	Ailments from Sulph. or Cinchona.*

Predomin. worse — **Predomin. better**

In wet weather, when assuming an erect position, from active motion, when walking, partic. walking out-doors, from bodily exertion, and after breakfast.

Predomin. better — **Predomin. worse**

In dry weather, when stooping, during rest, after sweat,† from eructation, from *passive* motion (riding), when crossing the limbs, on an empty stomach, and from rubbing and scratching.

N.B. Nitr. acid. very rarely has the over-sensitiveness of Sepia to pain, although sensitiveness to touch is common to both remedies.

---

* Both remedies are of service against the consequences of abuse of Mercury.
† Both remedies generally have aggrav. while perspiring.

Nitr. acid.	Sulphur.
Pain pressing inwards—Rending pain upwards.	Pain pressing outwards — Rending pain downwards.
Humid cutaneous eruptions	Eruptions predom. dry—Paralysis.
Pulse very irregular	Pulse accelerated, full, and hard; but sometimes imperceptible.
Sweat on suffering part	Cold on suffering part.
Thirst is wanting during chill	Thirst predom., but not constant.
Awaking too soon	Awaking too late.
Mood distrustful; malicious	Mood changing; gentle; indifferent; serious—Imbecility—Insanity.
Ailments from emotions generally . . .	Ailments from shame, mortification, hearing bad news, or vexation with fright, dread or fear, less frequently after anger.
Compl. predom. on under eyelids and on upper gum.	Compl. predom. on lower eyelids and on lower gum.
Appetite for fatty food	Aversion to fatty food.
Urine smelling sour *or* ammoniacal . . .	Urine sour; often, but scanty; sometimes (after material doses) copious.
Catamenia too soon and profuse	Catam. *generally* too late and scanty.
REMISSION of complaints forenoon . . .	REMISSION afternoon and before midnight.
Ailments from (Mercurius) Calc., or Digitalis.	Ailments from Nitr. acid., Metals, Sepia, Iodine, Cinchona, or Rhus.
Predom. worse when growing cold; better when growing warm.	*Generally* better when growing cold; worse when growing warm.
Worse (better) from cold *or* warmth . .	Predom. better fr. cold, worse fr. warmth.*
Worse before a thunder-storm	Worse during full moon, before or during a thunder-storm.
Worse when turning in bed	*Worse or* better when turning in bed
Predom. worse after getting out of bed .	Better *or* worse after getting out of bed.
Better on an empty stomach; worse after breakfast.	Worse (better) on an empty stomach *or* after breakfast.
Worse or better after meals	Worse after meals.
Worse after stool	Worse *or* better after stool.
Worse when sneezing	*Worse or* better when sneezing.
Worse from weeping	*Worse or* better from weeping
Predom. better when stooping; worse when rising.	*Worse or* better when stooping and when rising.
Worse from touch	*Worse or* better from touch.

Predomin. worse ⁀ **Predomin. better**

When growing cold, out-doors, from motion, when walking, when getting out of bed, & from pressure.

Predomin. better ⁀ **Predomin. worse**

When growing warm, in-doors,† during rest, when lying, in bed and from warmth of bed, after perspiring, when stooping, and when riding.

* Both remedies generally have improv. of symptoms in *cold* weather, aggrav. in warm air.
† Both remedies have aggrav. in *hot*, crowded rooms; with Sulph. we also find improv. by warmth of stove.

Nitrum.	Sepia.
Hæmorrhages, blood light-red—Very rarely paralysis.	Hæmorrhages, blood dark—Paralysis.
Apoplexy not yet observed	Apoplexy.
Complaints predominant in spleen, kidneys, upper arm.	Complaints predominant in liver, bladder, fore-arm.
Itching, relieved by scratching	Itching, aggravated by scratching.
Pulse accelerated, full, and hard; slow in the morning, frequent in the afternoon and evening.	Pulse accelerated, partic. by vexation and motion; frequent and full at night, also intermitting; slow during the day.
First chill, then heat	First heat, then chill.
Sleeplessness preval. after midnight . . .	Sleeplessness preval. before midnight.

Nitrum.	Sepia.
No unconsciousness—Delirium	Absent-mindedness—Fancies—Mental dullness—Insanity.
Vomiting predominantly slimy	Vomiting chiefly food.
Urine predominantly pale; too often and copious.	Urine dark—Discharge of urine too seldom.
Catamenia too soon	Catamenia generally too late.
Respiratio abdominalis	Respiratio thoracica.
Expectoration quite seldom; morning and evening.	Expectoration predominant, but not constant; is loosened night and morning and generally swallowed.

Nitrum.	Sepia.
Remission forenoon and before midnight .	**Remission** of complaints afternoon.
Worse during full moon	Worse during new moon.
Worse while perspiring	*Worse or* better while perspiring.
Worse on awaking from sleep	Better after sufficient sleep; but worse on awaking when roused.
Better when getting out of bed	*Better or* worse when getting out of bed.
Worse *or* better when assuming an erect position.	Predominantly better when assuming an erect position.
Worse from bodily exertion	*Generally* better from exertion.
Predominantly worse on inspiration, better on expiration.	*Generally* better on inspiration, worse on expiration.
Better *or* worse from pressure	Almost always aggravated by pressure.
Worse after meals	*Worse or* better after meals.
Worse when swallowing drink	Worse when swallowing food.

Predomin. worse — **Predomin. better**

In wet weather, when lying on painful side, when sitting erect, from bodily exertion, on inspiration, from cold diet, after breakfast, and after sleep.

Predomin. better — **Predomin. worse**

In dry weather, when lying on unpainful side, when sitting bent forward, after sweat, on expiration, from warm diet, on an empty stomach, and from rubbing and scratching.

N.B. Nitrum lacks the over-sensitiveness of Sepia to pain.

Nitrum.	Belladonna.
Upper right, lower left side—Very rarely paralysis.	Upper left, lower right side—Apoplexy.
Internal trembling; trembling sensation.	Trembling of external parts.
Complaints predominant in upper jaw and upper teeth, on soft palate and in the spleen.	Complaints predominant in lower jaw and lower teeth, on roof of mouth and in the liver.
Sleeplessness after midnight	Sleeplessness before midnight.
Thirst only during chill	Thirst not constant; most rare during chill; often *before* and *after* the attack of fever.
Chill lessened in bed	Chill increased in bed.

Sensitive disposition	Generally insensibility of disposition.
Complaints in abdomen worse when holding the breath.	Complaints in abdomen better when holding the breath.
Urine copious; pale	Urine generally scanty; dark oftener than pale.
Cough particularly in the morning . . .	Cough particularly in the evening and at night.
Expectoration in the morning and evening.	Expectoration from morning till evening.

REMISSION forenoon and before midnight .	REMISSION forenoon and after midnight.
Worse during wet cold weather	*Worse* during dry cold weather.
Better when and after getting out of bed.	*Worse* when getting out of bed, *better afterwards.*

Predomin. worse — **Predomin. better**

In wet weather, from cold* diet, when letting diseased limb hang down, during rest, when standing, lying, in bed, when sitting, partic. sitting bent forward, and when stooping.

Predomin. better — **Predomin. worse**

In dry weather, from warm diet, when lifting diseased limb, when moving, when sitting erect, and when getting out of bed.

N.B. Nitrum lacks the over-sensitiveness of Belladonna to pain.

*** Belladonna has also aggravation from "drinking cold water," because one of its symptoms (more prominently than with Nitrum) is: "Swallowing of drink is troublesome."**

Nitrum.	Phosphor.
Cramping pain in external parts . . .	Cramping pain in internal parts.
No apoplexy—Very rarely paralysis . .	Apoplexy—*Paralysis*.
Itching, relieved by scratching . .	Itching, *relieved or* aggrav. by scratching.
Pulse full, hard, and accelerated	Pulse various; irregular, intermitting.
Thirst predom. only during chill . . .	Want of thirst during all stages.
Chill lessened in bed	Chill increased in bed.
Sleeplessness after midnight; awaking too early.	Sleeplessness before midnight; awaking too late.

Complaints predom. in upper jaw, upper teeth, and in spleen.	Compl. predom. in lower jaw, lower teeth, and in liver.
Urine too often and copious	Urine often, but scanty.
Catamenia too profuse	Catam. too profuse *or* too scanty.
Nasal secretion watery	Nasal secretion thick or viscid, often yellow, like ochre.
Expectoration quite infrequent; morning and evening.	Expector. not constant; morning and during day.

REMISSION *forenoon* and before midnight .	REMISSION of complaints after midnight.
Worse during full moon	Worse before a thunder-storm or during a storm.
Worse when perspiring	*Worse or* better when perspiring.
Worse (better) when lying on painful *or* on unpainful side.	Predom. worse when lying on painful, better when lying on unpainful side.
Worse during sleep	Worse *or* better during sleep.
Worse when awaking from sleep	Better after sufficient sleep, but worse on awaking, when roused & after the siesta.
Predom. better after getting out of bed .	Worse *or* better after getting out of bed.
Worse when stooping	Better *or* worse when stooping.
Worse *or* better when assuming an erect position.	Almost always aggrav. when assuming an erect position.
Worse from touch	Almost always improv. by the touch.
Worse during and after meals	*Worse or* better during and after meals.
Worse after drinking	Almost always improv. after drinking.

Predomin. worse — **Predomin. better**

Out-doors, during rest, when standing, lying* and sitting, partic. sitting erect, from cold diet, after drinking, from the touch, and after sleep.

Predomin. better — **Predomin. worse**

In-doors,† from motion, when walking, when sitting bent forward, from warm diet, from change of posture, (when lying or standing), when getting out of bed, after perspiring, and when riding.

N.B. Nitrum lacks the over-sensitiveness of Phosphor. to pain, & generally also the sensation of numbness in suffering parts peculiar to Phosphor.

---

* The symptoms of both remedies are predom. aggrav. "*in bed.*"
† Both remedies have predom. aggrav. "*in hot room.*"

Nitrum.	Rhus.
Upper right, lower left side	Upper left, lower right side.
Tension or cutting pain in internal parts	Tension or cutting pain in **external parts.**
No apoplexy—Very rarely paralysis	Apoplexy—Paralysis.

Nitrum.	Rhus.
Compl. predom. on inside of nose, on upper jaw and upper teeth, and on upper arm.	Compl. predom. on outside of nose, on lower jaw, lower teeth, and on fore-arm.
Sleeplessness after midnight; awaking too early.	Sleeplessness predomin. before midnight; awaking too late.
Thirst only during chill	Thirst not constant.
Pulse sometimes slower than beating of heart; generally full, hard, & accelerated.	Pulse sometimes quicker than beating of heart; irregular; generally frequent, but faint and soft.
Nasal secretion watery	Nasal secretion thick.
Respiratio abdominalis	Respiratio thoracica.
Expectoration quite infreqent; morning & evening.	Expectoration not constant; oftener in the morning than in the evening.

Nitrum.	Rhus.
Remission forenoon and before midnight	Remission of compl. during day.
Worse during full moon	Worse during increase of moon.
Predominantly worse in bed	Generally better in bed.
Worse (better) when lying on painful *or* on unpainful side.	Predom. better when lying on painful side, worse when lying on unpainful side.
Better when getting out of bed	Worse *or* better when getting out of bed.
Predom. better after getting out of bed	*Worse or* better after getting out of bed.
Better when sitting down	*Worse or* better when sitting down.
Worse when rising from a seat	*Worse or* better when rising from a seat.
Better after rising from a seat	Worse *or* better after rising from a seat.
Worse when stooping	*Worse or* better when stooping.
Worse *or* better when assuming an erect position.	Almost always aggrav. when assuming an erect position.
Worse *or* better from pressure	Predom. better from pressure.
Worse after eating and drinking	*Worse or* better after eating and drinking.
Worse after stool	*Better or* worse after stool.
Worse when swallowing drink	Worse when swallowing food and when swallowing saliva.

Predomin. worse —— **Predomin. better**

From warmth of stove, in bed, when stretching out diseased limb or letting it hang down, when sitting erect, after breakfast, and after stool.

Predomin. better —— **Predomin. worse**

From change of position, after getting out of bed, when drawing up or lifting diseased limb, when sitting bent forward, before breakfast, and when riding.

N.B We very rarely find the sensation of numbness in suffering parts peculiar to Rhus with Nitrum.

Nitr. acid.	Thuya.
Dark hair—Muscles rigid	Light hair – Muscles lax.
Pain pressing inwards — Sore pain internally.	Pain pressing outwards—Sore pain in external parts.
In scars pain when the weather changes; break open.	In scars stinging and digging. C.Hg.
Spasms with full consciousness	Spasms with unconsciousness.
Pulse more irregular than with Thuya . .	Pulse slow and weak in the morning, accelerated and full at night.
Congestion of blood to ears	Congestion of blood to eyes.
Sweat on parts covered or lain on . . .	Sweat on parts uncovered, with dry heat of parts covered—Sweat general, with exception of parts lain on.
Complaints predominant on inside of nose, on upper gum, and on the hip-joint.	Complaints predominant on outside of nose, on lower gum, and on shoulder-joint.

Distrust	Seriousness—Haughtiness—Very rarely delirium.
Very rarely absent-mindedness	Very rarely unconsciousness — Insanity — Imbecility.
Urine scanty; cold *or* hot; sediment red or white.	Urine copious and often; hot; urinal sediment reddish.
Sexual desire decreased	Sexual desire increased.
Catamenia profuse	Catamenia scanty.
Respiration prevalently with moist sound .	Respiration with dry sound.
Expectoration not constant; morning and during day.	Expectoration constant; particularly in the evening.

REMISSION of complaints forenoon . . .	REMISSION forenoon and before midnight.
Rest in general improves; but yet worse after lying down.*	Rest in general aggravates; but yet better after lying down.
Better while riding, *worse after* riding .	*Worse* when riding.
Worse when swallowing food	Worse when swallowing saliva.
Throbbing in veins, better from drinking wine.†	Complaints from spirituous liquors.
Ailments from Mercur., Calc., or Digitalis .	Ailments from Mercur., Sulph., or Iod.

Predomin. worse — **Predomin. better**

From touch, from pressure, from washing, when bending diseased part backwards, when walking, from motion in general, but also after lying down and after stool.

Predomin. better — **Predomin. worse**

During rest, from warmth of bed, when stooping, and when riding.

---

* It is the change from an upright posture alone which causes this aggrav. with Nitr. acid., and improv. with Thuya.
† The inflammation of kidneys common to Nitr. acid., on the contrary, is aggravated by spirituous liquors.

Nitrum.	Sulphur.
Right side, particularly *upper right, lower left side.*	*Left* side, particularly *upper left, lower right side.*
Ulcerative pain in external parts	Ulcerative pain in internal parts.
Hæmorrhages, blood bright-red — Very rarely paralysis.	Hæmorrhages, blood dark—Paralysis.
Pulse slow in the morning, frequent in afternoon and evening.	Pulse frequent in the night and morning, slower during day and evening.
Chill lessened in bed	Chill increased in bed.
Sweat predominant on front part of body.	Sweat predominant on back part of body.
Thirst only during chill	Thirst mostly during heat; generally want of thirst during chill.
Sleeplessness after midnight; awaking too early.	Sleeplessness before midnight; awaking too late.

Hot spots on the head	A cold spot on the head.
Urine too often and copious	Urine often, but scanty; sometimes (after strong doses) copious.
Catamenia too soon, profuse, and of long duration.	Catamenia *generally* too late, scanty and of short duration.
Expectoration quite infrequent	Expectoration not constant.
Complaints predominant on upper arm . .	Complaints predominant on fore-arm.

Remission forenoon and before midnight .	Remission *afternoon* and before midnight.
Better after perspiring	*Worse or* better after perspiring.
Worse when lying on painful side, better when lying on unpainful side.	Better (worse) when lying on painful *or* on unpainful side.
Better when lying with the head high . .	Better when lying with head *high or* in a horizontal position.
Better from change of posture, (when lying or standing).	Better *or* worse from change of posture.
Predom. better after getting out of bed .	Better *or* worse after getting out of bed.
Better on an empty stomach; worse after breakfast.	Worse (better) on an empty stomach *or* after breakfast.
Worse when swallowing drink	*Worse or* better when swallowing, partic. worse when swallowing food and saliva.
Worse after drinking	*Worse or* better after drinking.
Worse after stool	Worse *or* better after stool.
Worse when taking a deep breath . . .	Worse *or* better when taking a deep breath.
Worse when stooping	Worse *or* better when stooping.
Worse from touch	*Worse or* better from touch.
Worse *or* better from pressure . . .	Predominantly better from pressure.

Predomin. worse ⁓ **Predomin. better**

From cold, out-doors, when lying on back, when sitting erect, when letting diseased limb hang down, and when holding the breath.

Predomin. better ⁓ **Predomin. worse**

From warmth, in-doors* when lying on side, when sitting bent forward, when lifting diseased limb, when riding, and after sweat.

N.B. Nitrum "very" rarely has the sensation of numbness in suffering parts peculiar to Sulphur.

*** Both remedies have aggravation "in a hot room;" Sulphur. has improvement from warmth of stove.**

Nux moschata.	Nux vomica.
Upper left, lower right side—Want of bodily irritability.	Upper right, lower left side — Increased irritability.
With the pains (headache, toothache, etc.), drowsiness.	With the pains, hot feeling; sometimes sweat, anxiousness, great weakness. C. Hg.
Dropsy of external parts; trembling in internal parts.	Dropsy of internal parts; trembling of external parts.
Dryness of skin—Very rarely paralysis	Dryness of skin *or* perspiring easily — Paralysis.
Predom. somnolence—Sleep after sweat .	Sleeplessness—Sleep between chill & heat.
Pulse somewhat accelerated as from ebullition of blood; sometimes trembling.	Pulse generally quick, full, & hard; sometimes intermitting or imperceptible.
Want of thirst during all stages of the fever.	Thirst, mostly dur'g chill; oft. *before* & *after* the attack of fever & betw. heat & sweat.
Mood cheerful; serious—Melancholy . .	Mood depressed; irritated; passionate; malicious; anxious — Ailments in consequence of fits of rage, partic. in the morn'g.
Over-estimating time and distance . . .	Often makes mistakes in speaking or in writing—Fancies.
Difficult comprehension	Rarely mental dullness.
Sensitiveness of the scalp in wet weather, to the touch, and when lain on; improv. by warmth.	Sensitiveness of scalp, partic. to the wind, cold, and touch, after lying down; better from warmth and external pressure.
Desire for drink without thirst	Thirst with aversion to drink.
Hunger predominant	Generally loss of appetite.
Diarrhœa predominant, painless	Constipation; when diarrhœa occurs, it is painful.
Urine dark	Urine generally light-colored.
Respiration predominantly slow; rattling.	Respiration generally quick; audible, without rattling of mucus.
Expector. quite constant; morning . . .	Expector. not constant; morning, during day or evening.
REMISSION morning and afternoon . . .	REMISSION evening till midnight.
Worse (better) when growing cold or warm.	Worse when growing cold; better when growing warm.*
Worse when lying on painful side, better when lying on unpainful side.	Worse (better) when lying on painful side *or* when lying on unpainful side.
Worse after sleep	Better after sufficient & not too long sleep; but worse on awaking when roused.
Predom. better after getting out of bed .	Worse *or* better after getting out of bed.
Better on an empty stomach; worse after breakfast.	Worse (better) when fasting *or* after breakfast.
Worse when eating	*Generally* better when eating.
Worse when stooping; better when rising.	*Better or* worse when stooping; almost always aggrav. when rising.
Generally worse from warmth of bed . .	Predom. better from warmth of bed.

Predomin. worse ——— **Predomin. better**

In wet weather, from washing and moistening diseased part, when sitting erect, but also when stooping, on inspiration,† when eating, from warmth of bed, and after sleep.

Predomin. better ——— **Predomin. worse**

In dry weather, when sitting bent forward, but also when rising from stooping, and on expiration.

* Both remedies have aggrav. from cold and in cold weather, predom. improv. from warmth and in warm air.
† Both remedies have aggrav. of compl. when taking a *deep breath*.

Nux moschata.	Pulsatilla.
Want of bodily irritability	Increased irritability.
With the pains (headache, toothache, etc.), drowsiness.	With the pains chilliness; sometimes heat or sweat, disposition to weep, weakness. C.Hg.
Aversion to open air	Inclination for open air.
Pulse somewhat accelerated; sometimes trembling.	Pulse predom. frequent, small, and weak, sometimes intermitting or imperceptible.
Chill increased out-doors, lessened in warm room.	Chill lessened out-doors, increased in warm room.
Want of thirst dur'g all stages of the fever.	Want of thirst predom., but constant only during chill.
Cheerfulness more frequent than melancholy.	Calm sadness of mild dispositions—Mood indifferent; peevish — Boldness — Avarice—Distrust.
Over-estimating time and distance . . .	Omitting letters when writing.
Rarely delirium—Imbecility	Fancies—Melancholy—Rarely mental dullness.
Saliva generally decreased	Saliva generally increased.
Catamenia too soon and profuse	Catamenia too late and generally scanty.
Stoppage of nose	Fluent coryza (partic. right side) more frequent than stoppage of nose.
Respiration predom. slow; rattling . . .	Respiration quick; preval. dry — Audible respiration.
Expectoration quite constant; morning .	Expector. predom., but not constant; morning and during day.
AGGRAVATION forenoon, evening, and night.	AGGRAVATION from noon till midnight.
Worse (better) when growing cold *or* warm.	Better when growing cold; worse when growing warm.
Worse after sleep	*Worse or* better after sleep.
Worse after meals	*Worse or* better after meals.
Worse after stool	*Better or* worse after stool.
Worse when stooping; better when rising.	*Worse or* better when stooping and when rising.
Worse when taking a deep breath . . .	Better *or* worse when taking a deep breath.
Worse or better from warmth of bed . .	Worse from warmth of bed.

Predomin. worse — **Predomin. better**

From cold and in cold weather, from uncovering, from washing and moistening diseased part, out-doors and when walking out-doors, from motion, when walking, from bodily exertion, on inspiration, when sitting erect, when lying on painful side, from drinking cold water and from cold diet generally, and after stool.

Predomin. better — **Predomin. worse**

From warmth and in warm air, from wrapping up, in-doors and from warmth of stove, during rest, when sitting, lying, in bed, on expiration, when lying on unpainful side, from warm diet, and when rising from stooping.

Nux moschata. — Rhus.

Nux moschata.	Rhus.
I. ⟶ R.	**R. ⟶ L.** C.Hg.
Compl. (cutting pain, etc.) predom. in internal parts.	Compl. (cutting pain, etc.) predom. in external parts.
With the pains (headache, toothache, etc.), drowsiness.	With the pains chilliness or feverish heat, anxiety, sadness, dejection. C.Hg.
Rarely paralysis	Paralysis of limbs.
Somnolence predominant	Sleeplessness.
Pulse somewhat accelerated, as from ebullition of blood.	Pulse irregular; generally frequent, faint, & soft; intermitting or imperceptible.
Want of thirst constant—Desire for drink without thirst.	Thirst not constant; thirst with aversion to drink.
Mood changing; *joyous or* melancholy .	Fear; sadness
Rarely delirium—Fancies	Rarely mental dullness.
Sensitiveness of the scalp in wet weather, to the touch, and when lain on; better from warmth.	Sensitiveness of scalp, partic. in the side not lain on & when growing warm in bed, to the touch, & when strok'g back the hair.
Sensation of a loose tooth as if pushed out fr. the shaking in going up or down stairs.	Sensation as if the teeth were drawn in. C.Hg.
Saliva generally decreased	Saliva generally increased.
Hunger predominant	Loss of appetite predom.
Painless diarrhœa	Diarrhœa generally painful.
Urine dark; scanty	Urine pale; too often and copious.
Impotency and sterility	Erections.
Menstrual blood generally dark . . .	Menstrual blood light-colored.
Stoppage of nose	Fluent coryza.
Respiration predominantly slow; rattling.	Respiration quick; with dry sound.
Expectoration quite constant	Expectoration infrequent.
Remission morning and afternoon . . .	Remission of complaints during day.
Worse or better from warmth of bed . .	*Better or* worse from warmth of bed.
Predom. better after getting out of bed .	*Worse or* better after getting out of bed.
Worse when stooping; better when rising.	Almost always aggrav. when stooping and when rising.
Worse *or* better from pressure	Predom. better from pressure.
Worse after meals.	*Worse or* better after meals.
Worse after stool	*Better or* worse after stool.
Worse (better) when growing warm or cold.	Better when growing warm, worse when growing cold.

Predomin. worse ⟵⟶ **Predomin. better**

From motion, when walking, walking out-doors,* when sitting erect, when lying on painful side, after breakfast, and after stool.

Predomin. better ⟵⟶ **Predomin. worse**

During rest, when sitting and lying, when sitting bent forward, when lying on unpainful side, after getting out of bed, on an empty stomach, and when rising from stooping.

N.B. Rhus lacks the over-sensitiveness of Nux moschata to pain, although sensitiveness to the touch is common to both remedies.

* Here the influence of motion decides for Rhus and not that of the open air; for out-doors in general both remedies have aggrav.

Nux vom.	Phosphor.
Hæmorrhages, blood dark — Scars aching .	Hæmorrh., blood light — Scars bleed. C.Hg.
Heat or sweat, with aversion to uncover* . .	Heat or sweat, with inclination to uncover.
Heat l. s.—Sweat on upp. or back part of body.	Heat r. s. — Sweat on lower or front part of [body.
Thirst predom.; mostly during cold stage . ,	Want of thirst.
Chill and heat lessened when sitting . . .	Chill and heat increased when sitting.
Sweat increased when eating	Sweat lessened when eating.
Sleeplessness preval. after midnight	Sleeplessness before midnight.

Nux vom.	Phosphor.
Loquacity—Sensitiveness	Taciturnity—Sensitiv. *or* insensibil. of dispos.
Mood depressed; irascible; malicious . . .	Mood changing; *cheerful or* depressed.*
Solicitude concerning the present	Solicitude concerning the future. C.Hg.
Difficult comprehension — Mental dullness — Absent-mindedness.	*Easy or* difficult comprehension — Mental excitability and active memory predom.
Pupils generally dilated—Far-sightedness . .	Pup. generally contracted—Short-sightedness.
Clear-sightedn.—Optic. illus. in bright colors.	Dim-sightedness—Opt. illus. in dark or prism. [colors.
Complaints predom. in inner ear	Compl. generally on external ear.
Gums and palate red	Gums and palate generally pale.
Costiveness predom.; diarrhœa painful . . .	Diarrhœa predom. painless.
Predom. aversion to sour things — Desire for, or aversion to beer.	Appetite for sour things—Aversion to beer.
Fetid flatus	Flatus scentless; passing easily; hot; loud.
Urine rare and scanty	Urine often, but scanty.
Catamenia too profuse and of long duration .	Cat. the same, *or* scanty and of short duration.
Nasal secretion watery	Nasal secret. thick or viscid, sometimes yellow
Complaints predom. on calf of leg	Complaints predom. on shin. [like ochre.

Nux vom.	Phosphor.
Remission evening till midnight	Remission of complaints after midnight.
Ailments from Arsenic., Plumb., Cuprum . .	Ailments from Iodine or Natr. mur.
Better from cold applications	Better from warm applications.
Generally better from pressure	*Generally* worse from pressure.
Generally worse when drawing up diseased limb, better when stretching it out.	Better when drawing up diseased limb; worse when stretching it out.
Predom. better in bed and from warmth of bed.	*Worse or* better in bed and fr. warmth of bed.
Worse (better) when lying on painful, *or* on unpainful side.	Worse when lying on painful side; better when lying on unpainful side.
Worse during sleep	Worse *or* better during sleep.
Worse after sleeping a *long* time	Worse after the *siesta.*
Better (worse) while fasting *or* after breakfast.	Pred. better while fasting, worse aft. breakfast.
Predom. better when eating	*Generally* worse when eating.
Almost always aggrav. *after* meals	*Worse or* better after meals.
Worse from drinking coffee	*Worse or* better from coffee.
Generally worse after drinking	Predom. better after drinking.
Generally better from eructation	Generally worse from eructation.
Better (worse) wh. opening or closing mouth.	Worse when opening, bett. wh. closing mouth.
Pred. worse opening, better closing the eyes .	Better (worse) wh. opening *or* closing the eyes.
Worse from shaking the head	*Worse or* better from shaking the head.
Worse or better from sneezing	Worse from sneezing.
Worse when swallowing food and saliva . .	Worse when swallowing food and part. drink.

Predomin. worse —————— **Predomin. better**

In dry weather, out-doors, from uncovering, from touch, when moving diseased part, when drawing up suffering limb, when lying on right side, from drinking cold water, from cold diet in general, from beer and spirituous liquors, after a satisfying meal, and after drinking.

Predomin. better —————— **Predomin. worse**

In wet weather, in-doors and from warmth of stove, from wrapping up, from pressure, from washing and moistening diseased part, when stretching out the suffering limb, when lying on left side, when eating, partic. from warm diet; from eructation, after perspiring, in bed and from warmth of bed, and when swallowing drink.

---

* Pulse with Nux vom. more equal than with Phosphorus.

† Ailments from indignation, mortification, disappointed love, or jealousy, have been relieved by Nux vom.; ailments in consequence of rage, irritable vehemence, or fright, have been relieved by Phosphor. as well as Nux vom.

Nux vom.	Pulsatilla.
pper right, lower left side—Aversion to open air.	Upper left, lower right side—Inclination for open air.
Dropsy, or cold sensation in internal parts .	Dropsy, or cold sensation in external parts.
Secretions of mucous membranes and ulcers generally decreased or suppressed.*	Secretions of mucous membranes and ulcers generally increased.
Plethora abdominalis, with congestion to the head.	Complaints from suppression of catamenia and other discharges, generally after wet feet.
Fixed, acute rheumatism	Shifting rheumatism in the joints.
Tonic spasms—Tetanic affections of single muscles.	Rheumatic stiffness of limbs—Hardness of the neuralgic portion of muscles.
Paralysis generally of both sides	Paral. generally one-sided; of rare occurence.
Compl. predom. on fore-arm and palm of hand.	Compl. pred. on upper arm, & on back of hand.
Pulse generally quick, full, and hard, partic. during hot stage; frequent in the morning, slow in the evening.	Pulse generally frequent, small, and weak; frequent in the evening, slow in the morning.
Heat left side—Sweat on diseased side . . .	One-sided heat, right side—Heat on diseased part.
Thirst during chill, before and after sweat† .	Want of thirst during chill.†
Sleeplessness after midnight	Sleeplessness before midnight.
Sanguine choleric temperament—Malicious.	Sanguine temperament—Good-naturedness.
Loquacity—Peevishness and irascibility . .	Taciturnity—Lachrymose *sadness* of mild dispositions—Changing mood—Indifference—Boldness—Avarice—Distrust.
Ailm. in consequence of contradiction, anger, indignation, disappointed love, or jealousy.	Ailments in consequence of excessive joy.
Vertigo, inclin. to fall sideways or backwards.	Vertigo, inclining to fall backwards.
Far-sightedness—Pupils predom. dilated . .	Short-sightedness—Pupils gener. contracted.
Generally things look too light	Dim-sightedness.
Food has a sour after-taste—No appetite . .	Food has a bitter after-taste—Hunger.
Desire for beer or aversion to it	Desire for beer.
Predom. aversion to sour things	Appetite for sour things.
A liking for fatty food, which disagrees . .	Aversion to fatty food (also disagreeing).
Nausea in stomach, less frequently in swallow.	Nausea in throat, stomach or abdomen.
Vomiting, first water, then food	Vomiting, food first, then water.
Constipation predom.—Strong urinal stream .	Diarrhœa predom. — Small urinal stream.
With Horses: Excrements in small balls . .	With Horses: Excrements in large balls.
Catam. too soon, profuse, and of long duration.	Cat. gener. too late, scanty & of short durat'n.
Painless stagnation of milk, from not sucking the child.	While nursing, the breasts swell and ache as if the milk rushed in. C.Hg.
Generally *stoppage* of nose, partic. out-doors; fluent in-doors.	Fluent coryza (partic. r. s.) oftener than stoppage; fluent out-doors, stopped in-doors.
Cough generally dry—Expectoration morning, during day, or evening.	Cough generally loose — Expectoration morning and during day.‡
Aggravation of symptoms after midnight, in the morning after sunrise, and during day.	Aggravation afternoon and evening, after sunset until midnight.
Ailments in consequence of dry cold, partic. from taking cold in the head, or from sitting on cold stones.	Ailm. in consequ. of taking cold in the head or feet during wet (cold or warm) weather
Worse during sweat, *better after* it	*Worse during* and after the sweat.
Better while eating; worse *afterwards*. . .	Better when drinking; worse afterwards.

Predomin. worse —— **Predomin. better**

Out-doors, from cold, uncovering, motion, bodily exertion, when opening the eyes, change of posture, tying the clothes tight, from drinking cold water, from cold diet generally, and from sour things (vinegar).

Predomin. better —— **Predomin. worse**

In-doors, from warmth, wrapping up, during rest, when standing, sitting and lying, when closing the eyes, after sleep, when bending diseased part backwards, from warm diet, and after perspiring.

* When the secretion of mucus is increased with Nux vom., it is watery and not critical.
† Comp. Capsicum—Nux vomica and Anacard.—Pulsatilla.
‡ Expectoration with Pulsat. sometimes putrid, sweet, sour, oftener salty, greasy, or tasting like old catarrh.

Nux vom.	Rhus.
Upper right, lower left side—Dark hair . .	Upper left, lower right side—Light hair.
Hæmorrhages, blood dark—Aversion to motion.	Hæmorrhages, blood bright-red—Inclination for motion.
Complaints of internal parts (pressure, cutting pain, etc.) predom.	Complaints of external parts predominant.
Painful ulcers—Sweat on right side . . .	Painless ulcers—Sweat on left side.
Sweat often confined to back part of body—Coldness on lower part of body.	Sweat often confined to front part of body—Chill on upper part of body.
Pulse predom. full and hard—Sleep between chill and heat.	Pulse predom. weak and soft—Sleep after sweat.
Chill or heat lessened when sitting	Chill or heat increased when sitting.
Heat increased by motion, lessened in-doors .	Heat lessened by motion, increased in-doors.
Sweat lessened during sleep	Sweat increased during sleep.
Thirst mostly during chill	Thirst not constant.
Bruised pain in side lain on, *or* in that not lain on.	Bruised pain in side not lain on.
Sleeplessness prevalent after midnight . . .	Sleeplessness preval. before midnight.
When intoxicated by wine: Sleep with drooping chin.	When intoxicated by beer: Sleep with head bent backwards and open mouth.

Nux vom.	Rhus.
Mood irritable, irascible, flying into a passion.	Mood sad, dejected.
Absent-mindedness	Rarely peevishness—Very rarely amorousness.
Vertigo, inclin'g to fall sideways or backwards.	Vertigo, inclin'g to fall forward or backwards.
Stupefying headache, in the morning, in the sun, when walking out-doors; better in-doors and in bed.	Stupefying headache with buzzing; in the morning, when sitting or lying; worse in the cold; better from motion and external warmth.
Sensitiveness of scalp, partic. to the wind, cold, touch; worse after lying down; *better* from pressure and warmth.	Sensitiveness (and swelling) of the scalp, partic. in side not lain on; when grow'g warm in bed, to the touch, and when strok'g back the hair.
Generally things look too light	Dim-sightedness.
Desire for wine, etc	Aversion to wine.
Desire for beer *or* aversion to it	Desire for beer.
Inguinal hernia, partic. large, of long standing.	Inguinal hernia, partic. small, of recent origin.
Constipation predominant	Diarrhœa predominant.
Urine seldom & scanty—Urinal stream strong.	U. often & copious—Urin'l stream spreads out.
Urinal sediment reddish	Urinal sediment white.
Generally stoppage of nose, partic. out-doors, while in-doors the coryza is fluent.	Fluent coryza.
Nasal secretion watery	Nasal secretion thick.
Expectoration from morning till evening . .	Expectoration in the morning.
Ailments in consequence of taking cold in dry weather.	Ailments in consequence of being wet through when the body was overheated.
Ailments in consequence of mental exertion .	Ailments in consequence of bodily exertion.

C. Hg.

Nux vom.	Rhus.
Remission evening till midnight	Remission of complaints during day.
Worse after sunrise	Some symptoms worse after sunset.
Generally better on an empty stomach, worse after breakfast.	Predominantly worse on an empty stomach, better after breakfast.

Predomin. worse —— **Predomin. better**

When moving, after stool, and in dry weather.

Predomin. better —— **Predomin. worse**

During rest, when standing, sitting and lying, in wet weather, from washing, and from wet applications.

N.B. With Nux vom. we rarely find the sensation of numbness in suffering parts peculiar to Rhus. On the other hand, Rhus lacks the over-sensitiveness of Nux vom. to pain. Sensitiveness to touch, however, is found with both remedies.

Nux vom.	Sulphur.
Right side, partic. *upper right, lower left side.*	*Left* side, partic. *upper left, lower right side.*
Increased irritability—Pinching internal . .	Want of bodily irritability—Pinch'g external.
Painful eruptions and ulcers	Painless eruptions and ulcers.
Sleeplessness predom. after midnight . . .	Sleeplessness before midnight.
Apoplexy	Very rarely apoplexy.
Sweat on suffering side	Coldness on suffering part.
Chill or sweat on right side	Chill or sweat predom. left side.
Sweat lessened while sleeping	Sweat increased while sleeping.
Coldness on lower part of body	Heat on lower part of body, or general, with exception of head.
Heat or sweat, with aversion to uncover . .	Heat or sweat, with inclination to uncover.
Thirst mostly during chill	Thirst wanted during chill; mostly dur. heat.

Maliciousness	Mood chang'g; solemn; sentimental; gentle.*
Ailments from indignation, grief, disappointed love, or jealousy.	Ailments from shame, or hearing bad news, less frequently from fright or anger.
Pupils gener. dilated—Clear-sightedness pred.	Pupils gener. contracted—Dim-sightedness.
Optic. illus. in bright colors—Far-sightedness.	Opt. ill. in dark colors—Short-sightedn. pred.
With the toothache, sweat	With the toothache, chill. C.Hg.
Saliva generally increased	Saliva generally diminished.
Desire for fatty things	Aversion to fatty things.
Urine too seldom and scanty — Sediment reddish.	Urine often, but scanty; sediment white oftener than red.
Catamenia too soon, profuse and of long duration.	Catamenia *generally* too late, scanty and of short duration.
Expectoration morning, during day, evening .	Expector. morning, during day; less at night.

Remission evening till midnight	Remission afternoon and before midnight.
Worse in the open air, better in-doors . . .	Predom. better in open air, worse in-doors.†
Worse when growing cold and in cold weather, better when growing warm and in warm air.	Better (worse) when growing cold and in cold air, or when growing warm and in warm air.
Better in bed	*Worse or* better in bed.
Generally worse lying on back, better on side,	*Generally* better lying on back, worse on side.
Worse (better) when lying on painful *or* on unpainful side.	Worse when lying on painful side, better when lying on unpainful side.
Worse in horizontal posture, better with head high.	Worse (better) in horizontal position, *or* with the head high.
Better after sufficient sleep. Comp. Borax .	Worse after sleep.
Pred. worse opening, better closing the eyes.	Better (worse) opening *or* closing eyes.
Worse when idle	Worse from being overhurried.
Worse when taking a deep breath	Worse *or* better when taking a deep breath.
Worse from touch and moving diseased part.	*Worse or* better fr. touch & moving the part.
Better (worse) when opening *or* closing mouth.	Better when opening mouth, worse closing it.
Alm. alw. aggr. when assuming erect position.	*Worse or* better when rising from stooping.
Better when sitting down	*Better or* worse when sitting down.
Predom. better when eating	Worse *or* better when eating.‡
Better *or* worse from eructation	Almost always improv. by eructation.
Worse after stool.	Worse *or* better after stool.

Predomin. worse — **Predomin. better**

In dry weather, from cold, from uncovering, in an extended posture, when lying on right side, when getting out of bed, when drawing up diseased limb or letting it hang down, from motion, and on expiration.

Predomin. better — **Predomin. worse**

In wet weather, from warmth, from wrapping up, in a contracted posture, when lying on left side, in bed and from warmth of bed, after sleep, when stretching out or lifting diseased limb, during rest, after lying down, when lying, sitting and standing, on inspiration, from washing and moistening the suffering part, and after perspiring.

N.B. With Sulphur we very rarely find the over-sensitiveness of Nux vom. to pain; but sensitiveness (to touch, &c.) is found with both remedies.

---

* Consequences of emotions, comp. Agaricus—Nux vom. and others, Antimon. crud.—Sulphur and others.
† Particularly in hot and crowded rooms. By the warmth of stoves the complaints of both remedies are improved.
‡ Both remedies have predom. aggrav. "*after* eating."

Opium.	Antim. tart.
Want of bodily irritability—Morbus coeruleus.	Increased irritability—Chlorosis.
Plethora—Predom. no pain (except bellyache. C.Hg.)	Anæmie—Sensitiveness in internal, numb sensation in external parts.
Pain pressing outwards—Sweat warm—When there is no fever, dryness of skin.	Pain pressing inwards—Sweat cold, sticky—When there is no fever, disposition to sweat easily.
Pulse is sometimes large, sometimes small, in the same person.	Pulse is sometimes accelerated, sometimes retarded, in the same person.
Pulse very various; sometimes intermitting; slow and full, with snoring respiration; quick and hard. with heat and quick, anxious respiration.	Pulse full, strong, and accelerated during the fever; often slow and weak during the remission; sometimes trembling.
Burning or sensation of coldness in the veins.	Sensation of coldness in the veins.
Distention of veins of hands	Distention of veins of feet.
Apoplexia sanguinea—Paralysis	Apoplexia nervosa and serosa.
Asphyxia neonatorum	Asphyxy of drowned persons.* C.Hg.
Somnolence, with sweating heat and snoring respiration.	Somnolence, with coldness.
Pleasant dreams predominant	Anxious dreams.
Joyousness	Dejection.
Mental excitability (ecstasies) *or* mental dullness.	Mental dullness.
Absent-mindedness—Fancies—Delirium—Insanity	Rarely unconsciousness.
Twitching trembling of the head and hands, with single jerks in the arms, with external coldness and somnolence; improved by motion and uncovering the head.	Wearisome trembling of the head and hands; aggravated when lying and by warmth of bed; improved by sitting up and by cold.
Eyes protruding	Eyes sunken.
Secretion of saliva diminished	Saliva predominantly increased.
Very rarely nausea	Nausea, partic. in stomach and abdomen.
Predominantly *bitter* vomit, with costiveness.	Predominantly *sour* vomit, with disposition to diarrhœa.
Urine seldom and scanty; sometimes copious.	Urine scanty.
Respiration generally slow	Respiration accelerated.
Short, inaudible inspiration, and long, audible expiration, with drawing in of abdomen.	Rattling of mucus.
Expectoration seldom; during day . .	Expectoration not constant; morning.
AGGRAVATION night and morning . . .	AGGRAVATION from evening till morning.
Ailments from Mercurius, Plumbum, Nux vom., or Tartar emetic	Ailments from Sepia or Baryt.
Predomin. worse	**Predomin. better**
During rest, when standing, and when stooping.	
Predomin. better	**Predomin. worse**
When moving.	

* Mechanical means, of course, not to be neglected. Opium has been given in 6 or 12; Tartar emetic in 30. C.Hg.

Opium.	Plumbum.
Upper left, lower right side—Light hair	Lower left, upper right side—Dark hair.
Muscles lax—Perspires easily	Muscles rigid—Dryness of skin.
Plethora—Heat descending	Anæmie—Heat ascending.
Pulse slow and full, *or* quick and hard	Pulse generally slow, small, & compressed.
Pulse irregular and unequal	Pulsus dicrotus, or undulating.*
Want of thirst predominant	Thirst predominant.
Gangræna—The bodies of the poisoned decompose rapidly.	Sphacelus—The bodies of the poisoned resist decomposition a long time.
No pain oftener than pain	Neuralgia predominant.
Very troublesome itching all over, fine pricking, rarely sensitive to touch.	Greatest sensitiveness to touch, to the air; rarely itching.*
Blue spots on skin	Dark spots on skin.*
Bruised pain of the whole right side	The left side goes to sleep.
Apoplexy more frequent than paralysis	Paralysis more frequent than apoplexy.
Paralysis painless	Paralysis predom. painful.
Jerks, only the flexores active	Jerks, flexores and extensores alternating.*
Screams, with convulsions	Rarely screams with the convulsion.*
Convulsion, with loss of consciousness	Convulsion, with consciousness.*
Somnolence and coma, day and night	Sleeplessness nights, drowsiness dur'g day.*
Joyousness — Rarely distrust — Indifference—Boldness—Loquacity.	Reserve—Taciturnity.
Turbul't audacity, follow'd by want of volit'n.	Gloom alternates with excitement.*
Absent-mindedness—Fancies—Ecstasies *or* mental dullness.	Very rarely unconsciousness—Mental dullness.
Memory oftener active than weak	Weak memory.
Congestion of blood to the brain	Vertigo, partic. before epilepsy.*
Great sensibility to sound, light, and the faintest odors.	Power of hearing and seeing lessened, and total loss of smell.*
Congestion of blood to ears	Congestion of blood to eyes.
Frequent alternation of great paleness of the face with redness or dark-red & light-red; face puffed up, veines swelled.	Livid, earthy fallow face, like a corpse, sunken in or swollen.*
Inability to swallow; paralytic dysphagia.	Diffic. of swallow'g, caused by constriction of œsophagus, or sensat. of a knot, a ball.*
Laxness of abdominal organs	Constriction of intestines.
During colic urging to stool and discharge of hard excrements.	During the colic retention of fæces & the emission of urine interrupted.*
Violent pain in rectum, pressing asunder	Contraction of sphincter ani.*
Urine seld'm & scanty; but somet. copious.	Urine seldom and scanty.
Pollutions	Prostatorrhœa.
Softness of uterus	Inabil. of uterus to expans. dur'g pregnancy.*
Catamenia with violent colicy pains; forcing to bend over, urging to stool.	With the colic the catamenia cease, or the catamenia appear and the colic ceases.*
Brought on labor-pains, the child was dark-blue, had convul., & died in ten minutes.	Abortion, or all children die within the first years.*
Stoppage of nose	Fluent coryza predominant.
Snoring	Puffing with lips.*
Cough generally dry	Cough generally with expectoration.
REMISSION during day and evening	REMISSION of complaints forenoon.
Predom. worse before and during sleep	Predom. worse after sleep.
Better from pressure and motion	*Better* from pressure; worse from motion.
Worse from bodily exertion	Bett. fr. exert'n, contract'g abdom. muscles.
Worse when looking sideways	Worse when looking up.

N.B. We often find over-sensitiveness to pain with Plumbum, but not with Opium.

*** marked are added by C.Hg.**

Opium.	Stramonium.
Apoplexia sanguinea—Paralysis oftenest one-sided.	Apoplexia nervosa — Paralysis generally of both sides.
Often indicated with old people	Often with children, partic. mania, chorea, fever.
Cannot bear the open air	Desire for the open air.
Fainting every fifteen minutes; shutting eyes; head hangs down; weak respiration; unconsciousness; pulse unaltered; spasmodic jerks; deep sighing; anxiousness.	Fainting forenoon; rolling eyes; dilated pupils; pale face; hanging of lower jaw; cool skin; dryness of mouth, pulse frequent and intermitting; difficult swallowing; snoring or imperceptible breath; no appetite.
During sleep lying on back	Lying on belly preferred.
Pulse slow and full, *or* quick and hard	Pulse very irregular; sometimes trembling or imperceptible.
Heat or sweat, with inclination to uncover	Heat or sweat, with aversion to uncover.
Dryness of skin predom.—Want of thirst	Disposition to sweat predom.—Thirst is wanting only during chill.
Typhus cerebralis	Typhus exanthematicus.
Suppurations painless	Suppurations with the most excessive pains (whitlow, abscesses, etc.) Raue.
Mood cheerful; bold; less frequently irritated or distrustful.	Mood cheerful *or* sad; malicious.
Ailm. fr. (fright, vexat'n) joy, anger, or shame.	Ailments from (fright, vexation) hearing bad news or jealousy.
Active memory predominant	Weak memory (confounding words*).
Imbecility more frequent than insanity	Insanity more frequent than imbecility.
Mania: sees spectres, distorted faces, devils, etc,	Mania: sees rats, mice, dogs, cats, etc.*
Delirium tremens in old emaciated, reduced persons; sees animals coming towards him; people want to hurt him, execute him; affrighted expression of face; creeping under the covers, or jumping out of bed.	Delirium tremens in young plethoric persons; sees animals moving towards objects he looks at, or hears voices scolding him; is full of distress, terrified; tries to run out of the house.†—*
Imagines parts of his body enormously large	Imagines one-half of his body has been cut off.*
Congestion to brain predom.	Vertigo predominant.*
Sometimes dim-sightedn., rarely seeing sparks.	Dim-sighted to blindness — Far-sightedness; sees everything awry, double.*
Mobility and hanging of lower jaw	Gnashing of teeth.*
Trismus rheumaticus, traumaticus	Prosopalgy—Singultus spasticus.*
Salivation predominant	Dryness of mouth predom.*
Costiveness following diarrhœa	Diarrhœa and costiveness alternating.*
Puerperal convulsions with sopor; mouth open, snoring.	Puerperal convulsions with copious sweating. Lippe.
Sopor in child-bed	Delirious mania.
Inspiration quick; expiration slow	Inspiration slow; expiration quick.
Expectoration infrequent	Expector. not yet observed.
Cough with difficult expectoration, gaping, or dry, tickling cough afterwards.	Cough hoarse, rough sounding, alternating with croup-like barking.*
Trembl'g sensat'n in the heart; beating double.	Angina pectoris.*
Worse when looking sideways	Worse when looking up, at something shining, or at running water.
Worse from light (candle-light); bett. in dark.	Better (worse) from light *or* in the dark.
Worse when fixedly looking at an object for any length of time.	Worse when straining the sight.
When drinking, cough	When drinking, spasm in œsophagus.*
Worse or better from spirituous liquors	Worse from spirituous liquors.
Worse *or* better after stool	Better after stool.
Worse from overheating	W. fr. cold water on erupt's, erysipelas, etc.*
Ailments from Lead or Charcoal vapors	Ailments from Mercurial vapors.

Predomin. worse — **Predomin. better**

From warmth, growing warm and in warm air, in-doors, in bed & from warmth of bed, fr. wrapp'g up, during rest, after lying down, when lying, sitting & standing, but also when moving diseased part.

Predomin. better — **Predomin. worse**

From cold, grow'g cold & in cold weather, out-doors, fr. uncover'g, fr. motion, walk'g, & fr. pressure.

N.B. Both are antidotes to Mercurius and Plumbum, partic. when the effects are long-lasting.*

† Compare Delirium tremens: Hyoscyamus—Stramon. —— * Added by C.Hg.

Opium.	Veratrum.
Want of bodily irritability—**Painless ulcers.**	Increased irritability—Painful ulcers.
Apoplexy more frequent than paralysis . .	Paralysis more frequent than apoplexy.
Paralysis oftener one-sided	Paralysis oftener of both sides.
Pulse slow and full, *or* quick and hard .	Pulse irregular; generally slow, small, and weak; sometimes trembling.
Heat more frequent than cold—Want of thirst.	Coldness predominant—Thirst not constant; rare during sweat.

Opium.	Veratrum.
Insensibility of disposition	Sensitive disposition.
Loquacity — Mood cheerful; indifferent; rarely irritable or distrustful.	Taciturnity—Mood cheerful *or* sad; malicious.
Ailments from (fright, anger, vexation) excessive joy or shame.	Ailments from (fright, anger, vexation, or) grief.
Active memory predominant	Weak memory.
Imbecility more frequent than insanity . .	Insanity more frequent than imbecility.
With Horses: Sleepy staggers	With Horses: Mad staggers (raving).
Eyes protruding — Pupils predominantly dilated.	Pupils predominantly contracted—Eyes generally sunken.
Very rarely nausea	Nausea in stomach, which, however, is often wanting when vomiting.
Costiveness predominant	Diarrhœa predominant.
Constipation, partic. with corpulent, even-tempered, good-humored children and women.	Constipation (or diarrhœa) with lean, choleric, or melancholy persons.
Respiration generally slow	Respiration quick.
Expectoration infrequent	Expectoration not constant.
Complaints predominant on fore-arm . .	Complaints predominant on upper arm.
Ailments from Nux vom., Tartar emetic, Mercurius, Lead or Charcoal vapors.	Ailments from Cinchona, Ferrum, or Arsenic vapors.

Opium.	Veratrum.
Worse from warmth, better from cold . .	Better (worse) from warmth *or* cold.
Worse from warmth of stove	*Better or* worse from warmth of stove.
Worse when growing warm; better when growing cold.	Better (worse) when growing warm *or* cold.
Worse in bed*	Worse *or* better in bed.
Better after getting out of bed	Better *or* worse after getting out of bed.
Worse or better from spirituous liquors .	Worse from spirituous liquors.
Worse after eating	Worse *or* better after eating.
Predominantly worse on inspiration, better on expiration.	Predominantly worse on inspiration and expiration.

Predomin **worse** ⏞ Predomin. **better**

In warm air, from warmth of stove,† when ascending, and from drinking milk.

Predomin. **better** ⏞ Predomin. **worse**

In cold weather, when descending, and from drinking cold water.

* Both remedies have predominant aggravation from "warmth" of bed.
† Both remedies have predominant aggravation in-doors, improvement of complaints out-doors.

Petroleum.	Calcarea.
Constriction in external parts	Constriction in internal parts.
Pulse slow during rest, but accelerated, full, and stronger by every motion.	Pulse quick and full; sometimes trembling.
Chill lessened after meals	Chill increased after meals.
Sweat often confined to back part of body.	Sweat often only on front part of body.
Chill without thirst; heat with thirst	Thirst during all stages of the fever.
First chill, then heat	First heat, then chill.
Apoplexy not yet observed	Apoplexy.
Complaints predom. in inner angle of eye, on outside of nose, on upper lip, on lower gum, and in hollow of knee.	Complaints predom. in external angle of eye, on inside of nose, on under lip, on upper gum, and on patella.
Mood dejected; undecided; malicious	Mood depressed *or* silly; peevish — Amorousness.
Cannot get rid of the same idea, in conversation.	Is obliged to think the same idea during the whole night. C.Hg.
Neither unconsciousness nor delirium	Fancies.
Did not know where she was in the street	Complete loss of memory. C.Hg.
Vertigo, inclining to fall forwards	Vertigo, inclining to fall backwards or sideways.
Predom. bitter vomit	Vomit sour oftener than bitter.
Painful diarrhœa	Generally painless diarrhœa.
Urine often, but scanty	Urine too often.
Sexual desire too weak—Erections, without desire for coition.	Sexual desire too strong—Impotence, with desire for coition.
Catamenia generally too scanty and too late.	Catamenia profuse and predom. too soon.
Expectoration infrequent; during day	Expectoration predom., but not constant; morning and during day.
REMISSION after midnight and during day.	REMISSION of complaints before midnight.
Worse before a thunder-storm, less frequently during full moon.	Worse during full moon.
Worse from light; better in the dark	Worse (better) from light *or* in the dark.
Worse when straining the sight	*Worse or* better when straining the sight.
Worse when looking up	Worse when looking up or down.
Worse on awaking from sleep	*Worse or* better after sleep.
Better after getting out of bed	Worse *or* better after getting out of bed.
Worse when rising from a seat	*Worse or* better when rising from a seat.
Better (worse) when stretching out diseased limb, *or* when drawing it up.	Worse when stretching out the limb, better when drawing it up.
Worse *or* better from touch	Better from touch.
Worse from smoking	*Worse or* better from smoking.

Predomin. worse — **Predomin. better**

In a horizontal position, when lying on painful side, from change of posture, when lying or standing, when lifting diseased limb, when standing, and from warmth of stove.*

Predomin. better — **Predomin. worse**

Lying with head high, lying on unpainful side, when bending the body backwards, and when letting diseased limb hang down.

N.B. Calcarea rarely has the over-sensitiveness of Petroleum to pain. The latter rarely has the sensation of numbness in suffering parts peculiar to Calcarea.

* Both remedies have predom. improv. "*in-doors*" in general, aggrav. of symptoms in the open air.

Petroleum.	Lycopodium.
Piercing pain inwards — Hæmorrhages, blood pale.	Pain piercing outwards — Hæmorrhages, blood dark.
Dry itch—No apoplexy	Humid itch—Apoplexy.
Pulse slow during rest, but accelerated, full, and stronger by every motion.	Pulse somewhat accelerated only in the morning and after meals.
Chill lessened after meals	Chill increased after meals.
Dejection	Mood depress. *or* cheerf.; chang'g; gentle; serious; peevish; haughty; amorous.
Neither unconsciousn., delirium nor fancies.	Parsimony—Distrust.
Did not know where she was in the street .	Cannot remember the meaning of the single letters; imitates in writing, without knowing the signification. C. Hg.
Ailments from vexation with fright . . .	Ailments in consequence of anger, mortification, grief or vexation with reserved displeasure, fear or vehemence.
Nasal complaints predominantly external .	Nasal compl. predom. internal.
Bitter vomit predominant	Vomit sour oftener than bitter.
Painful diarrhœa predominant	Painless diarrhœa predom.
Involuntary discharge of urine	Retent. of urine more freq. than incontinence.
Scrotum contracted	Scrotum relaxed. C.Hg.
Catamenia predom. too scanty	Catam. too scanty *or* too profuse.
Expectoration infrequent; during day . .	Expector. nearly constant; morn'g & even'g.
Aggravation morning and evening till midnight.	Aggravation morning and from *noon till midnight*.
Better when alone; worse in company . .	Worse (better) when alone *or* in company.
Worse before a thunder-storm, during a storm or during full moon.	Worse during new moon.
Predom. worse during cold weather, better in warm air.	Better (worse) in cold weather *or* in warm air.
Predom. worse when growing cold, better when growing warm.	Better (worse) when growing cold *or* when growing warm.
Worse after perspiring	Better *or* worse after perspiring.
Predom. worse in bed	Bett. *or* worse in bed & from warmth of bed.
Worse when getting out of bed or rising from a seat.	Worse *or* better when getting out of bed or rising from a seat.
Better when sitting down	Worse *or* better when sitting down.
Worse when stooping	*Better or* worse when stooping.
Better when assuming an erect position .	Worse *or* bett. wh. assum'g an erect posit'n.
Better (worse) when stretching out diseased limb *or* when drawing it up.	Worse when stretching out diseased limb; better when drawing it up.
Better *or* worse from touch	Almost always aggrav. by the touch.
Worse when looking up	Worse when looking at anything revolv'g.*
Worse or better when straining the sight .	Worse when straining the sight.
Worse after stool	*Worse or* better after stool.

Predomin. worse — **Predomin. better**

From cold, motion, walking, when moving suffering part, when lifting diseased limb, when ascending, out-doors and when walking out-doors, when stooping, and on an empty stomach.

Predomin. better — **Predomin. worse**

From warmth, during rest, after lying down, when lying and sitting, when letting diseased limb hang down, when descending, in-doors, from warmth of stove, and after breakfast.

* When walking on streets newly paved with bricks, on plaid carpets, when quickly passing picket fences. C.Hg.

Petroleum.	**Sepia.**
Light hair—Hæmorrhages, blood light-red.	Dark hair—Hæmorrhages, blood dark.
No apoplexy. Pressing pain inwards .	Apoplexy—Pressing pain outwards.
Pulse slow during rest, but accelerated by every motion; becoming full and strong.	Pulse often irregular or trembling; quick and full, also intermitt'g, at night; dur'g day accelerated only by vexat'n or mot'n.
Chill without thirst; heat with thirst . .	Want of thirst predom.; thirst appears dur'g chill & often also *before* & *after* the chill.
Indecision—Malice	Mood indiffer.; serious; peevish—Avarice.
Ailments from vexation with fright . . .	Ailments from shame or vexation with fear, rarely after fits of rage.
	Fancies—Insanity—Unconsciousness.
Pupils dilated	Pupils contracted.
Complaints predom. on upper lip . . .	Compl. predom. on under lip.
Hunger predominant—Urine too often, but scanty.	Generally loss of appetite—Urine not often enough.
Sexual desire lessened—Erections without desire.	Sexual desire changeable, with feeble ability.
Catamenia predominantly scanty	Catam. generally profuse, oft. also too scanty.
Respiration predom. with moist sound . .	Respiration predom. with dry sound.
Expectoration infrequent; during day . .	Expector. predom., but not constant; is loosened partic. night and morning, and generally swallowed.
Remission after midnight & dur'g the day.	**Remission** of complaints afternoon.
Worse in cold weather, better in warm air.	Worse (better) in cold weather *or* in warm air.
Worse before a thunder-storm or during a storm, and during full moon.	Worse during new moon.
Worse when looking up	Worse when looking over a large surface.
Worse or better when straining the sight .	Worse when straining the sight.
Predominantly worse from bodily exertion.	Improv. oftener than aggrav. by exertion.
Worse out-doors, better in-doors	Better (worse) out-doors *or* in-doors.
Worse from smoking	*Better or* worse from smoking.
Better from eructation	Almost always aggrav.
Predominantly worse in bed	Worse *or* better in bed.
Worse on awaking from sleep	Better after sufficient sleep, but worse on awaking when roused.
Worse when getting out of bed	*Better or* worse when getting out of bed.
Better *after* getting out of bed	*Better or* worse after getting out of bed.
Worse when rising from a seat	Worse *or* better when rising from a seat.
Better (worse) when stretching out diseased limb, *or* when drawing it up.	Worse when stretching out diseased limb; better when drawing it up.
Better *or* worse from touch	Almost always aggrav. by touch.

Predomin. worse — **Predomin. better**

In wet weather, when lying on painful side, when turning in bed, after sleep, when getting out of bed, from motion, when walking, when moving diseased part, from bodily exertion, and from smoking.

Predomin. better — **Predomin. worse**

In dry weather, when lying on unpainful side, during rest, when sitting & lying, from warmth of stove, and from eructation.

Petroleum.	Sulphur.
Right side—Ulcerative pain in external parts, pinching pain in internal par.s—Piercing pain inwards.	*Left* side—Ulcerative pain in internal, pinching pain in external parts—Piercing pain outwards.
Hæmorrhages, blood light-red	Hæmorrhages, blood dark.
Painful eruptions and ulcers	Painless eruptions and ulcers.
Pulse accelerated only by motion, becoming full and strong.	Pulse frequent, full, and hard; sometimes intermitting or imperceptible.
Chill without thirst; heat with thirst . . .	Thirst, mostly during heat; during chill generally want of thirst.
Chill lessened after meals	Chill increased after meals.
Excitability—Maliciousness.	Being wrapt in thought—Mood changing; gentle; indifferent; serious; peevish.
No memory for what is around or present. .	No memory for what recently transpired. CHg.
Ailments from (vexation or) fright	Ailments from (vexation) mortification, less frequently from anger or fright.
Neither unconsciousness, delirium, nor fancies.	Unconsciousness, delirium, and fancies.
Imbecility (more freq. than insanity. C.Hg.)	Insanity more frequent than imbecility.
Pupils dilated—Compl. predom. in inner angle of eye.	Pupils contracted—Complaints predom. in external angle of eye.
Hunger predominant.	Generally loss of appetite.
Desire for beer	Desire for *or* aversion to beer & spirituous liquors.
Vomit predominantly bilious	Vomit sour oftener than bitter.
Scrotum contracted	Scrotum relaxed. C.Hg.
Expectoration infrequent; during day . . .	Expector. not constant; morning and during day, less frequently at night.
Remission during day and after midnight . .	Remission *afternoon* and before midnight.
Worse when in company, better when alone .	Worse (better) when in company *or* alone.
Worse in cold weather, better in warm air .	Better (worse) in cold weather *or* in warm air.
Predom. worse when growing cold, better when growing warm.	Better (worse) when growing cold *or* warm.
Worse after perspiring	*Worse or* better after perspiring.
Worse out-doors, better in-doors	Predom. better out-doors; worse particularly in hot, crowded rooms.*
Worse when moving diseased part	Worse *or* better when moving diseased part.
Better *or* worse from touch	Predom. worse from touch.
Better (worse) when stretching out diseased part, *or* when drawing it up.	Predom. worse when stretching out diseased part, better when drawing it up.
Better when sitting down	*Better* or worse when sitting down.
Worse when stooping, better when rising . .	*Worse or* better when stooping & when rising.
Worse from change of posture (when lying or standing).	*Worse or* better from change of posture.
Worse when looking up	Worse looking down, partic. at runn'g water.
Worse when swallowing	*Worse or* better when swallowing.
Predom. worse on an empty stomach, better after breakfast.	Better (worse) on an empty stomach *or* after breakfast.
Worse or better after meals	Worse after meals.
Worse after drinking	*Worse or* better after drinking.
Worse after stool.	Worse or better after stool.

Predomin. worse — **Predomin. better**

From cold, out-doors, from motion, when walking.

Predomin. better — **Predomin. worse**

From warmth, in-doors,* dur'g rest, after lying down, when lying & sitt'g, & when lying after stoop'g.

N.B. Sulph. rarely has the over-sensitiveness of Petrol. to pain; the latter rarely has sensation of numbness in suffering parts.

* Both remedies have improv. of symptoms "*from warmth of stove.*"

Petroleum.	Thuya.
Right side—Constriction in external parts.	*Left* side—Constriction in internal parts.
Pulse slow during rest, but accelerated by every motion, full and strong.	Pulse slow and weak in the morning; accelerated and full in the evening.
Congestion of blood to the ears	Congestion of blood to the eyes.
First chill, then heat	First heat, then chill.
Small-pox when developing imperfectly, the pustules drying up.	Small-pox, during their first development, or pustules begin to fill up.
Indecision—Weak reasoning powers	Seriousness—Haughtiness – Absentmindedness – Day-dreaming—Mentally quick, *or* weak reasoning powers.
Pupils dilated	Pupils contracted.
Hunger predominant	Loss of appetite predominant.
Complaints predominant in the bladder	Complaints predominant in the kidneys.
Urine often, but scanty; sediment *white* or red	Urine too often and copious—Urinal sediment reddish.
Sexual desire generally too weak	Sexual desire prevalently strong.
Catamenia predominantly too late	Catamenia prevalently too soon.
Respiration generally with moist sound	Respiration with dry sound.
Expectoration infrequent; during day	Expectoration nearly constant; evening.
Complaints predominant on sole of foot	Complaints predominant on top of foot.
REMISSION during day and after midnight	REMISSION forenoon and before midnight.
Worse in cold weather, better in warm air.	Bett. (worse) in cold weather *or* in warm air.
Worse when growing cold, better when growing warm.	Better (worse) when growing cold *or* warm.
Worse on awaking from sleep	*Worse or* better after sleep.
Better after getting out of bed	Worse *or* better after getting out of bed.
Worse when turning in bed	*Worse or* better when turning in bed.
Worse or better after eating	Worse after eating.
Worse after stool	*Better or* worse after stool.
Worse *or* better from touch	Predominantly better from touch.
Worse from moving diseased part	Better *or* worse from moving the part.
Predom. worse when bending diseased part.	*Better or* worse when bending the part.
Better (worse) when stretching out diseased limb, *or* when drawing it up.	Predom. worse when stretching out the limb, better when drawing it up.
Worse or better when straining the sight.	Worse when straining the sight.
Worse when swallowing food	Worse when swallowing saliva.

Predomin. worse — **Predomin. better**

From cold, after sweat, from motion, when walking, when lifting diseased limb, when bending suffering part, on an empty stomach, and after stool.

Predomin. better — **Predomin. worse**

From warmth, partic. warmth of stove, during rest, when sitting and lying, when letting diseased limb hang down, and after breakfast.

N.B. We very rarely find the over-sensitiveness of Petroleum to pain with Thuya.

Phosphor.	Pulsat.
Upper right, lower left side — Hæmorrhages, blood pale—Blood uncoagulable.	Upper left, lower right side — Hæmorrhages, blood dark, coagulated.
Paralysis more frequent than apoplexy—Often indicated with old people.	Apoplexy more frequent than paralysis — Is often indicated with children and women.
Itching, lessen. oftener than aggr. by scratch'g.	Itching, aggrav. *or* unchanged by scratching.
Eruptions almost always dry — Wounds with injury of glands.	Humid eruptions — Wounds with injury of bones.
Pulse differs; irregular; quick, and at the same time generally full and hard.	Pulse generally frequent, small, and weak, sometimes imperceptible.
Sweat lessened during meals	Sweat increased during meals.
Sweat on lower or on front part of body—Want of thirst during all stages.	Chill on lower, sweat on back part of body — Want of thirst only during chill.
Compl. most frequent on *external* ear, on upper lip, upper part of chest, & in palms of hands.	Compl. most frequ. in *inner* ear, on lower lip, in lower part of chest, and on back of hand.
Apathy with occasional fits of passion . . .	Apathy with lachrymosity.
Disposition *insensible* or sensitive.	Sensitive disposition.
Dreads being alone — Cheerfulness *or* dejection—Haughtiness—Irritability.	Desire to be alone — Sadness — Gentleness — Boldness—Avarice.
Ailments from anger or vexation with vehemence.	Ailments from excessive joy, mortification, or vexation with fear.
Mental excitability—Active memory predom.	Mental dullness—Weak memory.
Insanity	Melancholy.
Stupefying headache, part. in the morning and when moving; bett. when lying & in cool air.	Stupef. headache, part. in the even'g, in-doors, & when lying; better wh. walking in cool air.
Optical illusions in dark or prismatic colors .	Optical illusions in light colors.
Growing black before the eyes when rising after lying.	Growing black before the eyes while lying down.
Putrid subjective smell predom.	Objective stench fr. nose; *subjective* pleasant odor, or like an old catarrh.
Aversion to herrings (salt-fish)	Appetite for herrings.
Nausea in stomach	Nausea in throat, stomach, or abdomen.
Pred. sour vomit — Pred. scentless, hot flatus.	Vomit bitter oftener than sour — Hot, fetid [flatus.
Diarrhœa generally painless	Diarrhœa generally painful.
Urine often, but scanty	Urine not often enough and scanty.
Catamenia predom. too soon; at the same time profuse and of long duration, *or* too scanty and of short duration.	Catamenia too late, of short duration, and generally too scanty.
Expectoration not constant	Expectoration predom., but not constant.
Remission of complaints after midnight . .	Remission from midnight till noon.
Ailments from abuse of Iodium or table-salt.	Ailm. from Sulphur, Sulph. ac., Ferr., Plat., [Stann., Argent.
Worse or better while perspiring	Worse while perspiring.
Worse *or* better during sleep	Worse during sleep.
Worse (better) when opening *or* closing eyes.	Better when opening, worse closing eyes.
Worse looking into light or at shining things.	Worse when looking up.
Worse when getting out of bed	*Better or* worse when getting out of bed.
Almost always improv. when sitting down. .	Worse *or* better when sitting down.
Worse wh. rising fr. a seat; bett. *afterwards.*	Worse *or* better when and after rising.
Better *or* worse when stooping	Predom. worse when stooping.
Alm. alw. aggr. when assum'g an erect posit'n.	Worse or better when assum. an erect posit'n.
Worse *or* better from eating bread	Worse from eating bread.
Worse after stool.	*Better or* worse after stool.
Worse when swallowing food and drink . .	Worse when swallowing saliva; often better when swallowing food, &c.

Predomin. worse — **Predomin. better**

From cold, from growing cold and in cold weather, from motion, when walking, when stretching out diseased limb, from bodily exertion, walking fast and running, from tying the clothes tight, when lying on back or on painful side, from pressure, from washing or moistening suffering part, from sour things, from vegetable diet, after stool, and when getting out of bed.

Predomin. better — **Predomin. worse**

From warmth, from growing warm and in warm air, during rest, when standing, sitting and lying, when drawing up diseased limb, from loosening the clothes, when lying on side, partic. when lying on unpainful side; from touch, from sweet things, from beer and spirituous liquors, after drinking in general, also after sleep, during twilight, from rubbing and scratching.

Phosphor.	Sulphur.
Right side, partic. *upper right, lower left side.*	*Left* side, partic. *upper left, lower right side.*
Ulcerative pain, or sensation as of a plug in external, pinching pain in internal parts.	Ulcerative pain, or sensation as of a plug in internal, pinching pain in external parts.
Hæmorrhages, blood pale— Vesicles around the joints.	Hæmorrhages, blood dark—Itching, erysipelas or vesicles around the joints.
Pulse differs; irregular	Pulse quick, full, and hard.
Sweat right s., on front or lower part of body.	Sweat left s., on back or upper part of body.
Itching *lessened or* aggrav. by scratching . .	Itching almost always relieved by scratching.
Sweat on lower part of body	Heat on lower, sweat on upper part of body.
Sweat often confined to front part of body .	Sweat often only on back part of body.
Chill increased in a warm room	Chill abating in a warm room.
Want of thirst during all stages	Thirst mostly during heat; during chill generally want of thirst.
Cures warts, &c., by suppuration	Causes atrophy of warts.
Complaints predom. in inner angle of eye, on external ear, on under lip, on shin.	Compl. pred. in external angle of eye, in inner ear, on upper lip, and on the calf of leg.
Disposition *insensible or* sensitive	Sensitive disposition.
Solicitude concerning the future	Solicitude concerning the present. C. Hg.
Joyousness *or* dejection—Haughtiness . . .	Mood sad; serious and solemn; gentle.
Ailments from fright, anger (grief), or vexation with vehemence.	Ailments from mortification, hearing bad news, or vexation with fear, less fr. fright or anger.
Easy or difficult comprehension	Difficult comprehension predom.
Mental excitability & active memory predom.	Mental dullness—Weak memory.
Hydrocephaloid of children	Hydrocephalus acutus in children. C. Hg.
Stye on lower lid	Stye on upper lid. C. Hg.
Putrid subjective smell predom.	Objective stench from nose predom.
Aversion to beer	Desire for, *or* aversion to beer & spir. liquors.
Predom. scentless flatus	Fetid flatus.
Urine often sour; smells often like Ammoniac.	Urine acid.
Catamenia predom. too soon	Catamenia generally too late.
Catam. suppressed, with milk in the breasts .	Catamenia suppressed, with hæmorrhoidal tumors. C. Hg.
Labor-pains too painful	Labor-pains weak or ceasing.
Milk generally increased	Milk decreased.
Nasal secretion thick or viscid	Nasal secretion watery.
Remission of complaints after midnight . .	Remission *afternoon* and before midnight.
Ailments from Iodium or table-salt	Ailments fr. metals or abuse of Cinchona, &c.
Generally worse when alone, bett. in company.	*Generally* better when alone, worse in comp.
Predom. worse when growing cold and in cold weather, better when growing warm and in warm air.	Better (worse) when growing cold and in cold weather, *or* when grow'g warm & in warm air.
Worse when sneezing, after perspiring, and from change of posture.	*Worse or* better when sneezing, after perspiring, and from change of posture.
Worse *or* better while perspiring, during sleep, after eating, partic. eating bread, and from eructation.	Worse while perspiring, during sleep, after eating, from eating bread, and from eructation.
Worse after stool	Worse *or* better after stool.
Almost always improv. by touch	*Worse or* better from touch.
Worse looking into light or at shining things.	Worse looking down, partic. at running water.
Worse when swallowing food and drink . .	Worse when swallowing food and saliva.

Predomin. worse — **Predomin. better**

From cold, but also from warmth of stove,* from warm diet, when alone, when lying on back, from motion, when walking, when getting out of bed, when letting diseased limb hang down, and from pressure.

Predomin. better — **Predomin. worse**

From warmth, from drinking cold water, from cold diet generally, when in company, when lying on side, during rest, when standing, sitting and lying, after† sleep, when lifting diseased limb, from touch, after drinking, from sweets, from beer and spirituous liquors.

N.B. With Sulphur we very rarely find the over-sensitiveness of Phosphor. to pain.

* Both remedies have aggrav. of symptoms *in hot crowded rooms.*
† Phosphor. also has an aggrav. after the siesta and on awaking when roused.

Phosph. acid.	Arsenic.
Tension in external parts — Hæmorrhages, blood dark.	Tension in internal parts — Hæmorrhages blood pale.
Paralysis generally one-sided	Paralysis often of both sides.
No putrid fever	Putrid fever.
Sweat on upper part of body, sensation of heat on lower part.	Sweat or chill on lower part of body.
Taciturnity, partic. during the sweating stage.	Talkativeness during the sweat. C.Hg.
Sweat increased when walking out-doors . .	Sweat lessened when walking out-doors.
Cold hands and warm feet	Cold feet and hot hands.
Want of thirst predominant; thirst appears almost only during sweat.	Least thirst during chill, most during sweat.
Complaints predominant on external ear, on soft palate, on fore-arm, on the outer side of thigh, and on shin.	Complaints predominant in inner ear, on roof of mouth, on upper arm, on inner side of thigh, and on the calf of leg.

Insensibility of disposition — Taciturnity— Mood gentle; less frequently irritated.	Sensitive disposition—Loquacity—Mood irritable; malicious—Avarice.
Ailments from shame, mortification, disappointed love or jealousy.	Ailments from fright or vexation with fear or vehemence.
Fancies	Insanity.
Eruption on under lip	Eruption on upper lip.
Dislike to bread	Appetite for bread, partic. rye-bread.
Urine too frequent and copious; less frequently scanty.	Urine scanty (with diarrhœa) *or* copious.
Sexual desire feeble, even with erections . .	Great sexual desire.
Voice nasal	Voice trembling.
Expectoration nearly constant; morning . .	Expectoration not constant; during day.

Remission afternoon and before midnight . .	Remission *during day* and before midnight.
Worse (better) from cold and when growing cold, *or* from warmth and when grow'g warm.	Worse from cold and when grow'g cold, better from warmth and when growing warm.*
Generally worse in-doors and from warmth of stove, better out-doors.	*Generally* better in-doors and from warmth of stove, worse out-doors.
Worse during and after sweat	*Worse or* better during and after sweat.
Predominantly worse after sleep	Better after sufficient sleep, but worse on awaking when roused.
Predominantly worse in bed	Better in bed (warmth) *or* (rest) worse.
Worse when rising from stooping	*Better or* worse when rising.
Better or worse when swallowing	Worse when swallowing.
Worse after stool and after urinating . . .	Worse *or* better after stool and after urinating.
Worse *or* better when straining the sight . .	Worse when straining the sight.
Worse from light, better in the dark . . .	Worse (better) from light *or* in the dark.

Predomin. worse — **Predomin. better**

In-doors and from warmth of stove, from warmth of bed, warm diet, when standing and sitting erect, when letting diseased limb hang down, when bending suffering part, after sleep, when getting out of bed, and when rising from stooping.

Predomin. better — **Predomin. worse**

Out-doors, when swallowing and eating, from cold diet,† when sitting bent forward, when lifting diseased limb, and from change of posture.

---

* Both remedies have predominant aggravation in cold weather, improvement in warm air. (But in cholerine it has been observed that Phosph. acid. is indicated more decidedly as soon as the weather becomes hot, while Veratrum corresponds to cholerine during cooler days, although this remedy is generally indicated after dry land-winds. C. Hg.)

† Both remedies have aggravation from drinking cold water.

Phosphor. acid.	Phosphor.
Upper l., lower r. side—Inclinat. for motion.	Upper r., lower l. side — Aversion to motion
Depression and exhaustion	Alternat'n of oppos. states; more vivid react'n.
Generally no pain	Congest'n of blood to upp. parts; acute pains.
Frequent aggrav. by depressing emotions .	Agrav., partic. by *external impressions*, odors, thunder-storms, change of weather.
Hæmorrhages, blood dark	Hæmorrhages, blood *light-red.*
Painless (cold) swelling of glands . . .	Hot swelling of glands.
Diseases of the periosteum	Diseases of the bones (diaphyses).
Wounds with injury of the bones . . .	Wounds with injury of the glands.
Emaciation, particularly of the feet . . .	Emaciation, particularly of the hands.
Somnolence	Sleepin. dur'g day & nocturnal restlessness.
Sensation of heat on lower part, sweat on back of body.	Sweat on lower part and front of body.
Heat, with aversion to uncover	Heat, with inclination to uncover.
Pulse generally frequent, small, and weak .	P. generally frequent or quick, full, & hard.
Thirst almost only during sweat	Constant want of thirst.
Eruptions, particularly on parts not covered.	Erupt's (petechiæ), partic. on parts covered.
Complaints predom. on lower eyelids, on upper jaw and upper teeth, in lower part of chest, and on tip of elbow.	Complaints predom. on upper eyelids, on lower jaw and lower teeth, in upper part of chest, and in the hollow of elbow.
Nerv. fevers with depress'n—No putrid fever.	Erethic typhus—Pneumo-typh.—Putr. fev'r.
Dejection predominant	Joyousness (predom.) *or* melancholy.
Taciturn indifference; cross; lachrymose .	Irritable disposition; irascibility.
Mood gentle; very rarely irritable . . .	Chang'g mood — Haughtiness—Amorousn.
Ailments from shame, mortification, disappointed love or jealousy, and from vexation with reserved displeasure.	Ailments in consequence of fright, anger, or vexation with vehemence.
Difficult comprehension—Mental dullness—Imbecility.	Easy *or* difficult comprehension — Mental excitability—Ecstasies — Insanity—Very rarely imbecility.
Eyes sunken, lustreless—Pupils mostly dilat.	E. protrud., bright—Pupils mostly contract.
Stye on upper lid	Stye on lower lid. C.Hg.
Repugnance for sour things—Appetite for milk or beer.	Appetite for sour things—Aversion to milk or beer.
Nausea in throat, less frequent in stomach .	Nausea in stomach.
Urine oft. & copious, only exception'y scanty.	Urine often, but scanty.
Not much sex. des.—Erect's without salacity.	Incr. sex. desire — Erect's with strong desire.
Catamenia profuse—Milk scanty or spoiled.	Catam. *profuse or* scanty—Milk increased.
Voice nasal—*Cough* partic. in the morn'g (with expectoration) and in the evening (without expectoration).	V. trembl'g or hiss'g—*Cough* partic. in the even'g & dur'g night, & then dry; in the morn'g & during day with expectoration.
REMISSION afternoon and before midnight .	REMISSION of complaints after midnight.
Worse before and when passing urine . .	*Worse when and after* passing urine.
Improved oftener than aggrav. by change of posture.	*Worse* from change of posture.
Ailments from Lachesis	Ailm. from abuse of table-salt or Iodium.

Predomin. worse — **Predomin. better**

After* sleep, during rest, when standing and sitting, in dry weather, from drinking cold water, and from uncovering.

Predomin. better — **Predomin. worse**

From motion, from change of posture (when lying or standing), in wet weather, & from wrapping up.

* On awaking, when roused from sleep, Phosphorus has aggravation; the same after the siesta.

Phosphor. acid.	Pulsatilla.
Inclination for motion—Shuns the open air .	Aversion to motion—Inclination for open air.
Want of bodily irritability—Painless swelling of glands.	Increased irritability—Painful, hot swelling of glands.
No apoplexy	Apoplexy.
Sweat increased when walking out-dors . .	Sweat lessened when walking out-doors.
Sensation of heat on lower part of body—Pulse more irregular than with Pulsat.	Heat on upper part of body; chill on lower part.
Pulse affected by coffee and tea	Pulse affected by beer and coffee. C. Hg.
Thirst almost only during sweat	Want of thirst predom., but constant only during chill.
Complaints most frequent on external ear, on upper jaw, upper teeth, on soft palate, on fore-arm, and on tip of elbow.	Complaints predom. on inner ear, on lower jaw, lower teeth, on roof of mouth, on upper arm, and in the hollow of elbow.
Disposition insensible	Disposition sensitive.
Ailm. from (grief, mortification) disappointed love or jealousy, from shame or vexation with reserved displeasure.	Ailments from (grief, mortification) excessive joy, fright or vexation with dread or fear.
Imbecility	Melancholy.
Vertigo, inclin'g to fall forwards or backwards.	Vertigo, inclining to fall backwards.
Pupils predom. dilated	Pupils generally contracted.
Appetite for milk	Aversion to milk.
Nausea, partic. in throat, less freq. in stomach	Nausea in throat, stomach or abdomen.
Sour vomit	Vomit bitter oftener than sour.
Diarrhœa painless	Diarrhœa generally painful.
Urine too often and copious; less freq. scanty	Urine not often enough and scanty.
Sexual desire weak—Erections without desire.	Sexual desire strong—Erections with desire.
Catamenia too soon and too profuse . . .	Catamenia too late, and generally too scanty.
Milk decreased	Milk generally increased.
Expectoration nearly constant; morning . .	Expect. not constant; morning & during day.
AGGRAVATION from midnight till noon, and in the evening.	AGGRAVATION from noon till midnight.
Worse (better) from cold and growing cold, *or* from warmth and when growing warm.	Better from cold & when growing cold; worse from warmth and when growing warm.
Worse when assuming an erect position, and when rising from a seat.	*Worse or* better when assuming an erect position and when rising from a seat.
Better *after* rising from a seat	Worse *or better* after rising from a seat.
Worse when getting out of bed	*Better or* worse when getting out of bed.
Worse *or* better *after* getting out of bed . .	*Generally* improved *after* getting out of bed.
Predom. better when sitting down	Better *or* worse when sitting down.
Worse when sitting erect, better when sitting bent forward.	*Generally* better when sitting erect, worse when sitting bent forward.
Generally better from change of posture, when lying or standing.	*Generally* worse from change of posture.
Better when moving diseased part	*Better or* worse when moving the part.
Worse when bending diseased part	Better *or* worse when bending the part.
Worse from bodily exertion, running, &c. . .	Predom. improv. by exertion.
Worse *or* better when straining the sight . .	Worse when straining the sight.
Predom. better when eating	Almost always aggrav. by eating.
Worse *after* eating	*Worse or* better after eating.
Worse from drinking cold water	*Generally* better from drinking cold water
Predom. better when swallowing	*Generally* worse when swallowing.
Worse after stool	*Better or* worse after stool.

Predomin. worse — **Predomin. better**

In cold dry weather, from uncovering, when lying on painful side, when sitting erect, when getting out of bed, from bodily exertion, after meals, after eating sour things, from drinking cold water,* after stool, and from tying the clothes tight.

Predomin. better — **Predomin. worse**

In warm and moist air, from wrapping up, when lying on unpainful side, when sitting bent forward, from change of posture (lying or standing), when swallowing† and eating, and from loosening the clothes.

* Both remedies have improv. from cold diet in general, and aggrav. of complaints from warm diet.

† Phosphor. has: worse when swallowing food; Pulsat.: worse when swallowing saliva.

Phosph. acid.	Sepia.
Complaints predom. in internal parts . . .	Complaints predom. in external parts.
No apoplexy—Paralysis generally one-sided .	Apoplexy—Paralysis generally of both sides.
First chill, then heat	First heat, then chill.
Thirst almost only during sweat	Thirst constant only dur'g cold stage of fever.*
Pulse generally frequent, small and weak . .	Pulse frequent and full at night; during day accelerated only by vexation or motion; sometimes trembling.
Pulse affected by coffee and tea	Pulse affected by drinking beer. C.Hg.

Phosph. acid.	Sepia.
Taciturnity—Gentleness	Loquacity—Irritable mood—Avarice.
Ailments from disappointed love or jealousy, from shame, mortification, grief, or vexation with reserved displeasure.	Ailments from vexation with fear; less frequently after anger or disappointed love.
Imbecility	Insanity *or* imbecility—No delirium.
Hair hanging down like flax, but greasy . .	Hair tangled.
Pupils generally dilated—Short-sightedness .	Pupils contracted—Far-sightedness.
Complaints most frequent on external ear . .	Complaints most frequent in internal ear.
Appetite for milk—Sour vomit.	Aversion too milk—Predom. bitter vomit.
Urine predom. pale; too often and copious .	Urine predom. dark—Discharge of urine too seldom.
Sexual desire weak—Erection without desire.	Sexual desire changeable — Ability feeble even with inclination.
Catamenia too soon	Catam. generally too late.
Expectoration almost constant; morning . .	Expector. not constant; is loosened, partic. night and morning, and generally swallowed.
Complaints predom. on shin.	Compl. generally on calf of leg.

Phosph. acid.	Sepia.
Remission afternoon and before midnight . .	Remission of compl. afternoon.
Worse in cold weather, better in warm air .	Worse (better) in cold weather *or* in warm air.
Worse (better) from cold and when growing cold, *or* from warmth and when grow'g warm.	Predom. worse from cold & when growing cold, better from warmth and when grow'g warm.
Worse when perspiring and after meals . .	*Worse or* better when perspiring & after meals.
Worse *or* better ween straining the sight . .	Worse when straining the sight.
Worse from bodily exertion	*Better or* worse from exertion.
Worse when closing the eyes, better when opening them.	Better (worse) when closing *or* when opening the eyes.
Predom. worse after sleep	Better after sufficient sleep, but worse on awaking when roused.
Worse when getting out of bed	Worse *or better* when getting out of bed.
Worse *or* better after getting out of bed . .	Predom. better after getting out of bed.
Worse when rising from a seat	Worse or better when rising from a seat.
Better when eating; worse *afterwards*. . .	Better when drinking, worse *afterwards*.

Predomin. worse — **Predomin. better**

From warmth of bed, after sleep, when lying on painful side, when sitting erect, when rising from stooping, from bodily exertion, after breakfast, from drinking cold water,† and when getting out of bed.

Predomin. better — **Predomin. worse**

When lying on unpainful side, when sitting bent forward, from pressure, on an empty stomach, when swallowing and eating.

N.B. Over-sensitiveness to pain is much more frequent with Sepia than with Phosph. acid.

---

* Want of thirst is predom. with both remedies.

† Both remedies have predom. improv. from cold diet in general, aggrav. from warm diet.

Phosphor. acid.	Sulphur.
External parts become black—Pinching pain in internal parts.	Red parts become white—Pinching pain in external parts.
Compl. predom. on lower eyelids, in inner angle of eye, on external ear, in lower part of chest, on tip of elbow, on outer side of thigh, and on shin.	Compl. predom. on upper eyelids, in external angle of eye, in inner ear, in upper part of chest, in hollow of elbow, on patella, on inner side of thigh, and on the calf.
Paralysis generally one-sided	Paralysis often of both sides.
Pulse generally frequent, small, and weak; irregular.	Pulse quick, full, and hard.
External chill, with internal heat	Internal chill, with external heat.
Heat or sweat, with aversion to uncover	Heat or sweat, with inclination to uncover.
Cold hands and warm feet	Hot hands and cold feet.
Want of thirst predom., except during sweat.	Thirst predom., but not constant.
Insensibility of disposition — Mood rarely irritable.	Sensitive disposition—Mood changing.
Ailments from disappointed love or jealousy, from grief, shame, or vexation with reserved displeasure.	Ailments from vexation with fright or fear; less frequently from anger.
Faculty of thinking is weak in the morning	Faculty of thinking is weak in the evening—Rarely unconsciousness.
Imbecility	Insanity more frequent than imbecility.
Hair too greasy, like flax; easily turns grey	Hair too dry.
Pupils generally dilated	Pupils generally contracted.
Eruption on lower lip	Eruption on upper lip.
Desire for beer and spirituous liquors	Desire for *or* aversion to beer and spirituous liquors.
Appetite for milk—Nausea in throat	Aversion to milk—Nausea in stomach.
Urine too often and copious; less frequently scanty.	Urine often, but scanty; copious only after large doses.
Catamenia too soon and profuse	Catam. generally too late and scanty.
Expectoration almost constant; morning	Expector. not constant; morning and during day, less frequently at night.
REMISSION *before midnight*	REMISSION before midnight, but much less important than the remission of Phosph. acid. symptoms.
Worse in cold weather, better in warm air	Better (worse) in cold weather or in warm air.
Worse (better) from cold or from warmth	Predom. better from cold, worse from warmth.
Predom. worse on expiration	Predom. worse on inspiration.
Worse when looking into the light	W. when look'g down, partic. at runn'g water.
Worse in warm rooms	Better from warmth of stove; but worse in hot, crowded rooms.
Worse when assuming an erect position and after sweat.	*Worse or* better when assuming an erect position and after sweat.
Generally better from change of posture (lying or standing).	*Generally* worse from change of posture.
Better when moving diseased part	*Worse or* better when moving diseased part.
Better on an empty stomach, worse after breakfast.	Worse (better) on an emyty stomach *or* after breakfast.
Predom. better when eating	Worse *or* better when eating.
Worse after stool	Worse *or* better after stool.

Predomin. worse — **Predomin. better**

In dry weather, from uncovering, when getting out of bed, when sitting erect, when letting diseased limb hang down, and from warm diet.

Predomin. better — **Predomin. worse**

In wet weather, from wrapping up,* when sitting bent forward, when lifting diseased limb, from cold diet,† when swallowing, and from change of posture (when lying or standing).

* Both remedies have predom. aggrav. from warmth of bed.

† Both remedies have aggrav. of symptoms from drinking cold water.

Platina.	Lycopodium.
Dark hair—Skin and muscles **rigid** . . .	Light hair—Skin and muscles lax.
Pains pressing inwards	Pain pressing outwards.
Neither apoplexy nor paralysis	Apoplexy—Paralysis.
Spasms with full consciousness	Spasms with unconsciousness.
Sleeplessness after midnight	Sleeplessness prevalent before midnight.
Pulse small and weak, often trembling . .	Pulse somewhat accelerated only in the evening and after meals.
External chill, with internal heat	Internal chill, with external heat.
Thirst, particularly during heat	Thirst is wanting only during chill.
Pains increase gradually, and decrease in in like manner.	Pains appear suddenly, and disappear in like manner.

Joyous or dejected; haughty; malicious .	Gentlen. *or* irritability—Distrust—Avarice.
Ailments from shame, indignation, or vexation with fright.	Ailments from grief or vexation with reserved displeasure.
Mental excitability—Ecstasies	Mental dullness predominant—Imbecility.
Complaints predominant in the spleen . .	Complaints predominant in the liver.
Catamenia too soon and profuse	Catamenia too late; at the same time scanty *or* profuse.
No expectoration with the cough	Expectoration almost constant; morning and evening.

AGGRAVATION evening and (after midnight).	AGGRAVATION morning and *from noon till midnight.*
Worse when growing warm and in warm air, better when growing cold and in cold weather.	Better (worse) when growing warm and in warm air, *or* when growing cold and in cold weather.
Worse when looking up	Worse when looking at anything revolving.*
Worse when stooping	*Better or* worse when stooping.
Worse when assuming an erect position, in bed, and from warmth of bed.	Worse *or* better when assuming an erect position, in bed, and from warmth of bed.
Almost always improved when getting out of bed or rising from a seat.	Worse *or* better when getting out of bed or rising from a seat.
Better when sitting down	Worse *or* better when sitting down.
Better *or* worse when eating	Predominantly worse when eating.
Worse after stool	*Worse or* better after stool.

Predomin. **worse** — Predomin. **better**

In the shade or dark, on an empty stomach, when ascending, and when stooping.

Predomin. **better** — Predomin. **worse**

From light, after breakfast, when descending, when rising from a seat, and after sleep.

N.B. Platina lacks the over-sensitiveness of Lycopodium to pain.

* Compare note to diagnosis of Petroleum and Lycopodium.

Platina.	Pulsatilla.
Complaints of external parts predominant .	Complaints of internal parts predominant.
Consequences of poisoning by lead . . .	Ailments from Copper vapors — *Apoplexy*—Paralysis.
Pains pressing inwards	Pains pressing outwards.
Insensibility of skin	Sensitiveness of skin. C.Hg.
Ulcers with scanty discharge	Ulcers with copious discharge of pus.
Pain increases and decreases gradually . .	P. appears suddenly, and disapp. gradually.
Sleeplessness after midnight	Sleeplessness before midnight.
Awaking too soon	Awaking too late.
Pulse sometimes trembling	Pulse sometimes intermitting; generally accelerated.
One-sided heat, left side	One-sided heat, right side.
Cold on suffering part	Heat on suffering part.
Thirst, particularly during heat	Want of thirst predominant, but is constant only during chill.
Chill increased in the open air	Chill abated in the open air.
Complaints of upper lip, spleen, upper part of chest, and fore-arm predominant.	Complaints of under lip, liver, lower part of chest, and upper arm predominant.
Joyousness *or* dejection — Haughtiness—Maliciousness.	Calm sadness of mild dispositions—Indifference— Boldness—Good-naturedness—Avarice—Distrust.
Mental excitability—Ecstasies—Insanity .	Mental dullness—Melancholy.
Ailments from shame, anger, or vexation with indignation.	Ailments from excessive joy, grief, or vexation with reserved displeasure.
Mania from onanism	M. from suppressed menstruat'n. Grauvogl.
Disturbed state of mind, also religious, with taciturnity, haughtiness, voluptiousness, and cruelty.	Melancholy, from suppressed catamenia or other secretions, with lachrymose sadness.*
Convulsions, particularly during catamenia, or *better* during catam.	Convulsions after suppressed catamenia.
Generally loss of appetite	Predominantly hunger.
Constipation predominant—When diarrhœa occurs, it is painless.	Diarrhœa predominant; generally painful.
Catamenia too soon and too profuse . . .	Catamenia too late and generally too scanty.
Cough without expectoration	Expectoration predominant, but not constant; morning and during day.
AGGRAVATION particularly evening and after midnight.	AGGRAVATION from noon till midnight.
Worse on an empty stomach	Sometimes better, but oftener aggravated after eating.
Better after sleep	Aggrav. oftener than improved after sleep.
Worse after *passive* motion (riding) . .	*Worse* after *active* motion.
Ailments from Plumbum	Ailments from Cuprum, Mercur., Sulph., etc

Predomin. worse — **Predomin. better**

On inspiration, when opening the eyes, when stretching out diseased limb, when lying on painful side, and from pressure.

Predomin. better — **Predomin. worse**

On expiration,† when closing the eyes, when drawing up diseased limb, when lying on unpainful side, from rubbing and scratching, from light and the sun, from eructation, and after sleep.

N.B. Platina lacks the over-sensitiveness of Pulsatilla to pain.

* Satiety of life, and at the same time dread of death, is found with both remedies.

† Pulsatilla has improvement as well as aggravation when "taking a deep breath."

Platina.	Rhus.
Inclination for open air—Pain pressing inwards.	Aversion to open air—Pain pressing outwards.
Anæmie	Generally plethora.
Dark hair—Hæmorrhages, blood dark . .	Light hair—Hæmorrhages, blood pale.
Pain increases and decreases gradually . .	Pain appears suddenly & disapp. gradually.
Insensibility of skin	Sensitiveness of skin. C.Hg.
Ulcers, with scanty discharge	Ulcers, with copious discharge, partic. on dropsical legs, with constant discharge of the water.
Pulse more regular than with Rhus . . .	Pulse not so regular as with Platina.
Sleeplessness after midnight—Awaking too early.	Sleeplessness more before midnight—Awaking too late.
Heat or sweat, with inclination to uncover.	Heat or sweat, with aversion to uncover.
Thirst, partic. during hot stage	Thirst not constant.
Mood changing; cheerful *or* depressed; malicious—Haughtiness.	Mood sad & despondent; rarely peevish—Rarely amorousness.
Mental excitability—Ecstasies—Insanity .	Mental dullness—Rarely insanity.
Apoplexy or paralysis not yet observed .	Apoplexy—*Paralysis.*
Costiveness predom.; when diarrhœa occurs, it is painless.	Diarrhœa generally painful.
There is no expectoration with the cough .	Expector. not constant; morning.
Compl. predom. in upper part of chest . .	Compl. predom. in lower part of chest.
Aggravation evening and after midnight.	Aggravation evening, night, and morning.
Worse when looking up	Worse when looking down.
Predom. better from light and in the sun; worse in the shade.	Worse from light; better in the dark.
Worse in bed	*Better or* worse in bed.
Generally better after sleep	*Generally* worse after sleep.
Generally worse when lying on side; better when lying on back.	Better when lying on side; worse when lying on back.
Predom. bett. when & after gett'g out of bed.	Worse *or* bett. when & after gett'g out of bed.
Better when sitting down	Worse *or* better when sitting down.
Predom. better when rising from a seat .	*Worse or* better when rising from a seat.
Better *after* rising from a seat	Worse *or* better after rising from a seat.
Worse when moving diseased part . . .	*Better or* worse when moving the part.
Worse when bending diseased part . . .	*Worse or* better when bending the part.
Worse after eating	Worse *or* better after eating.
Worse after stool	*Better or* worse after stool.
Consequences of mental exertion	Consequences of bodily exertion. C.Hg.
Ailments in consequence of poisoning with Plumbum.	Ailments from Bryonia, Ranunculus, Rhododendron, Tart. emet., etc.

Predomin. worse — **Predomin. better**

From warmth, from growing warm and in warm air, in-doors and from warmth of stove, in bed, when lying on painful side, lying on the side in general, when stretching out diseased limb or letting it hang down, when moving suffering part, from wrapping up, from pressure, after stool, in the shade, resp. in the dark.

Predomin. better — **Predomin. worse**

From cold, from growing cold and in cold weather, out-doors,* after sleep, when lying on unpainful side, when lying on back, when drawing or lifting up diseased limb, from uncovering, when rising from a seat, from eructation, and from light.

* When "*walking* out-doors" *Rhus* also has improv., principally in consequence of the motion.

Platina.	Sepia.
Inclination for open air — Pain pressing inwards.	Aversion to open air—Pain pressing outwards.
Spasms with full consciousness	Spasms with unconsciousness.
Neither apoplexy nor paralysis	Apoplexy—*Paralysis.*
Sleeplessness after midnight	Sleeplessness preval. before midnight.
Pulse small and weak; more regular than with Sepia.	Pulse quick and full, also intermitting, at night; during the day accelerated only by vexation and motion.
Cold on suffering part	Sweat on diseased part.
Thirst, partic. during the hot stage of fever.	Want of thirst; but during the chill thirst usually appears.
Taciturnity—Mood alternat.; cheerful *or* depress'd; haughty; malicious—Amorousn.	Loquacity—Mood sad and despondent; indifferent; irritable—Avarice.
Haughty contempt of one's family . . .	Indifference towards one's family. C.Hg.
Ailments from shame or mortification . .	Ailments from disappointed love, vexation.
Mania from onanism	Mania from profuse menstruation. Grauvogl.
Mental excitability; ecstasies; **insanity** .	Mental dullness—*Imbecility* or insanity—No delirium.
Short-sightedness	Far-sightedness.
Compl. predom. on upper lip, in the spleen.	Compl. predom. on lower lip & in the liver.
Urine predominantly pale	Urine predom. dark.
Sterility—Catamenia too soon	Impotence—Catam. generally too late.
No expectoration with the cough. . . .	Expector. predom., but not constant; is loosened night & morn'g, & is generally swallowed.
Remission morning, during day, and before midnight.	Remission of complaints afternoon.
Predom. better from light and in the sun; worse in the shade.	Worse from light; better in the dark.
Better in cold weather, worse in warm air.	Worse (bett.) in cold weather *or* in warm air.
Worse when lying down and in bed . . .	*Worse or* better when lying down & in bed.
Almost always improv. when and after getting out of bed.	*Better or* worse when & after getting out of bed.
Predom. better when rising from a seat .	Worse *or* better when rising from a seat.
Worse from bodily exertion	Improv. oftener than aggrav. by exertion.*
Worse on inspiration, better on expiration.	*Generally* better on inspiration, worse on expiration.
Better *or* worse when eating	Worse when eating.
Worse *after* eating	*Worse or* better after eating.
Costiveness from travelling in cars . . .	While travelling in cars headache, nausea, anxiousness, fainting. C.Hg.
Ailments from poisoning with Plumbum .	*Ailm.* fr. abuse of Sulph., Mercur., or Cinch.

Predomin **worse**	Predomin. **better**

From warmth and when growing warm, from warmth of bed, from wrapping up, when turning in bed, when lying on side, partic. lying on painful side, when rising from stooping, when moving diseased part, from bodily exertion, on inspiration, and in the shade, resp. in the dark.

Predomin. **better**	Predomin. **worse**

From cold and when growing cold, from uncovering, when lying on back or when lying on unpainful side, on expiration, from light, and from rubbing and scratching.

N.B. Platina lacks the over-sensitiveness of Sepia to pain; the latter almost always lacks the sensation of numbness in suffering parts peculiar to Platina.

* Both remedies have headache very much increased by the least motion. C.Hg.

Plumbum.	Lycopodium.
Dark hair—Skin & muscles predom. rigid.	Light hair—Skin and muscles lax.
Pain piercing inwards—Stitches in internal parts.	Pain piercing outwards—Stitches in external parts.
Compl. predom. on outside of nose, on lower gum, on upper arm, and thigh.	Compl. predom. on inside of nose, on upper gum, on fore-arm, and on leg.
The whole left side as if "gone to sleep" .	The whole right side "gone to sleep."
Paralysis more frequent than apoplexy . .	Apoplexy more frequent than paralysis.
Painful paralysis predominant	Painless paralysis.
Pulse generally slow, small, compressed; more irregular than with Lycop.; sometimes intermitting.	Pulse somewhat accelerated only in the evening and after meals.
Thirst constant	Thirst is wanting only during chill.
Rarely dejection—Rarely amorousness . .	Mood changing; peevish; irritable; malicious—Avarice—Haughtiness.
No fancies—Rarely unconsciousness . . .	Absent-mindedness – Fancies.
Imbecility more frequent than insanity . .	Insanity more frequent than imbecility.
Appetite for bread	Aversion to bread, partic. to rye-bread.
Vomiting bile	Vomit sour oftener than bitter.
Urine not often enough and scanty . . .	Urine too often, but scanty.
Prostatorrhœa	Seminal emissions predom.
Catamenia too soon	Catamenia too late.
Fluent coryza predominant	Coryza dry oftener than fluent.
Remission of complaints forenoon . . .	Remission after midnight and *forenoon*.
Worse when in company; better when alone.	Worse (better) when in company *or* alone.
Worse when looking up	Worse wh. look'g at anyth'g which revolves.
Worse (better) when ascending *or* descending.	Predom. better when ascending, worse when descending.
Worse when stooping and when rising . .	*Better or* worse when stooping; worse *or* better when rising.
Worse when sneezing	*Worse or* better when sneezing.
Worse when perspiring and in bed . . .	Worse *or* better when perspiring; the same when in bed.
Brandy is a relative preventive of lead-colic.	Complaints from spirituous liquors.
Worse or better from eructation	Better from eructation.
Generally better after stool	*Generally* worse after stool.
Better in cloudy weather	Worse in wet weather.
Better from exertion, tension of the abdominal muscles, etc.	Worse from exertion, drawing in the abdomen, etc.

Predomin. worse — **Predomin. better**

From motion, when walking, when sitting bent forward, when stooping, from eructation, in extended posture, and before breakfast.

Predomin. better — **Predomin. worse**

During rest, when standing, sitting erect, when lying, in contracted posture, after breakfast, from touch & pressure, from brandy, with a cold in the head, in cloudy weather & from bodily exert'n, after stool.

N.B. Plumbum lacks the sensation of numbness in suffering parts, which is frequent with Lycopodium.

Plumbum.	Pulsatilla.
Upper right, lower left side—**Aversion** to open air.	Upper left, lower right side—**Inclination** for open air.
Paralysis (particularly of extensores) much oftener than apoplexy.	**Apoplexy** oftener than paralysis.
Painful paralys.—**Painless** swell'g of glands.	**Painless** paralysis—**Painful** swell'g of glands.
Itching, relieved by sratching	**Itch'g**, unchanged *or* aggrav. by scratch'g.
Insensibility of skin	**Sensitiveness** of skin. C. Hg.
Pulse very different; unequal; generally slow, small, and compressed.	**Pulse** predom. frequent, small, and weak; sometimes imperceptible.
Cold on suffering part	**Heat** on suffering part.
Partial sweat on front part of body . . .	**Partial** sweat on back of body.
Chill, increased by motion & in the open air.	**Chill**, lessened by motion & in the open air.
Thirst constant	**Want of thirst** predom., but is constant only during chill.

Plumbum.	Pulsatilla.
Rarely dejectedness—**Rarely** amorousness.	**Mood** changing; indifferent; peevish —Boldness—Avarice.
Rarely unconsciousness — **Imbecility** more frequent than insanity.	**Absent-mindedness**—**Fancies**—**Melancholy**.
Subjective putrid smell	*Objective* stench from nose, or *subjective* pleasant odor, or smell of old catarrh.
Saliva generally diminished	**Saliva** generally increased.
Appetite for bread—**Constipation** predom.	**Aversion** to bread—**Diarrhœa** predom.
Retention of urine	**Incontinence** oftener than retention of urine.
Remission of colic after stool	**Bellyache** after stool.
Catamenia too soon and generally profuse.	**Catam.** too late and generally scanty.
Milk decreased	**Milk** generally increased.
Expectoration almost constant	**Expectoration** not constant.
Complaints predom. on thigh	**Complaints** predom. on leg.

Plumbum.	Pulsatilla.
Remission of complaints forenoon	**Remission** from midnight till noon.
Better with fluent coryza	**Worse** with cold in head.
Worse when taking a deep breath . . .	**Better** *or* worse when taking a deep breath.
Worse when stooping and when rising . .	*Worse or* better when stoop'g & when ris'g.
Worse *or* better when getting out of bed .	*Better or* worse when getting out of bed.
Better *after* rising from bed or a seat . .	*Better or* worse *after* ris'g fr bed or a seat.
Worse when bending suffering part . .	**Better** *or* worse when bend'g suffer'g part.
Worse when stretching out diseased limb, better when drawing it up.	*Generally* better when stretching out diseased limb, worse when drawing it up.
Worse when swallowing	*Worse or* better when swallowing; in the latter case worse *after* swallowing.*
Worse after eating	*Worse or* better after eating.
Lead-colic is relatively prevented by alcoholic drinks.	**Compl.** from brandy and other spirituous liquors.

Predomin. worse —— **Predomin. better**

From motion, when walking, on inspiration, when bending suffering part sideways, when stretching out diseased limb, from cold diet.

Predomin. better —— **Predomin. worse**

During rest, when stand'g, on expiration, when draw'g up diseased limb, from warm diet, fr. alcoholic drinks, with cold in the head (coryza), in cloudy weather, from touch,† from rubb'g & scratching.

N.B. Plumbum lacks the sensation of numbness in suffering parts peculiar to Pulsatilla.

---

* The aggravation with Pulsatilla is particularly when swallowing saliva.

† Both remedies have predom. improv. from pressure.

Plumbum.	Sulphur.
Right side, particularly *upper right, lower left side.*	*Left* side, particularly *upper left, lower right side.*
Piercing pain, inwards	Piercing pain, outwards.
Painful paralysis predominant; generally of the upper limbs.	Painless paralysis; generally of the lower limbs.
Somnolence predominant	Sleeplessness predominant; particularly before midnight.
Pulse generally slow, small, compressed, more unequal than with Sulph.	Pulse generally accelerated, full, and hard.
Sweat on front of body	Sweat on back of body.
Thirst constant	Thirst mostly during heat; during chill generally want of thirst.
Rarely sadness—Distrust	Mood changing; indifferent; peevish; irritable.
Imbecility more frequent than insanity . . .	Absent-mindedness — Fancies—Insanity more frequent than imbecility.
Subjective putrid smell	Predom. objective stench from nose.
Hunger predominant—Appetite for bread .	Generally loss of appetite—Aversion to bread, partic. rye-bread.
Vomiting bile	Vomit sour oftener than bitter.
Urine not often enough and scanty	U. often, but scanty; copious after strong doses.
Catamenia too soon	Catamenia generally too late.
Expectoration nearly constant	Expectoration not constant; morning and during day, less frequently at night.
Complaints predominant on upper arm and top of foot.	Complaints predominant on fore-arm and sole of foot.
Remission of complaints forenoon	Remission afternoon and before midnight.
Worse when looking up	Worse when looking down, partic. at running water.
Predom. better from exertion, tension of the abdominal muscles, etc.	Predom. worse from exertion, walking fast, running, etc.
Worse when taking a deep breath	Worse *or* better when taking a deep breath.
Worse while perspiring, in bed, from change of posture, when sneezing, when swallowing, after drinking, and after passing urine.	*Worse or* better while perspiring, in bed, from change of posture, when sneezing, when swallow'g, after drink'g, & after pass'g urine.
Predom. worse on an empty stomach; better after breakfast.	Better (worse) on an empty stomach *or* after breakfast.
Worse or better from eructation	Almost always improved by eructation.
Lead-colic is relatively prevented by alcoholic drinks.	Complaints from brandy and other spirituous liquors.
Worse *or* better when getting out of bed . . .	Better when getting out of bed.
Better after getting out of bed	Better *or* worse after getting out of bed.
Worse (better) when ascending *or* descending.	*Generally* worse when ascending, better when descending.
Worse when stooping and when rising . . .	*Worse or* better when stoop'g and when ris'g.
Predom. better from touch	*Worse or* better from touch.
Better with fluent coryza	Worse with a cold in the head.
Worse when idle	Worse from being overhurried.

Predomin. worse — **Predomin. better**

From motion, when walking, when letting diseased limb hang down, from eructation, and in extended posture.

Predomin. better — **Predomin. worse**

During rest, when standing, when lifting diseased limb, from bodily exertion, from alcoholic drinks, in a contracted posture, from touch,* with cold in the head (coryza), and in cloudy weather.

N.B. Plumbum lacks the sensation of numbness in suffering parts, which we find with Sulph.; the latter, on the other hand, rarely has the over-sensitiveness of Plumbum to pain.

* Both remedies have predominant improvement from "pressure."

Pulsatilla.	Rhus.
Compl. in internal parts—Rarely paralysis	Complaints in external parts—Paralysis.
Inclination for open air—Aversion to motion.	Aversion to open air—Inclination for motion.
Hæmorrhages, blood dark	Hæmorrhages, blood pale.
Pulse suppressed, with strong beat of heart	Pulse sometimes oftener than beating of heart.
Heat on diseased part—Heat on upper part of body, chill on lower part.	Sweat or coldness on diseased part—Chill or heat on upper part of body.
Chill on front part of body—Heat or sweat predom. right side.	Partial chill on back part of body—Heat or sweat predom. left side.
Local sweat on head	Sweat general, with exception of head.
Sweat often confined to back part of body	Coldness on back part of body; heat or sweat on front part of body.
Want of thirst predom., constant during chill.	Thirst not constant.
Chill lessened by motion—Heat lessened by washing.	Chill increased by motion.—Heat aggrav. by washing.
Itching, aggrav. *or* unchanged by scratching.	Itching, relieved by scratching.
Mood changing; indifferent—Boldness	Mood rarely peevish—Rarely amorousness.
Absent-mindedness	Rarely absent-mindedness.
Vertigo, inclining to fall backwards	Vert., inclining to fall forwards *or* backwards.
Pupils generally contracted	Pupils dilated.
Swelling of lower lip predom.	Swelling of upper lip predom.
Generally hunger—Appetite for spirit. liquors.	Generally loss of appetite—Aversion to wine.
Nausea in throat, stomach or abdomen	N. in œsoph. *or* stomach, less frequ. in throat.
Bellyache after stool	Bellyache better after stool.
Urine not often enough and scanty—Sediment red—Stream small.	Urine too often and copious—Sediment white—Stream spreading.
Catam. too late, of short durat. & gen. scanty.	Catam. too soon, of long duration, and profuse.
Expect. pred., not constant; morn. & dur. day.	Exp. not constant; sometimes in the morning.
Compl. predom. on upper arm and sole of foot.	Complaints pred. on fore-arm and top of foot.
AGGRAVATION afternoon & evening, after sunset until midnight.	AGGRAVATION from evening until *morning*.
Worse before a thunder-storm	Worse during increase of moon.
Worse when looking up	Worse when looking down.
Worse while perspiring	*Worse or* better while perspiring.
Predom. worse in bed	*Better or* worse in bed.
Generally better when getting out of bed and *after* getting up.	Better *or* worse when getting out of bed; *generally* aggrav. *after* getting up.
Generally worse lying on side, better on back.	Better lying on the side, worse on back.
Generally improv. after rising from a seat	Worse *or* better after rising from a seat.
Worse or better when assum'g an erect posit.	Alm. alw. aggrav. when rising from stooping.
Better *or* worse when taking a deep breath	Worse when taking a deep breath.
Generally better from exertion, running, &c.	Worse from bodily exertion.
Better when bending the head sideways	Better when bending the head backwards.
Generally worse when letting diseased limb hang down; better when lifting it	Better when letting diseased limb hang down; worse when lifting it.
Almost always aggrav. when eating	Worse *or* better when eating.
Worse after drinking	*Worse or* better after drinking.
Worse or better from eructation	Worse from eructation.
Worse when swallowing saliva	Worse when swallowing saliva or food.
Worse after mental exertion	Worse after bodily exertion. C. Hg.

Predomin. **worse** — Predomin. **better**

In-doors and from warmth of stove, from warmth, when growing warm and in warm air, from warm diet, from wrapping up, in bed, when lying on side, after perspiring, on expiration, when bending the head backwards, when letting diseased limb hang down, and from rubbing and scratching.

Predomin. **better** — Predomin. **worse**

Out of doors,* from cold, from growing cold and in cold weather, from cold diet, from uncovering, after getting out of bed, when lying on back, on inspiration, when washing and moistening the suffering part,† when lifting diseased limb, and from bodily exertion.

N.B. Rhus lacks the over-sensitiveness of Pulsat to pain.—Both remedies have sensitiveness to touch

* Both have improv. "when *walking* out-doors,"—Rhus more in consequence of motion than of the open air.

† Both have aggrav. from getting wet feet and in wet weather.

Pulsatilla.	Sepia.
Compl. (cramp'g pain, &c.) pred. in int. parts.	l. (cramp'g pain, &c.) pred. in ext. parts.
Inclination for open air—Rarely paralysis	Aversion to open air—Paralysis of limbs.
Hot and painful swelling of glands	Painless swelling of glands.
Itching, aggrav. *or* unchanged by scratching.	Itching, always aggrav. by scratching.
Eruptions more humid than dry	Eruptions mostly dry.
Sweat often confined to the head	Sw. on the head *or* general, with exc. of head.
Want of thirst predom., but is constant only during chill.	Want of thirst pred.; only during chill thirst is usual.
Heat or chill, lessened by motion & out-doors.	Heat or chill, increased by motion & out-doors.
Heat on suffering part	Sweat on suffering part.
Pulse generally small, weak, but *frequent*, partic. in the evening, slow in the morning.	Pulse quick and full or frequent during night, slow by day; irregular; somet. trembling.
Taciturnity	Loquacity.
Mood gentle; distrustful—Boldness	M. irritable—Rarely amorousn.—No delirium.
Mania from suppressed menstruation	Mania from profuse menstruation. Grauvogl.
Short-sightedness—Opt. illus. in bright colors.	Far-sightedness—Opt. illusions in dark colors.
Objective stench fr. nose; *subject.* pleasant od.	Subjective putrid odor predom.
Nose-bleed'g, with scanty or suppress. menstr.	Nose-bleeding, with pregnancy or with hæmorrhoids. C.Hg.
Bloated *under* the eyes	Bloated *above* the eyes.
Generally hunger	Generally loss of appetite.
Urinal sediment red	Urinal sediment *red or* white.
Catamenia of too short duration, and generally scanty.	Catamenia lasting too long, at the same time generally too profuse.
Fluent coryza of the right nostril	Fluent coryza of the left nostril.
Expectoration morning and by day	Expectoration is loosened night and morning, and is generally swallowed.
Milk mostly increased	Milk diminished.
Complaints predom. on upper arm	Complaints predom. on fore-arm.
Remission from midnight till noon	Remission of complaints afternoon.
Worse in warm air; better in cold weather	Better (worse) in warm *or* cold air.
Worse in-doors; better in the open air	Better (worse) in-doors *or* in the open air.
Worse while perspiring	*Worse or* better while perspiring.
Worse from warmth of bed	*Generally* better from warmth of bed.
Almost always aggrav. after lying down, when lying, and in bed.	*Worse or* better after lying down, while lying, and in bed.
Generally worse when lying on side; better when lying on back.	Predom. better when lying on side; worse when lying on back.
Mostly worse after sleep	Better after sleep; but worse when disturbed.
Worse or better from change of posture, when lying or standing.	Better when turning in bed.
Worse or better when rising from stooping	Almost always improv. when rising.
Worse *or* better when sitting down	Better when sitting down.
Better or worse after rising from a seat	Better after rising from a seat.
Better or worse when moving diseased part	Almost always improv. when moving the part.
Better *or* worse when bending the part	Worse when bending diseased part.
Mostly better from pressure	Predom. worse from pressure.
Worse before a thunder-storm	Worse dur. new moon *or* bef. a thunder-storm.
Worse when closing, better when opening eyes.	Pred. better when closing, worse when opening the eyes.
Worse or better when swallowing; partic. worse when swallowing saliva.	Worse when swallowing food.
Better or worse after stool	Almost always aggrav. after stool.

Predomin. better —— **Predomin. worse**

In wet weather, from warmth and when growing warm, from wrapping up, from warmth of bed, after sleep, when lying on side, when closing the eyes, when rising from stooping, when drawing up diseased limb, from change of posture, from smoking, and from loosening the clothes.

Predomin. worse —— **Predomin. better**

In dry weather, from warmth and cold and when growing cold, from uncovering, from washing and moistening diseased part, when lying on back, when opening the eyes, when stretching out diseased limb, from acids, after stool, from pressure,* from tying the clothes tight.

N.B. We rarely find the sensation of numbness in suffering parts peculiar to Pulsatilla with Sepia.

* The symptoms of both remedies are aggrav. "by *touch*."

Pulsatilla.	Stannum.
Right side—Complaints predominant in internal parts.	*Left* side—Complaints predominant in external parts.
Itching in external parts	Itching in internal parts.
Cutaneous eruptions predominantly humid.	Eruptions dry.
Complaints predominant in lower part of chest, in the liver, and in the hollow of elbow.	Complaints predominant in upper part of chest, in the spleen, and on tip of elbow.
First chill, then heat	First heat, then chill.
Heat abated by motion	Heat increased by motion.
Want of thirst predominant	Thirst predominant.
More thirst *before* the heat than *after* it .	Thirst particularly between heat and sweat.
Mood changing; indifferent; distrustful—Boldness – Avarice—Absent-mindedness.	Mood rarely peevish — Rarely amorousness—No delirium.
Apoplexy	No apoplexy.
Appetite for beer	Aversion to beer.
Diarrhœa predominant	Constipation predominant.
Catamenia too late and generally scanty .	Catamenia too soon and profuse.
Mostly fluent coryza, particularly right side.	Dry coryza predominant.
Expectoration morning and by day . . .	Expectorat'n particularly by day and even'g.
REMISSION from midnight till noon . .	REMISSION of complaints after midnight and during day.
Better *or* worse when taking a deep breath.	Better when taking a deep breath.
Worse or better when swallowing . . .	*Better or* worse when swallowing.
Better while drinking, worse *afterwards* .	Better while eating, worse *afterwards*.
Worse or better from eructation . . .	Worse from eructation.
Better or worse after stool	Worse after stool.
Worse or better after sleep	Worse after sleep.
Better or worse after rising from bed or a seat.	Better after rising from bed or a seat.
Better or worse when mov'g diseased part.	Better when moving diseased part.
Better *or* worse when bend'g suffer'g part.	Worse when bending suffering part.
Mostly worse when letting the limb hang down, better when lifting it.	*Mostly* better when letting the limb hang down, better when lifting it.
Mostly worse when drawing up diseased limb, better when stretching it out.	Better (worse) when drawing up diseased limb *or* when stretching it out.
Worse when swallowing saliva	Worse when swallowing drink.

Predomin. worse ——— **Predomin. better**

When swallowing and eating, when letting suffering limb hang down, and from loosening the clothes.

Predomin. better ——— **Predomin. worse**

After stool, when lifting diseased limb, when bending suffering part sideways, when washing or moistening it, when getting out of bed, from tying the clothes tight, and from weeping.

N.B. Stannum lacks the over-sensitiveness of Pulsatilla to pain.

Pulsatilla.	Sulphur.
Right side — Increased irritability — Inclination for open air—Pinching pain in internal parts.	*Left* side—Want of bodily irritability—Aversion to open air—Pinching pain in external parts.
Painful eruptions — Itching, aggrav. *or* unchanged by scratching.	Painless eruptions—Itching, predom. relieved by scratching.
Apoplexy more frequent than paralysis . .	Paralysis more frequent than apoplexy.
Complaints predom. on inner angle of eye or inner side of gums, in lower part of chest, and on upper arm.	Complaints predom. on external angle of eye, on outer side of gums, in upper part of chest, and on fore-arm
Pulse frequent, small, and weak; partic. frequent evenings, slow mornings.	Pulse frequent, full, and hard, partic. frequent night and morn'g, slower dur. day & even'g.
Heat on suffering part — Heat on upper part of body.	Coldn. on suffering part—Heat on lower part of body, or general, with exception of head.
Want of thirst predom.	Thirst predom., but not constant.
Heat lessened by washing	Heat increased by washing.
Sweat lessened when walking out-doors . .	Sweat increased when walking out-doors.
Satiety of life with fear of death—Boldness—Avarice—Distrust.	Satiety of life, with longing for death — Embarrassment—Mood serious, solemn.
Optical illusions in bright colors	Optical illusions in dark colors.
Swelling of lower lip predom.	Swelling of upper lip predom.
Generally increased secret. of saliva & hunger.	Gen. dimin. secret. of saliva & loss of appetite.
Desire for beer and spirituous liquors . . .	Desire for *or* aversion to beer & spirit. liquors.
Nausea in throat, stomach or abdomen . . .	Nausea in stomach, less frequently in throat.
Vomit bitter oftener than sour	Vomit sour oftener than bitter.
Urine not often and scanty; smells like Ammoniac; red sediment.	Urine often, but scanty, sometimes copious; sour; sediment white oftener than red.
During suppress. menstruation milk in breasts.	During suppressed menstruation hæmorrhoidal [tumors. C.Hg.
Milk mostly increased	Milk diminished.
Expectoration predom. (not constant) morning and during day.	Expectoration not constant; morning and during day; less frequently at night.
REMISSION from midnight till noon	REMISSION afternoon and before midnight.
Worse when looking up	Worse when look'g down, part. at runn. water.
Worse when sneezing; better from weeping .	*Worse or* better from sneezing or weeping.
Worse when closing, better opening the eyes.	Better (worse) when closing *or* opening eyes.
Pred. *worse* after sleep, and pred. better after getting out of bed.*	Worse after sleep; better getting out of bed.
Worse from touch	*Worse or* better from touch.
Mostly better from tying the clothes tight; worse from loosening them.	Worse from tying the clothes tight; better from loosening them.
Worse on empty stomach, better after breakf.	Better on empty stomach, worse after breakf.
Nearly always aggrav. when eating	Better *or* worse when eating.
Worse or better after meals	Worse after meals.
Better from vegetable diet; worse from meat.	Worse from vegetables *or* from meat.
Worse or better from eructation	Nearly always improv. by eructation.
Worse when growing warm and in warm air; better when growing cold & in cold weather.	Worse (better) when growing warm & in warm air, *or* when growing cold & in cold weather.

Predomin. worse ——— **Predomin. better**

From warmth of stove,† from warm diet, from **eructation**, in extended posture, when lying on unpainful side, when drawing up diseased limb or letting it hang down, *from loosening the clothes*, on expiration, and from scratching.

Predomin. better ——— **Predomin. worse**

From cold diet and from drinking cold water, from acids, from vegetable diet, in contracted posture, when lying on painful side, when stretching out or lifting diseased limb, *from tying the clothes tight*, on inspiration, from washing and moistening the suffering part, fr. bodily exertion, running, &c.

N.B Sulph. generally lacks the over-sensitiveness of Pulsat. to pain, but not the sensitiveness to touch.

* "Almost always improved when sitting down, and worse when rising from a seat; better afterwards," characterizes the Sulph.; Puls. has also the opposite; moving diseased part is pred. aggravating in Sulph., pred. improving in Puls.

† Both remedies have aggrav. "*in crowded rooms.*"

Pulsatilla.	Sulphur. acid.
Upper left, lower right side—The right side is generally affected.	Upper right, lower left side—Left side, principally, is affected. C.Hg.
Apoplexy	One-sided paralysis of limbs. C.Hg.
Complaints (pinching pain, etc.) predom. in internal parts.	Complaints (pinching pain, etc.) predom. in external parts.
Often indicated with children and young women.	Oftener indicated with old people than with children, (particularly old women. C.Hg.)
Pain pressing outwards	Pain pressing inwards.
Complaints predominant on lower jaw, in lower part of chest, and in the liver.	Complaints predominant on upper jaw, in upper part of chest, and in the spleen.
Itching aggravated *or* unchanged by scratching.	Itching changing its locality, less frequently relieved, by scratching.
Moles, freckles, particularly in young girls.	Blue spots after a fall, particularly in old women. C.Hg.
Sleeplessness before midnight	Sleeplessness after midnight.
Awaking late	Awaking too early.
Palpitation of heart, with fear	Palpitation of heart, without fear.
Pulse predominantly affected by beer & coffee.	Pulse affected by alcoholic drinks. C.Hg.
One-sided heat, right side	One-sided heat, left side.
Want of thirst predominant, but constant only during chill.	Thirst predominant.
Gentleness—Indifference—Boldness—Avarice—Rarely mental dullness—Fancies.	Seriousness—Rarely peevishness—Rarely amorousness—Mental excitability predominant—Rarely absent-mindedness—No unconsciousness.
Jerks in the head, particularly during hot stage and in-doors; better from motion in the open air.	Jerks in the head, better in-doors and from warmth, worse from motion in the open air.
Generally hunger	Loss of appetite predominant.
Nausea in throat, stomach, or abdomen	Nausea in stomach.
Vomiting, particularly first food, then water.	Vomiting, particularly first water, then food.
Diarrhœa predominant—Urinal sediment reddish.	Constipat'n of bowels predominant—Urinal sediment yellow.
Catamenia too late, generally scanty	Catamenia too soon and profuse.
Generally fluent coryza	Dry coryza predominant.
Expectoration predominant, but not constant; morn'g & dur'g day.	Expectoration predominant; morning.
AGGRAVATION from noon till midnight; partic. in the afternoon.	AGGRAVATION from midnight till noon, and evening; partic. dur'g forenoon C.Hg.
Ailments from Copper vapors and from spirituous liquors.	Ailments from smelling coffee and after taking brandy, but improv. by drink'g wine.
Consequences of a concussion, fall, or being bruised; partic. bruised pain in the bones, and sore pain when touched.	Consequences of pressure, concussion, or being bruised with a dull instrument; partic. soreness in young people, or blue spots in old people. C.Hg.

Predomin. worse ——— **Predomin. better**

In-doors, from warmth, during rest, on expiration, and from rubbing.

Predomin better ——— **Predomin. worse**

Out-doors, from cold, from motion,* from bodily exertion, and on inspiration.

N.B. Sulph. acid. lacks the over-sensitiveness of Pulsatilla to pain, but not the sensitiveness to touch.

* Yet Pulsatilla has aggravation "in the beginning of motion," either aggravation *or* improvement "when moving diseased part."

Pulsatilla.	Thuya.
Right side—(Coldness, heat, and other compl.)	*Left* side predom.—(Chill, coldness, and other complaints.
Sweating of uncovered parts; but sweat often disappears in bed.	Sweating of uncovered parts, but often also in bed.
Sweat only on head	Sweat general, with exception of heat.
First chill, then heat	First heat, then chill.
Fainting during the chill	Fainting during heat or sweat. C.Hg.
Generally want of thirst during hot stage . .	Thirst predom. during hot stage.
Chill, lessened in the open air	Chill, increased in the open air.
Complaints predom. in internal parts . . .	Compl. predom. in external parts.
Apoplexy — Nervous paralysis	No apopl.—Paralysis with atrophy of muscles.
Compl. predom. on inside of gums, in lower part of chest, on upper arm, back of hand, leg, and sole of foot.	Compl. predom. on outside of gums, in upper part of chest, on fore-arm, palm of hand, thigh, and top of foot.
Itching, aggrav. *or* unchanged by scratching.	Itching, relieved by scratching.
Hot, painful swelling of glands	Cold, painless swelling of glands.
Awaking too late	Awaking too early.
Mood changing; gentle; indifferent; distrustful—Avarice—Boldness.	Mood serious; haughty; irritable — Rarely amorousness.
Rarely mental dullness—Melancholy . . .	Rarely unconsciousness or delirium — Imbecility or mental excitability.
Eyes sunken	Eyes protruding.
Saliva mostly increased	Saliva mostly diminished.
Generally hunger	Loss of appetite predom.
Food tastes too salty	Food tastes as though salted too little.
Diarrhœa predom.—Urine too seldom & scanty.	Costiveness predom.—Urine too oft. & copious.
Catamenia too late	Catamenia predom. too soon.
Fluent coryza (partic. right side) oftener than dry.	Fluent coryza (partic. left side) in the open air; dry coryza in the room.
Expectoration predom., but not constant; morning and during day.	Expector. nearly constant; evening.
Remission from midnight till noon*	Remission forenoon† and before midnight.
Worse in the sun	Worse in the moon-light.
Worse in warm air; better in cold weather .	Better (worse) in warm *or* cold air.
Worse when closing, better when opening the eyes.	Better (worse) when closing *or* when opening the eyes.
Predom. worse in-doors, better in the open air.	*Generally* bett. in-doors, worse in the open air.
Predom. better from washing and moistening the part.	*Generally* worse from washing, etc.
Better or worse when getting out of bed . .	Worse when getting out of bed.
Worse or better when rising from a seat . .	Worse when rising from a seat.
Worse or better when swallowing, after eating, and from eructation.	Worse when swallowing and after eating; better from eructation.
Generally worse when lying on side, better when lying on back.	*Generally* better when lying on side, worse when lying on back.

Predomin. worse —— **Predomin. better**

In-doors, when lying on unpainful side, when drawing up diseased limb, from loosening the clothes, when bending the suffering part backwards, partic. the head, when sneezing, after perspiring, from eructation, on expiration, from touch, and from rubbing and scratching.

Predomin. better —— **Predomin. worse**

In the open air, when lying on the painful side, when stretching out diseased limb, from tying the clothes tight, when getting out of bed, from bodily exertion, from washing and moistening suffering part, from sour things, and on inspiration.

N.B. Thuya has neither the over-sensitiveness of Pulsatilla to pain, nor the sensation of numbness in suffering parts peculiar to the latter.

---

* Except diarrhœa. C.Hg.

† According to the Vienna provings with strong doses of the tincture, & Wolf's provings in Berlin with high potencies, the "forenoon remission" cannot be admitted, but in both remedies the afternoon is still the predominant part of the day. C.Hg.

Rheum.	Chamomilla.
Upper right, lower left side	Upper left, lower right side.
Bubbling, partic. in the joints, mostly elbow and knee.	Cracking of the joints, particularly lower extremities.*
Wrist and knee predominantly affected .	Finger-joints and toes predom. affected.*
Lameness	Weakness as if beaten.*
Anasarca	Chafing of skin.*
Pulse generally unaltered; only a little accelerated.	Pulse changed, generally frequent, small, & tense; sometimes irregular.
Pulse full & accelerated, partic. in the even'g.	Pulse accelerated, but not full.*
Want of thirst, partic. during hot stage	Thirst during all stages, partic. the heat.*
Disposition to sweat easily in diseases without fever.	Dryness of skin (following excessive sweating).
Children cry and toss about all night; delirious talking; full of fear.	Child. cannot remain in bed, will be carried about; inhalation shortened.
Child is pale, quarrels, frets in sleep; with convulsive startings in the fingers.	Child lies with open mouth, snoring in a hot, viscous sweat, partic. on fore-head, with a serious or vexed sad face.
During sleep heat, jerking motion of the muscles in the face or eyelids (similar to Bryonia), trembling, moving the limbs, bending head backwards.	During sleep starting, crying, tossing about, snoring, moaning, weeping.*
Arms and hands overhead during sleep	Lower limbs stretched or drawn up; knees spread asunder in sleep.*
Anxious fears—Fear of death—Indolence—Dislikes to talk.	Anxious feeling in the heart—Excitability—Seriousness—Is lost in thought.
Wants what is not to be had, and dislikes what is offered to him.	Undecided; impatient; obstinate; quarrelsome; vehement.*
Delirium predominant	Talking in sleep; rarely delirious.*
Vertigo, with heaviness or beat'g in the head.	Vert., with loss of sight, diarrhœa, fainting.*
Pupils dilated, with pressing headache; later contracted, with internal restlessness.	Pupils contracted; after consciousness returns, dilated.*
One or both cheeks pale, cool face, hot hands and feet; forehead perspiring from the least motion.	Pale or red face, partic. cheeks red; often one-sided; hot face, with general coldness.*
Pale face with the diarrhœa	Sweat on face with the colic.*
Salivation with the colic or diarrhœa . .	Salivation, with dryness of the mouth and tongue, and with thirst.*
Salivation with the toothache, & cold sensation in the teeth.	Salivation, with rheumatic toothache and swelling of cheeks.*
Bitter taste of food, even sweets	Bitter taste, partic. in the morning *
Sour taste in the mouth	Bread tastes sour.*
Insipid or nauseous taste in mouth . . .	Everything tastes like rancid fat.*
The child wants different things, but cannot eat them.	Child does not want anything.*
When eating, is very soon satisfied or as if he had overloaded his stomach.	Appetite comes while eating.*
Nausea in stomach or abdomen	Nausea in stomach.*
After dinner colic	After the meals distension of abdomen.*
Bellyache after dinner; worse when standing.	After dinner bellyache; worse when lying, partic. on the unpainful side.*
Colic from eating prunes	Colic from coffee or milk.*
Copious diarrhœa, with violent colic, tenesmus, vomiting, chill & fever, great thirst, general sweat, prostration, restlessness, and fear of death.	Pain around the navel when awaking from sleep, remission during day; child smells sour, also from the mouth.
Diarrhœa worse from change of weather	Diarrhœa from taking cold.*

(Continued.)

Rheum.	Chamomilla
With suckling children painless diarrhœa, bright-yellow, with much slime. The children are very fretful, cry much, stiffening themselves, stool like soap-sud, sour, mostly in the evening; during the night vomiting and great restlessness.	With suckling children bilious, slimy, yellow-greenish diarhœa, like curdled eggs, with rumbling, expansion of belly, cutting, griping pain, no appetite, restlessness, crying.*
Diarrhœa during dentition, with frequent urging, tossing about — Discharge sour, curdled or fermented, frothy, turning green, reddening the anus; with pale face and salivation; worse from walking, moving about, partic. while standing.	Diarrh. during dentition—Discharge white, hot, slimy, or watery; green or yellow, brown; smells like rotten eggs or scentless, with much wind; rumbl'g in bowels; no appetite, thirst, tongue furred; (bitter) belching; attempts to vomit; after it burning and biting in anus; dry mouth & tongue, thirst, expansion, hardness of abdomen; *worse after eating;* abdomen sore to the touch.*
Burning in bladder before & with urination.	Like labor-pain bef. urinat'n, burn'g in bladder & urethra, and anxiety dur'g urinat'n.*
Boring down in uterine region while stand'g.	Bearing down pain; worse when lying.*
In childbed watery diarrhœa, with great weakness.	In childbed milky-white diarrhœa, while the milk disappears from the breasts.*
Both nipples hurt, sting; she says from wind in the abdomen.	Nipples sore, inflamed, festering.*
Yellow, bitter milk	Spoiled milk.*
Expectoration not constant; morning . .	Expector. seldom; during day.*
Most weariness in thighs all day	Weariness most in feet and at night.*
Limbs fall asleep, mostly the lower, when putting one over the other.	Arms fall asleep when taking a firm hold the toes when sitting.*
Compl. predom. on top of foot	Compl. predom. on sole of foot.*
AGGRAVATION night and morning . . .	AGGRAVATION evening and night partic before midnight.
Bad effects from Cantharides†	Bad effects of Coffee, Senna, Valeriana (and narcotics, partic. Opium*).
Worse from cold, better from warmth . .	Generally better fr. cold, worse fr. warmth.
Worse from uncovering, better from wrapping up.	Better (worse) from uncovering *or* from wrapping up.
Worse after sleep	*Worse or* better after sleep.
Better after getting out of bed .	*Worse or* better after getting out of bed.
Worse (better) when drawing up diseased limb or when stretching it out	Predom. better when drawing up the limb, worse when stretching it out.
Worse while walking (headache, tenesmus, pressing in inguinal ring).	Worse when beginning to walk.*
Better when eating, *worse afterwards* . .	Predom. worse when and after eating.
Worse or better after stool	*Better or* worse after stool.

Predomin. worse — **Predomin. better**

From cold, from motion, when walking, when lying on painful side, and after stool.

Predomin. better — **Predomin. worse**

From warmth, during rest, after lying down, while lying and standing, when lying on unpainful side,‡ after getting out of bed, when swallowing and eating.

N.B. The over-sensitiveness of Chamomilla to pain has not yet been observed with Rheum. H. Gr. Likewise not its over-sensibility of all senses and also against cold air.*

† Both are useful in ailments caused by abuse of Magnesia, Rheum particularly in abdominal complaints; Chamom. partic. in neuralgies; both act complimentary to Magnesia carbonica; in both the direction is from l. to r.; both have symptoms worse on inspiration, and with both the wind seems to rise from below the ribs into the chest.*

‡ By Chamom. pain in left hip increases while lying on right side.*

* Added by C.Hg.

Rheum.	Nux vomica.
Left side Neither apoplexy nor paralysis.	*Right* side†—Apoplexy—Paralysis.
In the joints: lameness, most in wrists and knees; after sprains and dislocations.	Joints: cracking and dryness predom. in lower limbs, partic. knees and toes; *disposed* to sprain or dislocate them.*
Beating in joints, painful by moving . . .	Pressing pain in joints worse from moving.
Anasarca	No anasarca—Contraction of skin.*
Restless nights, with tossing about or starting; *takes the queerest position to be able to rest awhile.*	Restless nights; arms want to be uncovered, then covered; in the lower limbs constant stretching and drawing up.*
Walking in the sleep	During sleep nightmare.*
When asleep, arms and hands over head .	Hands under the head when asleep.*
Requires very little sleep and not much food.	Requires good, long sleep, and feels better after eating, partic. after breakfast.*
Pulse generally unchanged, only a little accelerated.	Pulse changed in quality and strength; generally hard, full, quick; sometimes intermitting or imperceptible.
Veins distended on hands	No distended veins.*
Want of thirst, partic. during hot stage . .	Thirst with chill; heat with or without thirst.*
Sweat on hairy scalp	Sweat general, except on the head.*
After abuse of Magnesia carb.	Abuse of wine, coffee, or aromatics.*
Grunting, groaning, screaming	Quarrelsome; over-conscientious; full of scruples.
Fear, as if he had done wrong	Anxious feeling in the chest and heart.
Fretful; disagreeable	Obstinate—Is in too great a hurry, or idles away the time.
Child asks for different things impetuously and with crying; dislikes even its favorite things.	Inclined to reproach others—Inconsolable, despairing; full of fears—Jealousy.
Silent, dislikes to talk; lazy—Fear of death with the diarrhœa.	Satiety of life; thinks of suicide; rarely fear of death.
At night during restl. sleep he imagines himself walking about semi-conscious; during the day as though he were half-asleep.	Coma vigil.—He speaks and writes wrong words.
Delirium predom.	Rarely delirium.*
Vertigo and heaviness, with beating in head; worse while standing.	Vertigo, with headache and loss of consciousness, &c.; better when standing.*
Pupils dilated, with pressing headache; later contracted, with inward restlessness.	Pupils contracted; later dilated, with very slow breathing.*
Bitter taste of the food, even of sweets .	Bitter taste in mouth, but neither food nor drink tastes bitter *
Sour taste in the mouth	Sour taste after eating bread or drinking [milk.*
Insipid and nauseous taste in mouth . . .	Putrid taste in mouth.*
Nausea in stomach or abdomen	Nausea in stomach, rarely in œsophagus.
Colic from eating prunes	Colic from acids, *coffee* or beer.*
Colic after dinner, worse when standing .	Colic after dinner; worse when lying on [painful side.*
Diarrhœa predom.	Constipation predom.
Diarrhœa during dentition, frequent urging; *sour*, curdled, or *fermented*, frothy stools, *turning green;* reddening anus, with *pale face*, salivation, tossing about, drawing up of legs; worse from walking and moving, partic. *while standing.*	Diarrhœa, frequent urging, with violent colic, dark-brown fœtid stools — three, four a day — with heaviness of head, thickly furred tongue, and thirst.*

† While Rheum-symptoms go from left to right, Nux vomica very probably acts in the opposite direction.*

Rheum.	Nux vomica.
(Continued.)	
Diarrhœa, with inflammatory rheumatism.	*Diarrhœa*, with comatose fever or after scarlet fever, fæces lumpy, with slime and blood.*
Dysentery: after the bloody stools have ceased, tenesmus with discharge of brown, mush-like fæces, mixed with slime, smelling sour.	*Dysentery:* bloody slime; sometimes small, hard, little lumps; violent tenesmus, with *pressure in sacrum and rectum; dry tongue, not much thirst.**
Chronic diarrhœa: sour, frothy, with a moist tongue, much thirst, and complete loss of appetite.	Chronic dysentery, every two hours; thin, greenish, bloody, putrid discharges; whitish, dry tongue; constant desire to eat; dry skin; feeble pulse.*
Bearing down while standing	Bearing down better when standing.*
Pressing to inguinal ring, worse when walking.	As if the hernia were incarcerated when lying in bed.*
Burning in kidneys	Burning heat in loins and kidneys, with abdominal congestions.*
Burning in bladder before and with urination.	Pain in bladder before; stitches and soreness in urethra and neck of bladder during urination.*
After abortus, urinary complaints . . .	In child-bed painful urination or retention of urine.*
Both nipples hurt, sting; she says from wind in the abdomen.	Nipples hurt, are sensible to the touch; tearing pain when suckling.*
Fluent coryza	Mostly dry coryza, partic. in the open air; in-doors, on the contrary, coryza is fluent.
Expectoration in the morning	Expectoration morning, by day, evening.
In thighs most weariness	In thighs heaviness and unsteadiness.*
Limbs fall asleep from lying on them, particularly the lower, in putting one over the other.	Arms and hands are "asleep" in the night; lower limbs, while sitting or standing, or after sitting.
Remission during day and evening . . .	Remission evening till midnight.
Worse when lying on painful side; better when lying on unpainful side.	Worse (better) when lying on painful side, *or* when lying on unpainful side.
Worse after sleep	Better after sufficient and not too long sleep; but worse on awaking when roused.
Better after getting out of bed . .	Worse *or* better after getting out of bed.
Worse when stooping	Better *or* worse when stooping.
Better when bending diseased part . . .	Generally worse when bending the part.
Worse when fixedly looking at an object for any length of time.	Worse when looking into the light.
Better when swallowing	*Worse or* better when swallowing.
Better when eating, worse *afterwards* . .	*Better or* worse when eating; *wor.* better *afterwards.*
Worse or better after stool.	Worse after stool.†

Predomin. worse — **Predomin. better**

After sleep, in bed, and when sitting erect.

Predomin. better — **Predomin worse**

When sitting bent forward, when bending the suffering part, and when swallowing.

N.B. Rheum appears to lack the over-sensitiveness of Nux vomica to pain.

† Passing fœtid flatus relieves colicky pains in both remedies.*

* Added by C.Hg.

Rhododendron.	Pulsatilla.
Complaints predom. in external parts . .	Compl. predom. in internal parts.
Want of bodily irritability—Inclination for motion.	Increased irritability—Aversion to motion.
Pains pressing inwards—No apoplexy . .	Pains pressing outwards—Apoplexy.
Cold swelling of glands	Hot, painful swelling of glands.
Sleeplessness after midnight; awaking early.	Sleeplessn. before midnight; awak'g too late.
Pulse often unchanged; generally slow, weak.	Pulse changed, sometimes intermitting; generally frequent, small, weak.
Want of thirst constant.	Want of thirst predom., but is constant only during cold stage—Thirst appears partic. *before & between* the different stages of the fever.
Chill or sweat increased when walking in the open air.	Chill or sweat abated when walking in the open air.
Insensibility of disposition.	Sensitive disposition—Delirium.
Loss of appetite predom.	Generally hunger.
Compl. of the spleen predom.	Compl. of liver predom.
Painless diarrhœa	Diarrhœa generally painful.
Sexual desire too weak	Sexual desire too strong.
Contracted scrotum	Relaxed scrotum. C.Hg.
Coryza dry oftener than fluent	Coryza fluent oftener than dry.
Expector. quite seldom; partic. at night .	Expector. predom., but not constant; morning and during day.
Complaints predominant on fore-arm . .	Compl. predom. on upper arm.
AGGRAVATION aft. midnight, morn'g, even'g.	AGGRAVATION from noon till midnight.
Worse (better) when growing cold *or* warm.	Better when growing cold, worse when growing warm.
Better after perspiring	*Worse or* better after perspiring.
Better or worse after sleep	*Worse or* better after sleep.
Worse when getting out of bed	*Better or* worse when getting out of bed.
Worse when rising from a seat, better *afterwards.*	*Worse or* better when rising from a seat, *better or* worse *afterwards.*
Better when moving diseased part, worse when bending it.	*Better or* worse when moving the part, worse *or* better when bending it.
Worse when swallowing and after eating .	*Worse or* bett. when swallow'g & after eat'g.
Better or worse from eructation	Predom. worse from eructation.
Worse after stool	*Better or* worse after stool.

Predomin. worse —— **Predomin. better**

From cold and in cold weather, from drinking cold water, from uncovering, when lying on painful side, from bodily exertion, after stool, and when getting out of bed.

Predomin. better —— **Predomin. worse**

From warmth and in warm air, from warmth of stove* and warmth of bed,† after perspiring, from wrapping up, when lying on the unpainful side, and after sleep.

N.B. Rhododendron lacks the over-sensitiveness of Pulsatilla to pain, which is in accordance with the constitutional characteristic of both remedies.

* Both remedies have predom. aggrav. *in-doors* generally and improv. of complaints in the open air.
† Both remedies have predom. aggrav. *in bed* generally.

Rhododendron.	Rhus.
Desire for open air—Pains press'g inwards.	Avers'n to open air—Pains press'g outwards.
Pains also in the bones, in small spots; radiating from place to place.	Pains chiefly in the joints; spreading a great deal; cramping pains. C.Hg
No apoplexy—Very rarely paralysis . .	Apoplexy—Paralysis of limbs.
Cold swelling of glands	Hot, painful swelling of glands.
Sleeplessness after midnight; awaking too early.	Sleeplessness predomin. before midnight; awaking too late.
Pleasant dreams predom.	Anxious dreams.
Pulse often unchanged; slow and weak .	Pulse generally small, weak, often weak & accel.rated, often irregular, sometimes intermitting or trembling.
Heat on upper part of body—Congestion of blood to the ears.	Chill or heat on upper part of body—Congestion to the eyes.
Thirst is generally wanting	Thirst not constant.
Compl. predom. on lower lip and on shin .	Compl. predom. on upper lip & on calf of leg.
Painless diarrhœa	Diarrhœa mostly painful.
Urine greenish	Urine whitish, muddy. C.Hg.
Sexual desire lessened at first, later increased.	Erections at night, towards morning. C.Hg.
Coryza oftener dry than fluent	Fluent coryza.
Expector. rather seldom; partic. at night.	Expector. not const.; partic. in the morn'g.
Remission during day and before midnight.	**Remission** of complaints during day.
Aggrav. before a thunder-storm	Aggrav. during increasing moon.
Worse or better in bed	*Better or* worse in bed.
Worse when getting out of bed; almost always improv. *afterwards.*	Better *or* worse when getting out of bed; *worse or* better *afterwards.*
After the least exercise, great dejection and painful weariness.	Pains relieved after moving. C.Hg.
Worse when rising from a seat; better *afterwards.*	*Worse or* better when rising from a seat; better *or* worse *afterwards.*
Better when sitting down	Better *or* worse when sitting down.
Better when moving diseased part, worse when bending it.	*Better or* worse when moving the part, *worse or* better when bending it.
Pains on moving during the transition from rest to motion.	Pains worse when reposing after motion. C.Hg.
Worse after eating and drinking	*Worse or* better after eating and drinking.
Better *or* worse from eructation	Worse from eructation.
Worse after stool	*Better or* worse after stool.

Predomin. worse — **Predomin. better**

In-doors, in bed, when lying on painful side, when descending, from warm diet, and after stool.

Predomin. better — **Predomin. worse**

In the open air,* after getting out of bed, when lying on unpainful side, when ascending, from cold diet, after sleep, from washing and moistening suffering part.

N.B. With both remedies the compl. of the limbs extend from the right to the left side, both have desire for motion with the pain, the patient cannot let the limb rest, and motion improv. somewhat; both have pain after taking cold, Rhus alone after gett'g wet through; Rhus alone also has compl. after over-lifting and spraining; Rhododendron alone, on the other hand, aggrav. of all complaints, even dysentery before a thunder-storm. C.Hg.

* Both remedies have predom. improv. when *walking* in the open air.

Rhus.	Lachesis.
Blood coagulates easily	Blood incoagulable.
Muscles rigid—Desire for motion	Muscles lax—Disinclination for motion.
Hæmorrhages, blood bright-red – Pale or scarlet-red swellings	Hæmorrh., blood dark-red—Blueish black swellings, (dark-blue blisters. C.Hg.)
Painless ulcers with copious discharge*. .	Painful ulcers with scanty discharge.
Cutting pain in external parts	Cutting pains in internal parts.
Anxious dreams—Awaking late	Pleasant dreams—Awaking too early.
Pulse pred.. affected by beer (brandy, coffee).	Pulse pred. affected by wine & brandy. C.Hg.
Thirst not constant	Want of thirst predom.; thirst particularly *before* the cold stage.
Complaints predom. on outside of nose, on back of hand, and on calf of leg.	Complaints predom. on the inside nose, in palm of hand, and on shin.
Sadness—Dejection—Very rarely amorousness.	Cheerfulness — Irritability — Malice — Distrust.
Difficult comprehension; rarely dullness .	Haughtiness—Easy comprehension—Mental excitability—Ecstasies.
Mania very seldom	Unconsciousness or fancies very seldom.
Ailments from vexation with dread or fear.	Ailm. from fright, disapp. love or jealousy.
Satiety of life with fear of death	Satiety of life with longing for death.
Dislike for wine; but appetite for beer . .	Generally desire for wine.
Aggrav. by spirituous drinks	Spirituous drinks aggrav. the complaints; in cases of poisoning, however, (bite of snake) they improve.
Diphtheria: awaking frequently, rising and complaining of pain in the throat; during sleep, bloody saliva runs out of the mouth; parotid or other glands swollen; transparent jelly-like discharges with or after the stool. Raue.	Diphtheria: worse after sleep, partic. in the morning; exsudative patches on the tonsils, particularly left side; cannot bear the throat to be touched; small, soft or thin, very offensive stools. C.Hg.
Diarrhœa generally painful	Diarrhœa painless.
Catam. too profuse and of long duration. With suppressed menstruation, milk in the breasts.	Catam. of too short duration and generally too scanty. With suppressed menstruation, toothache, or menstruation scanty and bleeding from anus. C.Hg.
Nasal secretion thick	Nasal secretion watery.
Respiration frequent and deep.	Respiration slow (with apoplexy it is blowing, puffing. C.Hg.)
Cough, partic. in the evening till midnight.	Cough loosens in the morning & during day.
Expector. not constant, partic. in the morn.	Exp. rather seldom, is generally swallowed.
AGGRAVATION from evening till morning .	AGGRAVATION from noon till midnight.
Worse during increasing moon	Worse before a thunder-storm.
Predom. worse when swallowing, partic. swallowing saliva and food; often better, however, when swallowing drink, if it is not cold.	Better *or* worse when swallowing, partic. worse when swallowing saliva and drink; often better, however, when swallowing solid food.
Worse in snowy air	Worse from heat of sun.

Predomin. **worse** ——— Predomin. **better**

From cold diet, from coffee, during sleep,† when taking a deep breath, from shaking the head, and when lying on unpainful side.

Predomin. **better** ——— Predomin. **worse**

From warm diet, from moderate pressure, when lying on the painful side.

N.B. Rhus never has over-sensitiveness to pain, which sometimes occurs with Lachesis; the latter never has sensation of numbness in suffering parts peculiar to Rhus. Sensitiveness to touch, however, is found with both remedies, (partic. with Lach. C.Hg.)

---

* Partic. on dropsical legs, with spontaneous, constant discharge of "the water," (the same as in Lycopod C.Hg.)

† Aggrav. as well as improv. occur with both remedies "*after* sleep," but yet aggrav. pred., (part. with Lach. C.Hg.)

Rhus.	Phosphor.
Upper left, lower right side — Light hair — Desire for motion.	Upper right, lower left side — Dark hair — Dislikes moving.
Sensitiveness or cutting pain in external parts.	Sensitiveness or cutting pain in internal parts.
Itching around the joints — Itching relieved by scratching.	Vesicles around the joints — Itching *lessened or* aggrav. by scratching.
Eruptions (idiopathic) mostly humid . . .	Eruptions (symptomatic) generally dry.
Wounds, partic. with straining of muscles . .	Wounds, partic. with injury of glands.
Hæmorrhages, blood coagulated already or coagulating quickly.	Hæmorrhages, blood incoagulable or coagulating imperfectly.
Causes atrophy of warts	Cures warts by suppuration.
Sweat, left side—Pulse mostly weak and soft.	Sweat, right side – Pulse mostly full and hard.
Heat or sweat, with aversion to uncover . .	Heat or sweat, with desire to uncover.
Typhoid fevers, with pain in limbs—Thirst not constant.	Typhoid fevers, without pain—Want of thirst constant.
Chill increased in the open air & by drinking.	Chill lessened in the open air and by drinking.
Fear of being poisoned	Fear of apoplexy or loss of reason.
Mood *sad* or despondent	Mood changing; cheerful *or* melancholy.
Ailments from vexation with dread or fear .	Ailm. fr. fright, anger. or vexation with vehem.
Weakness of memory — Diffic. comprehension.	Active memory—*Easy or* diffic. comprehens'n.
Mental dullness — After a fall on the head periodical mental confusion.	Mental excitability; ecstasies—Insanity.
Compl. predom. on upper lip, in lower part of chest, on calf of leg, on back of hand and top of foot.	Compl. predom. on under lip. in upper part of chest, on shin, in palm of hand, and on sole of foot.
Pupils predom. dilated—Styes on lower lid .	Pup. pred. contract'd—Stye on upp. lid. C. Hg.
Objective stench from nose — Appetite for sweets — Nausea in œsophagus or stomach.	Putrid subjective odor—Aversion to sweets—Nausea in stomach.
Diarrhœa mostly painful	Diarrhœa mostly painless.
Urine too often and copious—Urinal sediment white.	Urine often, but scanty—Sediment *white*, yellowish or reddish.
Catamenia too soon, profuse, and of long duration.	Catam. too soon, profuse, and of long duration, *or* too late, scanty, and of short duration.
Respiratio thoracica—Expectoration not constant, partic. in the morning.	Respiratio abdominalis — Expectoration not constant; morning and during day.
Remission of complaints during day	Remission after midnight.
Worse during increasing moon	Worse before a thunder-storm.
Worse when looking down	Worse when looking at shining objects.
Worse during sleep; afterwards; worse *or* better when getting out of bed, and when rising from a seat and after it.	Worse *or* better during sleep — Better after suffic. sleep; worse on awaking when roused, or after siesta, or when getting out of bed, and when rising from a seat; better after it.
Better *or* worse when sitting down; leaning against something.	Almost always improv. sitting down; leaning back.
Worse from shaking the head or stooping . .	*Worse or* bett. when shaking the head *or* stooping.
Worse *or* better when bending the part . .	Worse when bending diseased part.
Generally better from moderate pressure . .	*Generally* worse from pressure.
Better *or* worse when eating; w. eating bread or drinking coffee; *w. or b.* after drinking; w. when swallowing food and saliva; worse from eructation; bett. or worse after stool.	*Worse or* bett. wh. eating; b. *or* w. fr. bread; *w. or* b. fr. coffee; alw. bett. after drinking; w. wh. swallowing food & part. drink; worse *or* better from eructation; worse after stool.

Predomin. worse — **Predomin. better**

In the open air, "from uncovering," from touch, during rest, when standing, sitting, lying; when lying on unpainful side, when drawing up, lifting, or resting diseased limb on something; after sleep, on an empty stomach, from drinking cold water and from cold diet in general, from beer and spirituous liquors, after drinking generally.

Predomin. better — **Predomin. worse**

In-doors and from heat of stove, in bed, from warmth of bed, "from wrapping up," from moderate pressure, from motion, when walking, when lying on painful side, when stretching out diseased limb or letting it hang down, from being overheated, after perspiring, after breakfast, from warm diet, and after stool.

N.B. Rhus lacks the over-sensitiveness of Phosphor to pain.

Rhus.	**Sepia.**
Light hair—Hæmorrhages, blood light-red .	Dark hair—Hæmorrhages, blood dark.
Nervous paralysis — Itching, relieved by scratching.	Paralysis with atrophy of muscles—Itching, aggrav. by scratching.
Eruptions mostly humid—Skin hardened . .	Eruptions mostly dry—Skin chafed. C.Hg.
Hot, painful swelling of glands	Painless swelling of glands.
Pulse generally frequent, faint, & weak; sometimes trembling.	Pulse frequent and full at night, during day accelerated only by vexation or motion.
First chill, then heat—Heat abated by motion.	First heat, then chill—Heat increas'd by mot'n.
Thirst not constant	Thirstlessness predom. — Only during chill thirst is frequent.
Heat on front part, coldness on back part of body.	Heat on back part of body.
With the chill or the sweat aching of the teeth.	Toothache mostly during the hot stage. C.Hg.

Fear of being poisoned	Fear of apoplexy.
Delirium	Indifference—Irritability—Avarice.
Pupils dilated—Swelling under the eyes . .	Pupils contracted—Swelling above the eyes.
Objective stench from the nose	Subjective putrid odor predom.
Swelling or breaking out of upper lip predom.	Swelling or breaking out of under lip predom.
Aversion to wine; appetite for beer . . .	Appetite for wine or brandy.
Urine too often and copious—Sediment white.	Disch. of ur. too seldom—Sedim. *red* or whitish.
Catam. too soon—Milk mostly increased . .	Catam. mostly too late—Milk diminished.
Nasal secretion thick—Cough *generally* dry—Expectoration not constant, partic. in the morning.	Nasal secretion watery or viscid—Cough *generally* with expectoration; loosened night and morning, and generally swallowed.
Complaints predom. on patella and hollow of knee.	Compl. predom on tip of elbow and in hollow of elbow.

REMISSION of complaints during day. . . .	REMISSION afternoon.
Worse during increasing moon	Worse during new moon *or* in sultry air.
Worse in cold weather; better in warm air .	Worse (better) in cold weather *or* in warm air.
Worse when looking down	Worse when looking up or over a large surface.
Predom. worse in the open air, better in-doors.	Better (worse) in the open air *or* in-doors.
Generally better in bed	*Generally* worse in bed.
Predom. worse after sleep	Better after sufficient sleep, but worse on awaking when roused.
Worse *or* better when getting out of bed and after it; when rising from a seat & after it.	*Better or* worse when getting out of bed and after it; when ris'g from a seat; *better* after it.
Better *or* worse when sitting down	Better when sitting down.
Better *or* worse when leaning back against something.	Worse when leaning back against something.
Worse or better when bending diseased part.	Worse when bending diseased part.
Worse from exertion, running, dancing, etc. .	Predom. better from bodily exertion.
Worse when taking a deep breath	Better *or* worse when taking a deep breath.
Worse when hungry	Worse after a satisfying meal.
Better *or* worse when eating	Worse when eating.
Worse or better after drinking	Worse after drinking.
Better or worse after stool	*Worse or* better after stool.

Predomin. worse ——— **Predomin. better**

In wet weather, from bodily exertion, *on inspiration*, after sleep, after getting out of bed, when assuming an erect position, from stooping, when drawing up diseased limb, from change of posture, when lying or standing, from drinking cold water, from cold diet generally, after drinking, and from smoking.

Predomin. better ——— **Predomin. worse**

In dry weather, *on expiration*, in bed, when stretching out diseased limb, from warm diet, after stool, after perspiring, from moderate pressure, when bending back the head, from rubbing & scratch'g.

N.B. Rhus lacks the over-sensitiveness of Sepia to pain; Sepia generally has not the sensation of numbness in suffering parts peculiar to Rhus. But mere sensitiveness to the touch appears with both remedies.

Rhus.	Silicea.
Upper left, lower right side—Skin & muscles rigid.	Upper right, lower left side—Skin & muscles lax.
Itching, relieved by scratching	Itching, aggrav. or unchanged by scratching.
Painless ulcers	Painful ulcers.
Wounds, partic. with straining of muscles . .	Wounds, partic. with injury of the glands or bones.
Causes atrophy of warts	Cures warts, cystic tumors, etc., by suppurat'n.
Eruptions mostly humid	Eruptions mostly dry.
Sleeplessness predom. before midnight . . .	Sleeplessness predom. after midnight..
Heat increased in-doors	Heat abated in-doors.
Sweat often only on front part of body . .	Sweat often only on back part of body.
Pulse predom. soft (and accelerated) . . .	Pulse predom. hard (and accelerated).
Pulse predom. affected by drinking brandy, beer, or coffee.	Pulse affected by drinking wine. C. Hg.
Thirst not constant	Thirst constant in fevers.
Congestion of blood to eyes predom.	Congestion to ears predom.
Mood sad & depressed—Very rarely amorousness.	Mood gentle; indifferent; despondent; peevish.
Unconsciousness—Delirium	Rarely unconsciousness—No delirium.
Vertigo, inclin'g to fall backwards or forwards.	Vertigo, inclining to fall forwards.
Painful sensitiveness of the scalp (with swelling), partic. in the side not lain on, when growing warm in bed, to the touch, and when brushing back the hair.	Sensitiveness of the scalp to pressure, partic. in the side lain on, when growing warm in bed, and when scratching, after which there is a burning pain.
Pupils dilated	Pupils contracted.
Nasal compl. external oftener than internal .	Nasal compl. internal oftener than external.
Nausea in œsophagus or stomach, less frequently in throat.	Nausea, partic. in stomach, less frequently in abdomen.
Diarrhœa predom.—Urinal sediment white .	Costiveness predom.—Urinal sediment reddish or yellow.
Catamenia too soon and profuse	Catam. *generally* retarded and scanty.
Fluent coryza	Stoppage of nose oftener than fluent coryza.
Expector. not constant; partic. in the morn'g.	Expector. nearly constant; during day.
Compl. generally on top of foot	Compl. generally on sole of foot.
Remission of complaints during day . . .	Remission before midnight.
Worse during increasing moon	Worse during *full moon*, new moon, or *before a thunder-storm.*
Worse in wet weather, better in dry weather.	*Generally* better in wet weather, worse in dry weather.
Worse from washing and moistening suffering part.	*Worse or* better from washing, etc., the diseased part.
Worse when looking down	Worse when looking up.
Generally worse when opening, better when closing the mouth.	*Generally* better when opening, worse when closing the mouth.
Better or worse from warmth of stove . . .	Better from warmth of bed.
Worse *or* better when getting out of bed . .	Worse when rising from bed.
Worse or better when rising from a seat; worse *or* better *afterwards.*	Worse when rising from a seat; better *afterwards.*
Better *or* worse when sitting down	Better when sitting down.
Worse *or* better when bending diseased part.	Worse when bending diseased part.
Worse from bodily exertion	Worse *or* better from exertion.
Worse when hungry	Worse after a satisfying meal.
Better or worse after stool	Worse after stool.

Predomin. worse —— **Predomin. better**

In wet weather, when lying on unpainful side, when drawing up diseased limb, when rising from stooping, on an empty stomach, and from eructation.

Predomin. better —— **Predomin. worse**

In dry weather, when lying on painful side, when stretching out diseased limb, when walking in the open air,* after breakfast, after stool, from moderate pressure, after perspir'g, fr. rubb'g & scratch'g.

N.B. Rhus lacks the over-sensitiveness of Silicea to pain. But mere sensitiveness (to touch, etc.) appears with both remedies.

* Both remedies have aggrav. predom. *in the open air* generally, and improv. in-doors.

Rhus.	Sulphur.
Right side — Cutting pain in external parts— Hæmorrhages, blood pale.	*Left* side — Cutting pain in internal parts— Hæmorrhages, blood dark.
Eruptions generally humid—Skin disposed to harden.	Eruptions generally dry — Skin inclines to chafe. C. Hg.
Itching around the joints	Itch'g, erysipelas or vesicles around the joints.
Sweat on suffering side	Coldness on diseased part.
Pulse predominantly soft and weak	Pulse predom. hard and full.
Chill or heat on upper part of body . . .	Sweat on upper part of body.
Sweat sometimes general, with exception of the head.	Heat sometimes general, with exception of the head.
Sweat sometimes only on front part of body .	Sweat sometimes only on back part of body.
Chill predom. right side	Chill predom. left side.
Heat or sweat, with aversion to uncover . .	Heat or sweat, with inclination to uncover.
Rarely peevishness—Rarely mania	Mood changing; irritable; solemn—Insanity.
Pupils dilated—Stye on lower lid	Pupils contracted—Stye on upper lid. C. Hg.
Saliva predominantly increased	Saliva generally diminished.
Sensation as if the teeth were drawn in . .	As if the teeth were pulled out. C. Hg.
Dislike for wine—Appetite for beer	Appetite or disl. for beer & spirituous liquors.
Urine too often and copious—Sediment white.	Urine often, but scanty—S. white *or* reddish.
Catamenia too soon and profuse and of long duration—During suppressed menstruation milk in the breasts. C. Hg.—Milk generally increased.	Catamenia *generally* too late, scanty, and of short duration—During suppressed menstruation hæmorrhoidal tumors.. C. Hg.—Milk diminished.
Nasal secretion thick—Expectoration, partic. in the morning.	Nasal secretion watery—Expector. morning and during day, less frequently at night.
Frequent compl. in lower part of chest and on top of foot.	Compl. predom. in upper part of chest and on sole of foot.
Remission of complaints during day . . .	**Remission** afternoon and before midnight.
Worse during increase of moon	Worse during full moon and in sultry air.
Predom. worse from growing cold and in cold weather; better when growing warm and in warm air.	Better (worse) when growing cold and in cold weather, or when growing warm and in warm air.
Worse in the open air, better in-doors . . .	Better in the open air, worse in-doors (partic. in crowded rooms*).
Better after perspiring	*Worse or* better after perspiring.
Generally better in bed & from warmth of bed.	*Generally* worse in bed & from warmth of bed.
Worse when lying on back, better when lying on side.	*Generally* better when lying on back, worse when lying on side.
Worse *or* better when getting out of bed, when rising from a seat, and *afterwards.*	Better when getting out of bed; worse when rising from a seat, *afterwards* better.
Worse *or* better when sitting down	Predom. better when sitting down.
Worse when rising from stooping, from change of posture, when lying or stand'g, from sneezing, when tak'g a deep breath, & from touch.	*Worse or* better when rising, from change of posture, when sneezing, when taking a deep breath, and from touch.
Better or worse when moving diseased part .	*Worse or* better when moving the part.
Better when bending the head backwards . .	Worse *or* bett. wh. bend'g the head backwards.
Worse when hungry, on an empty stomach; better after breakfast; worse or better after meals; better or worse after stool.	Worse after a satisfying meal; better (worse) on an empty stomach *or* after breakfast; worse after meals; worse *or* bett. after stool.

Predomin. **worse** —— Predomin. **better**

In the open air, from cold, from uncovering, in extended posture, when lying on back or when lying on unpainful side, when drawing up diseased limb, and from eructation.

Predomin. **better** —— Predomin. **worse**

In-doors,* from warmth and from warmth of bed, from wrapping up, in contracted posture, when lying on side, partic. when lying on painful side, when stretching out diseased limb, & after perspiring.

* The symptoms of both remedies are improv. by heat of stove.

Ruta.	Pulsatilla.
Lef. side, partic. *lower left. upper right side.*	*Right* side, partic. *lower right. upper left side.*
Complaints predom. in external parts	Complaints predom. in internal parts.
Aversion to open air—Inclination for motion.	Inclination for open air—Aversion to motion.
Paralysis—No apoplexy	Apoplexy—Paralysis rather infrequent; generally painless and one-sided.
In periost. burning, gnawing, tension; in bones pressing, piercing, digging, as if broken; slow hardening after fractures.	In periost. scraping, tingling. tickling; in bones jerking, boring pain.* C.Hg.
Jaundice from liver complaints	Skin pale, rarely yellowish. C.Hg.
Itching, generally relieved by scratching	Itching, aggrav. or unchanged by scratching.
Copious discharge of ulcers	Ulcers; sometimes scanty discharge. C.Hg.
Pulse somewhat accelerated, but only during heat.	Pulse generally frequent, small, and weak; sometimes intermitting; accelerated in the evening, slow in the morning.
Chill (as well as other symptoms) appear particularly on left side of body.	Chill (as well as other symptoms), partic. on right side of body.
Thirst commonly wanting only during heat	Want of thirst predom., but is constant only during chill.
Optical illusions in dark colors	Optical illusions in bright colors.
Complaints mostly on external ear, and on outside of gums.	Complaints mostly on inner ear, and on inner side of gums.
Inclined to bring the tongue sideways between the molar teeth.	Tongue too large and too broad. C.Hg.
Loss of appetite predom.	Generally hunger.
Nausea, part. in stomach, less freq. in abdom'n.	Nausea in throat, stomach, or abdomen.
Stool like sheep dung	Stool soft, slimy. C.Hg.
Expectoration rather constant; evening	Expect. not constant; morning & during day.
Wrist giving way when lifting something heavy.	Wrist and hand cannot hold anything. C Hg.
Complaints predom. on thigh	Complaints predom. on leg.
Weariness, giving way in the knees when going up and down stairs.	Soft, shining white swelling of knee; weariness, tearing pain, jerks. C.Hg.
Antidote to Mercurius	Antidote to Sulphur and Ferrum. C.Hg.
Aggravation of complaints afternoon	Aggravation from noon till midnight.
Worse when looking into the distance	Worse when looking up.
Better after sufficient sleep; but worse on awaking when roused from sleep.	*Worse or* better after sleep.
Worse when getting out of bed	*Better or* worse when getting out of bed.
Worse when rising from a seat; better *afterwards.*	*Worse or* better when rising from a seat; *better or* worse *afterwards.*
Predom. better when sitting down	Worse *or* better when sitting down.
Mostly better when standing	Worse when standing.
Worse when moving diseased part	*Better or* worse when moving the part.
Worse when bending it	Better *or* worse when bending it.
Predom. worse from pressure	Generally better from pressure.
Worse after eating	*Worse or* better after eating.
Worse after stool	*Better or* worse after stool.

Predomin. worse — **Predomin. better**

In the open air, from cold, from growing cold and in cold weather, when lying on painful side, when getting out of bed, when stretching out diseased limb, when moving suffering part, from bodily exertion, from pressure, after eating, after stool, and after expectoration.

Predomin. better — **Predomin. worse**

In-doors, from warmth, growing warm and in warm air, when lying on unpainful side, after sleep, when drawing up diseased limb, when standing, from rubbing and scratching.

N.B. The over-sensitiveness of Pulsatilla to pain has not yet been observed with Ruta.

* Both Ruta and Pulsatilla have a sore pain in the bones, or as if laced and drawn together; in the periosteum a sensitiveness or as if bruised, a tearing or shooting, piercing pain, and either of them may be indicated in osteitis, softening and swelling of bones; also after abuse of Mercury, inflammation, and suppuration.

Ruta.	Sulphur.
Upper right, lower left side—Pinching pain in internal parts.	Upper left, lower right side—Pinching pain in external parts.
In periosteum burning pains or as if bruised; in bruises and after concussions; in bones as if broken, or a gnawing, digging, or a tensive, pressing, piercing pain.	In bones a cold sensation or a tingling, tickling, throbbing, or boring pain; as if the flesh was beaten off—Fragility—Necrosis.* CHg.
Cutaneous eruptions humid	Eruptions generally dry.
Copious discharge of ulcers	Ulcers, sometimes scanty discharge. C.Hg.
A large, painful wart, with a broad basis inside on the third finger of right hand; obliterates, peels off, and disappears, 15c. B.Fincke.	Small or hard and horny warts, with burning, throbbing, shooting pain. C.Hg.
Compl. generally on lower eyelids, in inner angle of eye, on external ear, on upper gum, and on upper arm.	Compl. generally on upper eyelids, in external angle of eye, in inner ear, on lower gum, and on fore-arm.
Pulse unchanged; somewhat accelerated only during heat.	Pulse generally hard and accelerated; sometimes intermitting or imperceptible.
Chill, increased in a warm room	Chill, abated in a warm room.
Thirst commonly wanting only during heat .	Most thirst during heat; generally want of thirst during chill.
Inclination to put the tongue between the molar teeth.	Sensation of quivering on the tongue. C.Hg.
Urine too seldom and scanty	Urine often, but scanty; increased only after strong doses.
Expectoration nearly constant; evening . .	Expector. not constant; morning and during day, less frequently at night.
In the wrist lameness or as if sprained; soreness and lame feeling, or rheumatic stiffness after luxations; stitches in wet cold weather.	In the wrists weariness, cutting pain, rhagades, stiffness; worse fr. slight mot'n; better after exertions; worse during rest, at night. C.Hg.
Lameness of the knee	Swell'g of the knee, inflamm., white, weakness, tension, when walk'g, going up stairs. C.Hg.
Sublocation of the ankle-joint	Spraining the back. C.Hg.

Ruta.	Sulphur.
Aggravation afternoon	Remission *afternoon* & before midnight.
Worse from growing cold and in cold weather, better when growing warm and in warm air.	Better (worse) from growing cold & in cold weather, *or* when grow'g warm & in warm air.
Predom. worse in the open air, better in-doors.	*Generally* better in the open air; worse (partic. in crowded) rooms.†
Worse when looking into the distance . . .	Worse when looking down.
Worse in bed and from change of posture .	*Worse or* bett. in bed & fr. change of posture.
Better after sufficient sleep, but worse on awaking when roused from sleep.	Worse after sleep.
Predom. better after getting out of bed . .	Better *or* worse after getting out of bed.
Generally better when standing	Worse when standing any length of time, but better when standing still after motion.
Worse when moving diseased part, from touch, and when stooping.	*Worse or* better when moving the part, from touch, etc.
Worse when eating and after stool	Worse *or* better when eating and after stool.
Worse after passing urine	*Worse or* better after passing urine.

Predomin. worse — **Predomin. better**

In the open air, from cold, when getting out of bed, on expiration, after expectoration, from boring in the ear & nose with the finger, when lett'g diseased limb hang down, when descend'g, & fr. pressure.

Predomin. better — **Predomin. worse**

In-doors, from warmth, after sleep, on inspiration, when lifting diseased limb, when ascend'g, & when standing.

---

* Both Ruta and Sulphur. have a sore pain in bones or as if laced together and constricted or boring; either of them may be indicated after fractures, if healing too slowly, in osteitis, exostoses, malacio, curvatures, caries, and partic. after abuse of Mercury.

† Sulphur. has improv. of symptoms from warmth of stove.

Sabadilla.	Nux vom.
Upper left, lower right side—Obesity	*Upper right, lower left s.* pred. — Emaciation.
Light hair — Muscles lax — No paralysis — Rarely apoplexy.	Dark hair — Muscles rigid — Paralysis—Apoplexy.
Sleeplessness before midnight—Sleep after the sweat.	Sleeplessness predom. after midnight — Sleep between chill and heat.
Pulse small, but somewhat spasmodic	Pulse predom. frequent, full, and hard; sometimes intermitting, or imperceptible.
Sweat on front part of body, or only on the head.	Sweat on back of body, or general, with exception of the head.
Chill lessened after eating—More sweat during sleep.	Chill increased after eating — Sweat lessened during sleep.
Want of thirst predom.*	Most thirst during cold stage.
Easy or difficult comprehension	Difficult comprehension — Absent-mindedness —Unconsciousness.
Complaints predom. on external ear.	Complaints predom. in inner ear.
Dislike for wine, but appetite for beer	Inclination for spirituous liquors—Inclination or dislike for beer.
Sexual desire too weak	Sexual desire too strong.
Catamenia too late, scanty, and of too short duration—Blood bright-red.	Catamenia too soon, copious, and of too long duration—Blood dark-red.
Nasal secretion thick	Nasal secretion watery.
Expectoration seldom; during day	Expectoration not constant; morning, during day, evening.
Heat in the fingers (during fever)	The hands become as though dead, and nails blue (during fever).
AGGRAVATION forenoon and night, part. before midnight.	AGGRAVATION after midnight, in the morning after sunrise, and during day.
Worse when lying on the side, better when lying on the back.	*Generally* better when lying on side; worse when lying on back.
Worse when lying on painful side; better when lying on unpainful side.	Worse (better) when lying on painful *or* on unpainful side.
Predom. worse from pressure	*Generally* better from pressure.
Worse from change of posture	*Worse or* better from change of posture, when lying or standing.
Worse after sleep	Better after sufficient and not too long sleep; but worse on awaking, when roused fr. sleep.
Worse when perspiring	*Worse or* better when perspiring.
Better after perspiring	*Better or* worse after perspiring.
Worse on an empty stomach; better after breakfast.	Better (worse) on an empty stomach *or* after breakfast.
Better or worse when swallowing	*Worse or* better when swallowing.
Worse after drinking	*Worse or* better after drinking.
Better from eructation	*Better or* worse from eructation.
Better *or* worse after stool	Worse after stool.
Generally worse when sitting erect; better when bending forward.	*Generally* better when sitting erect; worse when bending forward.
Better *or* worse when bending diseased part	*Worse or* better when bending the part.
Worse when sneezing	*Worse or* better when sneezing.
Generally worse on inspiration, better on expiration.	*Generally* better on inspiration; worse on expiration.
Worse when opening, better when closing the mouth.	Better (worse) when opening *or* when closing the mouth.
Better or worse when moving diseased part.	Worse when moving the suffering part.

Predomin. **worse** — Predomin. **better**

During rest, after lying down, when standing, sitting and lying, partic. sitting erect; when lying on the side, after sleep, on inspiration, and from pressure.

Predomin. **better** — Predomin. **worse**

From motion, partic. when moving the suffering part; when walking, when sitting bent forward, when lying on back, when rising, wh. getting out of bed, on expiration, when swallowing, & after eating.

N.B. The over-sensitiveness of Nux vom. to pain is very rarely found with Sabadilla.

* Sabadilla has the most thirst between chill and heat, N. vomica and others have it more between heat and sweat.

Sabadilla.	Pulsatilla.
Very rarely apoplexy—No paralysis . . .	Apoplexy—Paralysis.
Complaints most frequent on external ear, inside of nose, upper lip and on fore-arm.	Complaints most frequent in inner ear, on outside of nose, on under lip, and upper arm.
Pulse small, but somewhat spasmodic . . .	Pulse predom. frequent, small, and weak; sometimes intermitting or imperceptible.
Pulse affected by wine	Pulse affected by beer or coffee. C.Hg.
Partial sweat on front of body	Partial sweat on back of body.
Chill lessened after eating and in a warm room.	Chill increased after eating and in a warm room.
Want of thirst predom.	Want of thirst predom., but is constant only during the chill.

Sabadilla.	Pulsatilla.
Easy *or* difficult comprehension — Imbecility.	Difficult comprehension — Absent-mindedness — Unconsciousness — Melancholy.
Appetite for milk—Aversion to sour things .	Aversion to milk—Appetite for sour things.
Dislike for wine, but appetite for beer . . .	Desire for spirituous liquors.
Sexual desire too weak — Menstrual blood light-red.	Sexual desire too strong — Menstrual blood dark.
Expectoration seldom; during day	Expectoration predom., but not constant; morning and during day.
Heat in the fingers (during fever)	Fingers are like dead (during fever).

Sabadilla.	Pulsatilla.
Aggravation forenoon and night	Aggravation afternoon and evening after sunset until midnight.
Worse during full or new moon	Worse in sultry weather or before a storm.
Worse after sleep	*Worse or* better after sleep.
Worse from change of posture when lying or standing.	*Worse or* better from change of posture.
Better when getting out of bed	*Better or* worse when getting out of bed.
Worse when rising from a seat; better *afterwards.*	*Worse or* better when rising from a seat, *better or* worse *afterwards.*
Better when sitting down	Better *or* worse when sitting down.
Generally worse when sitting erect; better when bending forward.	*Generally* better when sitting erect; worse when bending forward.
Better when assuming an erect position . .	Worse *or* better when assuming an erect position.
Generally worse on inspiration, better on expiration.	*Generally* better on inspiration; worse on expiration.
Worse when taking a deep breath	Better *or* worse when taking a deep breath.
Predom. worse from pressure	Generally better from pressure.
Better or worse when swallowing	*Worse* or better when swallowing.
Worse on an empty stomach; better after breakfast.	Worse (better) on an empty stomach *or* after breakfast.
Almost always improv. after eating	*Worse or* better after eating.
Better from eructation	*Worse or* better from eructation.
Worse or better after stool	*Better or* worse after stool.

Predomin. worse ——— **Predomin. better**

In cold dry weather, from cold and when growing cold, from uncovering, in the open air and when walking in the open air, from bodily exertion, on inspiration, when sitting erect, when lying on the painful side, from pressure, and from sour things.

Predomin. better ——— **Predomin. worse**

In warm and damp air, from warmth and when growing warm, in bed and from warmth of bed, from wrapping up, in-doors and from warmth of stove, on expiration, when sitting bent forward, when lying on the unpainful side, after perspiring, when swallowing, while and after eating, from eructation, and from rubbing and scratching.

N.B. We very rarely find the over-sensitiveness of Pulsatilla to pain with Sabadilla; it also lacks the sensation of numbness in suffering parts peculiar to Pulsatilla.

Sabadilla.	Rhus.
Muscles lax—Pressure or sore pain in internal parts.	Muscles rigid—Pressure or sore pain in external parts.
No paralysis—Very rarely apoplexy . .	Paralysis—Apoplexy.
Pleasant dreams predom.	Anxious dreams.
Pulse small, but somewhat spasmodic .	Pulse irregular; generally frequent, faint, and soft; sometimes intermitting or imperceptible.
Pulse affected by wine	Pulse affected by beer, alcohol, coffee; fever increased. C.Hg.
Sweat only on the head	Sweat general, with exception of head.
Want of thirst almost constant	Thirst not constant.
Thirst often between chill and heat . . .	Thirst often already *before* the chill.
Chill lessened after eating	Chill increased after eating.
Ailments from fright—Easy *or* difficult comprehension—Imbecility.	Ailments from vexation with fear—Difficult comprehension—Unconsciousness—Mental confusion after a fall on the head.
Compl. of inner nose	Nasal compl. external oftener than internal.
Constipation of bowels most frequent . .	Diarrhœa predom.
Urine too scanty	Urine too often and copious.
Weak sexual desire	Erections.
Catam. too late, scanty, & of short durat'n.	Catam. too soon, profuse, & of long durat'n.
Expector. seldom; during day	Expect. not constant; partic. in the morn'g.
Compl. predom. on sole of foot	Compl. generally on top of foot.
AGGRAV. forenoon and before midnight. .	AGGRAV. from evening after sunset until morning.
Better in damp and warm air	Better in dry, warm air.
Worse during full or new moon	Worse during increase of moon.
Worse when looking upward, better when looking down.	Worse when looking down.
Better when getting out of bed	Worse *or* better when getting out of bed.
Worse when rising from a seat; better *afterwards*.	Worse *or* better when and *after* rising from a seat.
Better when sitting down	Better *or* worse when sitting down.
Generally worse when sitting erect, better when bending forwards.	*Generally* better when sitting erect, worse when bending forwards.
Better when leaning back against something.	Worse *or* better when leaning against something.
Better when eating; almost always improv. *afterwards*.	Worse *or* better when eating; *worse or* better *afterwards*.
Worse after drinking	*Worse or* better after drinking.
Worse *or* better after stool	*Better or* worse after stool.
Worse after mental exertion	Wore *after* bodily exertion. C.Hg.

Predomin. worse — **Predomin. better**

In dry weather, when *walking* in the open air,* when lying on the side, partic. the painful side, from pressure, and when sitting erect.

Predomin. better — **Predomin. worse**

In wet weather, when lying on the back or on unpainful side, when sitting bent forward, when assuming an erect position, when looking down, when swallowing, after meals, from eructation, from washing and moistening the diseased part.

N.B. Sabadilla lacks the sensation of numbness in suffering parts which Rhus has.

* Both remedies have aggrav. predom. *out-doors*, improv. in-doors.

Sambucus.	Arsenic.
Cutting pain in external parts — Apoplexia sanguinea.	Cutting pain in internal parts — Apoplexia serosa—Paralysis.
Pulse generally very frequent and small; often also slow and full.	Pulse frequent, small, and weak; sometimes trembling or imperceptible.
Creeping chills and *sweat* in alternation . .	Creeping chills and *heat* in alternation.*
Sweat appears early and very copious; sweat also after other attacks.	Sweat often long after the fever and rarely very copious.*
Hot sweat†	Cold sweat predom., also viscous, sour.*
Partial sweat on upper part of body (partic. face*) or general, with exception of head.	Sweat on lower part of body (and on back parts, occiput, neck, etc.*)
Sweat predominant night and morning . . .	Sweat predom. evening and night.*
Sweat before sleep, *lessened when falling asleep, disappears during sleep*, increased after awaking and still more after getting out of bed, on the whole *more when awake.*	Sweat increased before fall'g asleep, when fall'g asleep, when first asleep, part. *during sleep;* lessened after awaken'g & better after gett'g out of bed; walking in the open air.*
Cannot bear uncovering during the sweat . .	Indifference to being covered or not.*
Sweat predominant during motion, when lying, with or after the stool.	S. predom. after mot'n; better out-doors, when sitt'g, while eat'g, and after eat'g or drink'g.*

Sambucus.	Arsenic.
Sweat from anxiety	Anxiety with the sweat.*
With the sweat: Timidity, delirium	With the sweat: Indifference or despair.
With the sweat: Face sometimes bluish-red, predom. want of appetite, no thirst, stoppage of nose, cough predom. with expectoration, hands *blue and cold*, feet cold.	With the sweat: Face pale or red, nausea, bitter vomit, constant thirst, nose running, cough predom. with expectoration, fingers like dead, swelling of feet.*
Inability to sweat	Sweat too easily, or has been checked.*
Want of thirst constant	Drinks often, but little at a time.
Thirst, with disgust for drink	Desire for drink, without thirst.
Itching, relieved *or* unchanged by scratching.	Itching, aggravated by scratching.
Nausea in stomach or abdomen	Nausea, partic. in the throat.
Increased secretion of urine	Urine scanty (with diarrhœa) *or* copious.
Dry coryza	Fluent coryza.
Cough mostly dry, but often also with expect.	Expect. predom., but not constant; dur'g day.
Expectoration is yellow after Pneumonia . .	Expectoration is yellow after catarrh.*
Complaints predom. on fore-arm	Complaints predominant on upper arm.

Sambucus.	Arsenic.
Remission morning and during day	Remission of complaints *during day* and before midnight.
Worse while sweating, better *afterwards* . .	*Worse or* better during and after sweat.
Predom. worse in bed	Better in bed (warmth) *or* (rest) worse.
Worse or better during sleep	Worse during sleep.
Worse fr. change of posture (ly'g or stand'g).	Worse *or* better from change of posture.
Worse *or* better when getting out of bed; better *afterwards.*	Almost always improv. when getting out of bed; better *or* worse *afterwards.*
Worse when stooping, better when rising . .	Better *or* worse when stoop'g and when ris'g.
Ailments from abuse of Arsenic	Ailments from abuse of Cinchona, etc.
Worse from light, better in the dark . . .	Worse (better) from light *or* in the dark.

Predomin. worse — **Predomin. better**

From pressure, when bending the suffering part, when leaning against something, when standing, when sitting down.

Predomin. better — **Predomin. worse**

When rising from a seat, after sweat, from rubbing and scratching.

N.B. Over-sensitiveness to pain, which frequently occurs with Arsenic, has not yet been observed with Sambucus.

---

† Sambucus and Arsenic are both indicated in the so-called "Sudor anglicus;" both have fevers with "copious sweats," with both the sweat is better during motion, worse during rest, partic. in bed and "on awaking," worse when coughing; with both the concomitant complaints are: Unconsciousness, bodily restlessness; anxious, oppressed or short breathing; excessive weakness, etc. But the differences between these remedies are by far more essential, and to give both in alternation would be to depend on accidental cures.*

* added by C.Hg.

Sambucus.	Chamomilla.
Dropsy—Apoplexy—Delirium without fever .	No dropsy—Delirium during the hot stage.
Pulse generally very frequent. Comp. the next.	Pulse quick, small, and tense.
Sweat lessened during sleep	Sweat increased during sleep.
Sweat general, with exception of the head .	Sweat often confined to the head.
Sweat while awake; *disappearing on falling asleep.*	Sweat during sleep, *disappearing on awaking.*
Want of thirst constant	Thirst during all stages.
Pupils dilated	Pupils contracted.
Nasal complaints external	Nasal complaints predom. internal.
Hoarseness with hollow voice	Hoarseness with roughness or loss of voice.
Cough, partic. about midnight	Cough day & night; but often better dur. day.
Expectoration with sweetish or putrid taste .	Expector. with bitter, putrid, or sour taste.
Aggravation evening and night, partic. after midnight.	Aggravation evening and night, partic. before midnight.
Worse from uncovering, *better* fr. wrapping up.	Worse (resp. better) from uncovering *or* wrapping up.
Worse from pressure	Better *or* worse from pressure.
Better from moving diseased part	Generally aggrav. by moving diseased part.
Ailments from Arsenic	Ailments from Alumina or Borax.

Predomin. worse — **Predomin. better**

From cold,* when sitting bent forward, when lying on painful side, and from change of posture.

Predomin. better — **Predomin. worse**

From warmth, when sitting erect, lying on unpainful side, and from rubbing and scratching.

N.B. The over-sensitiveness of Chamomilla to pain seems to be wanting with Sambucus.

Sambuc.	Rhus.
Paralysis not yet observed	Paralysis of limbs.
Sleeplessness predom. after midnight . . .	Sleeplessness predom. before midnight.
Pleasant dreams	Anxious dreams.
Pulse generally very frequent & small; sometimes slow and full, sometimes intermitting.	Pulse generally accelerated, weak, faint, and soft; sometimes trembling or imperceptible.
Sweat lessened on falling asleep & during sleep.	Sweat increased on falling asleep & dur. sleep.
Want of thirst constant	Thirst not constant.
Nausea in stomach or abdomen	Nausea in œsophagus or stomach.
Milk diminished—Dry coryza	Secretion increased—Fluent coryza.
Aggravation evening and night, partic. after midnight.	Aggravation evening after sunset, night and morning.
Predom. worse in bed	*Better or* worse in bed.
Worse or better dur'g sleep; bett. after sleep.	Worse during and after sleep.
Better after getting out of bed, when and after rising from a seat, and worse when sitting down.	*Worse or* better after getting out of bed, when rising from a seat; better *or* worse *afterwards*, and when sitting down.
Worse when leaning against something, partic. against a sharp edge.	Worse *or* better when leaning against something, partic. better when leaning against something hard.
Worse when bending diseased part and after meals.	*Worse* or better when bending the part and after meals.

Predomin. worse — **Predomin. better**

In bed, when lying on painful side, and from pressure.

Predomin. better — **Predomin. worse**

After getting out of bed, when lying on unpainful side, after sleep, when rising from a seat, and when assuming an erect position.

---

* Chamomilla has aggrav. "in cold weather."

Sassaparilla.	Calcarca.
Upper left, lower right side—Rending pain downwards.	Upper right, lower left side—Rending pain upwards.
Muscles rigid—Inclination for open air . .	Muscles lax—Aversion to the open air.
Very rarely apoplexy—Itching, relieved by scratching	Apoplexy—Itching *relieved or* aggrav by scratching.
Miliary eruption breaks out in the open air.	Miliary eruption breaks out in-doors.
Anxious feeling in the head	Anxious feeling in the præcordia, in the region of the heart.

Sassaparilla.	Calcarca.
Compl. generally on external ear, on lower jaw and lower teeth, on lower gum, soft palate, in the spleen, on thigh, in the hollow of the knee, and on top of foot.	Compl. generally in inner ear, on upper jaw & upper teeth, on upper gum, hard palate, in the liver, on leg, on patella, and on the sole of the foot.
Pulse somewhat accelerated, partic. towards evening.	Pulse full and quick, particularly night and morning; often trembling.
Want of thirst—Want of appetite pred.—Appetite without hunger.	Thirst—Generally hunger, even without appetite.
Urine pale; too often and copious; sometimes scanty.	Urine dark; too often.
Catam. retarded and scanty	Catam. predom. too soon and profuse.
Cough without expectoration	Expectoration predom., but not constant; morning and during day.

Sassaparilla.	Calcarca.
REMISSION evening and night	REMISSION of complaints before midnight.
Ailments from abuse of Mercurius . . .	Ailments from Mercurius, Phosphor, Cinchona, Digitalis, or Nitric. acid.
Aggravation during new moon	Aggrav. during *full moon or* new moon.
Worse from light; better in the dark . .	Better (worse) from light *or* in the dark.
Worse from cold; better from warmth . .	Worse (better) from cold *or* from warmth.
Worse from warm diet, better from cold diet.	Worse (better) from cold *or* from warm diet.
Worse from smoking	*Worse or* better from smoking.
Worse when turning in bed	Better *or* worse when turning in bed.
Worse after sleep	*Worse or* better after sleep.
Worse when closing, better when opening the eyes.	Better (worse) when closing *or* when opening the eyes.
Better *or* worse when stooping	Worse when stooping.
Better when *sitting* bent forward; worse when sitting erect.	Worse (better) when sitting bent forward *or* erect.
Worse from bodily exertion	*Worse or* better from exertion, partic. worse from exertion on an empty stomach.
Worse from moving diseased part . . .	Better *or* worse when moving diseased part.

Predomin. **worse** ——— Predomin. **better**

In-doors, when lying on the painful side, from touch, when assuming an erect position, when sitting down, and after breakfast.

Predomin. **better** ——— Predomin. **worse**

Out-doors,* when lying on unpainful side, in bed, and before breakfast.

N.B. The sensation of numbness frequently found with Calcarea has not yet been observed with Sassaparilla.

---

* Both remedies have aggravation of symptoms predom. when "walking" out-doors.

Sassaparilla.	Mercur.
Dark hair—Muscles rigid—Sycosis . . .	Light hair—Muscles lax—Syphilis.
Emaciation—Pains pressing inwards . .	Emaciation *or* obesity—Pains pressing wards.
Is more disposed to paralysis (with atrophy of muscles) than to cramp.	Is more disposed to cramp than to para lysis.
Very rarely apoplexy—Inclination for open air.	Very rarely paralysis—Aversion to open air.
Cutaneous eruptions dry	Eruptions dry *or* humid.
Itching, lessened by scratching	Itching, aggrav. *or* lessened by scratching.
Ebullition of blood and protruding veins .	Throbbing in the veins.
Pulse frequent in the evening, slow in the morning.	Pulse frequent at night, slower during day; irregular; often trembling, intermitting or imperceptible.
Cheerfulness	Hopelessness.
Optical illusions, red color predominant .	Optical illusions, green color predom. C.Hg.
Palpitation of heart without fear	Palpitation of heart with fear.
Want of thirst predominant	Thirst predom., but not constant.
Nausea in stomach, less frequently in the throat.	Nausea in œsophagus or stomach, less frequently in throat.
Sour vomit	Bitter vomit.
Nose-bleeding, right side	Nose-bleeding, left side. C.Hg.
Complaints predom. in the spleen . . .	Compl. predom. in the liver.
Constipation predom.	Painful diarrhœa predom.
Urine often & copious, but sometimes scanty; pale; slimy; flaky, clayey or *sandy.*	Urine often and copious; dark; hot, fetid or *bloody.*
Catamenia too late, scanty, of short duration.	Catam. too profuse and of long duration; *or* too late, scanty, of short duration.
Coryza predominantly dry	Coryza oftener fluent than dry.
Cough without expectoration	Expector. not constant; during day.
AGGRAVATION (crescendo) in the morning on awaking, after getting out of bed, still more after breakfast, forenoon and afternoon.	AGGRAVATION (decrescendo) even'g, partic. in the night air, night & morning, partic. in the morn'g on awak'g; but *better* after getting up, & *still better* after breakfast.
Better in the open air, as long as one does not move about; *worse* in-doors.	*Worse* in the open air; *better* in-doors.
Worse from cold,* *better* from warmth . .	Worse *or* better from growing cold.
Worse when rising	*Worse* when stooping.

Predomin. worse — **Predomin. better**

After getting out of bed, after breakfast, from smoking, and in-doors.

Predomin. better — **Predomin. worse**

In bed,† on an empty stomach, and in the open air.

* Both remedies have aggrav. in wet cold weather, improv. in dry warm weather.
† A horizontal posture as well as rest, in general, improves with both remedies.

Secale corn.	Belladonna.
Emaciation—Painless cutaneous eruptions.	Obesity—Painful eruptions.
Insensibility of skin	Sensitiveness of skin. C.Hg.
Paralysis more frequent than apoplexy . .	Apoplexy more frequent than paralysis.
Paralysis generally of both side . . .	Paralysis often one-sided.
Heat or sweat, with inclination to uncover.	Heat or sweat, with aversion to uncover
Pulse often unchanged; generally slow and compressed; irregular.	Pulse generally quick, full, hard, and tense.
Thirst during all stages of the fever . . .	Thirst not constant; most rare during chill.

Secale corn.	Belladonna.
Indolence predominant — Very rarely unconsciousness.	Restlessness and hastiness predominant.
Weakness of memory	Memory very active *or* weak.
Eyes sunken	Eyes protruding.
Appetite for sour things	Aversion to sour things.*
Very rarely nausea†	Nausea in throat or abdomen, less frequently in stomach.
Urine pale—Retention of urine predominant.	Urine *dark or* light-colored—Retention of urine less frequent than incontinence.
Insufficient labor-pains,‡ particularly after loss of blood, or for want of the amniotic fluid.	Insufficient labor-pains, particularly in consequence of congestion of blood to the uterus.
Cramp-like labor-pains, with spasmodic hardness of the fundus uteri.	Spasmodic labor-pains, with constriction of the os tincæ.
Eclampsia parturentium, with opisthotonos.	Ecl. part., with ongest'ns to the head. C.Hg.
Incarceration of the placenta	Inclusion of parts of the child.
Diminished secretion of milk	Milk generally increased.
Complaints predominant on fore-arm . .	Complaints predominant on upper arm.

Secale corn.	Belladonna.
AGGRAVATION nocturnal	AGGRAVATION morning and from noon till midnight.
Worse when lying on the back, better when lying on the side.	Better (worse) when lying on back *or* on side.
Better when lying on painful, worse when lying on unpainful side.	Worse (better) when lying on painful *or* on unpainful side.
Worse when bending diseased part . . .	*Better or* worse when bending the part.

Predomin. worse — **Predomin. better**

From warmth, from growing warm and in warm air, from wrapping up, in bed, when lying on right side, and when sitting bent forward.

Predomin. better — **Predomin. worse**

From cold, from growing cold and in cold weather, from uncovering, but also when perspiring, when lying on left side, and when sitting erect.

N.B. Secale lacks the over-sensitiveness of Belladonna to pain; but Belladonna only very rarely has the sensation of numbness in suffering parts peculiar to Secale. Both remedies have sensitiveness to the touch. H.Gr.

---

* Compare Arsenicum—Belladonna.

† When nausea appears with Secale corn., it is in the stomach or oesophagus.

‡ According to Dr. Stens the Secale was decidedly of great use in pains of the sacrum, with a bearing down as if the parts should be forced out, worse when moving; as Belladonna has exactly the same symptoms, the decision can be made only by the characteristic differences given above, or the cure is merely an "accidental one." C.Hg.

Secale corn.	Veratrum.
Want of bodily irritability—Very rarely apoplexy.	Increased irritability—Apoplexy.
Painless eruptions and ulcers	Painful eruptions and ulcers.
Insensibility of skin	Sensitiveness of skin.*
Dry heat predom.—Pulse often unchanged .	Sweat predom.—Pulse sometimes trembling.
Beer increases the pulse	Beer lessens the fever.*
Thirst constant	Thirst predom., but not constant; most rare during sweat.

Secale corn.	Veratrum.
Rarely unconsciousness—Imbecility oftener than insanity.	Insanity oftener than imbecility.
Pupils generally dilated	Pupils generally contracted.
Hard of hearing after the cholera	Hard of hear'g, with (subjective) hear'g music or bells.*
Nose-bleeding: the blood is dark, runs continually, with great prostration, and a small, thread-like pulse; in old people or drunkards.	Nose-bleeding: pale face, cold skin, or small, slow, intermitting pulse; in nervous persons, subject to spasmodic complaints.*
Very rarely nausea	Nausea in stomach; vomiting without it.
Violent starting (jerking) of the body before and while vomiting bile.	Painful contraction of the belly while vomiting.*
Lumps and welts in the abdomen, in affections of the uterus.	Here & there hard knobs in the belly in colics *
Cholerine, with more retching than vomiting, chiefly with *loud noises in the belly*.	*Cholerine*, with more vomiting than retching, & less frequently rumbling in the intestines.*
Cholera Asiatica, with great collapsus and falling away of the whole body; face sunken, distorted, partic. the mouth; crawling sensation as of ants.	*Cholera Asiatica*, with very rapid loss of strength; face icy cold, disfigured, bluish, lips withered, bluish-black—Trismus.*
Cramps, with crawling sensation in the limbs, & partic. spasms, with the *fingers spread out*.	Cramps, partic. in the calves.*
In cholera Asiatica, *vain urging to urinate*.	Urging, with or without retention of urine.*
Urine pale	Urine dark.
Catamenia too soon—(Metrorhagia*) . . .	Catam. too soon *or* too late.—(Menostasia*).
Cough, with expectoration	Expector. not constant; during day.
Complaints predom. on fore-arm	Compl. predom. on upper arm.

Secale corn.	Veratrum.
Remission from morning till evening.	Remission during day and in the evening.
Worse from warmth and when growing warm,† better from cold and when growing cold.	Better (worse) from warmth and when grow'g warm, *or* from cold and when growing cold.
Better after getting out of bed	Worse *or* better after getting out of bed.
Worse when bending diseased part	Better *or* worse when bending the part.
Worse after eating, also after stool	Worse *or* better after eating, the same after stool.

Predomin. worse — **Predomin. better**

In warm air, when lying on the back or on unpainful side, when drawing up diseased limb, when walking, and from motion generally.

Predomin. better — **Predomin. worse**

In cold weather, when lying on side, partic. when lying on painful side, when stretching out diseased limb, during rest, after lying down, when sitting & standing, and when perspiring ‡

---

† Warm drinks, however, improve the cold feeling in the stomach, with Secale as well as many of the Veratrum complaints; the warmth of the bed aggravates pain in the limbs with both remedies.*

‡ This agrees fully with the predominance of dry heat as a symptom of Secale, & the heat with sweat of the Veratrum.

* added by C.Hg.

Sepia.	Aconitum.
Aversion to open air—Compl. predom. in external parts.	Inclination for open air—Compl. predom. in internal parts.
Itching, aggrav. by scratching — Vesicular erysipelas.	Itching, unchanged by scratching—Erysipelas with smooth skin.
Painless swelling of glands—Sweat on diseased parts.	Painful, hot swelling of glands—Heat on diseased parts.
Pulse frequent and full at night, during the day accelerated only by vexation or motion; sometimes trembling.	Pulse generally quick, full, and hard; but sometimes imperceptible.
Want of thirst; only dur'g chill thirst is usual.	Thirst during all stages of the fever.
First heat, then chill	First chill, then heat.

Sepia.	Aconitum.
Fear of apoplexy	Fear of loss of reason.
Mood serious; indifferent—Avarice	Mood malicious—Delirium.
Mental dullness	Ecstasies.
Nose-bleeding with pregnant or hæmorrhoidal persons.	Nose-bleeding with copious menstruation. C. Hg.
Complaints predom. on lower lip	Compl. predom. on upper lip.
Vomiting food	Vomiting mucus or worms.
Urinal sediment *reddish or* white — Incontinence predom.	Urinal sediment red—Retention oftener than incontinence.
Catamenia generally too profuse	Catam. generally too scanty.
Milk diminished	Milk increased—Galactorrhœa.
Nasal secretion generally watery	Nasal secretion thick.
Expectoration predom., but not constant; is loosened night and morning; is swallowed.	Expectoration very rare; morning and during day.
Complaints predom. on tip of elbow . . .	Compl. predom. on patella.

Sepia.	Aconitum.
Remission of complaints afternoon	Remission *during day* and before midnight.
Ailments from Sulph., or abuse of Mercurius or Cinchona.	Ailments from Sepia, Sulph., Chamom., Coffea, N. vom., Veratr., or Petroleum.
Worse in snowy air	Worse from the heat of the sun.
Worse (better) in cold *or* in warm air . . .	Worse in cold weather, better in warm air.
Worse (better) in the open air *or* in-doors .	Pred. worse in-doors, better in warm, open air.*
Better or worse from warmth of bed . . .	Worse from warmth of bed.
Worse or bett. dur'g sweat, worse *afterwards.*	Worse while sweating, better *afterwards.*
Better after sufficient sleep, but worse on awaking when roused from sleep.	Worse after sleep.
Better or worse when getting out of bed . .	Worse when getting out of bed.
Worse *or* better when rising from a seat . .	Worse when rising from a seat.
Worse when look'g up or over a large surface.	Worse when looking down.
Generally better on inspiration, worse on expiration.	Worse on inspiration, better on expiration.
Better or worse when taking a deep breath .	Worse when taking a deep breath.
Better or worse from exertion	Worse from bodily exertion.
Predom. worse during rest, better when moving, partic. the diseased part.	Better (worse) during rest *or* when moving, partic. the diseased part.
Worse when bending the suffering part . .	Better *or* worse when bending the part.
Worse or better after meals	Better *or* worse after meals.
Better from drinking cold water	Worse *or* better from drinking cold water.
Almost always aggrav. by eructation . . .	Better from eructation.
Worse or better after stool	Better *or* worse after stool.

Predomin. worse —— **Predomin. better**

On expiration, from uncovering, from washing and moistening diseased part, when lying on the back or on unpainful side, "after" sweat, when sitting, and from eructation.

Predomin. better —— **Predomin. worse**

On inspiration, from wrapping up, when lying on the side, partic. on the painful side, from warmth of bed, when turning in bed, after sleep, when getting out of bed, when assuming an erect position, from bodily exertion, and from smoking.

* Compare note to Aconit.—Bellad.

Sepia.	Belladonna.
Complaints predom. in external parts—Rending pain downwards.	Complaints predom. in internal parts—Rending pain upwards.
Paralysis with atrophy, generally of both sides.	Nervous paralysis, often one-sided.
Emaciation—Painless swelling of glands . .	Obesity—Painful swelling of glands.
Eruptions generally dry.	Humid eruptions.
Heat ascending—Sweat on suffering part . .	Head descending—Coldness on suffering part.
Want of thirst; only dur. chill generally thirst.	Thirst most rare during chill.
Mood serious; sad and despondent	Mood varying; silly—Cheerfulness or deject'n.
Weak memory—Mental dullness—Weakness of will.	Memory active *or* weak—Ecstacies or dullness.
Pupils contracted	Pupils generally dilated.
Eruption on under lip	Eruption on upper lip.
Appetite for sour things—Fetid flatus . . .	Aversion to sour things*—Scentless flatus.
Catamenia generally too late—Menstrual blood dark.	Catamenia too soon; blood generally light-colored.
Os tincæ swollen, with hardness	Os tincæ swollen, with heat. Lippe.
Secretion of milk diminished	Milk generally increased.
Fluent coryza of left side	Fluent coryza of right side.†
Respiration loud—Expectoration predom., but not constant; is loosened, partic. night and morning; is swallowed.	Respiration predom. low—Expectoration seldom with the cough; morning, during day, evening.
Complaints frequent on tip of elbow, in hollow of elbow, on fore-arm, and on calf.	Complaints frequent on patella, in hollow of knee, on upper arm, and on shin.
AGGRAVATION from evening till the next morning and during forenoon.	AGGRAVATION morning and noon till midnight.
Worse during new moon and in snowy air . .	Worse during full moon and from heat of sun.
Worse (better) in cold *or* in warm air	Worse in cold weather; better in warm air.
Worse or better after lying down and in bed.	Almost always improv. after lying down and in bed.
Predom. worse lying on back, better on side.	Better (worse) when lying on back *or* side.
Predom. better lying on painful, worse on unpainful side.	Better (worse) when lying on painful *or* on unpainful side.
Better after sufficient sleep; but worse on awaking when roused from sleep.	Predom. worse after sleep.
Better or worse when and after getting out of bed, and when rising from a seat.	Worse when getting out of bed; amost always improv. *afterwards* & when rising from seat.
Worse when leaning back	Worse *or* better leaning against something, partic. better against something hard.
Worse when bending the diseased part . .	*Better or* worse bending diseased part.
Worse when idle	Worse from being overhurried.
Worse after sweating	Worse during sweat.
Better (worse) in the open air *or* in-doors . .	Predom. worse in the open air, better in-doors,
Worse when looking up, or over a large surface.	Worse when looking sideways or at running water.
Worse when ascending; better descending .	Better (worse) when ascending *or* descending.
Worse when eating	Worse *after* eating.
Better when drinking; worse *afterwards* . .	Better (toothache) while eating; worse *afterwards*.
Complaints while swallowing food	Complaints, partic. while swallowing drink.

Predomin. worse — **Predomin. better**

During rest, after lying down, in bed, when lying, standing and sitting, partic. sitting bent forward; *when stooping*, when stretching out diseased limb, when bending the suffering part, partic. when bending the part or head backwards; when opening the eyes, on an empty stomach, from eructation, from pressure (from rubbing and scratching).

Predomin. better — **Predomin. worse**

When walking, from motion, partic. moving the suffering part; *from bodily exertion*, when sitting erect, *when rising* from stooping, when drawing up diseased limb, when closing the eyes, after sleep, when getting out of bed, after breakfast, and from drinking cold water.‡

* With the exception of desire for acid of lemons. Comp. Arsenic—Belladonna.

† Moreover Bellad. has predom. dry coryza, which also is not rare with Sepia.

‡ Both remedies have predom. improv. from cold diet in general, aggrav. from warm diet; but when drinking, *the difficulty of swallowing drink* peculiar to Bellad. must be taken into consideration.

Sepia.	China.
Complaints predom. in external parts . . .	Compl. predom. in internal parts.
Itching, aggrav. by scratching—Painless swelling of the glands.	Itching, unchanged by scratching — Painful, hot swelling of glands.
Pulse frequent & full at night, during the day accelerated only by vexation or motion; sometimes trembling.	Pulse quick and hard, but small; quieter after eating.
Pulse altered by beer	Pulse altered by alcohol, coffee, partic. tea. C. Hg.
First heat, then chill—Heat increas'd aft. eat'g.	First chill, then heat—Heat lessened aft. eat'g.
Sweat sometimes general, with except'n of head.	Sweat sometimes general, with except'n of feet.
Thirst only during chill and *before & after* it.	Thirst most prominent *before* and after the different stages of the fever.
Loquacity—Serious mood	Taciturnity—Amorousness
Ailments from vexation with fear, less frequently from fright, anger, or disappointed love.	Ailments from vexation.
Mental dullness—Imbecility—Insanity . . .	Mental excitability—Delirium.
Compl. most frequent in inside of ear, in liver, on fore-arm, on tip and in hollow of elbow, and on back part of thigh.	Compl. most frequent on outside of ear, in spleen, on upper arm, on patella & in hollow of knee, and on front part of thigh.
Far-sightedness	Short-sightedness.
Loss of taste—Predom. bitter vomit . . .	Delicate taste—Vomit oftener sour than bitter.
Urinal sediment *red or* white	Urinal sediment red.
Catamenia generally too late	Catamenia too soon.
Expectoration predom., but not constant; is loosen. night & morn'g & generally swallow'd.	Expector. not constant; during day & evening
REMISSION of complaints afternoon	REMISSION afternoon and evening.
Ailments from (Sulph., Mercurius, or) abuse of Cinchona, and from sting of insects.	Ailm. fr. (Sulph., Mercur.) Ferrum, Cuprum, Aurum, Arsenic, Asa fœt., Ipecac., Hellebor and Veratrum.
Spring diseases	Autumnal diseases.
Worse during new moon and before a thunderstorm.	Worse during increase of moon.
Better (worse) in the open air *or* in-doors . .	Worse in the open air, better in-doors.
Worse (better) in cold *or* warm air	Worse in cold weather, better in warm air.
Better or worse from warmth of bed . . .	Worse from warmth of bed.
Generally better when wrapping up the head, worse when uncovering it.	Worse from wrapping up the head, better when uncovering it.
Better or worse when and after getting out of bed.	Worse *or* better when getting out of bed, better *afterwards*.
Almost always improved when rising . . .	Worse *or* better when rising.
Better or worse from exertion	Worse from bodily exertion.
Almost always improv. when moving diseased part, worse when bending it.	Worse *or* better when moving the part and when bending it.
Worse from shaking the head	*Worse or* better from shaking the head.
Generally worse when opening, better when closing the eyes.	Better (worse) when opening *or* when closing the eyes.
Worse when grinding the teeth	Better *or* worse from biting.
Worse when eating, partic. eating meat . .	*Better or* worse when eating; *worse or* better from meat.

Predomin. worse — **Predomin. better**

In dry weather, from uncovering the head, when lying on the left or on the unpainful side, during rest generally, when bending back the suffering part, on an empty stomach, when eating, from rubb'g and scratching.

Predomin. better — **Predomin. worse**

In wet weather, from wrapping up the head, lying on right or on painful side, from warmth of bed, when turning in bed, from motion, from bodily exertion, after breakfast, and from smoking.

Sepia.	Graphites.
Hæmorrhages, blood dark—Apoplexy	Hæmorrh., blood light-red—No apoplexy.
Sensitiveness of external parts	Sensitiveness of internal parts.
Fainting spells in crowded rooms	Fainting spells in the open air.
The diseased parts are swollen	The diseased parts are emaciated.
Eruptions generally dry	Eruptions generally humid.
Pulse frequent and full at night, during day accelerated only by vexation or motion; sometimes trembling or intermitting; generally irregular.	Pulse full and hard, but only in the morning somewhat accelerated.
First heat, then chill	First chill, then heat.
Thirst only during chill & *before* & *after* it.	Want of thirst, partic. during hot stage.
Chill, increased in the open air	Chill, lessened in the open air.
Mood serious — Ailments from vexation with fear.	Mood changing—Amorousness—Ailments from grief.
Solicitude concerning bodily welfare	Solicitude concern'g spiritual welfare. C.Hg.
Fancies—Imbecility—Insanity	No unconsciousness.
Optical illusions in dark colors	Optical illusions in bright colors.
Eruption on under lip	Eruption on upper lip.
Coldness in the teeth	Burning in the teeth. C.Hg.
Generally loss of appetite	Generally hunger.
Vomit predominantly bitter	Sour vomit.
Urinal sediment *reddish* or whitish	Urinal sediment predom. whitish.
Catamenia of too long duration and generally profuse.	Catamenia of too short duration & scanty.
Expector. predom., but not constant; is loosened night and morning & generally swallowed.	Expector. almost constant; during day and in the evening.
Compl. predom. in hollow of elbow	Complaints predom. in patella.
REMISSION afternoon	REMISSION during day.
Ailments from Sulph., Mercurius, or abuse of Cinchona, also from sting of insects.	Ailments from abuse of Arsenic.
Worse during new moon	Worse during full moon.
Worse (better) in cold or warm air	Worse in cold weather; better in warm air.
Almost always worse when growing cold, better when growing warm.	Worse (better) when growing cold *or* warm.
Better or worse from warmth of bed	*Worse or* better from warmth of bed.
Better after sufficient sleep, but worse when roused from sleep.	Worse after sleep.
Better or worse when getting out of bed	Worse when getting out of bed.
Better *or* worse when rising from a seat	Worse when rising from a seat.
Better *or* worse when taking a deep breath.	Worse when taking a deep breath.
Worse when swallowing and after drinking.	*Better or* worse when swallowing and after drinking.
Worse after a satisfying meal	Worse when hungry.

Predomin. worse — **Predomin. better**

During rest, when standing, when lying on unpainful side, when riding, from pressure, after perspir'g, on an empty stomach, when swallowing, from warm diet, from spirituous liquors, after drinking, and from eructation.

Predomin. better — **Predomin. worse**

From motion, when walking, when lying on painful side, when turning in bed, after sleep, when gett'g out of bed, after breakfast, from cold diet.

Sepia.	Silicea.
Dark hair—Muscles rigid	Light hair—Muscles lax.
Itching, aggrav. by scratching	Itch'g, unchanged *or* aggrav. by scratch'g.
Vesicular erysipelas	Erysipelas with smooth skin.
Confluent small-pox. G. Bute.	Convulsions, abscesses or other suppurat's; eruptions, &c., after vaccination. C. Hg.
Painless swelling of glands	Painful swelling of glands.
Sleeplessness preval. before midnight	Sleeplessness preval. after midnight.
Pulse accelerated, part. by vexation or motion; sometimes trembling or intermitting.	Pulse generally quick, hard, but small.
Pulse altered by beer	Pulse altered by wine. C. Hg.
Sweat often general, with exception of head.	Sweat often confined to head.
Sweat on suffering part—Hands and fingers become like dead.	Coldness on suffering part—Heat in the fingers.
Want of thirst; only during cold stage there generally is thirst.	Thirst, part. during hot & sweating stages.
Compl. predom. in inner ear and in hollow of elbow.	Compl. generally on external ear and in hollow of knee.
Seriousness—Irritable mood	Gentleness—Amorousness.
Insanity—Imbecility	Very rarely mental dullness.
Solicitude concerning bodily welfare	Solicitude concern'g spiritual welfare. C. Hg.
Painful sensitiveness of the roots of the hair, in the evening, partic. on the *side not lain on*, when touched, during cold north-winds; burn'g sensat'n after scratching.	Sensitiveness of the scalp to the touch and to pressure, partic. in the evening, when growing warm in bed, and of the *side lain on;* burning sensation after scratching.
Eruption on under lip	Eruption on upper lip.
Discharge of urine too seldom—Sore pain in belly after stool.	Discharge of urine too often—Remission of bellyache after stool.
Urinal sediment red or white	Urinal sediment red or yellow.
Sexual desire changing, with impotence	Sexual desire generally increased.
Catam. generally profuse	Catam. generally too scanty.
Expector. predom., but not constant; is loosened night and morning and generally swallowed.	Expector. almost constant; during day.
REMISSION during afternoon	REMISSION before midnight.
Worse about the time of the new moon	*Worse* during new moon, and still oftener during full moon.
Improved oftener than aggravated when lying on painful side.	*Worse* when lying on painful side, better when lying on unpainful side.
Almost always improved by motion	Improved by continued moderate motion, but aggrav. by change of position.
Improv. oftener than aggravated by bodily exertion.	Aggrav. oftener than improved by bodily exertion.
Improved as often as aggrav. by walking in the open air; but always worse in crowded rooms.	*Worse* in the open air; better in-doors.

Predomin. worse —— **Predomin. better**

In company, after warm diet, on an empty stomach and in the side not lain on, therefore when lying on unpainful side.

Predomin. better —— **Predomin. worse**

From bodily exertion,* when alone, after cold diet, from smoking, after breakfast, and in the side lain on, therefore when lying on painful side.

* Both remedies have aggrav. after mental exertion. C. Hg.

Sepia.	Sulphur.
Ulcerative pain in external parts — Pinching pain in internal parts.	Ulcerative pain in internal, pinching pain in external parts.
Over-sensitiveness—Apoplexy	Insensibility—Very rarely apoplexy.
Painful eruptions and ulcers	Painless eruptions and ulcers.
Itching, aggrav. by scratching	Itching, predom. lessened by scratching.
Sweat on diseased part	Coldness on diseased part.
Sweat, somet. general, with exception of head.	Heat, often general, with exception of head.
Chill lessened after getting out of bed . . .	Chill increased after getting out of bed.
Thirstlessness; during chill generally thirst .	Thirst, mostly during hot stage; during the cold stage generally thirstless.
Irritable mood—No delirium	M. changing; gentle *or* irritable—Delirium.
Far-sightedness—Stye on lower lid	Short-sightedn. pred.—Stye on upp. lid. C.Hg.
Putrid subjective odor predom.	Objective stench from nose predom.
Swelling or eruption on under lip predom. .	Swelling or eruption on upper lip predom.
Sensation of weight in teeth	Sensation of looseness in the teeth. C.Hg.
Desire for spirituous liquors	Desire *or* dislike for beer & spirituous liquors.
Predom. bitter vomit	Vomit sour oftener than bitter.
Catam. of too long durat'n & gener'ly profuse.	Cat. generally of too short duration & scanty.
Expectoration predom., but not constant; is loosened, part. night & morn.; is swallowed.	Expector. not constant; morning and during day, less frequently at night.
Complaints predom. on tip of elbow . . .	Complaints predom. on patella.
Remission of complaints in the afternoon . .	Remission *afternoon* and before midnight.
Worse during new moon and when idle . .	Worse during full moon & when overhurried.*
Better or worse from exertion	Predom. worse from bodily exertion.
Alm. alw. improv. wh. moving diseased part.†	*Worse or* better when moving diseased part.
Almost always aggrav. by the touch . .	*Worse or* better from the touch.
Worse when stooping, almost always improv. when rising.	Better *or* worse when stooping; *worse or* better when rising.
Worse when growing cold; better when growing warm.	Better (worse) when growing cold *or* warm.
Worse after sweat	*Worse or* better after sweat.
Better or worse from warmth of bed . . .	Predom. worse from warmth of bed.
Predom. worse lying on back; better on side.	*Generally* better lying on back, worse on side.
Better when turning in bed	*Worse or* better when turning in bed.
Better after sufficient sleep; worse when roused from insufficient sleep.	Worse after sleep.
Better or worse getting out of bed	Better when getting out of bed.
Better or worse when rising from a seat . .	Worse when rising from a seat.
Predom. worse on an empty stomach; better after breakfast.	Better (worse) on an empty stomach *or* after breakfast.
Worse wh. eating; *worse or* bett *afterwards.*	Bett. *or* worse wh. eating; worse *afterwards.*
Predom. worse after stool and urinating . .	Worse *or* better after stool or urinating.
Worse when looking up or over a large surface.	Worse when looking down, partic. at running water.
Worse when sneezing	*Worse or* better from sneezing.

Predomin. worse ⸻ **Predomin. better**

In dry weather, from cold, from uncovering, when lying on back or on unpainful side, from scratching, from pressure, "on expiration," from warm diet, from eructation.

Predomin. better ⸻ **Predomin. worse**

In wet weather, from warmth, from wrapping up, when lying on side, partic. on painful side; from warmth of bed, after sleep, when turning in bed, "on inspiration," from drinking cold water and from cold diet generally, from smoking, when rising from stooping, when moving diseased part, from bodily exertion.

N.B. Sulph. rarely has the over-sensitiveness of Sepia to pain; the latter rarely the sensation of numbness in suffering parts peculiar to Sulph.—Both remedies have mere sensitiveness to touch.

* The complaints, when idle (Sepia) and from being overhurried (Sulphur), are only different expressions of the sam impatient mental state.

† Pains in thigh driving out of bed and to walk about "without relief" in Sepia, "with relief" in Sulphur (and Arsenic). C.Hg.

Silicea.	Sulphur.
Right side, partic. *upper right, lower left side.*	*Left* side, partic. *upper left, lower right side.*
Over-sensitiveness — Increased bodily irritability.	Insensibility or sensation of numbness—Want of bodily irritability.
Painful eruptions, ulcers, or swelling of glands.	Painless eruptions, ulcers, or swell'g of glands.
Cures wens or other tumors by suppuration .	Generally causes atrophy of warts.
Itching. aggrav. *or* unchanged by scratching.	Itching, lessened by scratching.
Sleeplessness prevalent after midnight . . .	Sleeplessness preval. before midnight.
Dreams of water, thieves, ghosts, business, diseases, or historical.	Dreams of fire, misfortunes, also merry, mentally exerting dreams, etc.
Pulse irregular; generally quick, hard, & small.	Pulse quick, hard, and full; sometimes intermitting or imperceptible.
Heat or sweat, with aversion to uncover . .	Heat or sweat, with inclination to uncover.
Apoplexy	Very rarely apoplexy.
Amorousness	Changing mood.
Faculty to think, weak; improved in the evening.	Faculty to think, weak, partic. in the evening; better in the morning.
Compl. generally in inner angle of eye, on external ear, and in lower part of chest.	Compl. generally in external angle of eye, in inner ear, and in upper part of chest.
Far-sightedness—Saliva predom. increased .	Short-sightedn.—Saliva generally diminished.
Bitter vomit—Bellyache better after stool .	Vomit sour oftener than bitter — Bellyache after stool.
Urinal sediment yellow or red	Urinal sediment white or red.
Catamenia generally of too long duration . .	Catamenia generally of too short duration.
Expectoration almost constant; during day .	Expector. not constant; morning and during day, less frequently at night.
REMISSION of complaints before midnight . .	REMISSION *afternoon* and before midnight.
Ailments from Sulphur. or Mercurius . . .	Ailm. from Mercurius & other metals, Nitric. acid., Iodine, Sepia, Cinchona, Rhus.
Worse when idle	Worse from being over-hurried.
Worse when alone, better when in company .	*Generally* bett. when alone, worse in company.
Worse when growing cold and in cold weather, better when growing warm and in warm air.	Better (worse) when growing cold and in cold weather, or when grow'g warm & in warm air.
Worse in the open air, better in-doors.	*Generally* better in the open air, worse in-doors (partic. in crowded rooms*).
Worse after sweat	*Worse or* better after sweat.
Worse during full *or* new moon	Worse during full moon.
Predom. worse when lying on back, better when lying on side.	*Generally* better when lying on back, worse when lying on side.
Worse from change of posture when lying or standing.	*Worse or* better from change of posture.
Worse when stooping, better when rising . .	*Worse or* better when stooping & when rising.
Worse when looking up	Worse when looking down, partic. at running water.
Worse from weeping, also after drinking .	*Worse or* better fr. weep'g, also after drink'g.
Better on an empty stomach, worse after breakfast.	Worse (better) on an empty stomach *or* after breakfast.
Better (worse) when opening *or* when closing the mouth.	Worse when opening, better when closing the mouth.
Worse *or* better from exertion	Almost always worse from bodily exertion, running, etc.
Worse when taking a deep breath	Worse *or* better when taking a deep breath.
Worse from the touch	*Worse or* better from the touch.

Predomin. worse ⏟ **Predomin. better**

In dry weather, in the open air, from cold, from uncovering, when alone, when lying on back, when gett'g out of bed, when resting the diseased limb on something, from pressure, and from rubb'g and scratching.

Predomin. better ⏟ **Predomin. worse**

In wet weather, in-doors,* from warmth, from wrapping up, in company, when lying on side, from warmth of bed, and when rising from stooping.

* Both remedies have improv. of complaints from warmth of stove.

Spigelia.	Belladonna.
Left side, partic. *lower left, upper right side.*	*Right* side, partic. *lower right, upper left side.*
Light hair—Compl. predom. in external parts.	Dark hair—Compl. predom. in internal parts.
Internal trembling sensation—No apoplexy .	Trembling of external parts—Apoplexy.
Complaints predom. on eyelids	Complaints predom. in the angles of the eye.
Compl. generally on upper jaw, in the spleen, in lower part of chest, on fore-arm, in hollow of elbow, on the calf and on top of foot.	Complaints generally in lower jaw, liver. upper part of chest, on upper arm, in hollow of knee, on shin and sole of foot.
Pulse slow and strong, more frequent in the evening; irregular; sometimes trembling.	Pulse generally frequent or quick, full, bard and tense.
Heat or sweat, with inclination to uncover .	Heat or sweat, with aversion to uncover.
Thirstless; during heat sometimes thirst . .	Thirst most rare during chill.

Spigelia.	Belladonna.
Weak memory	Memory very active *or* weak.
Easily irritated or offended; cannot bear to see pointy things; rarely indifferent.	All the senses over-sensitive or complete apathy. C.Hg.
Sensitive hearing in neuralgia	Over-sensit. to light pred. in neuralgia. C.Hg.
Stammering or looking cross-eyed in abdominal diseases.	Stammering or speechless in diseases of brain or spine. C.Hg.
Eyelids lame, relaxed, have to be lifted up with the fingers, or paralytic stiffness.	Eyelids heavy; they fall down or tremble; quivering or spasms, and ectropium. C.Hg.
Eyes gummy all day	Lids stick together in the morning. C.Hg.
Desire *or* dislike for beer	Dislike for beer.
Expectoration rather infrequent	Expectoration very infrequent; morning, during day, evening.

Spigelia.	Belladonna.
Remission of complaints after midnight . .	Remission after midnight and in the *forenoon.*
Ailments from abuse of Mercurius	Ailm. from Mercur., Platina, Cuprum, Plumbum, Ferrum, or from sting of insects.
Better *or* worse from washing and moistening the part.	Worse from washing, &c., the diseased part.
Worse or bett. in bed; worse fr. warmth of bed.	Better in bed and from warmth of bed.
Generally worse when lying on right side, better on left.	Better when lying on right side, worse when lying on left.
Worse when lying on painful, better when lying on unpainful side.	Better (worse) when lying on painful *or* on unpainful side.
Worse *or* better after getting out of bed . .	Alm. always improv. after getting out of bed.
Predom. worse when stooping; better when rising.	*Better or* worse when stooping; *worse or* better when rising.
Worse when ascending, bett. when descending.	Better (worse) when ascending or descending.
Worse when bending the diseased part . . .	*Better or* worse when bending the part.
Almost always improv. while eating; predom. better *after* meals.	*Worse or* better while eating; worse after meals.
Worse from spirituous liquors	*Worse or* better from spirituous liquors.
Better *or* worse from smoking	Worse from smoking.
Worse looking upwards, downw., or sideways.	Worse looking sideways or at running water.

Predomin. worse — **Predomin. better**

In wet weather, when growing warm, from wrapping up, in bed and "from warmth of bed," when lying on right side, when bending diseased part, when stooping, when stretching out suffering limb, when opening the eyes, when holding the breath, when fasting, and from cold diet* (or sweets, C.Hg.)

Predomin. better — **Predomin. worse**

In dry weather, when growing cold, from uncovering, also during sweating stage, when lying on left side, when rising from stooping, when drawing up suffering part, when closing the eyes, after breakfast, during and after meals, from warm diet, after drinking, and after stool.

---

* Belladonna, as well as Spigelia, has aggravation predom. from drinking cold water, because it is peculiar to Bellad. that "swallowing fluids" is difficult; with Spigelia we find more complaints when swallowing saliva.

Spigelia.	Pulsatilla.
Left side, partic. *lower left, upper right side.*	*Right* side, partic. *lower right, upper left side.*
Complaints (pinching pain, &c.) predom. in external parts.	Complaints (pinching pain, &c.) predom. in internal parts.
Dropsy of internal parts — Aversion to the open air.	Dropsy of external parts—Desire for the open air.
Itching, aggrav. *or* unchanged, *or* lessened by scratching.	Itching, aggrav. *or* unchanged, but never relieved by scratching.
Complaints generally on upper jaw, upper lip, in the spleen, fore-arm, palm of hand, patella, thigh, and top of foot.	Complaints generally on lower jaw, lower lip, in the liver, upper arm, back of hand, hollow of knee, leg, and on sole of foot.
No apoplexy	Apoplexy.
Pulse generally strong, but slow; irregular; trembling.	Pulse generally weak, but accelerated; sometimes intermitting or imperceptible.
Pulse often quicker than beating of heart . .	Pulse often suppressed, with strong beating of heart.
Thirst appears only sometimes during hot stage.	Want of thirst predom., but constant only during cold stage.
Irritable mood—Rarely unconsciousness . .	Gentleness—Good-naturedness—Delirium.
Pain like a sore in the head, evenings, when stooping and when moving the eyes; *better* when lying with head high, from pressure and when laying the hand on it; *worse when walking in the open air.*	Pain like a sore in the head, under the same conditions as Spigelia, but *better when walking in the open air.*
Pupils dilated—Far-sightedness	Pup. generally contracted—Short-sightedness.
Appetite for spirituous liquors; desire or aversion to beer.	Desire for beer and spirituous liquors.
Urine too often and copious—Sediment white.	Urine too seldom and scanty—Sediment red.
Expectoration rather rare	Expectoration predom., but not constant.
Palpitation of heart with trembling beats . .	Palpitation of heart with equal beats, rarely with intermissions.
Aggrav., partic. from morning till midnight .	Aggravation from noon till midnight.
Worse from bodily exertion	*Generally* better from exertion, running, &c.
Worse after perspiring	*Worse or* better after perspiring.
Generally worse when lying on right side; better when lying on left side.	Predom. better when lying on right side; worse when lying on left side.
Almost always improv. when sitting down .	Worse *or* better when sitting down.
Worse when looking sideways, up, or down .	Worse when looking up.
Predom. better after eating	*Worse or* better after eating.
Better *or* worse from smoking	Worse from smoking.
Almost always improv. after stool	*Better or* worse after stool.
Worse when assuming an erect position . .	Better *or* worse when assuming an erect position.
Worse when getting out of bed; worse *or* better afterwards.	*Better or* worse when and after getting out of bed.
Almost always aggrav. when rising from a seat; better afterwards.	*Worse or* better when rising from a seat; *better or* worse *afterwards.*
Worse when moving the part; worse when bending it.	*Better or* worse when moving diseased part; worse *or* better when bending it
Worse *or* better from washing and moistening the part.	Predom. better from washing and moistening diseased part.

Predomin. worse — **Predomin. better**

From cold and in cold weather, in the open air and when walking out-doors, from motion, when walking, from bodily exertion, when lying on right or on painful side, when getting out of bed, when opening the eyes, when bending suffering part sideways, when stretching out diseased limb, when sitting erect, from drinking cold water and from cold diet in general, when moving suffering part.

Predomin. better — **Predomin. worse**

From warmth and in warm air, in-doors, during rest, after lying down, when standing and lying, particularly lying on left or on unpainful side, when closing the eyes, when drawing up diseased limb, when sitting bent forward, while and after eating, after drinking, from warm diet, and when perspiring.

N.B. Spigelia lacks the numb feeling in suffering parts peculiar to Pulsatilla.

Spongia.	Bryonia.
Desire for open air	Aversion to the open air.
Rending pain upwards	Rending pain downwards.
Complaints predominant in external parts—Constriction in internal parts.	Compl. predom. in internal parts — Constriction in external parts.
Compl. predominant on upper jaw, fore-arm, on tip of elbow, and on shin.	Compl. predom. on lower jaw, on upper arm, on patella, and on calf.
Itching, unchanged *or* aggrav., or locality changed by scratching.	Itching, unchanged *or* relieved by scratching.
Pleasant dreams predominant	Anxious dreams.
No apoplexy—No paralysis	Apoplexy—Paralysis.
Cheerfulness—Satiety of life	Dejection—Despondency—*Irritability.*
Very rarely fancies or delirium . . .	Unconsciousness.
Catamenia too soon	Catamenia too soon *or* retarded.
Voice interrupted	Voice nasal.
Respiration predom. with dry sound . .	Respiration predom. with moist sound.
Cough generally dry, sometimes with expectoration, which is loosened in the morning and swallowed.	Expectoration not constant; morning and evening, less frequently during the day.
Aggravation *afternoon* and night, partic. before midnight.	Aggravation from evening till morning.
Worse during full moon	Worse in sultry air or during a storm.
Worse in cold weather, better in warm air .	Worse (better) in cold weather *or* in warm air.
Worse when closing the eyes, better when opening them.	Worse (better) when closing or when opening the eyes.
Worse when lying on painful side, better when lying on unpainful side.	*Generally* better when lying on painful, worse when lying on unpainful side.
Better *or* worse when stooping, worse when rising.	Worse when stooping, *worse or* better when rising.
Worse from eructation	Better *or* worse from eructation.

Predomin. worse —— **Predomin. better**

In contracted posture, when lying on right or on painful side, when lying generally, from warmth of bed, when sitting, particularly when sitting erect, when sitting down, after stool, from external pressure, from rubbing and scratching.

Predomin. better —— **Predomin. worse**

In extended posture, when lying on left or on unpainful side, when sitting bent forward, when and after rising from a seat, when walking out-doors, when swallowing and eating.

N.B. Spongia lacks the over-sensitiveness to pain which often occurs with Bryonia. Both remedies have sensitiveness to the touch.

Spongia.	**Phosphorus.**
Light hair—Skin and muscles lax	Dark hair—Skin and muscles rigid.
Complaints predominant in external parts	Compl. predom. in internal parts.
Often indicated with children and women	Often indicated with old people.
Complaints generally in external angle of eye, in upper jaw, on tip of elbow, in the thigh, partic. in front part of it.	Complaints generally in inner angle of eye, in lower jaw, hollow of elbow, and in thigh, partic. in back part of it.
Itching, aggravated or locality changed, or unchanged, by scratching.	Itching, *lessened or* aggravated by scratching.
When asleep, lying in a horizontal position or with head low.	When asleep, often a sitting posture.
Pulse more equal than with Phosphorus	Pulse irregular, sometimes intermitting.
Thirst predominant	Want of thirst.
Neither apoplexy nor paralysis	Apoplexy—*Paralysis.*

Difficult comprehens'n—Mental dullness—No unconsciousness—Rarely delirium or fancies.	*Easy or* difficult comprehension—Mental excitability—Ecstasies—Insanity.
Eyes protruding oftener than sunken	Eyes sunken.
Appetite for beer, *or* dislike for it	Dislike for beer.
Urinal sediment white or yellow	Urinal sediment *white*, yellow, or red.
Voice interrupted	Voice trembling or hissing.
Respiration predom. slow	Respiration generally quick.
Cough generally dry; expectoration not constant, is loosened in the morning and swallowed.	Expectoration not constant; morning and during the day.

Remission from midnight till noon and in the evening.	Remission after midnight.
Worse (better) when growing cold *or* warm.	Worse when growing cold, better when growing warm.
Worse when perspiring	*Worse or* better when perspiring.
Better or worse in bed	*Worse or* better in bed.
Generally worse when lying on side, better when lying on back.	*Generally* better when lying on side, worse when lying on back.
Worse after sleep	Better after sufficient sleep, but worse on awaking when roused and after the siesta.
Worse when closing, better when opening the eyes.	Better (worse) when closing *or* when opening the eyes.
Predom. worse after getting out of bed	Worse *or* better after getting out of bed.
Predom. better while eating, worse *afterwards.*	*Worse or* better while and after eating.
Worse from eructation	*Worse or* better from eructation.
Worse during full moon	Worse in sultry weather or dur'g a storm.

Predomin. worse ———— **Predomin. better**

In dry weather, when lying on side, partic. on "right" side, when sitting down, while sitting, partic. sitting erect, after sleep, lying with head high, from touch, from rubbing and scratching.

Predomin. better ———— **Predomin. worse**

In wet weather, when lying on back or on "left" side, when rising from a seat, when sitting bent forward, in bed, in a horizontal position or with head low, after perspiring, and after swallowing and eating.

N.B. Spongia lacks the over-sensitiveness of Phosphorus to pain.

Spongia.	Pulsatilla.
Complaints predom. in external parts . .	Compl. predom. in internal parts – Apoplexy—Paralysis.
Dropsy in the cavities of the body . . .	Anasarca.
Itching, aggrav. *or* unchanged, *or* locality changed by scratching.	Itching, aggravated or unchanged by scratching.
Ulcers, with scanty discharge	Ulcers, with copious discharge.
When asleep, horizontal position with head bent back.	When asleep, lying on the back, the arm above the head, *or sitting posture.*
Pulse quick, full, and hard	Pulse generally frequent, small, and weak; sometimes intermitting.
Thirst predom., but rarely dur'g cold stage.	Thirstlessn. predom., always dur'g cold stage.
Cheerfulness predom.—Stubbornness . .	Calm sadness of mild disposit'ns—Distrust—Avarice—Chang'g mood—Gentleness—Amorousness.
Very rarely fancies—Rarely delirium . .	Absent-mindedness—Unconsciousness.
Compl. generally in external angle of eye, on outside of ear, upper jaw, tip of elbow, fore-arm, and on thigh.	Compl. generally in inner angle of eye, on inside of ear, lower jaw, in hollow of elbow, on upper arm, and on leg.
Eyes protruding oftener than sunken . .	Eyes sunken.
Saliva predominantly diminished	Saliva generally increased.
Dislike for beer oftener than appetite for it.	Thirst for beer.
Constipation predominant	Diarrhœa predominant.
Urinal sediment white or yellow	Urinal sediment red.
Catamenia too soon	Catamenia too late.
Dry coryza predominant	Coryza fluent oftener than dry.
Respiration predominantly slow	Respiration predominantly quick.
Voice, as with Pulsatilla, but sometimes without resonance, hollow, interrupted.	Voice failing or rough and hoarse.
Cough generally dry	Cough generally with expectoration.
Expector. is generally swallowed, is loosened in the morning, and is like the coryza, viscous or hardened.	Expector. morning and during the day, is like the nasal secretion, thick mucus *or* like pus, yellow, and of a bad odor.
AGGRAVATION afternoon & before midnight.	AGGRAVATION afternoon and evening, after sunset till midnight.
Worse in dry cold weather	*Worse* in wet cold or warm weather.
Worse when moving	*Better* during continued moderate motion.
Better in a horizontal posture	Better when lying with head high.
Worse while perspiring, *better afterwards.*	*Worse while and after* perspiring.
Better while swallowing, *worse* when not swallowing.	Worse *or* better when swallowing.

Predomin. worse — **Predomin. better**

In dry weather, from cold, when lying on painful side, from tying the clothes tight, on inspirat'n, from bodily exertion, when sitting erect, when holding diseased limb bent, when bending the head sideways, from pressure, when lying with the head high, and from motion.

Predomin. better — **Predomin. worse**

In wet weather, from warmth, when lying on unpainful side, from loosening the clothes, on expiration, during rest, when standing, when sitting bent forward, in bed,* in a horizontal position, & after perspiring.

N.B. Spongia lacks the over-sensitiveness of Pulsat. to pain. Both remedies have sensitiveness to touch.

* Both remedies have aggravations from *warmth* of bed.

Stannum.	Lycopodium.
Left side, partic. *upper left, lower right side.*	*Right* side, partic. *upper right, lower left side*
Dark hair—Sensitiveness (internal or external).	Light hair—Numb sensation (internal or external).
Apoplexy not yet observed	Apoplexy.
Itching or pinching pain in internal parts .	Itching or pinching pain in external parts.
Dry eruptions	Eruptions generally humid.
Compl. generally on lower lip, in the spleen, on upper arm, on tip of elbow.	Compl. generally on upper lip, in the liver, on fore-arm, and in hollow of elbow.
Pulse quick and small	Pulse somewhat accelerated only after eating and in the evening.
External chill with internal heat	Internal chill with external heat.
Thirst, partic. between hot and sweating stage.	Thirst is wanting only during chill, and remains *after* the sweating stage.

Stannum.	Lycopodium.
Mood very rarely peevish or irritable . .	Mood changing; serious; haughty; malicious—Avarice—Distrust.
No delirium—Rarely unconsciousness—Imbecility.	Absent-mindedness—Insanity more frequent than imbecility.
Pupils contracted	Pupils dilated.
Nausea in throat, less frequently in stomach or abdomen.	Nausea in stomach.
Urine scanty	Urine often, but scanty.
Catam. too soon and profuse—Leucorrhœa mild.	Catam. too late; scanty or profuse—Leucorrhœa predom. acrid.
Expector. predom., but not constant; part. during day and evening.	Expector. nearly constant; morning and evening.

Stannum.	Lycopodium.
REMISS. after midnight and during the day	REMISS. after midnight and in the forenoon.
Worse from weeping	*Better or* worse from weeping.
Better when alone; worse when in company.	Worse (better) when alone or in company
Almost always aggrav. in bed	Better *or* worse in bed.
Generally worse when lying on left side, better when lying on right side.	*Generally* better when lying on left, worse when lying on right side.
Predom. worse when getting out of bed .	Better *or* worse when getting out of bed.
Worse (better) when drawing up diseased limb *or* when stretching it out.	Better when drawing up diseased limb, worse when stretching it out.
Worse when perspiring	Better *or* worse when perspiring.
Better *or* worse from exertion	Worse from bodily exertion.
Worse when stooping	*Generally* better when stooping.
Worse after stool	*Worse or* better after stool.

Predomin. worse — **Predomin. better**

When lying on left side, when stooping and when sitting bent forward, when lifting diseased limb, when ascending, on expiration, from weeping, and from eructation.

Predomin. better — **Predomin. worse**

When lying on right side, when sitting erect, when letting diseased limb hang down, when descending, on inspiration and when taking a deep breath, when swallowing and eating, and from pressure.

N.B. Stannum lacks the over-sensitiveness of Lycopodium to pain.

Stannum.	**Sulphur.**
Desire for open air	Aversion to the open air.
Pulse frequent and small	Pulse quick, full, and hard; sometimes intermitting or imperceptible.
External chill with internal heat	Internal chill with external heat.
Thirst, partic. between hot and sweating stages.	Thirst mostly during heat; during chill generally want of thirst.
Compl. predom. on lower lip, on upper arm, and on tip of elbow.	Compl. predom. on upper lip, on fore-arm, and in hollow of elbow.
Very rarely irritable mood	Mood changing, indifferent, serious, and solemn.
No delirium—Imbecility.	Absent-mindedness—Insanity—Very rarely imbecility.
Generally hunger	Generally want of appetite.
Aversion to beer	Desire for *or* aversion to beer and spirituous liquors.
Nausea in throat, less frequently in stomach or abdomen.	Nausea in stomach, less frequently in throat.
Urine too scanty	Urine often, but scanty.
Catam. too soon and profuse	Catam. *generally* retarded and scanty.
Spasmodic labor-pains—Leucorrhœa mild.	Weak or ceasing labor-pains—Leucorrhœa acrid.
Nasal secretion thick	Nasal secretion watery.
Voice hoarse *or* raised	Voice hoarse *or* deep.
Expector. predom., but not constant; partic. during the day and evening.	Expect. not constant; morning and during the day, less frequently at night.
AGGRAV. morning and evening till midnight.	AGGRAV. from midnight till noon and in the evening.
Worse when lying on side, better when lying on back.	*Generally* worse when lying on the side, better when lying on back.
Predom. worse when getting out of bed; better *afterwards*.	Better when getting out of bed, better *or* worse *afterwards*.
Better when moving diseased part . . .	*Worse or* better when moving the part.
Worse (better) when stretching out diseased limb or when drawing it up.	Almost always aggrav. when stretching out the limb, improved by drawing it up.
Worse when blowing the nose, but better *afterwards*.	Worse when blowing the nose.
Better when taking a deep breath . . .	Worse *or* better when taking a deep breath.
Better *or* worse from bodily exertion. . .	Almost always *aggrav.* by exertion, running, &c.
Worse when stooping; worse *or* better when rising.	*Worse or* better when stooping and when rising.
Worse from touch, from weeping, and after urinating.	*Worse or* better from touch, from weeping, and after urinating.
Worse when swallowing drink.	Worse when swallowing dry food and when swallowing saliva.
Better while eating	Worse *or* better while eating.
Worse after stool	Worse *or* better after stool.
Worse from eructation	Almost always improved by eructation.

Predomin. **worse** ——— Predomin. **better**

On expiration, when getting out of bed, and from eructation.

Predomin. **better** ——— Predomin. **worse**

On inspiration, when moving diseased part, and when swallowing.

Staphisagria.	Colocynthis.
Upper left, lower right side—Pain pressing inwards.	Upper right, lower left side—Pain pressing outwards.
Sensitiveness or inflammation of external parts.	Sensitiveness or inflammation of internal parts.
Dryness of the skin	Generally disposition to sweat.
Complaints generally on inside of ear, in the bladder, on back part of thigh, and on sole of foot.	Complaints generally on outside of ear, in the kidneys, on front part of thigh, and on top of foot.
Pulse frequent & small, sometimes trembl'g.	Pulse generally frequent, full, and hard.
Thirst is predom. only during hot stage .	Want of thirst predominant.

Indifference—Ailments from (shame, grief, mortification, or from vexation with indignation or reserved displeasure) misbehavior of others, or from disappointed love.	Ailments from (shame, grief, mortification, or from vexation with indignation or reserved displeasure) anger.
Fancies—Imbecility	Insanity.
Bellyache worse after stool and passing urine.	Bellyache abated after stool.
Urine often, but scanty	Urine diminished *or* increased.
Catamenia retarded and scanty	Catamenia too soon and profuse.
Expectoration nearly constant; is loosened partic. at night; is swallowed.	Expectoration quite seldom.

AGGRAVATIONS appear at all times of the day and night.*	AGGRAVATIONS during the day and evening.
Generally worse from cold	*Generally* better from cold.
Worse *or* better when growing cold . . .	Better when growing cold.
Better or worse in bed	Almost always aggravated in bed.
Worse from touch	Better *or* worse from touch.
Worse from pressure	*Better or* worse from pressure.
Worse or better when leaning against something.	Better when leaning against something, but worse *afterwards.*
Worse when smoking	*Better or* worse from smoking.
Worse after stool	Better *or* worse after stool.
Worse after urinating	*Worse or* better after urinating.
Ailments from Mercurius or Thuya . . .	Ailments from Causticum.

Predomin. worse — **Predomin. better**

From motion, from pressure, from cold, when lying on painful side, after perspiring, from smoking, from eructation, from rubbing and scratching.

Predomin. better — **Predomin. worse**

During rest, after lying down, when standing and lying, from warmth, in bed, when lying on the painful side.

N.B. The main characteristic of Colocynthis is that it produces cramp-like pains in internal and external parts; tonic spasms with jamming, pressive pains, and in such is Staphisagria its main antidote. Hahnemann.—Causticum, Colocynthis, and Staphisagria are nearly related, and often one, after its effects cease, will indicate the other. They may all be followed by Sepia, our great finishing remedy. C.Hg.

---

* Compare note ‡ to Mercurius—Staphisagria.

Staphisagria.	Lycopodium.
Upper left, lower right side—Anæmia . . .	Upp. right, low. left side—Plethora *or* anæmia.
Dark hair—Skin and muscles rigid	Light hair—Skin and muscles lax.
Pain pressing inwards—Pinching pain in internal parts.	Pain pressing outwards—Pinching pain in external parts.
No apoplexy — Paralysis generally one-sided.	Apoplexy—Paralysis often of both sides.
Scabs around the joints	Sweat around the joints.
Pleasant dreams predominant	Unpleasant dreams predominant.
Pulse frequent & small, sometimes trembling.	Pulse somewhat accelerated only in the evening and after eating.
Want of thirst predom.; only during hot stage there is more thirst.	Thirst is wanting only during chill, & remains *after* the fever attack.
Mood sad, rarely distrustful	Mood changing; sad *or* cheerful; gentle or irritable; haughty; malicious—Greediness.
Rarely unconsciousness—No delirium . . .	Unconsciousness—Delirium—Absent-mindedness.
Ailments from the misbehavior of others, from shame, disappointed love, or from vexation with indignation.	Ailments from fright, anger, or from vexation with fear or vehemence.
Swelling of upper lip predominant	Swelling of lower lip predom.
Nausea in throat—Hot fetid flatus	Nausea in the stomach—Scentless flatus pred.
Discharge of succus prostaticus predominant, partic. with the stool.	Pollutions predominant.
Catamenia too scanty	Catamenia too scanty *or* too profuse.
Fluent coryza predominant	Coryza dry oftener than fluent.
Expector. is loosened at night and swallowed.	Expector. morning and evening.
Complaints predom. in lower part of chest .	Compl. predom. in upper part of chest.
Trembling beating of the heart	Equal palpitation of the heart.
Complaints predom. on wrist	Compl. predom. on ankle.
Remission undecided	Remission after midnight and in the *forenoon*.
Worse in cold weather, better in warm air .	Better (worse) in cold weather or in warm air.
Worse (better) from uncovering *or* from wrapping up.	Predom. better from uncovering, worse from wrapping up.
Worse while and after perspiring	Worse *or* better while and after perspiring.
Worse (better) from light *or* in the dark . .	*Generally* worse from light, better in the dark.
Worse when getting out of bed; *worse or* better *afterwards*.	Worse *or* better when getting out of bed; almost always improved *afterwards*.
Better when sitting down	Worse *or* better when sitting down.
Worse when rising from a seat, when sneezing, and after stool.	*Worse or* better when rising from a seat, when sneezing, and after stool.
Better *or* worse when stooping; worse when rising.	Predom. better when stooping; worse *or* better when rising.
Worse or better when washing, etc., the part.	Worse from wash'g & moisten'g diseased part.
Worse *or* better when swallowing	Worse when swallowing.
Worse *or* better when eating	Almost always aggravated when eating.
Worse when gaping, but better *afterwards* .	Worse when gaping.

Predomin. **worse** ——— Predomin. **better**

From cold, in the open air & when walking out-doors, from motion, partic. moving diseased part, when walking, when ascending, on expiration, when closing the eyes, when fasting, from eructation, and in extended posture.

Predomin. **better** ——— Predomin. **worse**

From warmth, in-doors, during rest, after lying down, when lying, sitting and standing, when descending, on inspiration, when taking a deep breath, when opening the eyes, after breakfast, in contracted posture, and when resting diseased limb on something.

Staphisagria.	Nux vomica.
Upper left. lower right predominant . . .	*Upper right, lower left.*
Complaints (pulsating, sensation of **cold, etc.**) predominant in external parts — **Internal** trembling sensation.	Complaints (pulsating, sensation of cold, etc.) predom. in internal parts — Trembling of external parts.
Pain pressing inwards	Pain pressing outwards.
Paralysis generally one-sided	Paralysis generally of both sides—Apoplexy
Painless eruptions	Painful eruptions.
Pulse frequent & small; sometimes trembling.	P. generally full & hard; sometim. intermitt'g.
Heat or sweat, with inclination to uncover .	Heat or sweat, with aversion to uncover.
Chill increased after sleep, lessened by motion and out-doors.	Chill lessened after sleep, increased by motion and out-doors.
Want of thirst; only during **hot stage thirst is predominant.**	**Thirst mostly dur'g chill, but also between heat & sweat, and before & after the whole attack.**

Staphisagria.	Nux vomica.
Hypochondria, with apathy **and exhaustion** .	**Hypoch., with disconsolateness & over-sensitiv**
Suppressed irritability	Outbursts of anger—Malice.
Changing mood—Taciturnity	Loquacity.
Ailm. fr. the misbehavior of others & fr. shame.	Ailm. fr. fright, jealousy, anger, & contradict'n.
Rarely unconsciousness	Absent-mindedness—Delirium.
Dim-sightedness — Optical illusions in black, dark colors.	Predom. seeing objects too clearly — Optical illusions in bright colors.
Face peaked **and hollow-eyed—Gums white** .	Features puny, earthy-colored, yellowish, or red & puffed up—Gums & inner mouth red.
Hunger predominant	Generally loss of appetite.
Appetite for bread	Aversion to bread, partic. rye-bread.
Nausea in throat; **less frequently in stomach** or abdomen.	Nausea, partic. in the stomach; less frequently in œsophagus.
Horses: Ischuria, with the flanks drawn in and dung in large balls.	Horses: Spasmodic colic, with the flanks drawn in and dung in small, dry balls or black, covered with mucus.
Urine often, but scanty; dark oftener than light.	U. seldom & scanty; generally light-colored.
Urinal stream thin	Urinal streams large.
Catamenia too late and scanty	Catam. too soon and profuse.
Fluent coryza predom. — Secretion thick or viscid.	Generally stoppage of nose, partic. out-doors; but in-doors fluent coryza—Secretion watery.
Expector. quite constant; **at night; is generally swallowed.**	Expectoration not constant; in the morning, during day and evening.
Trembling beating of the heart	Beating of heart equal; rarely intermitting.
Complaints predom. **on wrist**	**Compl. predom. on ankle.**

Staphisagria.	Nux vomica.
Remission of complaints undecided* . . .	Remission evening till midnight.
Worse when gaping; *better afterwards* . .	*Worse while and after* gaping.
Worse after perspiring	*Worse while* perspiring, *better afterwards.*
Worse when swallowing drink	Worse when swallowing food and saliva.
Better (worse) from light *or* in the dark . .	Worse from light; better in the dark.

Predomin. worse —— **Predomin. better**

When sitting erect, in wet weather, from washing & moistening diseased part, from pressure, after sleep,† after perspiring, when swallowing drink, and when stretching out diseased limb.

Predomin. better —— **Predomin. worse**

When sitting bent forward, in dry weather, when drawing up diseased limb, and after gaping.

---

* Compare note † to Mercurius—Staphisagria.

† After sleeping *too long* Nux vomica has aggravation; likewise on awaking when roused from sleep; it has improvement only after sufficient, but not too long sleep.

Staphisagria.	Pulsatilla.
Aversion to the open air—Complaints of external parts predom.	Desire for open air—Complaints of internal parts predom.
No apoplexy—Pain pressing inwards . . .	Apoplexy—Pain pressing outwards.
Itching, aggravated *or* the locality changed by scratching.	Itching, aggravated *or* unchanged by scratching.
Painless eruptions—Awaking too soon . . .	Painful eruptions—Awaking too late.
Pulse sometimes trembling	Pulse sometimes intermitting or imperceptible.
	Want of thirst predominant, but constant only during chill.
Thirst is predominant only during hot stage .	Th. partic. *before* & betw. the different stages.
Rarely distrust	Mood changing; gentle — Boldness—Avarice.
Rarely unconsciousness—Imbecility	Absent-mindedness— Melancholy—Delirium.
Ailments fr. disappointed love, and fr. vexation with indignat'n or reserved displeasure.	Ailments from joy, fright, or vexation with fear or dread.
Optical illusions in black or in dark colors .	Optical illusions in bright colors.
Pupils dilated	Pupils generally contracted.
Nasal complaints generally internal	Nasal complaints generally external.
Swelling of upper lip predominant	Swelling of lower lip predominant.
Appetite for milk	Dislike for milk.
Urine often, but scanty	Urine seldom and scanty.
Trembling beating of heart	Palpitation of heart with equal, less frequently with intermitting beats.
Expectoration quite constant; is loosened at night; is swallowed.	Expectoration predominant, but not constant; in the morning and during the day.
Complaints predominant on fore-arm . . .	Complaints predominant on upper arm.
The horse does not allow any one to approach him while he eats his feed.	The horse is sensitive to touch, especially on the ears; does resist being bridled.
Aggravation at all times of the day or night.	Aggravation from noon till midnight.
Worse (better) when growing cold *or* growing warm.	Better when growing cold, worse when growing warm.
Worse (better) from uncover'g *or* from wrapping up.	Predominantly better from uncovering, worse from wrapping up.
Better or worse in bed	Predominantly worse in bed.
Worse when turning in bed, after sleep, after perspiring, and from eructation.	*Worse or* better from change of posture, after sleep, after perspiring, and from eructation.
Worse when getting out of bed; *worse or* better *afterwards.*	*Better or* worse when and after getting out of bed.
Worse when rising from a seat; better *afterwards.*	*Worse or* better when ris'g from a seat; *better or* worse *afterwards.*
Worse when sitting down	Better *or* worse when sitting down.
Better *or* worse when stooping	Predom. worse when stooping.
Better when assuming an erect position and when taking a deep breath.	Worse *or* better when assuming an erect position and when taking a deep breath.
Worse when moving diseased part and from exertion.	*Better or* worse when moving the part and from exertion.
Worse when bending diseased part	Better *or* worse from bending the part.
Worse from pressure and after stool . . .	*Better or* worse from pressure and after stool.
Worse on an empty stomach, better after breakfast.	Worse (better) on an empty stomach *or* after breakfast.
Better *or* worse when eating; worse *afterwards.*	Almost always aggravated when eating; *worse or* better *afterwards.*
Worse when gaping; better afterwards . .	Worse when gaping.
Worse when swallowing drink	Worse when swallowing saliva.

Predomin. **worse** —— Predomin. **better**

From cold and in cold weather, in the open air and when walking out-doors, from motion, partic. when moving diseased part, when walking, while and after getting out of bed, from bodily exertion, when stretching out diseased limb, when bending the suffering part sideways, when sitting erect, when lying on painful side, from pressure, from eating sour things, after stool, and from washing and moistening diseased part.

Predomin. **better** —— Predomin. **worse**

From warmth and in warm air, in-doors, during rest, after lying down, in bed, when standing, sitting and lying, partic. when sitting bent forward, when lying on unpainful side, and when drawing up diseased limb.

Staphisagria.	Sulphur.
Right side—Increased bodily irritability	*Left* side—Want of bodily irritability.
Pain pressing inwards — Pinching pain in internal parts.	Pain pressing outwards—Pinching pain in external parts.
Paralysis generally one-sided	Paralysis generally of both sides.
Itch'g, aggrav. *or* locality chang'd by scratch'g.	Itch'g, almost always improved by scratching.
Scabs around the joints—Itch predom. humid.	Itching, erysipelas, or vesicles around the joints—Itch predom. dry.
Awaking too early	Awaking too late.
Pulse frequent, small; often trembling	Pulse generally frequent, sometimes full and hard; intermitting or imperceptible.
Want of thirst, except hot stage	Thirst predom., but not constant.
Chill increased in a warm room	Chill abated in a warm room.
Solicitude concerning the future	Solicitude concerning the present. C.Hg.
Amorousness	Mood changing; gentle *or* irritable; rarely amorousness.
Ailments from the misbehavior of others, shame, grief, disappointed love, indignation, vexation with reserved displeasure.	Ailments from hearing bad news, shame, or vexation with fright, dread or fear; less frequently from anger.
No delirium—Imbecility	Absent-mindedn.—Insanity oft. th. imbecility.
Pupils dilated	Pupils contracted.
Compl. predom. on inside of gums—**Gums white.**	Compl. on outside of gums—Gums red.
Teeth: sensation as if pressed in	Teeth: sensation as if drawn out. C.Hg.
Saliva predominantly increased	Saliva generally diminished.
Hunger predominant	Generally loss of appetite.
Appetite for bread or milk	Aversion to bread, partic. rye-bread, & to milk.
Desire for spirituous liquors	Desire for or aversion to beer and spirituous liquors.
Nausea, partic. in throat	Nausea in the stomach.
Urine often, but scanty	Urine often, but scanty.
Nasal secretion thick *or* viscid	Nasal secretion watery.
Expector. nearly constant; is loosened, partic. at night, and swallowed.	Expector. not constant; in the morning and during the day, less frequently at night.
Compl. predom. in lower part of chest	Compl. predom. in upper part of chest.
Trembling beating of heart	Palpitation of heart, with accelerated, sometimes intermitting beats.
Remission of complaints undecided	Remission *afternoon* and before midnight.
Ailments from Mercurius or Thuya	Ailments from Mercurius and other metals, from Nitric. acid., Iodine, Sepia, Cinchona, or Rhus.
Worse in cold weather; better in warm air	Better (worse) in cold weather or in warm air.
Worse in the open air; better in-doors	*Generally* bett. in the open air, worse in-doors, partic. in crowded rooms.*
Worse *or* better from warmth of bed & when swallowing and eating.	Almost always worse from warmth of bed & when swallowing and eating.
Better *or* worse when biting	Worse when clenching the teeth.
Worse when swallowing drink	Worse when swallowing dry food and saliva.
Worse on an empty stomach, better after breakfast.	Better (worse) on an empty stomach *or* after breakfast.
Worse after stool	Worse *or* better after stool.
Worse when gaping, but better *afterwards*†	Worse when gaping.

Predomin. worse — **Predomin. better**

In the open air, from cold, but also from warmth of stove, on expiration, from motion, when getting out of bed, when sitting erect, from pressure, from rubbing & scratching, and from eructation.

Predomin. better — **Predomin. worse**

In-doors, from warmth, on inspiration, during rest, after lying down, in bed, when lying, standing and sitting, partic. sitting bent forward.

* Still we find "*improvement from warmth of stove*" with Sulphur.

† *Staphis.* has: Worse when turning in bed, after perspiring, when sneezing, from touch, when moving diseased part, when assuming an erect position, and after passing urine. — *Sulphur*: "Worse or" better under the same conditions.

Staphisagria.	Thuya.
Right side predominant—Dark hair . . .	*Left* side—Light hair.
Muscles rigid	Muscles lax.
Anæmia	Plethora.
Itching of the skin, aggrav. *or* locality changed by scratching.	Itching, lessened by scratching.
Scabs around the joints	Oedema around the joints.
Paralysis generally one-sided	Apoplexy—Paralysis often of both sides.
Pain pressing inwards	Pain pressing outwards.
Pulse frequent and small, often trembling .	Pulse slow and weak in the morning, accelerated and full in the evening.
Congestion of blood to the ears	Congestion of blood to the eyes.
Want of thirst is constant during sweating and cold stages.	Thirst is not constant during sweating stage.*
Chill lessened in the open air	Chill increased in the open air.
Complaints generally on inside of nose, on lower jaw, on inside of gums, in lower part of chest, in the bladder, on the hands, and on the soles of the feet.	Complaints generally on outside of nose, on upper jaw, on outside of gums, in upper part of chest, in the kidneys, on the feet, and on the instep.
Pleasant dreams predominant	Anxious dreams predominant.
Amorousness — Weakness of mental faculties.	Rarely amorousness—Excitability and ecstasies, *or* weakness.
Eyes predominantly sunken	Eyes protruding
Pupils dilated—Objects appear too large .	Pup. contracted—Objects appear too small.
Saliva predominantly increased	Saliva generally diminished
Hunger predominant	Loss of appetite predominant.
Urine often, but scanty	Urine often and copious.
Catamenia too late and scanty	Catamenia predom. *too soon* and scanty.
Expectoration predominant; is loosened partic. at night and generally swallowed.	Expectoration predominant; in the evening.
REMISSION undecided.—Comp. Mercurius—Staphisagria.	REMISSION in the forenoon and before midnight.
Many symptoms, except those on the scalp, are aggravated by cold, improved by warmth.	Many symptoms, excepting those of the skin, are aggravated by warmth and growing warm, and improved by cold.
Consequences of taking cold, also after getting warm out-doors.	Consequences of being overheated.
Better in a warm room	*Better* in-doors, but *worse* when the room is too warm.
Better when resting on diseased limb . .	*Worse* when rest'g on diseased limb or lett'g it hang down, *better* when lifting it.
Worse when swallowing drink	Worse when swallowing saliva.
Worse when rising	Worse when stooping.
Worse from touch and pressure	Generally improved by touch and pressure.
Ailments from Mercurius or Thuya . . .	Ailm. from Mercur., Sulphur or Iodine.

Predomin. worse — **Predomin. better**

From cold, from motion, on an empty stomach, after stool, after perspiring, from washing or moistening diseased part, from rubbing and scratching, "from touch and pressure."

Predomin. better — **Predomin worse**

From warmth, during rest, when standing, sitting, lying, in bed and when swallowing, on inspiration, and after breakfast (resting on diseased limb).

N.B. Thuya generally lacks the increased constitutional irritability of Staphisagria.

* **Both remedies have thirst predominant during hot and none during cold stage.**

Stramonium.	Plumbum.
Upper left, lower right side—Light hair	Upper right, lower left side—Dark hair.
Sensitiveness predominant in internal parts.	Sensitiveness of external parts.
Painless paralysis of limbs	Painful paralysis predominant.
Apoplexy more frequent than paralysis	Paralysis more frequent than apoplexy.
Plethora—Perspires easily	Anæmia—Dryness of skin.
Pulse generally quick, full, and hard; sometimes trembling or imperceptible.	Pulse generally slow, small, and contracted.
Sweat on suffering part	Coldness on diseased part.
Thirst is wanting only during chill	Constant thirst.

Stramonium.	Plumbum.
Loquacity—Haughtiness—Mood irritable; malicious.	Taciturnity—Rarely merriness or amorousness.
Fancies—Ecstasies	Rarely unconsciousness—No ecstasies.
Insanity more frequent than imbecility	Imbecility more frequent than insanity.
Itching, unchanged by scratching	Itching, lessened by scratching.
Vomiting mucus or bile	Vomiting food or bile.
As if the navel were pulled out by a string.	As if the navel were drawn in by a string to the backbone. Lippe.
Urine seldom and scanty; sometimes copious.	Urine seldom and scanty.
Catamenia too late	Catamenia too soon.
Secretion of milk increased	Secretion of milk diminished.
Dry coryza	Coryza predom. fluent.
Cough without expectoration	Cough generally *with* expectoration.
Complaints generally on fore-arm	Complaints predom. on upper arm.

Stramonium.	Plumbum.
Remission during day and evening	Remission of complaints during forenoon.
Better in the sunshine	Better in cloudy weather.
Worse when getting out of bed	Worse *or* better when getting out of bed.
Worse *or* better *after* getting out of bed	Better after getting out of bed.
Worse from spirituous liquors	Brandy is a relative preventive of lead-colic.

Predomin. worse — **Predomin. better**

In the open air, when alone, from drinking brandy, from touch and pressure, from rubbing and scratching.

Predomin. better — **Predomin. worse**

In-doors, in company,* after lying down, and in bed

N.B. Stramonium lacks the supersensitiveness of Plumbum to pain.

---

* Yet we also find "aggravation when among strangers" with Stramonium.

Stramonium.	Pulsatilla.
Left side—Want of bodily irritability—Aversion to the open air.	*Right* side—Increased irritability—Inclination for the open air.
Paralysis generally of both sides	Paralysis generally one-sided.
Itching, unchanged by scratching	Itching, aggrav. *or* unchanged by scratching.
Painless eruptions—Perspiring easily . . .	Painful eruptions—Dryness of the skin.
Pulse irregular; often quick, full, hard; sometimes trembling.	Pulse generally frequent, small, and weak.
Pulse predom. affected by alcohol or beer .	P. predom. affected by beer or coffee. C.Hg.
Heat, lessened in bed	Heat, increased in bed.
Thirst predom.; is wanting only during chill.	Want of thirst predom., but constant only during chill.
Coma predominant	Coma less frequent than sleeplessness.
Insensibility of disposition—Loquacity . .	Sensitive disposition—Taciturnity.
Dread of being alone—Satiety of live with longing for death.	Inclination to solitude—Satiety of life with fear of death.
Mood *cheerful or* sad; irritable; malicious—Haughtiness—Jealousy—Rage—Cruelty.	Mood changing; sad and despondent; gentle and good-natured; rarely irritable; indifferent—Boldness—Avarice.
Ailments from hearing bad news or from jealousy.	Ailments from excessive joy, grief, or from vexation with fright or fear.
Ecstasies—Insanity—Imbecility	Rarely mental dullness—Melancholy.
Horse getting restless from every noise, inclining to run off, biting and attacking with great agility.	The horse is sensitive to the touch, especially on the ears; does resist being bridled.
Eyes protruding—Pupils dilated oftener than contracted.	Eyes sunken—Pupils contracted oftener than dilated.
Optical illusions in dark or prismatic colors .	Optical illusions in bright colors.
Complaints predom. on soft palate — Saliva generally diminished.	Compl. predom. on roof of mouth — Saliva generally increased.
Diarrhœa painless—Urine seldom and scanty; sometimes copious.	Diarrhœa generally painful — Urine seldom & scanty.
Retention of urine oftener than incontinence.	Retent. of urine less frequent th. incontinence.
Catamenia of too long duration and profuse .	Catam. of too short durat'n & generally scanty.
Dry coryza—Cough without expectoration .	Coryza generally fluent—Expector. predom., but not constant; in the morn'g & dur'g day.
Complaints predom. on fore-arm	Compl. predom. on upper arm.
Remission during day and evening	Remission from midnight till noon.
Worse after sleep	*Worse or* better after sleep.
Worse when getting out of bed	*Better or* worse when getting out of bed.
Worse *or* better after getting out of bed . .	*Better or* worse after getting out of bed.
Worse when rising from a seat	Worse *or* better when rising from a seat.
Better when sitting down	Better *or* worse when sitting down.
Worse when stooping and when rising . . .	*Worse or* better when stooping & when rising.
Better when moving diseased part	*Better or* worse when moving the part.
Worse from pressure	*Generally* better from pressure.
Worse when swallowing	*Worse or* better when swallowing.
Better after stool	*Better or* worse after stool.

Predomin. worse —— **Predomin. better**

From cold, from growing cold and in cold weather, in the open air and when walking out-doors, from uncovering, when lying on right side, when gett'g out of bed, from motion, when walking, from pressure, and from drinking cold water.

Predomin. better —— **Predomin. worse**

From warmth, from growing warm and in warm air, in-doors, from wrapping up, during rest, after lying down, when standing, sitting and lying, in bed and from warmth of bed, when lying on left side, and after perspiring.

N.B. Stramonium lacks the over-sensitiveness of Pulsatilla to pain.

Sulphur.	**Apis.**
Want of bodily irritability — Aversion to the open air.	Increased irritability—Inclination for open air.
Paralysis more frequent than apoplexy	Apoplexy more frequent than paralysis.
Paralysis generally of both sides (& painless).	Paralysis generally one-sided (often painful).
Painless cutaneous eruptions	Painful eruptions.
Eruption general, with exception of the face.	Eruption general, with exception of feet.
Sleeplessness, partic. before midnight	Coma predominant.
Chill abated in a warm room	Chill increased in a warm room.
Thirst rare during chill, mostly during heat	Thirst is wanting only during sweat.
Mood changing, anxious and sad; serious & solemn.	Exaggerated merriment; (less frequently despondency); flighty restlessn. & inconstancy.
Ailments from shame or mortification, less frequently from anger.	Ailments from anger, fright, or jealousy.
Anxious feeling in the præcordia	Anxious feeling in the head.
Fancies — Insanity more frequent than imbecility.	Imbecility more frequent than insanity.
Hydrocephalus developing slowly. after psoric eruptions; head drops backwards; likes to lie with head low; face changing often red or pale; nausea while lifting the head up; breath sour; urine as if mixed with flour.	Hydrocephalus suddenly, after erysipelatous eruptions; prostration; unconscious; one side lame or jerking; big toe turning up; squinting; nausea while lying; breath offensive; tongue sore. C. Hg.
Pupils generally contracted	Pupils generally dilated.
Compl. predom. in external angle of eye and on inside of ear.	Compl. predom. in inner angle of eye and on outside of ear.
Saliva generally diminished	Saliva predom. increased.
Vomit predominantly sour	Vomit bitter, bilious.
Catamenia *generally* too late and scanty	Catam. too soon; at the same time profuse *or* scanty.
Expector. not constant; in the morning and during the day, less frequently at night.	Cough awakens before midnight & ceases as soon as something is loosened, which is swallowed.
Remission afternoon and before midnight	Remission of complaints during day.
Ailments from Metals, Nitric. acid., or Iodine.	Ailments from animal poisons.
Worse in snowy air	Worse from the heat of the sun.
Worse or better when rising	Better when rising.*
Better (worse) in cold *or* in warm air	Worse in cold weather, better in warm air.
Better from warmth of stove, but worse in crowded rooms.	Worse in a warm room.
Better or worse from pressure.	*Worse or* better from pressure.
Worse when looking at running water	Worse when looking at something white.
Worse when swallowing dry food	Worse when swallowing *drink* or food.

Predomin. worse — **Predomin. better**

During rest, when assuming an erect position, from washing & moistening the suffering part, and after eating.

Predomin. better — **Predomin. worse**

From motion & pressure, when sitting down & after rising from a seat, & when holding the breath.

N.B. We very rarely find the over-sensitiveness of Apis to pain with Sulphur., but both remedies have sensitiveness to touch.

* *Apis* has aggravations in bed and from warmth of bed, after getting out of bed & when stooping, when sitting down, moving the diseased part, from touch, when sneezing. — *Sulphur:* "worse or better" under the same conditions.

Sulphur.	Graphites.
Upper left, lower right side—Pinching pain in external parts.	Upper right, lower left side — Pinching pain in internal parts.
Hæmorrhages, blood dark	Hæmorrhages, blood light-red.
Itching, erysipelas, or vesicles around the joints.	Rhagades around the joints.
Eruptions generally dry	Eruptions generally humid.
Painless eruptions and ulcers	Painful eruptions and ulcers.
Dreams of fire, vexation, misfortunes, business of the day, or merry dreams.	Dreams of water, misfortunes, embarrassment, &c.
Pulse frequent, full, and hard; sometimes intermitting or imperceptible; quick *night* and morning; slow *during the day* & even'g.	Pulse full and hard; only in the morning somewhat accelerated.
Internal chill and external heat predom.	External chill with internal heat.
Chill worse after drinking	Chill better after drinking. C.Hg.
Heat or sweat, with inclination to uncover	Heat or sweat, with aversion to uncover.
Sweat often only on back part of body	Sweat often only on front part of body.
Thirst predom., mostly during heat	Want of thirst, partic. during heat.

Sulphur.	Graphites.
Mood gentle *or* irritable—Rarely amorousness.	Mood depressed oftener than irritable.
Ailments from hearing bad news, from shame, mortification, or from vexation with fright or fear.	Consequences of grief.
Fancies—Insanity	*Neither* unconsciousn., delirium, nor insanity.
Complaints predom. on external angle of eye.	Complaints predom. on inner angle of eye.
Optical illusions in dark colors	Optical illusions in bright colors.
Complaints predom. on outside of gums	Complaints predom. on inside of gums.
Secretion of saliva generally diminished and loss of appetite.	Saliva and hunger predom. increased.
Appetite for beer or aversion to it	Desire for beer.
Urine often, but scanty	Urine scanty.
Expectoration not constant; in the morning and during the day; less frequent at night.	Expectoration nearly constant; during the day and evening.

Sulphur.	Graphites.
Remission *afternoon* and before midnight	Remission of complaints during day.
Ailments from metals, Nitric. acid., Iodine	Ailments from abuse of Arsenic.
Worse (better) in warm air *or* in cold weather.	Better in warm air, worse in cold weather.
Worse in crowded rooms; but better from warmth of stove.	Worse in a warm room.
Worse or better after perspiring	Better after perspiring.
Almost always aggrav. by warmth of bed	Worse *or* better from warmth of bed.
Worse *or* better when turning in bed, from touch, from weeping, and when sneezing.	Worse when turning in bed, from touch, from weeping and sneezing.
Worse *or* better when stooping, when taking a deep breath, and after stool.	Worse when stooping, when taking a deep breath, and after stool.
Worse (better) on an empty stomach *or* after breakfast.	Better on an empty stomach; worse after breakfast.
Worse after a satisfying meal	Worse when hungry.
Better *or* worse when eating; worse *afterwards.*	Almost always aggrav. when eating; worse or better *afterwards.*
Predom. worse from spirituous liquors	Better from wine.
Worse when looking down, partic. at running water.	Worse when looking up.

Predomin. worse ⁓ **Predomin. better**

From warmth, from wrapping up, after perspiring, during rest, after lying down, when lying and standing, when riding, when swallowing, from drinking wine, and *after* drinking generally.

Predomin. better ⁓ **Predomin. worse**

From cold, from uncovering, when getting out of bed, from motion, and when resting diseased limb on something.

N.B. Sulphur very rarely has the over-sensitiveness of Graphites to pain.

Sulphur.	Thuya.
Pinching pain in external parts, sensitiveness in internal *or* external parts.*	Pinching pain or sensation of numbness in internal parts, sensitiveness in external parts
Pain is sometimes excited by moving distant parts.	Pain often spreads to most distant parts.
Dry skin	Greasy skin.
Itching, erysipelas or vesicles around the joints.	Oedema around the joints.
Hot, but generally painless swelling of the glands.	Cold, painless swelling of the glands.
Pulse accelerated, full, and hard; partic. frequent *night* and morning, *during the day* & evening slower, sometimes intermitting or imperceptible.	Pulse slow & weak in the morn'g, accelerated and full in the evening.
Pulse affected mostly by beer, next by alcohol, least by coffee.	Pulse affected mostly by wine, next by tea or beer. C.Hg.
Sweat increased when walking in the open air.	Sweat lessened when walking in the open air.
Heat often general, with exception of the head; sweat sometimes only on the parts which itch.	Sweat often general, with exception of head; sometimes only on the inner surfaces of the limbs.
Awaking too late	Awaking too soon.
Changing mood—Gentleness	Haughtiness.
Insanity more frequent than imbecility . . .	Imbecility more frequent than insanity.
Eyes generally sunken	Eyes protruding.
Styes on upper lid	Styes on lower lid. C.Hg.
Vomit sour oftener than bitter	Bitter vomit predominant.
Urine often, but scanty; copious only after massive doses.	Urine too often and copious.
Sediment *white* or red.	Urinal sediment red.
Catamenia generally too late	Catamenia predominantly too soon.
Expectoration not constant; morning and during day, less frequently at night.	Expectoration nearly constant; evening.
Complaints generally on sole of foot . . .	Complaints predom. on top of foot.
REMISSION afternoon and before midnight . .	REMISSION *forenoon* and before midnight.
Ailments from metals, Nitric. acid., Iodine .	Ailments from abuse of Mercury.
Worse in the sunshine	Worse in the moon-light.
Worse when looking at running water . . .	Worse when looking at moving objects.
Worse when looking down	Worse when looking up, sideways or downwards.
Generally better in the open air, worse in-doors, partic. in crowded rooms; better from warmth of stove.	Predominantly worse in the open air, better in-doors, but worse from warmth of stove.
Worse or better after perspiring	Better after perspiring.
Worse after sleep.	*Worse or* better after sleeping.
Worse or better from touch	*Better or* worse from touch.
Better *or* worse when stooping	Worse when stooping.
Worse *or* better after stool	Predom. better after stool.
Worse or better after passing urine . . .	Worse after passing urine.
Worse *or* better when bending back the head.	Better when bending back the head.
Generally worse when lying on side, better when lying on back.	*Generally* better when lying on the side, worse when lying on the back.

Predomin. worse — **Predomin. better**

In-doors, after perspiring, when lifting diseased limb, when bending the suffering part, partic. when bending it backwards, from touch, from drinking cold water, and from cold diet generally.

Predomin. better — **Predomin. worse**

In the open air, but also from warmth of stove, when letting diseased limb hang down or when resting it on something, when getting out of bed, and from warm diet.

---

* Sulphur has sensitiveness as well as sensation of numbness "in external parts."

Sulphur.	Valeriana.
Want of bodily irritability—Rending pain downwards.	Increased irritability — Rending pain upwards.
Painless eruptions	Painful eruptions.
Complaints generally on upper lip, in upper part of chest, on fore-arm, and on back and inner surface of the thigh.	Complaints generally on lower lip, in lower part of chest, on upper arm, and on front and outer surface of thigh.
Pulse sometimes intermitt'g or imperceptible, generally frequent, full, and hard.	Pulse various, in general much more irregular than with Sulphur.
Chill, cold shudders, or heat, ascending . .	Chill, cold shudders, or heat, descending.
Internal chill, with external heat predom. .	External chill, with internal heat.
Fainting during the hot or sweating stage .	Fainting during the cold stage. C.Hg.

Sulphur.	Valeriana.
Wrapt in thought — Mood gentle; predominantly *sad & despondent;* anxious; indifferent; peevish; serious and solemn.	Being beside one's self—Cheerfulness.
Difficult comprehension—Mental dullness—Absent-mindedness.	Easy comprehension — Ecstasies — Rarely delirium.
Insanity	Insanity not yet observed.
Dim-sightedness—Optical illusions in dark colors.	Clear-sightedness—Optical illus'ns in bright colors.
Nausea in stomach, less frequently in throat.	Nausea in throat, less frequently in stomach or abdomen.
Urine too often, but scanty; increased only after massive doses.	Urine too often and copious.
Cough with *or* without expectoration . .	Cough not yet observed.

Sulphur.	Valeriana.
REMISSION afternoon and before midnight	REMISSION after midnight.
Generally worse in-doors, (particularly in crowded rooms); better in the open air, but also better from warmth of stove.	Better in-doors; worse in the open air.
Worse or better when mov'g diseased part, from change of posit'n, & after perspir'g.	Better when moving diseased part, from change of position, and after perspiring.
Worse or better from touch	Worse from touch.
Worse *or* better when bending the head back, when taking a deep breath, and after stool.	Worse when bending the head back, when taking a deep breath, and after stool.
Better (worse) on an empty stomach or after breakfast.	Predom. worse on an empty stomach; better after breakfast.
Worse after eating	Better or worse after eating.

Predomin. worse ——— **Predomin. better**

In-doors, from light, after perspiring, when moving diseased part, from change of position when lying or standing, when lifting the suffering limb, and when rising from a seat.

Predomin. better ——— **Predomin. worse**

In the open air, in the dark, from pressure, when resting on diseased limb or when letting it hang down, when getting out of bed, and when sitting down.

N.B. We very rarely find the over-sensitiveness of Valeriana to pain with Sulphur. Valeriana, on the other hand, lacks the sensation of **numbness** in suffering parts peculiar to Sulphur.

Sulphur.	Veratrum.
Left side—Want of bodily irritability . .	*Right* side—Increased irritability.
Pinching pain predom. in external parts .	Pinching pain predom. in internal part. .
Painless eruptions and ulcers, sometimes with proud flesh.	Painful eruptions and ulcers.
Pulse predominantly accelerated, full, and hard, particularly night and morning.	Pulse irregular; generally slow, small, and weak; sometimes slower than the beat'g of the heart; sometimes trembling.
Chill ascending	Chill descending.
Chill increased after getting out of bed . .	Chill lessened after getting out of bed.
Heat on lower part of body	Sweat, sometimes cold, only on lower part of body, *or* confined to upper part of body or forehead.
Drinking beer lessens the fever; coffee accelerates the pulse.	Drinking beer increases the fever and the pulse. C.Hg.
Thirst most rare during chill	Thirst most rare during sweat.
Seriousness — Being wrapt in thought—Embarrassment.	Jesting — Being beside one's self — Boldness.
Mood changing; predominantly depressed; indifferent—Rarely amorousness.	Cheerfulness more frequent than deject'n—Haughtiness—Maliciousness—Distrust.
Ailments from hear'g bad news, from shame, or fr. vexat'n with fright—Rarely apopl.	Ailments from fright, anger, or grief—Apoplexy.
Optical illusions in dark colors	Optical illusions in bright colors.
Objective stench from the nose predominant.	Subjective putrid odor.
Lameness, and sensation as if loose, in the teeth (while eating).	Heaviness in the teeth, sensation as if they were filled with lead. C.Hg.
Vomit sour oftener than bitter	Vomit predom. bitter.
Catamenia generally last'g too short a time and late.	Catamenia lasting too long; at the same time too soon *or* retarded.
Expectoration in the morning and during day, less frequent at night.	Expectoration, particularly during day.
Complaints predominant on fore-arm . .	Complaints predominant on upper arm.
Aggravation from midnight till noon and in the evening.	Aggravation night and morning.
Ailments from metals, Iodine, Nitric. acid.	Ailments from Ferrum, Cinch., or Arsenic.
Better (worse) in cold *or* in warm air . .	Worse in cold weather; better in warm air.
Predom. worse on inspiration, better on expiration.	Predominantly worse on inspiration and expiration.
Worse or better from weeping	Worse from weeping.
Worse or better after perspiring	Better after perspiring.
Better when getting out of bed	Better *or* worse when getting out of bed.
Worse when rising from a seat	Worse *or* better when rising from a seat.
Worse or better when assuming an erect position.	Worse when assuming an erect position.
Worse *or* better when bend'g back the head.	Better when bending back the head.
Predom. worse when bend'g diseased part .	Better *or* worse when bending the part.
Worse or better from touch.	Worse from touch.
Worse (better) on an empty stomach, *or* after breakfast.	Predom. better on an empty stomach, worse after breakfast.
Better *or* worse when eat'g, worse *afterw.*	Worse when eat'g, worse *or* better afterw.
Worse from being overhurried.	Worse when idle.

Predomin. worse — **Predomin. better**

When sitting bent forward, when ascending, after perspiring, and when bending diseased part backwards.

Predomin. better — **Predomin. worse**

When sitting down, when sitting erect, and when descending.

Sulphur. ac.	Phosphor.
Light hair—Compl. (sensitiveness or pinching pain, etc.) predom. in external parts.	Dark hair — Compl. (sensitiveness, pinching pain, etc.) predom. in internal parts.
Itching, locality changed by scratching, less frequently unchanged *or* lessened.	Itching, *lessened or* aggravated by scratching.
Humid cutaneous eruptions	Eruptions almost always dry.
In scars stinging	In scars contraction; they break open, bleed. C.Hg.
Disposition to sweat predominant	Dryness of skin predom.
Sweat, particularly on upper part of body .	Sweat, partic. on lower part of body.
Sweat appears or disappears when moving .	Sweat during sleep or while eating; sometimes also it disappears while eating.
Sweat increased by eating	Sweat abated by eating.
Pulse accelerated, small, and weak	Pulse various, irregular; generally frequent, full, and hard; sometimes intermitting.
One-sided heat, left side	One-sided heat, right side.
Chill or heat descending	Chill or heat ascending.
Distention of veins of feet	Distention of veins of hands.
Thirst mostly during hot stage	Want of thirst during all stages.

Sulphur. ac.	Phosphor.
Mood serious; depressed	Mood *cheerful or* despondent; indifferent.
Weak memory—Rarely delirium	Active memory predom.—Unconsciousness.
Compl. generally on lower eyelids, in upper jaw, and in the spleen.	Compl. generally in upper eyelids, in lower jaw, and in the liver.
Urine too seldom—Sediment yellow	U. often, but scanty—Sed. *white*, yellow or red.
Catamenia too profuse	Catam. too profuse *or* too scanty.
Expector. infrequent; morning & evening .	Expector. not constant; morn'g & dur'g day.

Sulphur. ac.	Phosphor.
Remission *afternoon* and before midnight . .	Remission of compl. after midnight.
Ailments from abuse of Cinchona	Ailments from Iodine or table-salt.
Worse in the evening twilight	Better in the twilight.
Worse after lying down	Better *or* worse after lying down.
Worse during sleep	Worse *or* better during sleep.
Worse on awaking from sleep	Better after sufficient sleep, but worse when roused from sleep and after the siesta.
Worse or better when getting out of bed . .	Worse when getting out of bed.
Predom. better after getting out of bed . .	Worse or better after getting out of bed.
Worse *or* better when standing	Predom. better when standing.
Worse when stooping	Better *or* worse when stooping.
Worse (better) when lifting the limb *or* when letting it hang down.	Predom. better when lifting the limb, worse when letting it hang down.
Worse after meals	Worse *or* better after meals.
Better from eructation	Worse *or* better from eructation.

Predomin. worse ——— **Predomin. better**

In the open air, in the twilight, after sleep, when sitting, from touch, when resting diseased limb on something, and from drinking cold water.*

Predomin. better ——— **Predomin. worse**

In-doors, after perspiring, from external pressure, and when swallowing.

N.B. Sulphur. ac. lack the over-sensitiveness of Phosphor. to pain.

---

* Both remedies have predom. improvement from cold diet generally, aggravation of complaints from warm diet.

Sulphur acid.	Sepia.
ght hair—Pinching pain in external parts.	Dark hair—Pinching pain in internal parts.
Pain piercing inward—No apoplexy . . .	Pain piercing outward—Apoplexy.
Paralysis generally one-sided	Paralysis often of both sides.
Itching. locality changed by scratching, less frequently unchanged or relieved.	Itching aggravated by scratching.
Humid eruptions	Eruptions generally dry.
Sleeplessness after midnight	Sleeplessness predom. before midnight.
Pulse frequent, small, and weak	Pulse frequent and full at night, during the day accelerated only by vexation or motion; unequal; trembling or intermitting.
Thirst mostly during hot stage	Want of thirst; but dur'g chill thirst is usual.
Chill or heat descending	Chill or heat ascending.
Chill abated by motion and in the open air .	Chill increased by motion and in the open air.
Mood changing; distrustful; rarely irritable .	Mood indifferent; peevish, irritable—Avarice.
Mental excitability—Rarely mental dullness .	Mental dullness—Fancies—Insanity.
Delirium, but quite rare	Unconsciousness.
Short-sightedness	Far-sightedness.
Sour vomit	Vomit predominantly bitter.
Affections of the spleen predom.	Liver complaints predom.
Urinal sediment generally yellow	Urinal sediment reddish *or* white.
Erections	Sexual desire changeable—Impotence, with inclination.
Catamenia too soon	Catamenia generally too late.
Fluent coryza, right side*—Secretion thick .	Fluent coryza, left side—Secretion watery or viscid.
Expectoration seldom; *morning* and evening.	Expectoration predom., but not constant; is loosened night and morning; is swallowed.
REMISSION *afternoon* and before midnight . .	REMISSION of complaints afternoon.
Ailments from abuse of Cinchona	Ailments from Cinchona, Mercurius, or Sulphur, and from mosquito bites.
Worse in cold weather; better in warm air .	Worse (better) in cold weather *or* in warm air.
Pred. worse in the open air; better in-doors.	Better (worse) in the open air *or* in-doors.
Predom. worse after lying down; worse *or* better while lying.	*Worse or* better after lying down and while lying.
Worse on awaking from sleep	Better after sufficient sleep; but worse when roused from sleep.
Worse *or* better when getting out of bed . .	*Better or* worse when getting out of bed.
Better *or* worse when standing	Worse when standing.
Worse or better when sitting	Worse when sitting.
Worse from bodily exertion	*Better or* worse from exertion.
Worse on inspiration, better on expiration .	*Generally* better on inspiration, worse on expiration.
Better or worse when swallowing	Worse when swallowing.
Better *or* worse when eating; worse *afterwards.*	Worse when eating; *worse or* better *afterwards.*
Complaints of brandy-drinkers—Symptoms are palliated by the use of wine.	Complaints from spirituous liquors and from beer.

Predomin worse — **Predomin. better**

In wet weather, after sleep, when assuming an erect position, from motion, when walking, from bodily exertion, on inspiration, from smoking, from drinking cold water,† and after breakfast.

Predomin. better — **Predomin. worse**

In dry weather, after perspiring, during rest, on expiration, when swallowing, from eructation, *before* breakfast, from pressure, from rubbing and scratching.

N.B. Sulphur acid. lacks the over-sensitiveness of Sepia to pain. Mere sensitiveness to touch occurs with both remedies.

* Both remedies also have "dry coryza;" with Sulphur acid. it is even predominant.
† The symptoms of both remedies are improved by "cold diet" in general, and predom. aggravated by warm drink.

Sulph. acid.	Sulphur.
Right side, partic. *upper right, lower left side.*	*Left* side, partic. *upper left, lower right side.*
Ulcerative pain in external parts — Pain piercing inwards.	Ulcerative pain in internal parts—Pain piercing outwards.
Paralysis generally one-sided	Paralysis generally of both sides.
Itching, locality changed, rarely unchanged or relieved.	Itching, almost always relieved by scratching.
Humid eruptions	Eruptions generally dry.
Sleeplessness after midnight	Sleeplessness before midnight.
Pulse frequent, small, and weak	Pulse frequent, full, and hard; sometimes intermitting or imperceptible.
Chill, cold shudders or heat descending	Chill, shudders or heat ascending.
Sweat often brought on by the least motion, but often also disappears when moving.	Sweat increased by motion.
Wine lessens the sweat	Beer (brandy) or coffee increase the pulse.
	C.Hg.

Sulph. acid.	Sulphur.
Mood distrustful; rarely irritable	Mood gentle *or* irritable; indifferent.
Mental excitability—Rarely delirium	Fancies—Insanity.
Complaints predominant on lower eyelids	Compl. predom. on upper eyelids.
Secretion of saliva predominantly increased	Saliva *generally* diminished.
Desire for brandy	Des. for *or* avers. to beer & spirituous liquors.
Urine too seldom—Sediment generally yellow.	Urine often, but scanty—Sed. *whitish* or red.
Catamenia too soon and profuse	Catam. generally too late and scanty.
Nasal secretion thick	Nasal secretion watery.
Expectoration seldom; *morning* and evening.	Expector. not constant; morning and during day, less frequently at night.
Ailments from abuse of Cinchona	Ailm. from Cinchona, Rhus, and metals.

Sulph. acid.	Sulphur.
Worse from growing cold and in cold weather, better from growing warm & in warm air.	Better (worse) from growing cold and in cold weather, *or* fr. grow'g warm & in warm air.
Predom. worse in the open air, better in-doors.	*Generally* bett. in the open air, worse in-doors (partic. in crowded rooms), but better from warmth of stove.
Better after perspiring	*Worse or* better after perspiring.
Better *or* worse when lying	Worse when lying.
Worse *or* better when getting out of bed	Better when getting out of bed.
Predom. better *after* getting out of bed	Better *or* worse after getting out of bed.
Better *or* worse when standing	Worse when continuing to stand, but better when standing still after motion.
Worse when stooping	Worse *or* better when stooping.
Worse (better) when lifting diseased limb *or* when letting it hang down.	Predom. worse when lifting diseased limb, better when letting it hang down.
Worse from touch	*Worse or* better from touch.
Predom. better on an empty stomach, worse after breakfast.	Worse (better) on an empty stomach *or* after breakfast.
Compl. of brandy-drinkers — Symptoms are palliated by the use of wine.	Predom. worse from spirituous liquors.
Worse after stool	Worse or better after stool.

Predomin. worse —— **Predomin. better**

In the open air, from cold, from motion, when resting diseased limb on something, & from warm diet.

Predomin. better —— **Predomin. worse**

In-doors, from warmth, during rest, after perspiring, when swallowing, and from cold diet.*

---

* Both remedies, however, have aggravations from *drinking cold water.*

Thuya.	Apis.
Muscles lax—Want of bodily irritability . .	Muscles rigid—Increased irritability.
Generally aversion to open air	Inclination for open air.
Dislike to move, but motion improves . . .	Desire to move, but motion aggravates.
Sensation of numbness in internal parts . .	Sensation of numbness in external parts.
Emaciation *or* swelling of diseased part . .	Swelling of diseased part.
Oedema around the joints — Diseases of the bones.	Redness around the joints—Inflammation of the periosteum.
Cold, painless swelling of glands	Painful swelling of glands.
Paralysis more frequent than apoplexy . .	Apoplexy more frequent than paralysis.
Paralysis often of both sides	Paralysis often one-sided.
Sleeplessness predom. — Awaking too early .	Coma predom.—Awaking too late.
Chill without thirst — Thirst is wanting only during chill.	Chill with thirst—Thirst is wanting only during sweat.
Sweat abated in-doors	Sweat increased in-doors.
Seriousness — Haughtiness — Anxious feeling in præcordia.	Exaggerated merriment — Fickleness — Jealousy—Anxious feeling in head.
Fancies — Very rarely delirium — Reserve—Fear of loss of reason.	Talkativeness—Fear of apoplexy.
Ailments from vexation or anger	Ailm. from hearing bad news, from vexation with fright or vehemence, & from jealousy.
Complaints predom. on inside of ear, on foot, and on instep.	Compl. predom. on outside of ear, on hand, and on sole of foot.
Pupils generally contracted	Pupils generally dilated.
Objects appear too small.	Objects appear too large.
Saliva generally diminished	Saliva predom. increased.
Very rarely nausea	Nausea.
Urine often and copious	Urine often, but scanty; sometimes copious.
Involuntary emission of urine	Retention of urine.
Catam. predom. too soon; at the same time scanty and of short duration.	Catam. too soon; at the same time scanty or profuse.
Coryza dry in-doors, fluent in the open air .	Fluent coryza.
Cough, partic. night and morning—Expector. quite constant; evening.	Cough which loosens with difficulty, rouses from sleep before midnight, and ceases as soon as the least particle is loosened, which is swallowed—Expectoration seldom.
Aggrav. partic. afternoon & after midnight.	Aggravation from evening till morning.
Remission forenoon and before midnight . .	Remission during the day.
Complaints from the moon-light	Complaints from heat of sun.
Generally *aggrav.* in the open air	*Better* in the open air.
Generally improved by touch and pressure .	Worse from touch — Worse from pressure, with exception of headache.
Better *or* worse after lying down and after getting up.	*Worse* after lying down and after getting out of bed.
Worse from washing	Better *or* worse from washing.
Better *or* worse from moving diseased part .	*Worse* from moving the suffering part.
Generally *aggrav.* when letting diseased limb hang down or when resting it on something, better when lifting it up.	*Better* when letting diseased limb hang down, worse when lifting it.
Worse when swallowing saliva	Worse when swallowing *drink* or food.
Ailments from abuse of Mercurius, Iodine, or Sulphur.	Ailments from animal poisons, from Iodine, or abuse of Cinchona.

Predomin. worse — **Predomin. better**

When getting out of bed, during rest, from spirituous liquors, with leucorrhœa, when letting diseased limb hang down, and in the open air.

Predomin. better — **Predomin. worse**

When moving, when sitting down, after rising from a seat, from drinking cold water, from vomiting, from touch, when lifting diseased limb, and in-doors.

Thuya.	Argent. nitr.
Muscles lax—Pain pressing outward . .	Muscles rigid—Pain pressing inward.
Complaints predom. in external parts . .	Complaints predom. in internal parts.
Sensitiveness of external, insensibility of internal parts.	Insensibility (numbness) of external parts.
Apoplexy	Apoplexy not yet observed.
Heat, with inclination to uncover	Heat, with aversion to uncover.*
Thirst is wanting only during chill . . .	Thirstlessness predom.

Thuya.	Argent. nitr.
Fear of loss of reason — Mood serious; haughty — Absent-minded dreaminess — Insanity.	Fear of apoplexy — (Hypochondrical and gloomy mood—Apathy, with great weakness).
Pupils generally contracted	Pupils unequal; light does not act on them.
Short-sightedness	Far-sightedness.
Urine increased	Secretion of urine diminished.
Sexual desire increased oftener than decreased	Sexual desire too weak.
After drinking cold water: panting for breath, with palpitation, hiccoughing, and prostration.	After drinking: cannot bear the handkerchief coming near the nose, it threatens to suffocate (even in cholera). C.Hg.
Expectoration quite constant	Expectoration quite rare.

Thuya.	Argent. nitr.
AGGRAVATION *after midnight* and morning, as well as *afternoon* and evening.	AGGRAVATION after midnight, morning and afternoon.
Generally worse in the open air, better indoors.	*Generally* better in the open air, worse indoors.†
Generally better from cold; worse from warmth.	Predom. better from warmth,† worse from cold.
Predom. worse from washing and moistening.	Better from washing or bathing with cold water.
Worse or better after sleep	Worse on awaking from sleep.
Worse (better) when opening *or* when closing the eyes.	Better when opening, worse when closing the eyes.
Better *or* worse after getting out of bed .	Worse after getting out of bed.
Better *or* worse when moving diseased part.	Worse when moving the part.
Predom. worse when stretching out diseased limb; better when drawing it up.	Better (worse) when stretching out the limb *or* when drawing it up.
Better *or* worse from sneezing	Worse when sneezing.
Worse or better when taking a deep breath.	Worse when taking a deep breath.
Worse after meals	Worse *or* better after meals.
Predom. worse from spirituous liquors . .	Better from drinking wine.
Worse from light; better in the dark . .	Better (worse) from light *or* in the dark.

Predomin. worse — **Predomin. better**

In the open air, from warmth, during rest, when standing and lying, from washing and moistening with cold water, when letting diseased limb hang down, from warm diet, from spirituous liquors, and from acids.

Predomin. better — **Predomin. worse**

In-doors, from cold, from motion, when walking, when lifting diseased limb, from cold diet, partic. drinking cold water, from eructation, from touch, and from rubbing and scratching.

---

* This refers to the sensation of the skin; in regard to respiration, on the other hand, Argent. nitr. favors uncovering.
† Both remedies have aggravation predominant in "hot rooms" and from "warmth of bed."

Thuya.	Arsenic.
Left side—Plethora—Muscles lax	Right side—Anæmia—Muscles rigid.
Complaints (gnawing, tension, heaviness, &c.) in external parts.	Complaints (gnawing, tension, heaviness, &c.) in internal parts.
Sensitiveness of skin predom. also in external parts.	Insensibility of internal parts predom.
Apoplexy — Paralysis, partic. after spasms .	No apoplexy — Paralysis of limbs that before were painful, sometimes oedematic.
Oedema around the joints	Erysipelas around the joints.
Swelling of the extreme phalangies of the fingers, even with general emaciation.	General emaciation, partic. atrophy of the extreme phalangies of the fingers.
Warts on the finger-tips	Vesicles filled with blood on the tips of the fingers; ulcers, with crusts under the nails.
Stinging and digging in the scars	Burning in scars. C.Hg.
Itching, improved by scratching	Itching, aggrav. by scratching.
Pulse quick and full in the evening, slow and weak in the morning.	Pulse quick in the morning, slow in the evening; irregular.
Heat or sweat, with inclination to uncover	Heat or sweat, with aversion to uncover.
Sweat often disappears on awaking	Sw. sometimes disappears when falling asleep and sometimes on awaking.
First heat, then chill	First chill, then heat.
Heat in the forenoon, chilliness in the aftern.	Chill during day, sweat at night.
Clonic spasms during the heat or sweat . .	Clonic spasms during the chill.
Inclinat. for solitude—Taciturnity—Haughtiness — Absent-mindedness — Dreaminess — Rarely delirium.	Fear of solitude — Loquacity — Malice — Avarice—Delirium.
Costiveness predom.	Diarrhœa predom.
Urine too often and copious	Urine scanty (with diarrhœa) *or* copious.
Catamenia too scanty and of short duration .	Catamenia too profuse and of long duration.
Expectoration quite constant; evening . .	Expectoration not constant; during day.
Complaints predom. on instep.	Complaints predom. on sole of foot.
REMISSION *forenoon* and before midnight . .	REMISSION during day and before midnight.
Ailments from abuse of Mercurius	Ailments from Cinchona, Strychnine, Iodine, Digitalis, Plumb., Phosphor., or from contagious Anthrax.
Complaints of tea-drinkers	Complaints of brandy-drinkers. C. Hg.
Generally better fr. cold, when growing cold; worse from warmth and when growing warm.	Worse from cold and when growing cold; better from warmth and when growing warm.
Worse (better) in warm *or* cold air	Better in warm air; worse in cold weather.
Predom. worse in bed	Better in bed (warmth) *or* worse (rest).
Worse or better after sleep	Better after sufficient sleep, but worse when roused from sleep.
Worse from light, better in the dark . . .	Worse (better) from light or in the dark.
Worse or better when moving, and bending the diseased part.	Predom. better when moving or bending the part.
Worse *or* better when sneezing or taking a deep breath.	Worse when sneezing or taking a deep breath.
Better or worse after stool	*Worse or* better after stool.
Worse after passing urine	Better *or* worse after passing urine.

Predomin. worse — **Predomin. better**

From warmth and when growing warm, from warmth of stove and of bed, from wrapping up, after sleep, when getting out of bed, from washing and moistening the suffering part, when letting diseased limb hang down, when standing, when riding, after a satisfying meal, from warm diet.

Predomin. better — **Predomin. worse**

From cold and when growing cold, from uncovering, after perspiring, after stool, from touch, from rubbing and scratching, when lifting diseased limb, from cold diet, partic. drinking cold water.

N.B. Thuya lacks the over-sensitiveness of Arsenic. to pain as well as its sensation of numbness in suffering parts.

Thuya.	Phosphor.
Left side, partic. *upper left, lower right side.*	*Right* side, partic. *upper right, lower left side.*
Light hair—Muscles lax—Often indicated with children.	Dark hair — Muscles rigid — Often indicated with old people.
Compl. predom. in external parts, particularly sensitiveness in external, numbness in internal parts.	Compl. predom. in internal parts, particularly sensitiveness in internal, numbness in external parts.
Spasms, with unconsciousness	Spasms, with full consciousness.
Paralysis, with atrophy of muscles	Nervous paralysis.
Emaciation *or* swelling of the suffering parts.	Swelling of the suffering parts.
Oedema around the joints	Vesicles around the joints.
Cold, painless swelling of glands	Hot swelling of the glands.
Pain in the middle of the long muscles	Compl. in the middle of the long bones.
Itching, relieved by scratching	Itching *relieved or* aggrav. by scratching.
Causes atrophy of warts	Cures warts, etc., by suppuration.
In scars stinging and digging	Scars pinching contraction, break open, bleed. C. Hg.
Awaking too early	Awaking too late.
Pulse frequent and full in the evening, slow & weak in the morning.	Pulse various, irregular, sometimes intermitting; generally frequent, full, and hard.
One-sided chill, predom. left side	One-sided chill, predom. right side.
First heat, then chill	First chill, then heat.
Heat in the forenoon, chilliness in the afternoon,	Coldness in the morning, heat in the evening.
Thirst is wanting only during chill	Want of thirst constant.
Chill, increased out-doors — Sweat, lessened in-doors.	Chill, lessened out-doors — Sweat, increased in-doors.
Desire for solitude and dreaminess	Fear of solitude.
Despondency	*Cheerfulness or* despondency.
Rarely unconsciousness or delirium	Unconsciousness—Delirium.
Mental dullness—Imbecility	Insanity more frequent than imbecility.
Weak memory	Active memory predom.
Compl. predom. on inside of ear, on upper jaw, upper lip, and on instep.	Compl. predom. on outside of ear, on lower jaw, on lower lip, and on sole of foot.
Eyes protruding—Objects appear too small	Eyes sunken—Obj. predom. appear too large.
Vomit predominantly bitter	Vomit predom. sour.
Urine too often and copious	Urine often, but scanty.
Catamenia scanty & of short duration; blood dark at first, then watery.	Catam. profuse and of long duration, *or* scanty and of short duration; blood watery at first, then dark.
Labor-pains weak or ceasing	Labor-pains spasmodic, too painful.
Expector. quite constant; evening	Expector. not constant; morning & dur'g day.
REMISSION *forenoon* and before midnight	REMISSION of complaints after midnight.
Ailments from abuse of Mercurius	Ailments from Iodine or table-salt.
Worse when stooping. after meals, and during sleep.	Worse *or* better when stooping, after meals, and during sleep.
Predom. worse after sleep	Better after sufficient sleep, but worse when roused from sleep and after the siesta.
Better *or* worse when sneezing, when bending the part, and from change of position.	Worse when sneezing, when bending the part, and from change of position.
Better from eructation	Worse *or* better from eructation.
Generally better from pressure	*Generally* worse from pressure.
Worse from swallowing saliva	Worse when swallowing food and partic. when swallowing drink.

Predomin. worse — **Predomin. better**

In the open air, from warmth and when growing warm, during rest, after sleep, when standing, sitting and lying, when resting diseased limb on something, after a satisfying meal, from sweets, from wine, and after drinking generally.

Predomin. better — **Predomin. worse**

In-doors,* from cold and when growing cold, from motion, when walking, after perspiring, when bending diseased part backwards, from pressure, and after stool.

N.B. Thuya rarely has either the over-sensitiveness of Phosphor. to pain nor its sensation of numbness in suffering parts.

* Both remedies have predom. aggrav. in "hot rooms."

Valeriana.	Ignatia.
Upper left, lower right side—Pain piercing outwards.	Upper right, lower left side—Pain piercing inwards.
Red parts become white	External parts become black.
Apoplexy or paralysis not yet observed .	*Apoplexy*—Paralysis.
Pulse generally quick and somewhat tense; very irregular, without extrinsic causes.	Pulse generally frequent, full, and hard; very variable from extrinsic causes.
Fainting during the chill	Fainting during the heat or sweat. C.Hg.
Heat increased when eating	Heat abated while eating.
Thirst, particularly during hot stage . . .	Thirst only during cold and after sweating stage.

Valeriana.	Ignatia.
Being beside one's self—Cheerfulness predominant—Irritable mood.	Being wrapt in thought Mood changing; predom. sad; gentle; indifferent; peevish — Amorousness — Consequences of hearing bad news, shame, reserved mortification, of grief or disappointed love.
Easy comprehension—Ecstasies . . .	Difficult comprehension—Mental dullness—Absent-mindedness—Insanity.
Clear-sightedness predominant . . .	Dim-sightedness.
Catamenia retarded and scanty . . .	Catamenia too soon and scanty.
Cough not yet observed	Cough, generally without expectoration.
Complaints predominant on the front part of thigh.	Complaints predominant on back part of thigh.

Valeriana.	Ignatia.
Remission after midnight	Remission of complaints before midnight
Worse when lying on painful side, better when lying on unpainful side.	*Generally* better when lying on painful, worse when lying on unpainful side.
Worse on awaking from sleep	*Worse or* better after sleep.
Worse when getting out of bed	Worse *or* better when getting out of bed.
Generally better from light	Worse from light, better in the dark.
Worse from washing	Better from washing the head.
Almost always aggravated when stooping .	Better *or* worse when stooping.
Worse when eating	*Better or* worse when eating.
Worse *or* better after eating	Almost always improved after eating.

Predomin. worse — **Predomin. better**

In the dark, on inspiration and when taking a deep breath, when stretching out diseased limb or when resting it on something, when eating, from drawing in the abdominal muscles, from pressure, from washing, and when lying on painful side.

Predomin. better — **Predomin. worse**

From light, on expiration, when drawing up diseased limb, when moving diseased part, after perspiration, and when lying on unpainful side.

Valeriana.	Nux vomica.
Left side, particularly *upper left, lower right side.*	*Right* side, particularly *upper right, lower left side.*
Sleeplessness before midnight	Sleeplessness predominant after midnight.
Pulse very irregular; generally quick and somewhat tense.	Pulse generally frequent, full, and hard; sometimes intermitting or imperceptible.
Sensation of cold in external parts . . .	Sensation of cold internal.
Fainting during the chill	Faint'g dur'g hot (or sweat'g) stage. C.Hg.
Thirst mostly during hot stage	Thirst mostly during cold stage.

Valeriana.	Nux vomica.
Changing mood—Cheerfulness	Mood anxious; sad; peevish; vexed; irritable; passionate; malicious—Amorousness.
Easy comprehension—Mental excitability—Rarely unconsciousness or delirium.	Difficult comprehension — Absent-mindedness—Melancholy.
Apoplexy or paralysis not yet observed .	Apoplexy—Paralysis.
Short-sightedness	Far-sightedness.
Nausea in throat—Affections of the spleen predominant.	Nausea in stomach—Liver complaint predominant.
Diarrhœa.	Costiveness predominant.
Urine too often and copious—Sediment *red* or white.	Urine seldom and scanty—Sediment generally red.
Catamenia too late and scanty.	Catamenia too soon and profuse.
Cough not yet observed.	Cough *dry or* with expectoration.
Complaints predominant on upper arm. .	Complaints predominant on fore-arm.

Valeriana.	Nux vomica.
Remission of complaints after midnight .	Remission evening till midnight.
Generally better from light, worse in the dark.	Worse from light, better in the dark.
Worse on inspiration, better on expiration.	*Generally* better on inspiration, worse on expiration.
Worse when lying on painful, better when lying on unpainful side.	Worse (better) when lying on painful *or* when lying on unpainful side.
Almost always improved by change of position.	*Worse or* better when turning in bed.
Worse on awaking from sleep	Better after sufficient and not too long sleep, but worse when roused from sleep.
Predominantly worse on an empty stomach, better after breakfast.	*Generally* better on an empty stomach, worse after breakfast.
Worse when eating	*Generally* better when eating.
Worse from external pressure, from washing, & when bend'g the part backwards.	Generally better from pressure, from wash'g, & when bend'g diseased part backwards.
Worse when stretching out diseased limb, better when drawing it up.	*Generally* better when stretching out diseased limb, worse when drawing it up.

Predomin. worse — **Predomin. better**

In the dark, on inspiration, during rest, when sitting down and while sitting, when standing, after lying down and while lying, in bed, after sleeping, from pressure, when resting diseased limb on something, when bending the suffering part backwards, from washing, when eating, and in contracted posture.

Predomin. better — **Predomin. worse**

From light, on expiration, from motion, particularly when moving the suffering part, when walking, when rising from a seat, from change of posture, when lying or standing generally, and in extended posture.

Veratrum.	Belladonna.
Light hair—Skin & muscles predominantly lax.	Dark hair predominant—Skin and muscles rigid.
Inclination for motion—Rend'g pain downwards.	Aversion to motion*—Rending pain upwards.
Paralysis more frequent than apoplexy . .	Apoplexy more frequent than paralysis.
Dry eruptions	Humid eruptions.
When the pulse becomes slow, it is weak .	When the pulse becomes slow, it is strong and full.
Pulse irregular; generally slow, small, and like a thread; sometimes intermitting, trembling, or imperceptible.	Pulse generally quick, full, and hard and tense.
Thirst most rare during sweating stage . .	Thirst most rare during chill.
Heat or sweat, with inclination to uncover.	Heat or sweat, with aversion to uncover.
Heat abated by drinking beer	Heat increased by drinking beer.

Veratrum.	Belladonna.
Sensitive disposition	Generally insensibility of disposition.
Satiety of life, with fear of death	Satiety of life, with longing for death.
Fear of solitude—Haughtiness	Inclination for solitude—Mood changing; indifferent—Amorousness.
Ailments from grief	Ailments from vexation with fright.
Easy *or* difficult comprehension—Memory weak—Rarely imbecility.	Difficult comprehension—Memory active *or* weak—Imbecility.
Horse strikes, bites, snaps at its tail, resists being bridled.	Horse stares restlessly, resists having fore-feet examined, refuses to be mounted, or "capsizes."
Cold spots on the scalp	Hot spots on the scalp.
Pupils generally contracted	Pupils generally dilated.
Eyes generally sunken	Eyes protruding.
Appetite for sour things—Nausea in stomach.	Aversion to sour things†—Nausea in throat or abdomen.
Catamenia too soon *or* retarded	Catamenia too soon.
Expectoration not constant; chiefly during day.	Expectoration infrequent; morning, during day, evening.
Complaints generally on calf	Complaints generally on shin.

Veratrum.	Belladonna.
AGGRAVATION night and morning . . .	AGGRAVATION morning and *from noon till midnight.*
Worse when idling	Worse from being overhurried.
Better (worse) when growing cold *or* warm.	Predom. worse when growing cold; better when growing warm.
Better after perspiring	Worse *or* better after perspiring.
Worse *or* better in bed	Predom. better in bed.
Worse when lying on side; better when lying on back.	Better (worse) when lying on side or on back.
Worse when lying on painful side; better when lying on unpainful side.	Better (worse) when lying on painful *or* on unpainful side.
Better *or* worse when and after getting out of bed.	Worse when getting out of bed; almost always improved *afterwards.*

---

* Belladonna also has inclination for motion in single or suffering parts.

† In the beginning of a recovery, after Belladonna had been taken, there appears in some cases a great longing for lemons or lemonade; then, a moderate use of it will promote the cure very much. Comp. Ars. and Bellad. C.Hg.

Veratrum. Belladonna.

(Continued.)

Veratrum	Belladonna
Better *or* worse when rising from a seat	Worse when rising from a seat.
Worse when assuming an erect position	*Worse or* better when assuming an erect position.
Better when ascending; worse when descending.	Worse (better) when ascending *or* when descending.
Worse when eating; worse *or* better *afterwards.*	Worse *or* better when eating; worse *afterwards.*
Worse from spirituous liquors	*Worse or* better from spirituous liquors.
Worse *or* better after stool	Worse after stool.
Ailments from Ferrum, Arsenic, or Cinchona.	Ailments from Ferrum, Plumbum, Cuprum, Mercurius, Platina, Aconite, or Hyoscyamus.

Predomin. worse — **Predomin. better**

In wet weather, in-doors, from warmth of bed, from wrapping up, during rest, when sitting down and while sitting, when standing, after lying down and while lying, when stooping, when bending suffering part inwards, when stretching out diseased limb, and from cold diet.*

Predomin. better — **Predomin. worse**

In dry weather, in the open air, from uncovering, from motion, particularly when moving diseased part, when walking, when drawing up diseased limb, and from warm diet.

N.B. Both are often indicated in typhoid fevers, it is true, in widely different cases, but sometimes the choice is difficult, particularly as Belladonna is equally applicable in apparently opposite states. Both have: Apathy, stupor, unconsciousness or great sensibility to noise and also to light; dislike to talk, except in delirium, the latter sometimes is furious (Veratrum, "tearing his clothing," Belladonna, "tearing their breasts awfully"), great fearfulness; eyes dim and glazy, face pale or by turns red and hot, distorted features, sudden startings in sleep, grinding of teeth; both have much thirst, frequent drinking, but only little at a time; the mouth dry, saliva lessened; diarrhœa; involuntary discharge of the fæces and the urine; both have nymphomania and other uterine affections in common; with both the head is often burning hot, while the limbs are cold; both have an aversion to being covered, both indicated particularly in children and women, etc. VERATRUM has a great similarity with Lycopodium in typhoid complaints of children; *Belladonna* with Rhus or Calcarea.—*Veratrum* predom. violent headache, the head is hot and covered with sweat; hands are often put on the head, children rub the head, *cannot bear being left alone;* dim eyes, are full of tears, eyelids livid, blue edges around the eyes; *face collapsed*, pale, bluish; the nose more pointy; boring in the nose, rubbing the mouth; lips bluish or hanging down; nausea, vomiting food or slime, violent colic with the diarrhœa; urine scanty, red-brown; breathing short, frequent, difficult; dry cough, or with a rattling noise, but no expectoration; *skin shrinking*, relaxed, without "turgor;" temperature sinking; coldness, cold viscous sweat; burning heat of head and trunk, with limbs alternately hot and cold; cannot bear being covered during the heat; pulse frequent, small and hard, or down to 48 beats, soft and intermitting; frequently indicated in cholera season. — *Belladonna:* Violent temper; morose or depressed and sad mood; *delirium*, mostly violent, raging (imagining enemies or animals), *in alternation with an apparently deep sleep;* desire to jump out of bed, run away, or picking the bed clothes; body in constant motion, jerking with hands, move hands about in the air; sudden starting from sleep with screams; convulsive motions of the limbs; giddiness, dizziness or fullness, heaviness, rush of blood to the head; throbbing, shooting on top of head alternately, with stitches in decayed teeth; cannot bear others walking through the room; eyes fiery, staring, rolling, sparks before the eyes; pupils first oversensitive, later not reacting by light; face puffed up, shining; hearing very acute or hard of hearing, buzzing in the ears; difficult speech, stammering, lisping, or speechlessness; twitching when attempting to talk; tongue white, smooth or cracked, red and dry, with a burning thirst; *spasmodic difficulty in swallowing*, cannot swallow but a few drops; breathing either frequent or *slow, hardly perceptible, interrupted by deep sighing; sleepless with great longing for sleep;* skin burning hot, rarely cold; heat often appears on upper part of body, with objective cold feet; pulse at first frequent, full and large, later quick, hard and suppressed; in violent rage they uncover themselves. Often indicated in hot summers, or in fevers from solar influence. C.Hg.

N.B. The supersensitiveness to pain is much more with Belladonna than with Veratrum. H.Gr.—But "pains driving to madness" is a characteristic indication for Veratrum. C.Hg.

*** Both remedies have predominant aggravation of symptoms from "drinking cold water," because it is peculiar to Belladonna to occasion difficulty in "swallowing drink."**

Veratrum.	Bryonia.
Upper left, lower right side—Constriction in internal parts.	Upper right, lower left side—Constriction in external parts.
Painful ulcers	Painless ulcers.
Fainting in the evening when trying to go to sleep, with cold sweat on the forehead.	Fainting in the morning when getting up.
Pulse irregular; generally slow, small, and weak.	Pulse accelerated, full, hard, and tense.
Chill increased by drinking	Chill lessened by drinking.
Drinks often, but little at a time	Drinks seldom, but much at a time.

Mood *cheerful or* sad; haughty; distrustful .	Dejection—No amorousness.
Ailments from grief	Ailments from mortification.
Easy *or* difficult comprehension — Absent-mindedness—Insanity.	Difficult comprehension.
Nausea in the stomach	Nausea in abdomen, rarely in stomach or œsophagus.
Diarrhœa, often painless	Costiveness; when diarrhœa occurs, it is generally painful.
Urine seldom and scanty; sometimes copious.	Urine often, but scanty; exceptionally copious.
Expectoration particularly during the day . .	Expectoration morning and evening, less frequently during day.
Complaints predominant in upper part of chest and on back part of thigh.	Complaints predominant in lower part of chest and on front part of thigh.

AGGRAVATION night and morning	AGGRAVATION evening, night, and morning.
Ailments from Cinchona, Ferrum, or Arsenic.	Ailments from Rhus or Alumina.
Worse in cold weather, better in warm air .	Worse (better) in cold weather *or* in warm air.
Worse *or* better in bed	Predominantly better in bed.
Worse when lying on painful, better when lying on unpainful side.	*Generally* better when lying on painful, worse when lying on unpainful side.
Worse after sleep	*Worse or* better after sleep.
Better *or* worse when and after getting out of bed.	Worse when getting out of bed; *afterwards* predominantly worse.
Better *or* worse when rising from a seat . .	Worse when rising from a seat.
Worse when assuming an erect position . .	*Worse or* better when assuming an erect position.
Worse *or* better when bending the diseased part.	Worse when bending the part.
Worse from touch and after drinking . . .	Worse *or* better from touch and after drinking.
Worse *or* better after eating	Predominantly worse after eating.
Better from eructation	Worse *or* better from eructation.
Worse *or* better after stool	Almost always better after stool.
Children are easier when carried about, but quickly.	Children dislike to be carried. C. Hg.

Predomin. worse — **Predomin. better**

In wet weather, from warmth of bed, when lying on painful side, during rest, when standing, when sitting down and while sitting, after lying down and while lying, when descending, when sitting erect, from drinking cold water, and from cold diet generally.

Predomin. better — **Predomin. worse**

In dry weather, when lying on unpainful side, from motion, particularly moving diseased part, when walking, after rising from a seat, when ascending, when sitting bent forward, from bending the head back, from warm diet and drinking milk.

Veratrum.	Nux vom.
Upper left, lower right side—Light hair—Skin and muscles predom. lax.	*Upper right, lower left side predom.* —Dark hair—Skin and muscles rigid.
External dropsy—Desire for motion	Internal dropsy—Aversion to motion.
Spasms generally with unconsciousness	Spasms generally with full consciousness.
Veratrine paralyses the muscles *through the blood*, not the nerves.	Strychn. paralyses the motory nerves directly, leaving the sensation unimpaired.
Sleeplessness before midnight	Sleeplessness predom. after midnight.
Pulse irregular; generally slow, small, and weak.	Pulse accelerated, full, and hard, partic. during hot stage.
Heat or sweat, with inclination to uncover	Heat or sweat, with aversion to uncover.
Chill lessened after getting out of bed	Chill increased after getting out of bed.
Thirst oftener during heat than sweat	Thirst oftener during chill than heat.
Beer lessens the fever	Alcohol, wine (beer), and coffee accelerate the pulse. C.Hg.

Veratrum.	Nux vom.
Taciturnity—*Cheerfulness* or dejection	Loquacity—Dejection.
Easy *or* difficult comprehension	Difficult comprehension.
Mental excitability or dullness	Mental dullness.
Pupils generally contracted	Pupils predom. dilated.
Saliva generally diminished	Saliva generally increased.
Appetite for sour things	Predom. aversion to sour things.
Diarrhœa predom., watery, copious, often painless.	Costiveness predom.; when diarrhœa occurs, it is scanty and painful.
Urine predom. dark; seldom and scanty, sometimes copious.	Urine generally light-colored; seldom and scanty.
Catamenia too soon *or* retarded	Catamenia too soon.
Breath cold	Breath hot.
Expectoration chiefly during day	Expectoration morning, during day, evening.
Complaints predom. on upper arm	Complaints predom. on fore-arm.

Veratrum.	Nux vom.
Remission during day and evening	Remission evening till midnight.
Worse (better) from cold and growing cold, *or* from warmth and growing warm.	Worse from cold and when growing cold; better from warmth and when growing warm.
Worse *or* better in bed	Almost always improved in bed.
Almost always aggrav. by warmth of bed	*Better or* worse from warmth of bed.
Worse when lying on side, better when lying on back.	Generally better when lying on side, worse when lying on back.
Worse when lying on painful, better when lying on unpainful side.	*Generally* worse when lying on painful, better when lying on unpainful side.
Worse after sleep	Better after sleep.*
Worse *or* better when getting out of bed, rising from a seat, or after stool	Worse when getting out of bed or rising from a seat, or after stool.
Worse when swallowing and after drinking	*Worse or* better when swallowing and after drinking.
Worse *or* better after meals	Almost always aggrav. after meals.
Better from eructation	Better *or* worse from eructation.
Worse when opening the mouth; better when closing it.	Better (worse) when opening *or* when closing the mouth.
Better *or* worse when bending diseased part	Predom. worse when bending diseased part.

Predomin. worse —— **Predomin. better**

In wet weather, in-doors, from warmth of bed, from wrapping up, during rest, when standing, when sitting down and while sitting, partic. sitting erect; after lying down and while lying, "when lying on side," partic. on "painful" side; after sleep, "when lifting or stretching out diseased limb," when descending, and when eating.

Predomin. better —— **Predomin. worse**

In dry weather, in the open air, from uncovering, from motion, partic. moving suffering part; when walking, when sitting bent forward, "when lying on back" or on "unpainful" side, "when letting diseased limb hang down or when drawing it up," when ascending, from eating meat or salty things.

N.B. Sensitiveness to pain is greater with Nux vomica than with Veratrum.

---

* If sufficient, but not too long; worse when the sleep is interrupted.

Veratrum.	Rhus.
Skin and muscles lax—Compl. predom. in internal parts.	Skin and muscles rigid—Compl. predomin. in external parts.
Painful ulcers, with scanty discharge	Painful ulcers, with copious discharge, partic. on dropsical legs, with constant discharge of water.
Dry eruptions	Eruptions generally humid.
Pulse generally slow, small, and weak; sometimes slower than beating of heart.	Pulse generally accelerated, weak, faint, and soft; sometimes quicker than beat'g of heart.
Heat, abated by drinking beer	Heat, increased by drinking beer.
Heat or sweat, with inclination to uncover	Heat or sweat, with aversion to uncover
Dread of solitude—Fear of being poisoned or of apoplexy.	Longing for solitude—Fear of being poisoned.
Mood *cheerful* or sad; haughty; distrustful; irritable & malicious—Amorousness.	Mood predomin. sad and dejected—Rarely amorousness.
Easy *or* difficult comprehension	Difficult comprehension.
Mental excitability or dullness	Mental dullness—Rarely mania.
Pupils generally contracted	Pupils dilated.
Nasal complaints predom. internal	Nasal compl. generally external.
Subjective putrid odor	Objective stench from nose.
Saliva generally diminished	Secretion of saliva predom. increased.
Nausea in stomach	Naus. in *œsophagus* or stomach, less frequently in the fauces.
Urine dark; infrequent and scanty, sometimes copious.	Urine pale; too often and copious.
Catamenia too soon *or* retarded	Catamenia too soon.
Dry coryza predominant	Fluent coryza.
Expectoration chiefly during day	Expector. chiefly in the morning.
Compl. predom. in upper part of chest and on upper arm.	Compl. predom. in lower part of chest and on fore-arm.
Remission during day and evening	Remission of complaints during day.
Ailments from Cinchona, Ferrum, or Arsenic.	Ailments from Bryonia, Rhododendron, or Tartar emetic.
Worse (better) from cold and when growing cold, or from warmth & when grow'g warm.	Worse from cold and when growing cold; better from warmth and when grow'g warm.
Predom. worse from warmth of bed	*Better or* worse from warmth of bed.
Predom. worse on inspiration & expiration	Worse on inspiration; better on expiration.
Better when moving diseased part	*Better or* worse when moving diseased part.
Better when bending diseased part backwards.	*Worse or* better when bending part backwards.
Predom. worse when sitting down	Worse *or* better when sitting down.
Worse when sitting erect, better when sitting bent forward.	*Generally* better when sitting erect, worse when sitting bent forward.
Predom. better after rising from a seat	Better *or* worse after rising from a seat.
Worse when eating	Worse *or* better when eating.
Worse after drinking	*Worse or* better after drinking.
Worse *or* better after stool; partic. bellyache after stool.	*Generally* better after stool; partic. bellyache better after stool.

Predomin. worse —— **Predomin. better**

In-doors, from warmth of bed, when lying on side, partic. when lying on painful side, when sitt'g erect, from wrapping up, when stretching out diseased limb, when descending, & after breakfast.

Predomin. better —— **Predomin. worse**

In the open air, when lying on back or on unpainful side, when sitting bent forward, from uncovering, when drawing up diseased limb, when ascending, when bending the suffering part backwards, on an empty stomach, and from drinking milk.

Zinc.	Mercur.
Dark hair — Want of bodily irritability . .	Light hair—Increased irritability.
Pressing inwards — Constriction in external parts.	Pressing outwards — Constriction in internal parts.
Itching, relieved, *or* locality changed, or unchanged by scratching.	Itching, relieved *or* aggravated by scratching.
Paralysis—No apoplexy	Apoplexy—Very rarely paralysis.
Pulse small and frequent in the evening, slow in the morning and during the day.	Pulse irregular, generally full and accelerated, partic. quick at night, slower dur'g the day.
Pulse affected by drinking wine	Pulse affected by drinking coffee. C.Hg.
Sweat lessened when eating	Sweat increased when eating.

Zinc.	Mercur.
Mood changing; cheerful; indifferent . . .	Mood serious; anxious; despondent.
Ailments from fright or vexation	Ailments from mortification.
Mental excitability	Mental dullness—Absent-mindedness—Unconsciousness—Fancies—Imbecility.
Complaints generally on inside of nose or roof of mouth, in lower part of chest, in hollow of elbow, on outer side of thigh, and on patella.	Complaints generally on outside of nose, on soft palate, in upper part of chest, on tip of elbow, on inner side of thigh, and in hollow of knee.
Optical illusions in bright colors	Optical illusions in dark colors.
With the toothache sweat breakes out . .	Toothache during the sweating stage; after toothache chill. C.Hg.
Urine predom. light-colored	Urine predom. dark.
Catamenia too scanty	Catamenia scanty *or* profuse.
Dry coryza predom.—Nasal secretion thick or viscid.	Generally fluent coryza — Nasal secretion watery.
Expectoration nearly constant; partic. in the morning.	Expectoration not constant; during the day.

Zinc.	Mercur.
Aggravation afternoon and evening, less frequently at night.	Aggravation from evening till morning.
Ailments from Baryta	Ailments from Arsenic or Copper vapors, from Aurum, Sulphur., etc.
Worse when growing cold, better when growing warm.	Better (worse) when growing cold or warm.
Worse after lying down	Better *or* worse after lying down.
Better from change of position when lying or standing.	Worse when turning in bed.
Better when getting out of bed	Better *or* worse when getting out of bed.
Worse when assuming an erect position . .	Worse *or* better when assum'g an erect posit'n.
Better *or* worse from touch	Worse from touch.
Worse on inspiration and expiration . . .	Worse on inspiration, better on expiration.
Generally better when swallowing	*Generally* worse when swallowing.
Worse when swallowing food, often better when swallowing drink.	Worse when swallowing saliva and drink, often better when swallowing food.
Almost always improved when eating; worse *afterwards.*	Worse *or* better when and after eating.

Predomin. worse ——— **Predomin. better**

In-doors, when drawing up diseased limb, when sitting and standing, and when swallowing food.

Predomin. better ——— **Predomin. worse**

In the open air, when stretching out diseased limb, from change of position, from pressure, when swallowing, partic. when swallowing drink, therefore from drinking cold water.

N.B. We very rarely find the over-sensitiveness of Zinc with Mercur.; apparently in contradiction to the constitutional character of both remedies; but compare the preface.

Zinc.	Pulsatilla.
Left side—Want of bodily irritability . . .	*Right* side—Increased irritability.
Pain pressing inwards — Hæmorrhages, blood light-red.	Pain pressing outwards—Hæmorrhages, blood dark.
Compl. predom. in external parts, dropsy in internal parts.	Compl. predom. in internal parts, dropsy in external parts.
Paralysis of the limbs—No apoplexy . . .	Apoplexy more frequent than paralysis.
Dry eruptions	Humid eruptions.
Itching, relieved, *or* locality changed, *or* unchanged by scratching.	Itching, aggrav. *or* unchanged by scratching.
Sweat on lower part of body	Chill on lower part of body.
Pulse more irregular than with Pulsatilla . .	Pulse irregular, but less so than with Zinc.
Wine affects the pulse	Beer or Coffee affects the pulse. C. Hg.
Chill, increas'd in the open air—Sweat, lessened when eating.	Chill, lessened in the open air — Sweat, increased when eating.
Compl. generally on inside of nose, on upper lip, on fore-arm, on patella and instep.	Compl. generally on outside of nose, on lower lip, on upper arm, in hollow of knee, and on sole of foot.
Mood cheerful; irritable	Calm, lachrymose sadness — Distrust — Boldness—Avarice.
Mental excitability	Mental dullness — Absent-mindedness — Fancies—Unconsciousness.
Vertigo, inclining to fall sideways (left side) .	Vertigo, inclining to fall backwards, less frequently sideways or forwards.
Stupefying headache in the morning . . .	Stupefying headache in the evening.
Generally costiveness; when diarrhœa occurs, it is generally painless.	Generally painful diarrhœa.
Urinal sediment yellow	Urinal sediment red.
Scrotum contracted	Scrotum relaxed. C. Hg.
Catamenia more copious during the night .	Catam. only dur'g the day while walk'g. C. Hg.
Dry coryza predominant	Coryza fluent oftener than dry.
Diminished secretion of milk	Milk generally increased.
Larynx dry	Larynx full of mucus.
Expectoration quite constant; partic. in the morning.	Expector. predom., but not constant; morning and during day.
Aggravation afternoon and evening . . .	Aggravation from noon till midnight.
Worse from exertion, running, etc.	*Better or* worse from bodily exert'n (but worse, on the other hand, fr. mental exert'n. C. Hg.)
Worse on inspiration and expiration . . .	Better on inspiration, worse on expiration.
Worse in bed and after sleep	*Worse or* better in bed and after sleep.
Better when and after getting out of bed, and after rising from a seat.	*Better or* worse when and after getting out of bed, etc.
Worse when sitting erect, better when sitting bent forward.	*Generally* better when sitting, worse when sitting bent forward.
Better *or* worse when lying and from touch .	Worse when lying and from touch.
Worse when moving or bending diseased part.	Better *or* worse when mov'g or bend'g the part.
Generally better when swallowing	Generally worse when swallowing.
Worse when swallowing food	Worse when swallowing saliva.
Better on an empty stomach; worse after breakfast.	Worse (better) on an empty stomach or after breakfast.
Worse after eating	*Worse or* better after eating,
Better when eating; worse *afterwards* . . .	Better when drinking; worse *afterwards*.
Bellyache ceases after stool	Bellyache after stool.

Predomin. worse — **Predomin. better**

From cold, from growing cold & in cold weather, from washing & moistening the suffering part, when opening the eyes, when sitting erect, from bodily exertion, running, etc., and after stool.

Predomin. better — **Predomin. worse**

From warmth, from growing warm & in warm air, when blowing the nose, when closing the eyes, when sitting bent forward, from change of position when lying or standing, when eating, from rubb'g and scratching.

Zincum.	Sepia.
Pain pressing inwards—Hæmorrhages, blood light-red—No apoplexy.	Pain pressing outwards—Hæmorrhages, blood dark—Apoplexy.
Itching, lessened, *or* locality changed *or* unchanged, by scratching.	Itching, aggravated by scratching.
Pulse small and frequent in the evening, slower in the morning and during day.	Pulse frequent, and full at night, during day accelerated only by vexation or motion; sometimes trembling.
Drinking wine accelerates the pulse	Drinking beer accelerates the pulse. C.Hg.
Thirst during heat, none during chill	Thirst *only* during the chill and *before* and *after* it.
Sweat lessened while eating	Sweat increased while eating.
Sweat often confined to lower part of body	Sweat often confined to upper part of body.

Zincum.	Sepia.
Mood changing; cheerful—Amorousness	Mood serious; anxious; sad; despondent—Avarice.
Ailments from fright	Consequences of vexation with fear.
Mental excitability — Delirium	Mental dullness — Absent-mindedness — Fancies—Imbecility—Unconsciousness.
Optical illusions in bright colors	Optical illusions in dark colors.
Eruption on upper lip	Eruption on lower lip.
Burning in the teeth	Coldness in the teeth. C.Hg.
Urine generally light-colored; sediment yellow.	Urine predominantly dark; sediment reddish or white.
Catamenia too scanty—Leucorrhœa thick	Catamenia generally too profuse—Leucorrhœa watery.
Nasal secretion *thick* or viscid	Nasal secretion *watery* or viscid.
Expectoration quite constant; particularly in the morning.	Expectoration not constant, is loosened particularly night & morn'g, and is swallowed.
Complaints on patella	Complaints generally on tip of elbow.

Zincum.	Sepia.
REMISSION night, morning, and forenoon	REMISSION of complaints afternoon.
Ailments from Baryta	Ailments from Sulphur, Mercurius, or abuse of Cinchona.
Worse in cold weather, better in warm air	Worse (better) in cold *or* in warm air.
Better in the open air, worse in-doors	Better (worse) in the open air *or* in-doors.
Worse after lying down and in bed	Worse *or* better after lying down and in bed.
Worse on awaking from sleep	Better after sufficient sleep, but worse when roused from sleep.
Better when and after getting out of bed	*Better or* worse when and after getting out of bed.
Worse from bodily exertion	*Better or* worse from bodily exertion.
Better *or* worse from touch	Almost always aggravated by touch.
Generally better when swallowing	Worse when swallowing.
Better while eating, worse *afterwards*	Better while drinking, worse *afterwards*.
Worse after meals	*Worse or* better after meals.
Cessation of bellyache after stool	Sore as if scraped in the belly after stool.

Predomin. worse — **Predomin. better**

In wet weather, when alone, after sleep, when rising, from bodily exertion, when moving the suffering part, when drawing up diseased limb, when sitting erect, after breakfast, and from loosening the clothes.

Predomin. better — **Predomin. worse**

In dry weather, when in company, when stretching out diseased limb, when sitting bent forward, from blowing the nose, on an empty stomach, when swallowing* and eating, from tying the clothes tight, from pressure, from rubbing and scratching.

---

* However, we find aggravation when swallowing "food" with both remedies.

Zincum.	Sulphur.
Hæmorrhages, blood light-red—Pain pressing inwards.	Hæmorrhages, blood dark—Pain pressing outwards.
Pinching pain in internal parts, ulcerative pain in external parts.	Pinching pain in external parts, ulcerative pain in internal parts.
Itching, lessened, *or* locality changed *or* unchanged, by scratching.	Itching, *lessened* by scratching, rarely aggrav. or locality changed.
Sweat on lower part of body	Heat on lower part of body, sweat on upper part of body.
Pulse small and frequent in the evening, slower during day and in the morning.	Pulse frequent (full, hard), partic. *night* and morning; slower during *day* and evening.
Pulse affected by drinking wine	Pulse affected by drinking beer. C.Hg.
Shudders descending	Shudders ascending.
External chill, with internal heat*	Internal chill, with external heat.
Mood cheerful—Amorousness	Mood serious and solemn; gentle; anxious; sad and despondent.
Ailments from fright or vexation	Ailments from hearing bad news, shame, mortification, or vexation with fear.
Repeats all questions before answering them.	Repeats the words spoken to him on account of difficulty in comprehending.
Hydrocephaloid	Hydrocephalus. C.Hg.
Optical illusions in bright colors	Optical illusions in dark colors . . . . .
With the toochache sweat	With the toothache chill. C.Hg.
Saliva generally increased	Saliva generally diminished.
Desire for beer	Des. *or* dislike for beer and spirituous liquors.
Wine disagrees	Beer disagrees. C.Hg.
Urinal sediment generally yellow	Sediment red or whitish.
Scrotum contracted	Scrotum relaxed. C.Hg.
Nasal secretion thick or viscid	Nasal secretion watery.
Larynx dry	Larynx full of mucus.
Expectoration quite constant; particularly in the morning.	Expectoration not constant; morning and during day; less frequently at night.
Complaints generally in lower part of chest, on outer side of thigh, and on instep.	Complaints generally in upper part of chest, on inner side of thigh, & on sole of foot.
Sweat on feet of a bad odor, causing soreness.	S. on feet cold, generally on the soles. C.Hg.
AGGRAVATION afternoon and *evening* . . .	REMISSION *afternoon* and before midnight.
Ailments from Baryta	Ailments from Metals, Nitric. acid., Iod.
Worse when looking up	W. when look'g down, partic. at runn'g water.
Worse when alone, better when in company .	*Generally* bet. when alone, worse in company.
Worse from growing cold and in cold weather, better when growing warm and in warm air.	Better (worse) when growing cold and in cold weather, *or* fr. grow'g warm & in warm air.
Better *or* worse when lying	Predominantly worse when lying.
Worse in bed and after passing urine . . .	*Worse or* better in bed & after passing urine.
Better fr. change of posit. when ly'g or stand'g.	*Worse or* better when turning in bed.
Better after getting out of bed	Worse *or* better after getting out of bed.
Worse when opening, better when closing the eyes.	Better (worse) when opening *or* when closing the eyes.
Worse when sneezing. when stooping, when rising, and when moving diseased part.	*Worse or* better when sneezing, stooping and rising, and when moving diseased part.
Better *or* worse from touch	*Worse or* better from touch.
Generally better when swallowing	Predom. worse when swallowing.
Better on an empty stomach, worse after breakfast.	Worse (better) on an empty stomach *or* after breakfast.
Almost always improved when eating . . .	Worse or better when eating.
Cessation of bellyache after stool	Bellyache after stool.
Eruptions worse in a warm room	Eruptions worse in the open air. C.Hg.

Predomin. **worse** — Predomin. **better**

When alone, from cold, when sitt'g erect, from warm diet, from eructation, & from loosen'g the clothes.

Predomin. **better** — Predomin. **worse**

In company, from warmth, when sitting bent forward, from change of position, when swallowing, from drinking cold water, from cold diet generally, and from tying the clothes tight.

N.B. The over-sensitiveness of Zincum to pain is very rarely found with Sulphur.

---

* This corresponds exactly to the influence of the external temperature in one case, and that of cold or warm diet in the other. Compare Ignatia—Phosph acid.

APPENDIX,

CONTAINING

The collateral symptoms, during stool, during urination. during menstruation, and during cough.

Translated from the Original by Doctor Conrad Wesselhœft, Dorchester, Mass.

LIST OF ABBREVIATIONS.

B., D., A.,	signify :	*Before, During, After.*	*Mens.*	signifies :	*Menses.*
St.	"	*Stool.*	*Cgh.*	"	*Cough.*
Ur.	"	*Urination.*	*l. and r.*	"	*left and right*
Beg.	"	*Beginning.*			

ACONITUM.

B. St.—Nausea, perspiration, flatulency.
Dur. St.—Colic, straining, flow of urine.
A. St.—Nausea, perspiration.
Dur. Ur.—Pain in glans penis; sensation of splashing of fluid in region of bladder; pinching about navel.
At beg. of Mens.—Cramps.
Dur. Mens.—Disturbance of mind.
Dur. Cgh.—Heat, thirst; fright, anxiety, restlessness; oppression; danger of suffocation; burning and constriction in the throat

AGARICUS.

Dur. Cgh.—Burning in the chest; stitches in l. side; palpitation, anxiety with perspiration.
B. St.—Cramps in abdomen; — urgent tenesmus; — painful straining in rectum.
Dur. St. Colic and passage of flatus; — burning soreness and cutting in anus; — perspiration; pain in loins extending into the legs, also continuing till after stool.
A. St.—Biting pain in anus; straining in rectum; griping in hypogastrium.
B. Ur.—Urgent desire to urinate.
At beg. of Mens.—Nocturnal restlessness on account of troublesome rigors.— Nocturnal wakefulness and toothache.
Dur. Menstr.—Headache and toothache; pain and itching in left ear, lessened by boring; pain in belly and back, like labor-pains; — pains in the l. arm; — itching here and there, particularly about the genitals; — rigors; palpitation; running of water from the mouth; awaking at night with headache and toothache.
A. Mens. Pain as if from exhaustion; palpitation; headache and dizziness; — interrupted sleep at night, with anxiety.

ALUMINA.

B. St.—While straining: involuntary passage of urine; straining and pressure; colic.
Dur. St.—Discharge of prostatic juice; in rectum feeling of dryness and contraction. — Chills.

A. St.—Throbbing in the spine; stinging and rawness in anus.
A. Ur.—Burning with discharge of urine, and desire to discharge stool.
B. Mens.—Congestions; palpitation and headache; — leucorrhœa.
D. Mens.—Bloatedness; diarrhœa and frequent discharge of excoriating urine; — leucorrhœa; running coryza.
A. Mens.—Lassitude of body, mind and temperament; — leucorrhœa.
D. Cgh.—Clawing sensation in the throat, soreness in the chest; pressure in occiput; pain in the nape of the neck; stitches in region of spleen.

AMMONIUM CARB.

B. St.— Cutting pain in belly.
D. St.—Straining and cutting pain in belly.
A. St.—Scratching and burning in anus; discharge of blood and prostatic juice; cutting pain in belly
A. Ur.—Drawing in urethra.
B. Mens.—Pain in belly and back.
D. Mens.—Labor-like pains in belly and back, exhaustion, coryza, toothache.
D. Cgh.—Soreness in the larynx, hoarseness; taste of blood in the mouth; asthma, constriction, rawness and soreness in the chest; pain and stitches in the sternum; exhausted feeling about chest and head; heat in the head; pain in the jaws; stitches in epigastrium and back.

AMMONIUM MUR.

B. St.– Flatulency, colic.
D. St.—Stinging, burning and soreness in anus; — colic.
A. St.—Pain in belly.
D. Mens.—Pains in belly, back, and loins; pressing in abdomen; vomiting and diarrhœa; bloody stools.
D. Cgh.—Stitches in chest and in region of the spleen.

ANACARDIUM.

D. St.—Pain in belly; discharge of prostatic juice.
A. St.—Abdominal pain; — gaping and eructations.
A. Ur.—Discharge of prostatic juice.
D. Cgh.—Scratching and soreness in the throat; difficulty of respiration; gaping; congestion to the head and headache; vomiting of food; pain in abdomen.

ANTIMON. CRUD.

D. St. – Burning itching; scraping and drawing in the anus; stitching, scraping, soreness, and prolapse of rectum.
D. Ur.—Burning and cutting.
D. Cgh.—Constriction and feeling as if there were a plug in the throat; hot breath; burning and stinging in chest.

ANTIMON. TART. (Tartar emetic).

B. St.—Motion of flatus and pain in abdomen.
D. St.—Vomiting; palpitation; thirst.
A. St.—Burning in anus; thirst.
At the cessation of urination—Pain in the bladder.
A. Ur.—Burning.
D. Cgh.—Rolling, catching of breath; stitches in the chest and hypochondriac regions: blueness of the face, warm perspiration about the head and hands; trembling of the head; convulsions; gaping; vomiting, first of food, then of mucus; or first of mucus, then bile.

APIS.

B. St.—Straining.
D. St.—Straining, pinching, nausea, vomiting, frontal headache, backache.
A. St.—Exhaustion, approaching faintness.
B. Ur.—Burning.
D. Ur.—Burning, soreness, and feeling of constriction in urethra; uneasy sensation in spermatic cord.
A. Ur.—Burning.
B. Mens.—Eruption; labor-like pains in the abdome.
D. Mens.—Eruption; labor-like pains in abdomen, particularly in right ovarian region; constipation; heat of the head.
D. Cgh.—Painful concussions in the head

ARGENTUM FOL.

B. and D. St.—Painful straining.
A. St.—Contracting pain in abdomen.
D. Ur.—Burning.
D. Cgh.—Hoarseness and soreness in the throat.

ARGENTUM NITRICUM.

B. St.—Abdominal pains.
D. St.—Flatus, straining to vomit; vomiting of slime, cramp of stomach; drawing in abdomen, difficult respiration.
A. St.—Pain in stomach.
D. Ur.—Itching, tickling, heat and burning in urethra.
A. Ur.—Cutting pain in posterior portion of urethra, extending into anus.
A. Ur.—Burning and straining;—dribbling of urine.
D. Mens.—Labor-like abdominal pains;—headache.
D. Cgh.—Straining to vomit; salivation; night-sweat.

ARNICA.

B. St.—Distention of abdomen.
D. St.—Rumbling and pressure in abdomen;—headache.
B. Ur.—Pressure in bladder.
D. Ur.—Burning.
At the end of Ur.—Cutting pain in the orifice of urethra.
A. Ur.—Stitches.
D. Mens.—Nausea in epigastrium.
D. Cgh.—Scratching in the throat; tickling in trachea; rawness and stitches in the chest; asthma; catching of breath; congestions and heat; bruised feeling in the ribs; vomiting; frontal pain; pressure and stinging in the head; prickling upon the head.

ARSENICUM.

B. St.—Chilliness, anxiety, fainting, cutting in abdomen; vomiting; thirst.
D. St.—Chilliness, nausea, vomiting, backache, straining and burning in anus and rectum.
A. St.—Cessation of acute abdominal pains;—distention, straining about the navel; burning in rectum; oppression, eructations, weakness with trembling and faintness, with desire to lie down; palpitation, perspiration.
D. Ur.—Burning in urethra; constriction in left groin.
A Ur.—Feeling of weakness in upper part of abdomen, with trembling.
D. Mens.—Stitches in rectum, extending into anus and vulva; stinging, cutting pain, extending from epigastrium into hypogastrium, sides of abdomen and back;—toothache.
A. Mens.—Discharge of bloody slime,—or stinking watery discharge from vagina and anus.
D. Cgh.—Catching of breath; soreness in the chest, stitches in the sides or in epigastrium,—heat of the head,—collection of water in the mouth.

ASA FŒTIDA.

D. St.—Discharge of flatus;—pain in abdomen.

AURUM

D. St.—Pinching pain in abdomen;—burning in rectum.
B. Mens.—Swelling of glands in the arm-pits.
D. Mens.—Colic; prolapse of rectum.
D. Cgh.—Pressure in the chest and abdomen;—pleuritic stitches in left side.

BARYTA.

B. St.—Colic.
D. St—Burning in anus and rectum.
A. St.—Burning in anus; moisture exuding from piles;—eructations.
B. Ur.—Urgent desire to urinate.
D. Ur.—Burning in urethra; pinching in hypogastrium.
A. Ur.—Renewed straining, with dribbling of urine.
B. Mens.—Toothache; swelling of cheeks; pain in abdomen and back; leucorrhœa heaviness of the feet.
D. Mens.—Colic; backache resembling bruise; pressing weight above os pubis.
D. Cgh.—Sore pain in the chest;—vomiting.

BELLADONNA.

B. St.—Constriction in the rectum; — sore aching in upper part of abdomen; perspiration.
D. St.—Shuddering; nausea and pressing pain in stomach.
A. St.—Tenesmus.
D. Ur.—Burning;—drawing in spermatic cord.
A. Ur.—Itching in prepuce.
B. Mens.—Colic; cramp of the stomach; loss of appetite, tiredness; clouded vision.
D. Mens.—Bearing down towards the genitals; pain in back and limbs; heat of the head, anxiety; disturbance of the mind;—chills, thirst; perspiration of the chest at night.
A. Mens.—Cramps of the stomach.
D. Cgh—Rattling, pain in the sternum; constriction of the throat; pain in the nape of the neck; stitches in the chest or uterine region; pains in the head, abdomen, hips, or legs; reversed action of the stomach; vomiting of mucus; bloody taste in the mouth; bleeding from the ear or nose; heat of the face; redness or blueness of the face; pressure in epigastrium; secessus; stiffening of the body; convulsions.

BORAX.

B. St.—Mental indisposition; indolence
B. Ur.—Burning.
A. Ur.—Soreness or burning tension in urethra; sore pain in meatus or in orifice.
B. Mens.—Oppression; catching of the breath; rushing sound in the ears.
D. Mens.—Throbbing in the head and rushing in the ears; nausea, pinching and griping in abdomen, pain extending from stomach into the back; bearing down and stinging in the groin; tiredness; perspiration after midnight.
A. Mens.—Pressing in region of liver, extending into right shoulder-blade; cramp-like pain in stomach and back, and vomiting afterwards.
D. Cgh.—Stitches in right side of chest and lumbar region, lessened by pressure; mouldy taste in the throat.

BROMINE.

B. St.—Rumbling and cutting pain in abdomen.
D. St.—Much flatus; painful hæmorrhoids; pressing in stomach and abdomen.
A. Ur.—Dribbling with burning.
B. Mens.—Stitches in abdomen; backache; feeling of weakness and want of appetite.
D. Mens.—Abdominal cramps, with subsequent soreness in abdomen; frontal pain, with feeling as if the eyes would drop out while stooping.
D. Cgh.—Feeling like sulphurous vapor in the throat, whistling inspiration; sore pain in the chest; dullness and pressing headache; watering and contraction of the eyes.

BRYONIA.

B. St.—Colic; nausea.
D. St.—Burning in anus; prolapse of rectum; motion like fermentation in abdomen; pain in stomach; vomiting; coldness and rigors; thirst; drowsiness.
A. St.—Burning in rectum; heat; sleepiness.
B. Ur.—Burning and cutting.
D. Ur.—Burning and constricted feeling in urethra;—abdominal pains.
At other times—Burning, pressing, drawing, and tearing in urethra.
D. Mens.—Pain in back and loins; tearing in the limbs; headache.
D. Cgh.—Scratching in the throat; shortness of breath; catching of the breath; thoracic pains lessened by pressure;—bruised feeling in hypochondriac regions, lessened by pressure;—pressing in the head;—bursting pain in head and chest;—stitches in head, throat and chest, sides and epigastrium, or hypochondria; pains in abdominal muscles; nausea and vomiting of food; sore pain in epigastrium;—lachrymation; toothache.

CALCAREA.

B. St.—Irascible irritability.
D. St.—Burning, tearing, and tenesmus in rectum; prolapse of rectum; piles; succus prostaticus; rolling in abdomen; pallor.
A. St.—Pressure in rectum;—erections;—lassitude; oppression of breath with anxiety; in epigastrium stitches during pressure.
B. Ur.—Burning.
D. Ur.—Cutting, burning, sore pain.
A. Ur.—Renewed desire with burning.
B. Mens.—Indisposition; disposed to frights; amorous dreams; headache; heat of the head; chills and nocturnal colicky pains; aching of back and hips; pain in the arm-pits; pain and swelling of the breasts; leucorrhœa.
At the beginning of Mens.—Cramps.
D. Mens.—Labor-like pains in abdomen and back, pain in the hip-bones or in the arms; heat of the head; headache and toothache; hardness of hearing; painful deglutition; nausea and ineffectual straining at stool; difficulty of breathing; anxiety and restlessness followed by faintness; nocturnal agglutination of eyelids; lachrymation in the morning; swelling of the feet.
A. Mens.—Leucorrhœa; toothache; inflammation of the eyes.
D. Cgh.—Rawness in the chest; pain like tearing off something in the throat; catching of breath; inclination to vomit and vomiting of sweetish matter: headache; pressure in the stomach; pain and extension of inguinal hernia; palpitation and throbbing of arteries; perspiration; convulsions.

CAMPHORA.

B. and D. St.—Pinching in abdomen.
B. and A. Ur.—Burning and cutting
D. Ur.—Burning in urethra.
D. Cgh.—Pain in trachea.

CANNABIS.

B. St.—Colic in upper part of abdomen.
D. St.—Soreness in anus.
D. Ur.—Burning, biting, stinging, or soreness.
At the end of Ur.—Dropping of blood from urethra.
B. and A. Ur.—Burning.
D. Cgh.—Pressure and stitches in the chest; palpitation; **erections.**

CANTHARIDES.

B. St.—Straining; colicky pains; cutting.
D. St.—Cutting colicky pains; burning in anus; prolapse of rectum.
A. St.—Remission of abdominal pains; burning, biting, and stinging in anus; straining; faintness; external coldness with internal warmth.
B. Ur.—Burning and cutting.
D. Ur.—Much burning; biting, cutting in kidneys, ureters, bladder and urethra;—drawing in spermatic cords.
At the end of Ur.—Cutting, dropping of blood.
A. Ur.—Burning, cutting, crawling, tickling in urethra; burning in the bladder.
B. Mens.—Burning of urine.
A. Mens.—Discharge of bloody mucus.
D. Cgh.—Shortness of breath; pain in abdomen; **erections.**

CAPSICUM.

B. St.—Flatulent colic.
D. St.—Burning or biting, stinging in anus; straining; twisting, cutting pain about the navel.
A. St.—Straining; thirst.
B. Ur.—Burning in urethra; pressure in the bladder.
D. Ur.—Burning or prickling.
A. Ur.—Burning or burning cutting.
D. Mens.—Nausea; pressure in epigastrium.
D. Cgh.—Drawing or stinging in the sides of chest; stitches in the back; pressing, ulcerative pain in neck or ear; bursting pain in the head, chest, and bladder; pressure about the thighs; inclination to vomit, or vomiting; offensive breath.

CARBO ANIMALIS.

B. St.—Rigors about the head; colicky pains; **bearing down toward the os pubis;** drawing from the anus through the vulva.
D. St.—Stitches in and about the groins; cutting pain in hæmorrhoids; tearing in abdomen proceeding upwards from the vulva; backache; bloatedness.
A. St.—Scratching in rectum; weakness and twisting feeling in the bowels; rigors;—desire to urinate, with exhaustion; sleepiness without sleep; ringing in the ears, and shaking chills.
D. Ur.—Burning and sore pain.
A. Ur.—Burning and voluptuous tickling.
B. Mens.—Heat with anxiety;—bruised feeling of thighs.
D. Mens.—Colic; pressing in the groins, back, and thighs, with ineffectual eructation, chilliness and gaping;—weariness with gaping and stretching; bloatedness.
D. Cgh.—Soreness in hypogastrium.

CARBO VEGETABILIS.

B. St.—Cutting and drawing in abdomen.
D. St.—Burning and cutting in anus; stitches in rectum; succus prostaticus;—epistaxis.

A. St.—Burning in anus; straining in the back, rectum, and bladder; feeling of emptiness; jamming or pinching stitches in abdomen; bloatedness; trembling weakness, anxiety with trembling feeling and involuntary motions.
D. Ur.—Burning, soreness; itching and stinging in the vulva.
A. Ur.—Tearing and drawing in urethra.
B. Mens.—Leucorrhœa; — cramp-like drawing in hypogastrium, extending into the back;—headache;—itching eruption on the nape of the neck and between the shoulder-blades.
D. Mens.—Headache and colicky pains;—headache and toothache;—vomiting;—burning in the hands and soles of the feet;—general soreness.
D. Cgh.—Burning, rawness, or feeling as if the chest were crushed; larynx feels sore and as if ulcerated;—stitches through the head;—retching, vomiting, flushes of heat and perspiration;—stitches in epigastrium, back, or loins; feeling of concussion in the abdomen; pains in the hips or in the legs; coryza, sneezing, lachrymation;—asthma; palpitation.

CAUSTICUM.

B. St.—Anxiety;—twisting abdominal pains.
D. St.—Discharge of mucus.
A. St.—Biting and burning in anus; succus prostaticus; pinching in the hypochondria; anxiety with heat of the face, nausea; running of water from the mouth.
D. Ur.—Burning and gnawing.
A. Ur.—Pain in the urethra and upon the crown of the head.
B. Mens.—Anxious dreams, melancholy; colic and backache;—cramp-like spasms.
D. Mens.—Pressing in the stomach, labor-like pains in loins and back, diarrhœa, stitches beneath the left breast, yellowness of the face, whirling dizziness and headache; dejection, tiredness, perspiration.
D. Cgh.—Soreness in the chest, stitches in left side, asthma, rattling of mucus, pain in abdomen and hips.

CHAMOMILLA.

B. St.—Anxiety; colic.
D. St.—Colic; eructation; nausea, retching, thirst, vertigo; perspiration with anxiety; flatus.
A. St.—Stitches in rectum; heat.
D. Ur.—Anxiety; biting (itching) in urethra; burning in urethra and neck of the bladder.
B. Mens.—Colic with drawing pain in thighs; toothache.
On appearance of Mens.—Cross, willful, quarrelsome temper; cramps.
D. Mens.—Labor-like pains in abdomen and back; ovarian pain;—diarrhœa; thirst; coldness of the limbs; derangement of the mind.
D. Cgh.—Hoarseness; inflammation and pain in the throat, tickling in trachea, rattling of mucus; salivation; convulsions.

CHINA.

B. St.—Colic.
D. St.—Stitches and acrid feeling in anus; thirst.
A. St.—Renewed desire; creeping in rectum as if caused by worms; headache; stiffness in the nape of the neck; backache; exhaustion.
D. Ur.—Burning in urethra; biting in the orifice.
A. Ur.—Burning.
B. Mens.—Leucorrhœa.
D. Mens.—Colic; asthma; swelling of the face; congestion of the head, with darkness before the eyes and loss of consciousness; clonic spasms.

D. Cgh.—Hoarseness, pressure on the chest, stitches in chest and back; sore pain in larynx; pain in trachea and sternum; snoring respiration; retching and vomiting.

CICUTA VIROSA.

D. St.—Vomiting; — cramps in abdominal muscles.

CINA.

D. Cgh.—Pain behind upper part of sternum, concussions in the trachea, gurgling in the same; cessation of breathing with rigidity of the body, cramps of the chest, gasping for breath; rising up in bed, trembling, loss of consciousness; jerking of the limbs; hoarseness; sneezing; lachrymation; colic.

CLEMATIS.

B. St.—Colic.
D. St.—Burning in rectum;—swelling of piles;—heat.
A. St.—Alleviation of bloatedness and headache; — itching in anus; — burning in anus and rectum.
B. Ur.—Biting tickling in orifice of urethra.
D. Ur.—Biting and burning in urethra, stirring and turning in orifice; drawing in spermatic cord; stitches, extending from abdominal cavity up into the chest; general feeling of heat.
A. Ur. – Burning in urethra;—tickling, itching, stinging in the orifice.
D. Cgh.—Nocturnal dryness of the mouth and feeling of constriction in the throat.

COCCULUS.

B. St.—Colic.
A. St.—Straining in rectum: – faintness.
B. Ur.—Pain in urethra.
B. Mens.—Colic, nausea, lassitude, anxiety; cramps of the chest; convulsions.
Dur. Mens.—Pain in abdomen and back; pressure in abdomen as if caused by a stone, contraction in the rectum; distension, spasm of stomach, headache; convulsions, leucorrhœa.
A. Mens.—Piles.
Dur. Cgh.—Nocturnal dryness of the mouth and feeling of constriction in the throat.

COFFEA.

During the straining of stool—Nosebleed.
B. and dur. the onset of Mens.—Cramps.
D. Mens. – Derangement of the mind.
D. Cgh.—Stitches in the sides; anxiety; dimness before the eyes and vertigo.

COLÇHICUM.

B. St.—Feeling like diarrhœa in anus; — flatulency; — pinching in the abdomen.
D. St.—Stinking flatus; rending pain in anus, backache; — vomiting, vertigo, faintness, cardial stitches.
A. St.—Remission of intestinal pains and of sensorial complaints; increase of pelvic pains; stinking flatus, feeling of diarrhœa in rectum, and sore biting in anus; renewed desire to go to stool.
B. Ur.—Burning in urinary passages.
D. Ur.—Burning in urethra; constriction in the neck of the bladder.
A. Ur.—Tickling in the fossa navicularis; tickling burning in urethra and discharge of a few drops.
D. Mens.—Tiredness and heaviness of the feet.
D. Cgh.—Spirting out of urine.

COLOCYNTHIS.

D. St.—Flatus, colic, nausea, feeling of coldness

A. St.—Remission of colic; — distension; — lassitude.

At the end of Ur.—Burning in the orifice of urethra.

A. Ur.—Burning or contused pain.

D. Cgh.—Stitches in the head; pains in the head, abdomen, hips, and legs.

CONIUM MACULATUM.

B. St.– Cutting abdominal pain.

D. St.—Burning, cutting, and straining in rectum; — flatus; — succus prostat.; — rigors.

A. St.—Intermittent palpitation of the heart; — trembling weakness necessitates recumbent posture.

D. Ur.—Burning, cutting, drawing; — pressure upon uterus.

A. Ur.—Burning;—stitches about neck of bladder; biting tenesmus; jamming pressure.

B. Mens.—Anxious dreams; heat without thirst; general bruised feeling, with inclination to weep; restlessness and anxious apprehensiveness; pains in the breasts; stitches in the liver; — distension.

D. Mens.—Labor-like abdominal pains, extending into thigh; — stitches in the chest; headache; eruption.

D. Cgh.—Stitches in head or chest; oppression and constriction of the chest; colic; vomiting of mucus.

CUPRUM.

B. St.—Colic; chilliness.

D. St.—Abdominal ache, nausea, vomiting, thirst, pains in the limbs.

A. St.—Lassitude.

D. Ur.—Burning, cutting pain or stinging at the meatus urinarius.

B. Mens.—Abdominal pains, headache, cramps of the chest, arterial excitement;—cramp

D. Mens.—Want of appetite, discomfort; asthma; cramps.

A. Mens. – Cramps.

D. Cgh.—Catching of breath; rigidity of the body, chills, heat of the head, blowing of blood from the nose, retching, vomiting of food, involuntary discharge of stool and urine;—twitching of the limbs.

CYCLAMEN.

B. St.—Nausea; rumbling and pinching in abdomen

D. St.– Straining and burning in anus;—colic; palpitation.

A. St.—Ineffectual straining at stool; pinching in abdomen, dullness and forgetfulness.

B. Ur.—Stitches in urethra; pressing in the bladder.

D. Ur.—Stitches in end of urethra; pains extending from bladder into urethra; pressure upon rectum and bladder.

B. Mens.—Melancholy;—straining and warmth in abdomen with sleeplessness.

D. Mens.—Improvement in temper and of the heaviness of the feet; labor-like pains in back and abdomen;—headache; vertigo; darkness before the eyes.

A. Mens.—Swelling of the breasts.

DIGITALIS

B. St.– Colic; vomiting.

D. St.—Cutting pain in abdomen.

A. St.—Renewed desire;—faintness.

B. Ur.—Cutting.

D. Ur.—Cutting and pressing burning in urethra; constriction in the bladder.

A. Ur.—Cutting and burning in urethra; pressure in the bladder.

B. Mens.—Labor-like pains in abdomen and back.

D. Cgh.—Contracting pain in the chest; asthma;—tensive pressure in arm and shoulder; vomiting;—heat;—perspiration.

DROSERA.

B. and A. St.—Tensive pain in upper part of abdomen while holding the breath.
A. St.—Ineffectual straining; abdominal and dorsal pains.
D. Cgh.—Constricting pains in chest, abdomen, and hypochondriac regions, ameliorated by pressure; — thoracic stitches; hoarseness; offensive breath; — nausea, retching and vomiting, first of food, then of mucus;—bleeding from nose and mouth;—rising up in bed with fear and trembling;—face pale or bluish.

DULCAMARA.

B. St.—Perspiration; nausea; rumbling and offensive flatus; pains in abdomen and back.
D. St.—Biting about the anus or prolapse of the same;—abdominal and dorsal pains;—eructation;—vomiting;—heat; perspiration; thirst.
A. St.—Remission of abdominal pains; - heat of the face; thirst.
B. Ur.—Burning in hips.
D. Ur. Burning in urethra.
B. Mens —Rash.
D. Cgh.—Stitches in the sides; hoarseness.

EUPHRASIA.

B. St.—Flatus.
A. St.—Burning in anus;—feeling of warmth.
D. and A. Cgh.—Tensive pressure in the chest;—oppression.

FERRUM.

B. St.—Flatulency;—paleness of the face.
D. St.—Cramp-like pain in abdomen, back, and anus; pains in the stomach.
A. St.—Lassitude.
B. Mens.—Discharge of vaginal mucus; motion in the bowels; stitches in head; singing in ears.
D. Cgh.—Stitches and bruised pain in chest; want of breath; pains in occiput;—paleness of face; sour vomiting of food.

FLUOR. ACID.

B. St.—Stinking flatus;—abdominal pain.
D. St.—Burning and protrusion of anus or piles;—pinching abdominal pain.
A. St.—Tenesmus; abdominal pain.
B. and A. Ur.—Vesical pain.
D. and A. Ur.—Burning.
D. Ur.—Stinging and burning.
A. Ur.—Elastic feeling in urinary organs, with subsequent pleasurable sensation.

GELSEMINUM.

Compare Dr. E. M. Hale's "New Remedies," published by Dr. Lodge, Detroit, 1866.

GLONOINUM.

B. and A. St.—Cutting pain in abdomen.
B. St.—Headache, vomiting.
D. and A. St.—Nausea; rumbling in hypogastrium; flatus; feeling of tightness of anus.

B. D., or instead of Mens.—Rush of blood to the head, with throbbing and tearing pains.

GRAPHITES.

B. St.—Loathing and pains in abdomen.
D. St.—Straining and burning in anus.
A. St.—Distension, uneasiness, and pinching in abdomen.
B. Ur.—Cutting straining in ureters.
D. Ur.—Tickling in urethra;—pain in coccyx.
A. Ur.—Burning in meatus urinarius.
B. Mens.—Itching of vulva.
D. Mens.—Labor-like pains in abdomen and back; excoriation about vulva; pains in varicose veins, strangury, hæmorrhage from anus; — eructation; nausea, with weakness and trembling; vomiting; — headache and toothache; — obscured vision; — erysipelas of one cheek; — oppression and pressure in the chest; — coryza, with fever and cough; — palpitation; — pains, numbness or formication in the limbs; swelling of the feet; — aggravation of the condition of present ulcers.
A. Mens.—Cutting pain in abdomen and diarrhœa; — chills.
D. Cgh.—Thoracic pains, heat of the head and coryza.

HELLEBORUS NIGER.

B. St.—Abdominal pain.
D. St.—Cutting stinging in rectum upwards; nausea and abdominal pain.
A. St.—Burning biting in anus.
D. Cgh.—Tension in region of the spleen.

HEPAR S. C.

B. St.—Pinching in the abdomen.
D. St.—Abdominal pain, straining, pressing, rumbling, and nauseous feeling in abdomen; — succus prostaticus; — heat in hands and cheeks; — inclination to lie down.
A. St.—Sore pain in anus and sanious secretion; — tympanitis; — obstruction of the nose.
D. Ur.—Burning, cutting, and soreness;—in the right shoulder-blade feeling as if something were running or creeping.
A. Ur.—Succus prostaticus.
B. Mens.—Constricting headache.
D. Mens.—Itching of the vulva.
D Cgh.—Stitches, burning, and swelling in the throat; burning in chest and stomach; catching of breath; — nausea, retching, vomiting; — reverberation in the head, throbbing in the forehead and temples;—dullness;—sneezing;—chills;—anxiety and bending backwards of the body in lying.

HYOSCYAMUS.

D. St.—Pain in anus; flatulency.
A. St.—Tiredness.
D. Mens. - Labor-like abdominal pains; headache and toothache; lockjaw; — stiffness of joints; — convulsive trembling; — cramps;—delirium; nausea; perspiration; flow of urine.
B. Mens.—Labor-like abdominal pains;—much loud laughing;—hysterical spasms.
D. Cgh.—Loss of breath; stitches in the head; soreness in abdominal muscles, vomiting of mucus.

IGNATIA.

B. St.—Cutting abdominal pains.

D. St.—Flatus; soreness of rectum and prolapse of the same; — succus prostaticus;—erections.

A. St.—Contraction of anus; pressing in rectum; painful piles;—lassitude.

D. Ur.—Burning, biting, soreness.

D. Mens.—Constricting abdominal pains; backache; vomiting;—pains, heat, and heaviness in the head; palpitation, anxiety, raving;—lassitude approaching faintness.

D. Cgh.—Nauseous feeling in epigastrium; concussions in hypogastrium; pain in penis; convulsions.

IODINE.

D. St.—Abdominal pains;—bearing down in genital organs;—painful pressure on the crown of the head.

A. St.—Burning in anus;—soreness in rectum;—pressing in hypogastrium.

B. Mens.—Uprising of heat, with palpitation; tension and swelling in the throat;—abdominal pains.

D. Mens.—Pains in back and ovaries; lassitude; coughing up of blood.

A. Mens.—Palpitation.

D. Cgh.—Tickling and burning pain in throat; oppression, pressing, burning and stitches in the chest;—rattling;—anxiety;—nausea.

IPECACUANHA.

B. St.—Abdominal pain, nausea, vomiting.

D. St.—Abdominal pain, uneasiness in abdomen, nausea, vomiting, lassitude, coldness, paleness of face.

A. St.—Tenesmus; lassitude; twitching of face.

D. Ur.—Burning in urethra;—pains in back and epigastrium.

D. Cgh.—Sore pain in the chest; paroxysms of suffocation, with rigidity of the body;—painful concussions (shocks) in stomach and head; pains in epigastrium and umbilical region;—bleeding from mouth and nose;—nausea, retching, vomiting;—perspiration of forehead; blueness of face; jarring of the body; — loss of consciousness and falling down; inflammation of the throat.

KALI CARB.

B. St.—Stitches in anus;—abdominal pains;—anxiety.

D. St.—Pinching abdominal pain, painful straining extending into genitals;—cramps of the stomach, nausea, eructation; rigors and watery vomiting, with staggering and shaking of hands and feet;—then anxiety, general heat, and remission of abdominal pains;—paleness of the face;—piles.

A. St.—Burning and biting sore pain in anus;—pressure in abdomen.

D. Ur.—Burning.

A. Ur.—Burning, renewed desire to pass water; dribbling;—succus prostaticus.

B. Mens.—Rigors, trembling, cramp-like sensation in abdomen;—heat, thirst, and nocturnal restlessness;—increased sexual desire; itching of vulva.

D. Mens.—Pain in back, loins and abdomen, pain in head, ears and teeth;—itching of the skin, nettle-rash;—lassitude, sleepiness; restless, dreamful sleep; foul taste in the mouth, eructation, nausea, vomiting, distension and rumbling in abdomen;—excoriation between the legs;—coryza

A. Mens.—Cutting abdominal pains;—coldness in the back in the evening, and after midnight awaking with a cramp-like pain and coldness in stomach.

D. Cgh.—Scratching and stinging in throat and chest; pain in abdomen and in hæmorrhoidal tumors; stitches in rectum; nausea, retching, vomiting; asthma; sparks before the eyes.

KALI BICHROMICUM.

B. St.—Abdominal pains;—erections.

D. St.—Burning and straining in anus; succus prostraticus;—gnawing about the navel, pain in the region of the spleen; metallic taste in the mouth; offensive breath; confusion in the head.

A. St.—Remission of complaints;—tenesmus;—burning soreness or drawing in the anus with nausea.

B. Ur.—Pain in coccyx, extending into urethra.

D. Ur.—Burning in fossa navicularis or in balbus of the urethra;—backache.

A. Ur.—Transient stitches in urethra;—burning, particul. in the anterior and posterior part of urethra.

D. Mens.—Febrile conditions, nausea, vertigo and headache.

D. Cgh.—Bloody taste in the mouth; nausea; ulcerative pain in the throat; pressure in sternum and in larynx, extending into os hyoides; burning pain in sternum, extending into the shoulders;—heaviness, sensitiveness and pains in the chest; palpitation and rattling (in the throat); pains in the sides and loins, alleviated by pressure.

KREOSOTUM.

B. St.—Flatulency.

While straining at stool—The pains pass from the lumber vertebræ into the right groin and hip-joint.

D. St.—Pressure towards the genitals;—thirst;—paleness of the face.

B. Ur.—Discharge of fluor albus.

D. Ur.—Burning in the vulva.

B. Mens.—Hardness of hearing; foamy eructation or vomiting of mucus; bloatedness; griping about the navel; burning in the back; leucorrhœa;—excitement and restlessness.

D. Mens.—Hardness of hearing; rushing sound in the ears; humming and pressing outwards in the head; stitches in the side, cutting pain in abdomen, borborygmi, flatus, diarrhœa, chills; sweat on chest and back.

A. Mens.—Labor-like abdominal cramps;—constricting pain in vagina, followed by fluor albus.

D. Cgh.—Scratching in the throat, stitches and bruised pain in the chest, asthma, jarring of the abdomen, retching, discharge of urine; chills and heat; sleepiness.

LACHESIS.

B. St.—Rumbling in abdomen;—cramp-like pains in anus and rectum.

D. St.—Burning in anus;—cramp-like pain in abdomen;—coldness; thirst.

A. St.—Extension of rectum; painful hœmorrhoidal tumors;—thirst.

B. Ur.—Renewed desire and discharge of urine.

B. Mens.—Leucorrhœa;—cutting abdominal pains;—pressing gastralgia;—eructations; cramps of the chest;—nose-bleed, vertigo, headache.

D. Mens.—Ovarian pain;—labor-like pains in abdomen, loins, and back;—discharge of blood or mucus from the anus;—throbbing in the head, toothache.

A. Mens.—Diarrhœa.

D. Cgh.—Tension in the head;—pains in epigastrium, abdomen and anus;—burning in chest;—ulcerative pain above and along the ribs;—stitches in chest;—running of water from the mouth; vomiting discharge of urine.

LYCOPODIUM.

D. St.—Biting or burning in anus, burning and stinging in rectum, pain in back as if broken, bursting pain in abdomen, pain in the stomach, headache, rushing in the ears.

A. St.—Burning in rectum; constriction in perineum; ineffectual straining. distension, rolling, and cramp-like pain in hypogastrium, tiredness, particularly in the thighs,—heat and pressure in the thighs,—heat and pressure in the head.

D. Ur.—Soreness; —burning in urethra and glans; — jammed feeling in perineum; cutting pain in abdomen.

A. Ur.—Crawling burning in urethra and bladder.

B. Mens.—Pain in abdomen;—melancholy, delirium with weeping; dilated pupils, rigors with discomfort and uneasiness, distension, coldness and heaviness of the feet.

D. Mens.—Pain in abdomen, back, and loins; itching of vulva; nausea, acid in the mouth;—headache, tiredness and faintness;—swelling of the feet.

A. Mens.—Leucorrhœa;—stitches in the head.

D. Cgh.—Jerking in the teeth; stitches in the throat, soreness in the chest, asthma and rattling, jarring of the chest and temples, pains in the head, gastric region, and sides of abdomen;—gaping;—palpitation, heat, irritable temper.

MAGNESIA CARB.

B. St.—Abdominal pain and diffusion of heat over the body.

A. St.—Tiredness.

D. St.—Tearing in rectum, extending into abdomen.

D. Ur.—Burning and soreness.

A. Ur.—Burning;—pinching below the navel, extending into loins and left hip.

B. Mens.—Labor-like pains in abdomen and back; voracious appetite; pain in stomach, nausea and eructation.

D. Mens.—Pain, heaviness, and heat in the head,—eyes are dull, dry, burning, and the lids stick together in the morning; — stopped coryza, chilliness, paleness of the face; -- flat taste and accumulation of water in the mouth; want of appetite; nausea; pains in abdomen and back, diarrhœa and trembling in the legs, lassitude and perspiration.

A. Mens.—Backache;—leucorrhœa.

D. Cgh.—Scratching in the throat; burning and cutting in the chest.

MAGNESIA MUR.

B. St.—Pinching pain in abdomen.

D. St.—Burning and soreness in anus;—pain in hæmorrhoidal tumors.

A. St.—Itching, burning and soreness in anus; — renewed desire to stool and discharge of mucus; — borborygmi, pain in abdomen, drawing in the loins; nausea and accumulation of water in the mouth.

D. Ur.—Burning;—erections.

A. Ur.—Burning.

B. Mens.—Excitement.

D. Mens.—Pain in abdomen, back, and thighs; lassitude;—gaping.

D. Cgh.—Burning, soreness, or ulcerative pain in chest.

MERCURIUS.

B. St.—Cutting. pinching, or twisting pain in abdomen;—rigor, anxiety, and trembling.

D. St.—Burning in anus; piles;—eructation, nausea, faintness; colic; heat, perspiration.

A. St.—Exhaustion; rigors; discharge of blood, tenesmus, prolapse of rectum, and trembling.

B. Ur.—Pressing in genital organs.

A. Ur.—Burning and stinging.

D. Ur.—Biting, burning, cutting, stinging;—nausea.

B. Mens.—Heat, with excitement of circulation and congestion to the head;—cramps.

D. Mens.—Dryness, redness and burning of the tongue, salty taste in the mouth; dullness of the teeth; discolored swollen gums; — anxiousness; weariness of life; inclination to commit murder.

A. Mens.—Leucorrhœa.

D. Cgh.—Stitches in occiput, chest, back, and scapula;—epistaxis;—offensive breath;—nausea, retching, vomiting;—secessus.

MEZEREUM.

B. St.—Creeping in the anus as if caused by worms;—abdominal pains; urgent desire to go to stool;—lassitude, rigors, chills, thirst.

D. St.—Prolapse of anus.

St.—Alleviation;—biting in anus and creeping as if from worms;—soreness and incarceration of prolapsed rectum; tenesmus, straining, and colic;—itching of inner surface of prepuce;—lassitude, rigors, chills, thirst.

D. Ur.—Burning, biting or soreness in anterior extremity of urethra;—pressure in abdominal ring, better on bending the knee.

A. Ur.—Cutting;—secretion of drops of blood.

D. Cgh.—Exhaustion, perspiration, anxiety, paleness, chills; — salivation, retching or scratching in the throat as if something sweet were sticking there; vomiting of food; scratching in lower part of sternum, and stitches in right frontal protuberance; — stitches in the side; — sore pain in the chest; tightness across the chest.

MOSCHUS.

B. St.—Rumbling and straining.

D. St.—Pressing in anus, cutting pain in abdomen, drawing in of the stomach.

D. St.—Painful drawing in hypogastrium.

MURIATIC. ACID.

D. St.—Rumbling, rolling and straining, cutting pain and nauseous feeling in abdomen; flatus;—cutting in anus;—constriction, burning and stinging in rectum;—soreness in anus and rectum.

A. St.—Burning in anus.

D. Ur.—Burning and cutting.

A. Ur.—Straining in urethra;—stinging biting in orifice.

D. Mens.—Colic;—dejection of spirits.

D. Cgh.—Catching of breath;—burning in the throat;—scratching, soreness, bruised feeling and bursting pain in the chest;—rolling in the chest.

NATRUM CARB.

B. St.—Cutting in abdomen and back; pinching abdominal pain and clawing in anus with chills.

D. St.—Cutting in anus and rectum; succus prostaticus; bearing down towards the genitals.

A. St.—Burning in rectum, burning and biting in anus.

D. Ur.—Burning, soreness, stinging;—succus prostaticus.

A. Ur.—Dribbling.

B. Mens.—Leucorrhœa; cutting in hypogastrium;—headache and stiffness in the nape of the neck.

D. Mens.—Distension with colic and diarrhœa; backache;—tearing and bruised pain in the hips;—tearing and throbbing in the head;—tearing and stitches in various places;—tired feeling with nausea;—shaking chills at night.

D Cgh.—Soreness in the chest, hoarseness, coryza, burning heat, particularly in the hands and soles of feet;—night-sweat;—bruised feeling;—loss of appetite and nausea.

NATRUM MUR.

B. St.—Pressure upon the bladder and rectum; contraction in urethra and rectum;—cutting abdominal pain; soreness in hypogastrium.

D. St.—Scratching and burning in rectum; labor-like abdominal pains, relieved by pressure;—succus prostaticus.

A. St.—Burning, tearing and itching about the anus;—pinching abdominal pain and ineffectual straining;—stupefaction, nausea, vertigo.

B. Ur.—Contraction in urethra and rectum.

D. Ur.—Biting, burning;—pressing in hypogastrium.

B. Mens.—Burning, cutting, tearing;—sore burning in vagina; leucorrhœa;—contraction in hypogastrium.

B. Mens.—Anxiousness, melancholy or irritability;—stitches from the loins into uterus; headache, lassitude, and trembling; twitching of eyelids; pressing headache; scraping faceache;—toothache.

Mens.—Dryness of vagina and aversion towards coition;—leucorrhœa; milky urine; colic; diarrhœa; difficult respiration, palpitation, accelerated pulse, dullness, stinging and cutting in the head, paleness; twitching before falling asleep.

D Cgh.—Pain in the head, throat, trachea, chest, testicle, spermatic cord; cutting and stinging in the chest; catching of breath; retching, vomiting of food; shocks in hypogastrium; shocks and bursting pain in the head; discharge of leucorrhœa.

NITRIC. ACID.

B. St.—Colic.

D. St.—Spasmodic contraction of the anus;—biting or tearing pain in rectum;—stinging, cutting and straining in anus and rectum; piles.

A. St.—Burning in anus; scratching and stinging in anus and rectum;—succus prostaticus;—ineffectual straining at stool;—colic, nausea, lassitude, anxiousness and indisposition

B. Ur.—Cutting pain in abdomen.

D. Ur.—Cutting, burning, soreness or sore pain in urethra;—stitches in the bladder;—rigors.

A. Ur.—Burning, renewed desire; discharge of mucus.

B. and D. Mens.—Bruised pain in the limbs.

D Mens.—Labor-like pains in abdomen and back; — eructation; — palpitation, heat, anxiety and trembling; tiredness; — burning in the eyes; — toothache and swelling of the gums.

D. Cgh.—Rattling;—sneezing; pains in the head, chest, upper abdomen, hypochondria and kness;—stitches in throat, chest, back, and rectum.

NITRUM.

B. St.—Pinching about the navel; pain in abdomen and back;—stitches in anus and groins.

D. St.—Swelling of anal piles or protrusion of rectum;—stitches in vulva;—thirst; cold feet.

A. St.—Burning and soreness in anus; discharge of blood.

B. Ur.—Burning and biting in urethra, burning at the orifice, itching in the glans;—soreness about the prepuce, stitches in the prostate.

At the end of Ur.—Burning.

D. Mens.—Thirst,—sensitiveness in the stomach and collection of water in the mouth; pain in abdomen and back;—burning in right groin;—tiredness and pains in the legs.

D. Cgh.—Scratching and burning extending up into the throat;—cutting and feeling of looseness in the chest, or tension and constriction; — heat and pressing pain behind the sternum, afterwards sore pain and mucous rattling in that place;—backache;- palpitation; redness of the face; headache.

NUX MOSCHATA.

D. St.—Stitches in anus;—acrid feeling in rectum;—painful constriction in anus and rectum;—pressing in hypogastrium;—distended feeling;—sleepiness

A. St.—Painful constriction in anus and rectum;—feeling as if more evacuations were to take place;—sleepiness.

D. Ur.—Burning and cutting.

D. Mens.—Lassitude, headache, pressing in stomach with running of water from the mouth;—pain in the liver;—straining in hypogastrium and drawing pain in the limbs.

D. Cgh.—Sore pain in trachea; rawness in the chest; catching of breath;—sleepiness.

NUX VOMICA.

B. St.—Pressing in rectum;—backache;—griping in upper abdomen.

During straining at stool—Increased pressure in the stomach.

D. St.—Stitching and constriction in rectum; colic.

A. St.– Stinging, biting, soreness or burning excoriated feeling in anus;—ineffectual straining; abdominal pain.

B. Ur.– Pressing in the bladder; pain in the neck of the bladder;—stinging in the urethra.

D. Ur.– Burning in the urethra or neck of the bladder.

A. Ur.—Soreness and pain in meatus urinarius;—pressing in the neck of the bladder.

B. Mens.—Pain in abdomen and back.

D. Mens.—Pains in back, abdomen and limbs; headache;—lassitude, particularly after stool;—in the morning attacks of faintness; vertigo; pressing and burning in the stomach;—chills.

D. Cgh.—Sharp pain in the pit of the throat;—sore pain in the chest;—rattling; paroxysms of suffocation;—nausea, retching, vomiting;—retraction of testicles;—bluish-red color of the face;—heat, pain in the head and limbs;—bursting pain in the head;—epistaxis;—pain as if bruised in hypochondria and upper abdomen.

OPIUM.

B. St.–Aching in abdomen and stomach; nausea; rush of blood to the head.

D. Ur.—Cutting in urethra, and feeling as if the passage to the bladder were closed.

D. Cgh.—Retching, vomiting; cough alternates with gaping.

PETROLEUM.

B. St.—Abdominal ache.

D. St.—Ascarides; foul eructations.

A. St.—Ravenous appetite, loathing, distension;—staggering & darkness before the eyes.

B. Ur.—Pressure upon the bladder.

D. Ur.—Burning and itching in urethra;—burning and cutting in the neck of the bladder

A. Ur.—Dribbling.

B. Mens. —Heat, throbbing and pressing in the head; boiling (waving) in epigastrium, abdominal pains

D. Mens.—Abdominal pains; tearing in the thigh; sensitive places on the lower legs;—heat in the hands and soles of the feet;—singing and roaring in the ears;—lassitude and exhaustion.

D. Cgh.—Dryness ef the throat;—pain in the sternum and inguinal hernia;—nausea.

PHOSPHORUS.

B. St.—Chills and heat; thirst for cold drinks;—flatulency; colic; contraction and stitches in rectum.

D St.—Chills;—cold sweat;—itching, creeping and soreness in rectum;—piles;—pain, extending from coccyx through the spine into the crown of the head.

A. St.—Soreness and scratching in anus; – pressing in rectum;—tenesmus and burning in anus and rectum, with burning desire to urinate; extrusion of painful piles, discharge of acrid mucus; erections; retching or sour vomiting;—thirst, lassitude, vertigo, and fainting.

D. Ur.—Burning and soreness;—discharge of mucus, with pain in perineum.

A. Ur.—Stitches in penis; biting in glans; – lassitude.

B. Mens.—Much weeping; swelling of the gums; - desire to urinate; leucorrhœa; bleeding of present ulcers.

D. Mens.—Pains in the ovary, abdomen, back, and limbs;—headache and toothache;—stinging itching of the skin, particularly about the hæmorrhoids;—leucorrhœa;—cramps in the calves;—rolling in abdomen;—nausea and vomiting;—gaping, relaxation, dullness;—chills, heat, cold perspiration on the forehead.

A. Mens.—Leucorrhœa;—exhaustion and blue circles around the eyes.

D. Cgh.—Hoarseness;—roughness, burning and stitches in the throat, and a sensation as if a piece of flesh were to be thrown up;—pain in the chest, alleviated by pressure;—hoarseness, burning, scraping, and soreness in the chest;—pressing or stinging in epigastrium;—stitches in the hypochondria or rectum; colic; secessus;—stitches or bursting pain in the head;—trembling;—night-sweat.

PHOSPHORIC ACID.

B. St.—Flatulency.

D. St.—Piles; colic; cutting in urethra.

A. St.–Biting in anus;—tearing down and tenesmus in rectum.

B. Ur.—Cutting and ineffectual straining to urinate;—anxiety and restlessness

D Ur.—Cutting, burning, and heat in urethra.

At the end of Ur.—Heavy pressure of hypogastrium.

B. Mens—Leucorrhœa.

D. Mens.—Pains in the liver.

A. Mens.–Leucorrhœa, with itching.

D. Cgh.—Pain in the chest.

PLATINA.

B. St.—Straining in anus

D. St.—Burning and pressing in rectum;—attacks of fainting.

A. St.—Straining and stinging in anus, with spasmodic contraction of nates toward the spine;—itching in rectum;—pain and sensation of weakness about the navel;—rigors, particularly about the upper part of body.

A. Ur.—Rigors.

B. Mens.–Labor-like abdominal pains; downward pressure.

At the beginning of Mens.—Pinching and bearing down in hypogastrium;—headache; depression of spirits;—restlessness; weeping; spasms (or also intermissions of the usual spasms during menstruation).

A. Mens.—Lassitude.

D. Cgh.—Spasms.

PLUMBUM.

B. St.—Colic.

D. St.—Pain in abdomen; burning in anus.

A. St.—Cessation of colic.

D. Ur.—Burning.

A. Ur.—Burning in urethra; abdominal pains.

PULSATILLA

B. St.—Movement in abdomen;—headache.

D. St.—Burning and cutting in rectum;—pain in abdomen, back, and head;—eructation, nausea; attacks of faintness, shaking chills.

A. St.—Sore pain in anus; pressing, stinging, and cutting in rectum; colic; pressing in epigastrium; stiffness of the neck; backache; chills, particularly in the back.

B. Ur.—Burning in urethra; pressing in the bladder; colicky pains.
D. Ur.—Burning, cutting, stinging; — discharge of acrid mucous stools, with sensation of weakness in the loins.
D. Ur.—Burning;—pressing and creeping in the glans or meatus ur.;—spasmodic pain of the neck of the bladder, extending into thighs.
At the end of Ur.—Dropping of blood.
B. Mens.—Leucorrhœa; desire to urinate; spasms of the stomach, also with running of water from the mouth, or vomiting;—pain in abdomen, liver, back;—asthma;—stitches in the sides;—vertigo and eructation;—chills, gaping and stretching;—convulsions.
D. Mens.—Labor-like pains in abdomen and back; — ineffectual straining at stool; spasms of the stomach; nausea and vomiting;—running of water from the mouth at night; stitches in the chest;—sick headache, obscured vision;—toothache;—chills and paleness of the face;—sadness and weeping;—convulsions.
In the beginning and at the end of Mens.—Headache or toothache.
A. Mens.—Leucorrhœa; difficult respiration.
D. Cgh.—Dryness, sensation of being swollen, constriction, and feeling like that caused by sulphurous vapors in the throat;—hoarseness;—catching of the breath;—palpitation;—stitches in the side;—shocks and bruised painfulness in abdomen;—concussions of the body;—turning of the stomach, retching and vomiting of mucus, bile, or food; — spasms of the stomach; cutting in the region of the spleen;—pains in the head, back, lumbar region, shoulder and arms;—epistaxis;—perspiration; gaping.

RHEUM.

B. St.—Anxiousness; cutting pain in abdomen and ineffectual straining to urinate.
D. St.—Cutting and constricting, pinching in abdomen; lassitude, rigors, paleness.
A. St.—Ineffectual straining; colic; perspiration; thirst.

RHODODENDRON.

B. St.—Ineffectual straining.
D. St.—Sensation of weakness in stomach and nausea.
A. St.—Sensation of emptiness in abdomen, afterwards pinching.
B. and D. Ur.—Burning.
A. Ur.—Burning, dribbling, rigors.
At beginning of Mens.—Febrile excitement and headache.
D. aud A. Mens.—Toothache.
D. Cgh.—Hoarseness in the throat;—oppression and pressing in lumbar vertebræ;—pressure in epigastrium.

RHUS TOX.

B. St.—Burning in rectum; pinching in abdomen; coxalgia; nausea; shortness of breath.
D. St.—Jamming in anus; — burning urine; — pains in head, abdomen and limbs;—epistaxis;—coldness.
A. St.—Remission of abdominal pains;—tenesmus.
B. Ur.—Stitches in bladder;—erections.
D. Ur.—Biting;—burning at the root of urethra;—eructation.
A. Ur.—Biting in urethra.
B. Mens.—Labor-like pains.
D. Cgh.—Bloody taste in the mouth; dryness and bitterness in the throat;—asthma;—tension and loathing (uneasiness) in the chest; stitches in the side; jarring of the chest;—concussion and shocks in the head;—pains in the hips and lower limbs;—anxiety;—gastralgia; vomiting of food.

RUTA.

B. St.—Nausea in abdomen;—ineffectual straining, also with prolapse of rectum.
D. St.—Prolapse of rectum.
B. Ur.—Urgent desire to urinate.
D. Ur.—Burning in the organs of parturition.
A. Ur.—Continued desire to pass urine; sensation of fullness and fluctuation in the bladder; pressure upon the neck of the bladder;—burning in the organs of parturition.
A. Mens.—Leucorrhœa.
D. Cgh.—Scratching and sensation of weakness in the chest after expectoration;—reversed action of the stomach

SABADILLA.

B. St.—Rolling, flatus, pinching in abdomen; drawing in spermatic cords; burning in anus;—shuddering.
A. St.—Burning in abdomen.
B. Ur.—Burning and straining in urethra.
D. Ur.—Burning.
A. insufficient urination—Increased desire to urinate.
B. Mens.—Painful (bearing down) pressure downwards.
D. Cgh.—Shortness of breath, pains in the chest, stitches in the chest and crown of the head; spasms of the stomach, vomiting; tears; heat and perspiration.

SAMBUCUS NIGRA.

D. Cgh.—Hoarseness, catching of the breath, stitches in the sides; straining to urinate; vomiting of food; — bloatedness of the face; — chills alternating with heat;—local perspiration with cool skin.

SASSAPARILLA

D. St.—Cutting, rolling and working in abdomen;—flatus;—corroding acridity, with tearing and cutting in rectum; pressing in epigastrium;—attacks of faintness.
A. St.—Straining, jamming and burning in anus.
D. Ur.—Scratching, burning and cutting in urethra.
A. Ur.—Burning and itching tearing about the glans down to the root of the penis.
B. Mens.—Desire to urinate; — itching eruption on the forehead, with burning and moisture after friction.
D. Mens. Griping in epigastrium; pinching in abdomen; pain in the thighs.
At the commencement of Mens.—Desire to urinate, acridity and sore pain in genitals.
D. Cgh.—Roughness in the throat;—headache.

SECALE CORN.

B. St.—Pain in abdomen and back.
D. St.—Colic;—failing of strength; heat;—coldness of the ears.
A. St.—Renewed desire;—lassitude; - heat, thirst; contortion of the face
D Ur.—Burning in urethra.
B. Mens.—Aggravation of all complaints.
D. Mens.—Pain in abdomen, back, and loins;—paleness, coldness of the limbs, cold perspiration;—cramps.

SEPIA.

B. St.—Chilliness; nausea; colic; perspiration.
D. St.—Chilliness;—contraction in abdomen and anus;—piles;—prolapse of rectum;—

succus prostaticus; stitches in genitals;—perspiration;—bearing down in the organs of parturition.

A. St.—Discharge of bloody slime;—tension in anus; sensation of emptiness and soreness in abdomen;—tension in epigastrium, with oppression;—sensation of hardness in the back;—headache.

D. Ur.—Biting and soreness.

A. Ur.—Succus prostaticus.

B. Mens.—Burning excoriation and swelling about the vulva;—sensation of distension of genitals; — leucorrhœa; — soreness about the perineum; — pain in abdomen, with faintness;—incarceration of flatus;—spasms of the stomach; foul odor and taste in the mouth;—rigors.

D. Mens.—Depression of spirits, lassitude; sleeplessness, febrile action, darkness before the eyes; pains in the stomach, abdomen, groins, head, teeth, and limbs; foul taste and odor from the mouth;—coughing up of blood.

D. Cgh.—Sore pain in the throat; hoarseness, burning, pressing, stinging, scraping, and emptiness in the chest; pain in sternum;—stitches in back and sides of abdomen; nausea and retching; — asthma; vomiting of food or bile; — pain in epigastrium, stitches in abdomen;—sneezing.

SILICEA.

D. St.—Itching and stinging in rectum; piles; succus prostaticus.

A. St.—Remission of abdominal pains;—pressing and burning in anus; burning in prepuce; eructation.

D. Ur.—Burning and soreness in urethra; — pressure in the bladder; — Itching of vulva.

A. Ur.—Involuntary discharge of urine.

B. Mens.—Pressing pain in forehead;—diarrhœa or constipation.

D. Mens.—Cold feet, pain in abdomen, burning and soreness about vulva; eruption on the inside of thighs;—drawing between the shoulders, paronychia;—chlorosis;—melancholic anxiety and weariness of life.

A. Mens.—Bloody mucous discharge from vagina.

D. Cgh.—Pressing, scratching, soreness or bruised pain in the chest; catching of the breath;—vomiting.

SPIGELIA.

B. St.—Flatulency, colic.

D. St.—Pinching pain in abdomen, coldness, faintness; — headache; — bruised pain of the ribs.

A. St.— Ineffectual straining;—pressing shocks in the forehead.

D. Ur.—Burning in urethra;—pressure upon the bladder.

D. Cgh.—Sore pain in the chest; headache.

SPONGIA.

B. St.—Snarling noises in abdomen;—stitches in anus.

D St.—Straining and sore pain in anus;—pressing in the lumbar region;—flatulency.

B. Mens.—Backache, afterwards palpitation.

D. Mens.—Drawing in the legs.

D. Cgh.—Hoarseness, roughness in the throat; pain in trachea and chest; burning, rawness, sore pain and contraction in the chest; paroxysms of suffocation; contortions of the face; pressure in hypochondria;—perspiration.

STANNUM.

B. St.—Motion, pinching and distension in abdomen.

D. St.—Cutting in anus;—drawing from the back through the thighs;—rigors.

A. St.—Discharge of mucus;—sore pain, excoriation and stinging in anus; pressing in rectum; burning pain in region of liver.

D. Ur.—Burning in urethra.

A. Ur.—Pressing in urethra and neck of bladder, with a feeling as if more urine were to come.

B. Mens.—Anxiety and melancholy;—pain like a blow in os zygomaticum.

D. Mens.—Improvement of mental condition.

D. Cgh.—Expectoration; soreness and stitches in the chest;—oppression; sore pain in trachea; colic.

STAPHISAGRIA.

B. St.—Digging and cutting in abdomen.

D. St.—Much flatus; succus prostaticus; chills about the head.

A. St.—Straining, jamming, contused pain and excoriating soreness in rectum; increased cutting pain in abdomen.

D. Ur.—Burning and cutting in urethra;—burning in neck of bladder;—pressure upon the bladder;—ineffectual straining at stool;—erections.

A. Ur.—Increased cutting;—pain like dislocation (or sprain) behind the os pubis;—colic.

D. Cgh.—Collection of water in the mouth;—excoriation and tearing pain in the throat; pain like ulceration behind the sternum;—pains in an inguinal hernia;—discharge of urine.

STRAMONIUM.

B. St.—Twisting in the bowels.

D. St.—Colic, distension of abdomen, rolling in abdomen;—vomiting; paleness

D. Ur.—Rolling in abdomen; rigors.

D. Mens.—Talkativeness;—voluptuous odor of body.

A. Mens.—Sobbing and whining; erysipelas of the left cheek.

D. Cgh.—Palpitation, anxiety; constriction of the chest;—convulsions.

SULPHUR.

B. St.—Eructation; pinching in abdomen and flatus, causing pain in anus;—itching. straining, cutting and sensation like prolapsus in anus;—pains in the bladder.

D. St.—Burning, sore pain and excoriating cutting in anus;—burning, pressing, cutting and prolapse of rectum;—piles;—succus prostaticus;—cutting in urethra;—pains in abdomen and head;—accumulation of water in the mouth;—nausea, vomiting;—catching of breath;—palpitation; congestions to the head;—chills, particularly about the lower part of body;—heat;—perspiration.

A. St.—Discharge of blood;—sensitiveness, contraction, burning and sensation of soreness and prolapse of anus;—straining. jamming and throbbing in rectum; pressing and stinging in anus and rectum;—succus prostaticus;—cramp-like pains in glans and in the angle of lower jaw;—cramp-like twitching about the orifices of the ears;—bruised pain and pinching in abdomen;—chills and lassitude;—thirst.

B. Ur.—Cutting pain in abdomen;—impatience.

D. Ur.—Burning in urethra;—feeling as if there were an obstruction about the neck of the bladder; stitches in neck of bladder and anus;—voluptuous pressure extending into anus;—itching of vulva; pains in back and limbs.

A. Ur.—Dribbling of blood;—succus prostaticus;—cutting and stinging in urethra;—straining in the bladder;—anxiousness and discomfort.

B. Mens.—Leucorrhœa;—itching of vulva;—lumbar pains;—cramp in splenic region; restlessness and anxiety;—epistaxis;—headache and toothache;—heart-burn;—cough in the evening in bed;—night-sweat.

D. Mens.—Irritability;—day-sleepiness;—congestion to the head;—pressure in the forehead;—vertigo;—excitement of circulation; palpitation; epistaxis; sore throat;—lassitude and heaviness of the feet;—pressure in epigastrium;—labor-like pains of abdomen and back, with heat and chills and ineffectual straining o stool.

A. Mens.—Leucorrhœa;—itching about the nose.

D. Cgh.—Hoarseness;—soreness in trachea;—constriction of air-passages;—sensation as if the lungs come in contact with the back;—pressing, tension, cramp-like pain, cutting, stinging, soreness and bursting pain in the chest;—pain in the chest;—pain in the sternum;—jarring of the chest and abdomen;—reverberation in the crown of the head;—bursting pain in the head, relieved by pressure, during cough;—cervical pain, epistaxis, palpitation; rattling;—retching and vomiting; paleness and cold hands;—sleeplessness and night-sweats; hypochondriac pains; pains in abdomen, back, lips, and legs;—secessus; convulsions.

SULPHURIC ACID.

B. St.—Stitches in anus.

D. St.—Burning and tearing pain in rectum; pinching in hypochondria; rolling in bowels and flatus.

A. St.—Sensation of emptiness and bruised feeling in abdomen.

D. Ur.—Burning, cutting;—pinching in abdomen.

A. Ur.—Bearing down in genitals and loins;—pinching in abdomen.

B. Mens.—Nightmare.

D. Mens.—Stitches in abdomen and vagina;—thirst and dry tongue.

A. Mens.—Increased sexual desire.

D. Cgh.—Pain as if caused by a blow in the edge of the right orbit.

THUYA.

B. St.—Pressing in hypogastrium;—erections; succus prostaticus.

D. St.—Painful contraction of anus;—piles;—succus prostaticus;—backache; rawness and sore pain in rectum; flatus.

A. St.—Burning and drawing in of anus;—weariness;—drippling of blood.

D. Ur.—Itching, cutting, or excoriating burning, particularly in the fossa navicularis;—biting, itching, soreness of vulva.

A. Ur.—Burning;—dribbling.

B. Mens. Excitement and pulsation of arteries, heat of the head, headache and toothache, labor-like abdominal pains, tenesmus and faintness;—much perspiration.

D. Mens.—Tiredness, palpitation, spasmodic weeping;—restlessness in the legs;—retching, pressing in the stomach, distension, pain in abdomen and back; bearing down out of the genital organs;—burning in the varicose veins of genitals, sensitiveness and swelling of the breast;—general coldness.

A. Mens.—Tiredness; rush of blood upwards; toothache; sleeplessness; nightmare.

D. Cgh.—Scratching, burning and constricted feeling in the throat; stitches in the sides; running of water from the mouth; vomiting; whistling respiration.

VALERIANA.

A. St.—Tenesmus.

D. Ur.—Prolapse of rectum.

VERATRUM ALBUM.

B. St.—Chilliness, anxiousness, nausea, vomiting; colic; weakness in hypogastrium like faintness.

D. St.—Chills and shivering; anxiety, nausea, vomiting; colic, tiredness, approaching faintness; burning in anus and cold perspiration on forehead.

A. St.—Improvement of cervical pains;—squalmishness in epigastrium; nausea, vomiting;—colic;—fainting.

D. Ur.—Burning.

A. Ur.—Stitches in meatus urinarius.

B. Mens.—Vertigo and perspiration;—epistaxis;—**nausea; – diarrhœa.**

D. Mens.—Disturbance of the mind; — gnashing of the teeth and **bluish color of the face;**—headache; roaring in the ears;—**diarrhœa, thirst;—pains in the limbs.**

A. Mens.—Backache.

D. Cgh.—**Pains in the chest, oppression, rattling, danger of suffocation with blueness of the face; — collection of saliva; — slimy or watery vomiting; — discharge of urine; — stitches, extending out of abdominal ring; — pains in spermatic cord or in inguinal hernia;—headache.**

ZINCUM.

B. St. - Protracted tenesmus;—**colic.**

D. St.—**Pressing, rolling, burning and stinging in anus;—pressing, rolling and pains in abdomen;—succus prostaticus;—vertigo and roaring in the ears.**

A. St.—Cessation of abdominal pains; — **increased tenesmus, with burning in anus;** — vertigo and roaring in the ears.

B. and dur. Ur. – Burning in urethra.

A. Ur.—**Burning and bleeding from urethra;—renewed desire to urinate.**

D. Mens.—**Indisposition, chilliness;** headache and toothache; **ophthalmia;—oppression, caused by the clothes in the epigastrium; — cramps in hypogastrium; — scalding urine;**—drawing in the knees; heaviness in the feet;**—lassitude in hand and feet.**

A. Mens.—**Discharge of bloody mucus, which causes itching of the vulva.**

D. Cgh.—**Stitches in head and chest;—heaviness, burning, soreness, or bursting pain in the chest, and after expectoration a feeling of hollowness or coldness in the chest.**